Progress in Oncology 2003

Edited by

Vincent T. DeVita, Jr.
Yale Cancer Center
New Haven, Connecticut

Samuel Hellman
Department of Radiation Oncology
University of Chicago
Chicago, Illinois

Steven A. Rosenberg
National Cancer Institute
National Institutes of Health
Bethesda, Maryland

JONES AND BARTLETT PUBLISHERS
Sudbury, Massachusetts
BOSTON TORONTO LONDON SINGAPORE

World Headquarters
Jones and Bartlett Publishers
40 Tall Pine Drive
Sudbury, MA 01776
info@jbpub.com
www.jbpub.com

Jones and Bartlett Publishers
Canada
2406 Nikanna Road
Mississauga, ON L5C 2W6
CANADA

Jones and Bartlett
Publishers International
Barb House, Barb Mews
London W6 7PA
UK

ISBN 978-0-7637-2064-3

Acquisitions Editor: Christopher Davis
Production Editor: Elizabeth Platt
Cover and Interior Design: Anne Spencer
Cover Image: © Photodisc
Manufacturing Buyer: Amy Bacus
Composition: Modern Graphics, Inc.
Printing and Binding: Malloy Lithographing
Cover Printer: Malloy Lithographing

Printed in the United States of America
07 06 05 04 03 10 9 8 7 6 5 4 3 2 1

Contents

Controversies in Oncology

List of Contributors

Harry Bartelink, MD, PhD
Radiotherapy Department, The Netherlands Cancer Institute, Amsterdam, The Netherlands

Mark D. Bednarski, MD, PhD
Lucas MRS Research Center, Department of Radiology, Stanford University School of Medicine, Stanford, California

Nancy Berliner, MD
Internal Medical Hematology, Yale University, New Haven, Connecticut

Tony Hsiu-Hsi Chen, PhD
Institute of Preventive Medicine, National Taiwan University, Taipei, Taiwan

Edward Chu, MD
Comprehensive Cancer Center, VA Connecticut Medical Center, West Haven, Connecticut

Suzanne D. Conzen, MD
Hematology/Oncology Section, Dept. of Medicine, University of Chicago, Chicago, Illinois

Abraham Dachman, MD
Department of Radiology, University of Chicago, Chicago, Illinois

Dominique Delbeke, MD, PhD
Department of Radiology, Vanderbilt University Hospital, Nashville, Tennessee

Bruce Dezube, MD
Department of Medicine, Beth Israel Deaconess Medical Center, Boston, Massachusetts

Stephen W. Duffy, PhD
Department of Mathematics, Statistics and Epidemiology, Cancer Research UK, London, United Kingdom

Warren E. Enker, MD
Department of Surgery, Beth Israel Medical Center, New York, New York

Douglas B. Evans, MD
University of Texas M.D. Anderson Cancer Center, Houston, Texas

Samira Guccione, PhD
Lucas MRS Research Center, Department of Radiology, Stanford University School of Medicine, Stanford, California

Robin M. Joyce, MD
Department of Medicine, Beth Israel Deaconess Medical Center, Boston, Massachusetts

Noah Kauff, MD
Clinical Genetics Service, Department of Medicine, Memorial Sloan-Kettering Cancer Center, New York, New York

John M. Kirkwood, MD
Department of Medicine, University of Pittsburgh Medical Center, Pittsburgh, Pennsylvania

Ana Kostic, MD
Division of Pediatric Hematology/Oncology, Fred Hutchinson Cancer Research Center, Seattle, Washington

King C. P. Li, MD, MBA
Radiology and Imaging Sciences Program, National Institutes of Health, Bethesda, Maryland

Kevin Lye, MD
Department of Surgery, Yale University, New Haven, Connecticut

Irvin M. Modlin, MD, PhD
Department of Gastroenterology, Yale Cancer Center, Yale University School of Medicine, New Haven, Connecticut

Jonathan P. Myles, PhD
Department of Mathematics, Statistics and Epidemiology, Cancer Research UK, London, United Kingdom

Kenneth Offit, MD, MPH
Clinical Genetics Service, Department of Medicine, Memorial Sloan-Kettering Cancer Center, New York, New York

Stanley R. Riddell, MD
Division of Clinical Research, Fred Hutchinson Cancer Research Center, Seattle, Washington

Charles L. Sawyers, MD
University of California, Los Angeles, Los Angeles, California

John Schmitz, PhD
Comprehensive Cancer Center, VA Connecticut Medical Center, West Haven, Connecticut

Robert A. Smith, PhD
American Cancer Society, Atlanta, Georgia

Lynne E. Spitler, MD
Northern California Melanoma Center, Tiburon, California

Làszló Tabár, MD
Department of Mammography, Central Hospital, Falun, Sweden

Anthony Tolcher, MD
Institute for Drug Development, San Antonio, Texas

Marc van de Vijver, MD
Department of Pathology, The Netherlands Cancer Institute, Amsterdam, The Netherlands

Laura van't Veer, MD
Department of Pathology, The Netherlands Cancer Institute, Amsterdam, The Netherlands

Bedrich Vitak, MD
Department of Diagnostic Radiology, University of Linköping, Linköping, Sweden

Jane Warwick, PhD
Department of Mathematics, Statistics and Epidemiology, Cancer Research UK, London, United Kingdom

Ming-Fang Yen, MSc
Department of Mathematics, Statistics and Epidemiology, Cancer Research UK, London, United Kingdom; Department of Statistical Science, University College, London, United Kingdom

Chapter 1

Antisense Attack on Bcl-2

Anthony W. Tolcher MD FRCPC

Normal tissue homeostasis requires a precise balance of cellular proliferation balanced with cell death. Agents that target aberrant cellular proliferation have largely been the focus of targeted drug development in oncology during the past two decades. However, the biochemical pathways that regulate cell apoptosis are being increasingly recognized as therapeutic targets for the treatment of malignant diseases. This chapter reviews the function of the Bcl-2 protein family in the dynamic regulation of apoptosis and an antisense oligonucleotide therapy as a strategy to target *bcl*-2 expression.

THE PREDOMINANT ROLE OF THE BCL-2 FAMILY OF PROTEINS IS TO REGULATE CASPASE ACTIVATION

Similar to proliferation, the apoptosis is a highly regulated biochemical process. The final common pathway that executes the process of apoptosis requires the activation of proteases named caspases. Caspases (*c*ysteine *asp*artyl–specific pro*teases*) are a family of intracellular cysteine proteases that exist as inactive zymogens, which, once activated, lead to a cascade of proteolysis downstream that is mediated through the recruitment and activation of other caspase family members.[1,2] Caspase-induced proteolysis is not indiscriminate; rather, a restricted set cellular proteins are substrates for degradation selected by both the presence of aspartate residues and specific adjoining amino acid sequences.[1] Although not all caspases are involved in apoptosis, caspase 3, 6, 7, 8, and 9 have well-described functions in cell death pathways. Once activated, the downstream effector caspases (e.g., caspase 6 and 7) mediate cellular destruction of "housekeeping" cellular processes through the cleavage of protein kinases and other signal transduction proteins, cytoskeletal proteins, chromatin-modifying proteins (e.g., polyADP ribosyl polymerase), DNA repair proteins, inhibitors of apoptosis (e.g., Bcl-2 protein), and inhibitory subunits of endonucleases (cell death–inducing DFF45-like effectors [CIDE] family of proteins). This process is both rapid and methodical, thereby eliminating the biochemical processes necessary for cellular viability.[1,2]

Because the activation of effector caspases represents the final common and irreversible pathway to apoptosis, initial caspase activation represents pivotal junction for the regulation and governance of apoptosis. The upstream activation of caspases is tightly regulated through the intrinsic and extrinsic pathways of apoptosis (Fig. 1.1). Although these pathways are often described separately, this division is both simplistic and arbitrary because several lines of evidence indicate important links between the two pathways that further co-regulate proapoptotic/antiapoptotic equilibrium.[3,4] Each pathway utilizes a separate upstream caspase family member to activate a common caspase, caspase 3, that subsequently activates common downstream effector caspases.

The extrinsic pathway is mediated by the ligands and membrane receptor proteins of the tumor necrosis receptor family that include tumor necrosis factor, tumor necrosis factor receptor apoptosis-inducing ligand, Fas ligand, and death and decoy death receptors 3, 4, and 5. The extrinsic pathway activates the upstream caspase, caspase 8, whereas the intrinsic pathway activates caspase 9 and is regulated through the dynamic interactions of members of the *bcl*-2 gene family of proteins that localize to the mitochondrial membrane.

The Bcl-2 Family of Proteins

The *bcl*-2 gene was originally identified at the chromosome breakpoint of the t(14:18) translocation found in follicular B-cell non-Hodgkin's lymphoma cells.[5-7] Bcl-2 protein is now part of a larger family of proteins that share considerable homology and include both death antagonists (e.g., Bcl-2, Bcl-XL, Bcl-w, Bfl-1, A1, and Mcl-1) as well as death agonists (Bax, Bak, Bok, Bad, Bcl-Xs, Bid, Bmf, Bik, BNIP3, Noxa, and Puma). Most family members, including the apoptosis agonists and antagonists, have Bcl-2 homologous (BH) regions, designated BH1 to BH4, which determine their capacity to interact with other Bcl-2 family members and the mitochondrial membrane. Structure and function studies indicate that the presence of the homologous regions BH1 and BH2 on Bcl-2 is required for the antiparallel homodimerization of Bcl-2 proteins, whereas the BH3 domain on the death agonists Bax and Bak is required both for heterodimerization with Bcl-2 and for a functional pro-apoptotic effect.[8,9] Most proteins encoded by genes of the Bcl-2 family localize to the outer mitochondrial membrane, and most

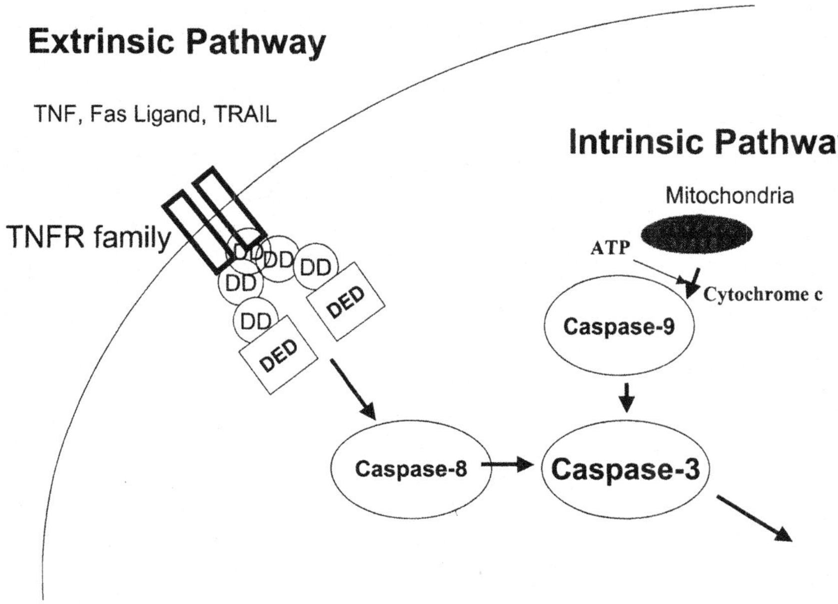

FIGURE 1.1 Schematic representation for the intrinsic and extrinsic pathways of apoptosis. The intrinsic pathway regulates caspase activation via mitochondrial interacting proteins, whereas the extrinsic pathway regulates caspases via the transmembrane tumor necrosis factor (TNF) receptor family. DD, death domain; DED, death effector domains.

members, with the exception of Bid and Bad, possess a carboxy-terminal transmembrane region that is responsible, at least in part, for subcellular localization and interaction with the mitochondria.[10]

The homeostatic control of the intrinsic pathway of cell death occurs through the competitive dimerization between selective pairs of antagonists and agonists (Fig. 1.2).[11] Bax is the prototypic protein capable of inducing apoptosis in the intrinsic pathway, although the exact mechanism whereby an apoptotic stimuli initiates Bax localization to the mitochondrial membrane is not currently known.[12] Several members of the protein family, including Bax and Bid, share structural similarity to pore-forming bacterial toxins.[13-15] These proapoptotic proteins interact with the mitochondrial membrane. This is followed by the first universal manifestation of the apoptotic process, disruption of mitochondrial membrane integrity. As a consequence, loss of the transmembrane potential occurs with release of cytochrome *c*, protease activators (including caspase 2, 3, 9), and apoptosis-inducing factors.[1] The functional protein that is external to the mitochondria membrane, apoptotic protease activating factor-1, exists as an inactive monomeric protein that, once bound to mitochondrial-released cytochrome *c* and in conjunction with adenosine triphosphate, undergoes a

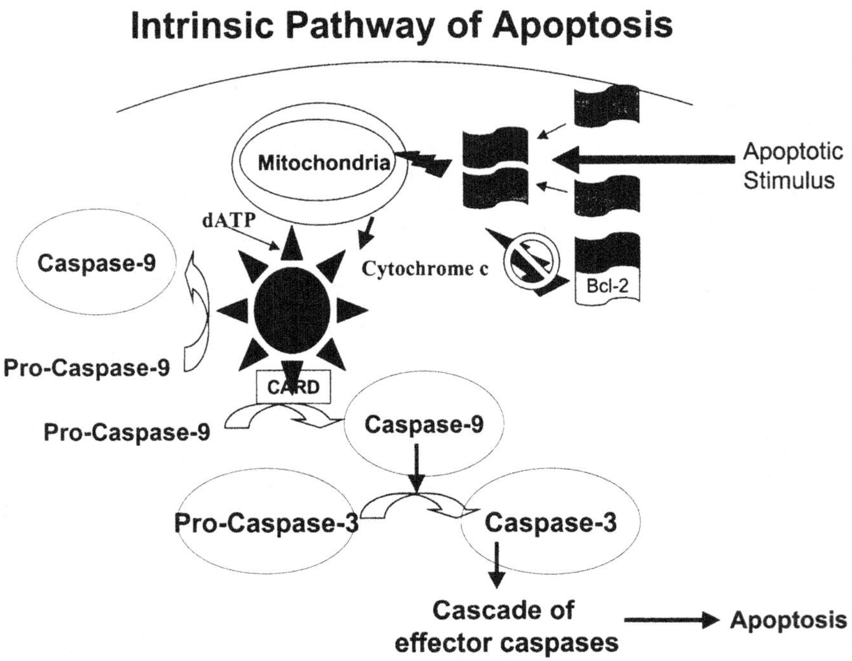

FIGURE 1.2 Schematic representation of the intrinsic pathway of apoptosis. Proapoptotic proteins of the Bcl-2 family (e.g., Bax) homodimerize and localize to the mitochondrial membrane after an apoptotic stimuli. Disruption of the mitochondrial membrane integrity occurs with release of protease activators and cytochrome *c*. Apoptotic protease activating factor-1 (Apaf-1) undergoes oligomerization in the presence of cytochrome *c* and deoxyadenosine triphosphate (dATP). Caspase recruitment domains (CARDs) of the apoptosome bind CARDs of procaspase 9 and activate and release caspase 9. Antiapoptotic members of the Bcl-2 family (e.g., Bcl-2) heterodimerize with Bax, prevent Bax homodimerization and mitochondrial localization, and thereby inhibit caspase activation.

conformational change with oligomerization to form a functional "hub" for biochemical activation of caspase-9. This oligomeric hub structure has been termed the *apoptosome*. Caspase recruitment domains at the center of the apoptosome bind caspase recruitment domains of pro–caspase 9 molecules, thereby activating caspase 9, and initiate activation of caspase 3 and the downstream pathway of proapoptotic caspase effectors.

The mitochondrial membrane alteration and biochemical trigger therefore initiates and irreversibly commits the cell to the apoptotic process through to the activation of caspase 9 and executes the active process of cellular destruction. Bcl-2 has a central role in the inhibition of this process through competitive heterodimerization with Bax and other apoptosis agonist proteins (e.g., Bid), sequestering and thereby restricting the interaction of these proapoptotic proteins at the mitochondrial membrane.[8] Heterodimerization-independent effects of Bcl-2 protein may also inhibit Bax-induced apoptosis; however, the underlying mechanism by which this occurs remains obscure.[8]

Dysregulation of the intrinsic pathway, either mediated through overexpression of apoptosis antagonists or diminished function or expression of apoptosis agonists, may contribute to the malignant transformation of human cells. In many normal epithelial tissues, Bcl-2 protein is ubiquitously expressed at low levels in the basal proliferative cell population but is diminished in fully differentiated cells.[16-18] Bcl-2 protein is also normally expressed in both pre–B cells and quiescent memory B cells, but it is down-regulated in differentiated B cells.[19] However, overexpression of Bcl-2 protein, secondarily to the t(14:18) chromosomal translocation, is associated with extended cellular survival and follicular lymphoproliferation in transgenic murine models and is also associated with indolent clonal proliferation of B cells in follicular non-Hodgkin's lymphoma.[6,20] This observation has implications for several malignancies in which Bcl-2 protein is overexpressed (Table 1.1). Dysregulation of apoptosis may be a common, and potentially a critical, mechanism during the neoplastic transformation of a broad array of malignancies. Further evidence of the importance of aberrant apoptosis is the finding that alternate mechanisms of apoptosis dysregulation, beyond

TABLE 1.1 Frequency of Bcl-2 Expression in Selected Human Malignancies

Malignancy	Prevalence (%)	Ref.
Hematologic Malignancies		
Acute myelogenous leukemia	34	98
Chronic myelogenous leukemia	57	99
Chronic lymphocytic leukemia	[a]100	100
Myeloma	71	101
Solid Tumors		
Melanoma	100	102
Localized prostate cancer	27–31	28,30
Hormone-refractory prostate cancer	33–100	103–105
Colorectal carcinoma	22–60	29,106,107
Non–small cell lung carcinoma	46–59	108,109
Small-cell lung carcinoma	110,111	
Breast carcinoma	26–85	18
Gastric carcinoma	54	17
Non-Hodgkin's lymphoma	89	27
Astrocytoma	92	26
Medulloblastoma	25	26
Neuroblastoma	100	26

[a]Small sample size.

Bcl-2, occur in several common malignancies. Similar to Bcl-2 overexpression, reduced *bax* gene expression leads to a dysequilibrium of apoptotic forces and a reduction in cellular apoptosis.[21] Mutations in the *bax* gene that impair normal Bax function occur at high frequency in carcinomas of the colon that possess the microsatellite mutator phenotype, whereas diminished Bax expression occurs in approximately 40% of ovarian and breast cancers.[21-25] These findings illustrate the important, albeit complex, relationships of the cell death pathway to carcinogenesis and also indicate that overexpression Bcl-2 may represent but one of many potential molecular targets governing aberrant apoptosis in malignant cells.

Several common solid and hematologic malignancies exhibit overexpression of Bcl-2 protein overexpression (Table 1.1). These include the B-cell malignancies (non-Hodgkin's lymphoma, chronic lymphocytic leukemia, and multiple myeloma), melanoma, gliomas, and prostate, ovarian, gastric, colorectal, and lung carcinomas.[17,26,27] Furthermore, Bcl-2 overexpression is a negative prognostic factor in several malignancies, including intermediate-grade non-Hodgkin's lymphoma, prostate cancer, and colorectal cancer, and it is associated with early relapse, or decreased survival, or both.[28-32] However, this finding is not universal, and some clinicopathologic studies indicate either no prognostic influence or an improved prognosis associated with Bcl-2 protein expression.[33-35]

Bcl-2 protein expression confers resistance to a diverse array of cytotoxic chemotherapeutic agents and hormone therapies in several tumor models. This includes the alkylating agents topoisomerase I and II inhibitors; mitomycin C; antimetabolites, including cytosine arabinoside, methotrexate, 5-fluorouracil, cisplatin, vincristine, and dexamethasone.[36-40] In the estrogen-sensitive MCF-7 human breast carcinoma cell line, estrogen up-regulates Bcl-2 expression and confers increased resistance to doxorubicin.[39] In contrast, androgen depletion increases Bcl-2 expression in the hormone-sensitive human prostate carcinoma (LNCaP) cell line.[41] Furthermore, increased resistance to the growth-inhibitory effects of androgen or estrogen withdrawal can be conferred experimentally to LNCaP and MCF-7 cells, respectively, by transfection and overexpression of the *bcl*-2 gene.[41-43] These studies indicate that the relative expression of Bcl-2 protein to proapoptotic proteins has a critical role in the realization of cellular apoptosis, irrespective of the therapeutic strategy (e.g., chemotherapy or hormone therapy) used to induce cell death.

In addition to regulation of apoptosis through the relative expression and heterodimerization of Bcl-2 expression with other proapoptotic partners, Bcl-2 function is further regulated, at least in part, through a dynamic equilibrium between phosphorylated and hypophosphorylated states. Phosphorylation of serine and threonine residues between the BH3 and BH4 regions of the Bcl-2 protein inhibits successful dimerization with Bax protein, thereby promoting apoptosis. A hierarchy may exist with respect to specific serine or threonine sites within these BH regions and their relative impact on Bcl-2 function. Mutations, particularly at threonine 56 and serine 87, appear to markedly impair the ability of Bcl-2 to inhibit glucocorticoid-induced apoptosis, whereas mutations of serine 70 and threonine 74 have less impact.[44-50] Regulation of function may also occur because of perturbations in phosphatases that lead to Bcl-2 dephosphorylation. This appears to be one mechanism by which chemotherapeutic agents, particularly antimicrotubule agents, mediate their anti-tumor therapeutic effect. Paclitaxel, docetaxel, and estramustine inhibit cytosolic phosphatases and shift the equilibrium to favor Bcl-2 in an inactivated phosphorylated state, resulting in an enhanced propensity for cellular apoptosis.[51,52]

Although frequently viewed as separate pathways, cellular proliferation and apoptosis are intrinsically linked. In experimental models, withdrawal of growth factor stimulation induces apoptosis that is mediated through selective Bcl-2 phosphorylation. Nerve growth factor regulates memory B-cell apoptosis through the selective trafficking of p38 mitogen-activated protein kinase.[45] After nerve growth factor stimulation, p38 mitogen-activated protein kinase is dephosphorylated and localizes to the cytosol of memory B cells. In contrast, after nerve growth factor withdrawal, p38 mitogen-activated protein kinase selectively localizes to the mitochondria and phosphorylates Bcl-2; apoptosis is induced. The partitioning of p38 mitogen-activated protein kinase by growth factor receptor activation represents an intriguing mechanism for apoptosis regulation.

Because of the pivotal role Bcl-2 has in the regulation of cellular apoptosis in a diverse spectrum of malignancies and also in the ability to confer resistance to a broad array of chemotherapeutic and hormone therapies, Bcl-2 protein therefore represents an attractive therapeutic target in the treatment of malignant diseases. Although preclinical development is ongoing with specific small molecule inhibitors of Bcl-2/Bax interaction, the clinical development of these agents has so far been elusive.[53,54] In contrast, antisense oligonucleotide strategies to inhibit Bcl-2 expression are presently in late-stage clinical development.

ANTISENSE OLIGONUCLEOTIDE AS THERAPEUTICS

Antisense oligonucleotides were originally described as experimental tools to inhibit specific gene expression.[55-58] Antisense oligonucleotides are short strands of ribose or deoxyribose nucleic acids that are synthesized to hybridize by Watson and Crick pairing to the complementary sequence within the messenger RNA (mRNA) of a specific gene. Hybridization results in RNAse H-mediated scission of the mRNA/oligonucleotide pairing, thereby inhibiting translation and protein expression.[55-59] On the basis of the marked selectivity that antisense oligonucleotides possess to inhibit gene expression, the potential for therapeutic uses were quickly recognized.[60] However, several physiochemical barriers associated with both oligonucleotide chemistry and the target mRNA/oligonucleotide hybridization impeded the clinical development of antisense oligonucleotide therapeutics.

Unmodified oligonucleotides are unsuitable for therapeutic purposes. Rapid degradation of the phosphodiester linkage occurs in vivo by ubiquitous plasma and cellular nucleases. To surmount this obstacle, the phosphodiester backbone is modified to incorporate sulfur substitutions for nonbridging oxygen atoms.[61] Because these modifications also reduce the affinity of an antisense oligonucleotide to hybridize with the target mRNA, strand lengths of 16 to 20 bases are used to optimize the binding kinetics and target specificity.[61]

Not all regions within an mRNA are suitable for antisense attack. The conformational structure of mRNA is not linear but instead exists as a three-dimensional structure with sequence-specific folding. These steric conformations hinder successful mRNA-antisense oligonucleotide hybridization. As a result, there can be a striking diversity in the potency of mRNA scission between different sequences of antisense Bcl-2 oligonucleotides, even though they may target regions in close proximity to one another or may even partially overlap target mRNA regions.[62] The absence of uniformity between antisense molecules with seemingly similar or partially overlapping sequences necessitates the screening of numerous oligonucleotide sequences to determine an optimal candidate for therapeutic use.[61] For the *bcl*-2 mRNA, several regions exhibit superior sensitivity antisense oligonucleotide–mediated cell kill, including codons 1–6, codons 141–147, and the termination region.[62]

OBLIMERSEN SODIUM

Oblimersen sodium (Genasense, formerly known as G3139, sequence 5′-TCTCCCAGCGTGCGCCAT-3′) is an 18-mer phosphorothioate antisense deoxynucleotide directed to the first six codons of the open reading frame of the Bcl-2 mRNA. Extensive preclinical studies across a broad spectrum of human tumor cell lines in vitro have demonstrated that oblimersen sodium induces nucleotide sequence–specific degradation of the *Bcl-2* mRNA that subsequently inhibits Bcl-2 protein expression.[63-66] In contrast, a reduction in Bcl-2 expression was not observed with either a two-base-pair mismatch control oligonucleotide (5′-TCTCCCAGCATGTGCCAT-3′) or a reverse-polarity control oligonucleotide (5′-TACCGCGTGCGACCCTCT-3′).[41,63,64] Furthermore, the inhibitory effects are dose dependent, with concentrations of 1–5 μg/mL being necessary for Bcl-2 protein expression inhibition in vitro.[41] In experimental time course studies in human tumor cell lines, oblimersen sodium reduced Bcl-2 protein expression to undetectable levels within 24 hours, although this effect was reversible and protein expression recovered to baseline values 48 hours after washout.[41]

Oblimersen has demonstrated dose-dependent tumor growth inhibition of several human tumor cell lines and implanted xenograft models. This includes the myeloid leukemia cell lines (KG1a and HL-60), bladder (T24), and both androgen-dependent and androgen-independent prostate carcinoma cell lines (LNCaP and PC3).[64,65,67] Because Bcl-2 overexpression confers intrinsic resistance to the apoptotic effects of cytotoxic agents experimentally, oblimersen has been combined with several chemotherapeutic agents to examine whether inhibition Bcl-2 expression enhances the apoptotic and therapeutic effectiveness of these agents. To this end, oblimersen markedly enhances the anti-tumor effectiveness of various chemotherapy agents in several human xenograft models, including dimethyltriazeno-imidazole carboxamide (dacarbazine) in a melanoma cell line (518A2), cyclophosphamide in a lymphoma cell line (DoHH2), docetaxel both for an androgen-independent prostate cell line (PC3) and non–small cell lung cancer NCI-H460.[63,68-71] The enhancement of apoptotic and therapeutic effect by oblimersen extends to combinations with nonchemotherapeutic strategies, such as androgen withdrawal in mice bearing the androgen-responsive prostate carcinoma cell line (LNCaP), estrogen withdrawal in mice bearing Bcl-2–transfected MCF-7 breast carcinoma cell line, and with rituximab in an Epstein-Barr virus–transformed lymphoblastoid cell line.[41,72]

Because cell proliferation and cell death pathways are inherently interrelated, Bcl-2 protein is an attractive target in malignancies where a direct link exists between an aberrant signal transduction pathway that mediates proliferation and Bcl-2 expression. In BCR-ABL transformed cells, the BCR-ABL tyrosine kinase mediates a clonal proliferation, at least in part, through increased Bcl-2 protein expression and inhibition of apoptosis.[73] Consistent with these findings, inhibition of Bcl-2 by oblimersen induces single-agent tumor regressions in an imatinib-resistant BCR-ABL transformed cell line.[74] The clinical implications of these results indicate that oblimersen may have a role as a single agent in the treatment of imatinib-resistant chronic myelogenous leukemia, as well as front-line treatment of chronic myelogenous leukemia to enhance the effectiveness of imatinib therapy.

Because oligonucleotides have the potential for nonspecific anti-tumor and immunostimulatory effects that may confound the interpretation of preclinical results, careful use of controls is necessary to appropriately interpret the results. The polyanionic charge of most antisense oligonucleotides represents an important barrier to the effective uptake and biologic activity in vitro. To overcome this physiochemical obstacle, cationic lipids are routinely used in vitro to permit sufficient cellular uptake to examine the biochemical and biologic properties of antisense treatment. In the absence of cationic lipids, the uptake of oblimersen in vitro is limited; therefore, the nonspecific effects become apparent, and caution must be used in the interpretation of these nonspecific effects.[75] In contrast, although the mechanism or mechanisms are not fully elucidated, cellular uptake is much greater in vivo, and cationic lipids are unnecessary for competent transfection and inhibition of target protein.[41] For in vivo studies, oligonucleotides with CpG motifs have nonspecific and nonantisense immunostimulatory properties, and for the oblimersen sequence, two such motifs are present. However, several lines of evidence indicate that the principal in vivo effects of oblimersen sodium, down-regulation of Bcl-2 protein and enhancement of cytotoxic anti-tumor activity, are specific to the anti–Bcl-2 properties and are not related to non-specific oligonucleotide or immunostimulatory properties. This includes both in vitro and in vivo evidence that oblimersen, but not a two-base-pair mismatch or reverse-polarity control oligonucleotide (the latter also containing two CpG motifs), enhance the anti-tumor activity of cytotoxic chemotherapy agents.[63,68,76] In addition, the anti-tumor effects observed occur in both nude and severe combined immunodeficiency disease mice models, both of which have limited host immune competency.[41,63] Lastly, modifications to oblimersen that silence the immunostimulant effects of CpG motifs maintain anti-tumor activity. Wacheck et al[77] abrogated the immunostimulatory properties of oblimersen sodium by selectively methylating cytosine amino acids present in the CpG motifs and found enhancement of anti-tumor and apoptosis activity with the modified oligonucleotide that was comparable to that observed with oblimersen in a xenotransplanted human melanoma model. Taken together, the results of these studies strongly support the targeted anti–Bcl-2 mechanism of action for oblimersen.

Preclinical evaluation of the distribution, metabolism, and excretion of oblimersen sodium have been performed in mice. After a single intravenous bolus injection of ^{35}S-labeled oblimersen sodium, the radioactivity rapidly distributed from the plasma to the tissues.[78] Accumulation of oblimersen in specific organs was observed with tissue-to-plasma ratios of 87, 17, 5, 3.5, and 2.5 for the kidney, liver, spleen, gut, and heart and lung, respectively. Notably, radiolabeled oblimersen sodium was not detectable in the brain. Initially, most oblimersen sodium (98%) was plasma protein bound, although at 24 hours only a small amount of radioactivity (23%) was associated with plasma proteins. The plasma concentration-time curve fit to a three-compartment model, with a terminal elimination half-life averaging 11 hours. Parent compound represented the vast majority of radioactivity detected initially (98% at 15 minutes) but was rapidly reduced to 36% at 6 hours and 25% at 48 hours. Although most of the radioactivity detected in the kidney was parent compound, only trace amounts of parent drug were detected in the urine. After the subcutaneous continuous 7-day route of administration, rapid distribution to tissues was again noted at tissue-to-plasma ratios comparable to those occurring with intravenous administration. With the 7-day continuous subcutaneous administration, radioactivity accumulated in the previously described organs between days 3 and 7, followed by undetectable radioactivity at day 14 (7 days after discontinuation of infusion). Subcutaneous administration was also associated with a more prolonged elimination half-life, which averaged 22 hours. Two main metabolites were detected, both of which appeared to be shortened oligonucleotide fragments, presumably derived from plasma and tissue exonucleases, and these were excreted in the urine and feces.

Oblimersen appears to distribute preferentially in xenotransplanted tumor tissue compared with normal murine host tissue. The ratio of oblimersen distributed to implanted tumor tissue versus normal tissue ranged from 2.5- to

3.8-fold. Furthermore, the accumulation of oblimersen in tumor tissue appears to be, at least in part, independent of steady-state plasma concentrations in xenograft models.[79] These preclinical pharmacokinetic studies indicate that oblimersen sodium distributes widely and accumulates preferentially in kidney, liver, and tumor tissues at concentrations anticipated to possess biologic activity.

EARLY CLINICAL TRIALS WITH OBLIMERSEN SODIUM

There is considerable clinical experience with oblimersen sodium therapy both as a single agent and in combination with chemotherapeutic agents. Oblimersen sodium has been examined in three single-agent phase I studies. The first clinical study administered oblimersen sodium by continuous subcutaneous 14-day infusion at doses that ranged from 4.6 to 195.8 mg/m^2/day for 14 days.[80,81] The population consisted exclusively of heavily pretreated low-grade and diffuse large-cell non-Hodgkin's lymphoma patients. The principal toxicities consisted of hyperglycemia, transient hepatic transaminase elevations, fever, fatigue, and local skin inflammation at the infusion site. Thrombocytopenia accompanied by both fever and fatigue was dose limiting in two of three patients treated at the highest dose level, with the maximum tolerated dose (MTD) determined to be 147.2 mg/m^2/day (approximately 4.1 mg/kg/day). Steady-state concentrations reached within 48 hours were proportional to dose. There was considerable interpatient variability with respect to steady-state concentrations, with a range of 0.96 to 6.67 μg/mL at the MTD. In a multivariate analysis of covariates that potentially influenced steady-state concentrations, only dose and renal function were significant.[81] Thrombocytopenia was the predominant dose-limiting toxicity and was related to both dose and steady-state concentrations. The plasma elimination half-life averaged 7.46 hours when this continuous subcutaneous infusion route of administration was used. One patient achieved a durable complete response lasting 36 months, whereas two other patients experienced minor responses.[80,81]

A continuous intravenous administration schedule was examined in the second single-agent dose-escalation study. The study population consisted of patients with advanced solid malignancies, and most of these patients had either hormone-refractory prostate carcinoma or renal carcinomas.[82] Doses up to and including 10 mg/kg/day could be feasibly administered for 14 days, and severe dose-limiting toxicity was rarely observed. The principal toxicities included fatigue, hepatic transaminitis, diarrhea, modest (grade 1 and 2) thrombocytopenia and leukopenia, and hyperglycemia. Steady-state G3139 plasma concentrations were attained within 10 hours, they were dose-proportional, and the mean elimination half-life was 2.1 hours. Although the clearance of oblimersen sodium was greater with the intravenous route of administration than with the subcutaneous route, this result was consistent with preclinical pharmacokinetic evaluations.[78] Average steady-state concentrations, which were 4.28 and 7.58 at the 5.3-mg/kg/day and 6.9-mg/kg/day dose levels, respectively, were comparable to those with subcutaneous administration.[78,81] Preliminary evidence from Bcl-2 quantification assays in peripheral blood mononuclear cells indicated that a marked reduction of Bcl-2 protein expression occurred by day 8, and Bcl-2 protein was undetectable at days 15 and 21. No objective responses were observed in this advanced solid tumor population.

Currently, only preliminary data from a single-agent dose-escalation study of oblimersen sodium performed exclusively in patients with chronic lymphocytic leukemia is available. In this patient population, a constellation of side effects, including fever, fatigue, and tumor lysis syndrome, have been observed.[83] In this study, 3 mg/kg/day of oblimersen sodium was feasibly administered to patients with chronic lymphocytic leukemia (CLL); however, for patients who did not experience evidence of dose-limiting toxicity, dose escalation to 4 mg/kg/day was possible. The discrepancy between the MTDs defined in these three single-agent studies is intriguing. Patients with lymphoproliferative malignancies may be less tolerant to single-agent oblimersen therapy, partly because of the release of inflammatory cytokines as part of the antilymphocytic effects, or in the case of CLL, because of byproducts of tumor cell death leading to tumor lysis syndrome.[83]

The observation of single-agent antilymphoma and antileukemic responses with oblimersen sodium is presumably due, at least in part, to the pivotal role that Bcl-2 expression has in the etiology of these diseases. The responses observed in non-Hodgkin's lymphoma and CLL provide important clinical "proof of concept" that Bcl-2 inhibition restores failed apoptosis.[6,84] However, for most other malignancies, Bcl-2 protein expression may be part of a larger number of molecular genetic changes associated with carcinogenesis and cellular proliferation, and Bcl-2 protein may not be fundamental to cell survival. In these malignancies, targeting Bcl-2 to enhance chemotherapy-mediated apoptosis is a sound rationale.

The established role for Bcl-2 protein expression conferring resistance to the cytotoxic effects of chemotherapy in laboratory models, combined with the evidence that inhibition of Bcl-2 protein expression by oblimersen enhances the effectiveness of several chemotherapeutic agents in vitro and in vivo, provides a strong impetus for the evaluation of oblimersen in combination with antineoplastic agents in clinical trials. Complete and preliminary results with several chemotherapy agents indicate that oblimersen sodium can be combined with full doses of several cytotoxic agents (Table 1.2).

Combination studies first examined oblimersen in combination with dacarbazine in patients with advanced malignant melanoma. This combination was chosen because of the intrinsically chemoresistant nature of melanoma and several intriguing features of melanocyte development. Bcl-2 protein has an integral role in the development of normal skin melanocytes. In *bcl*-2 knock-out mice, loss of dark hair color occurs after birth as a result of the rapid degeneration of hair bulb melanocytes.[85] In most melanoma tumor biopsy specimens, Bcl-2 protein is expressed, and overexpression of Bcl-2 protein is a negative prognostic

TABLE 1.2 Tumor Site-Specific Phase I/II Studies of Oblimersen in Combination with Cytotoxic Agents (completed)

Tumor Site	Maximum Tolerated Dose Oblimersen Dose/ Chemotherapy Dose	Reference
Melanoma	Oblimersen, 6.5 mg/kg/day CIV × 14 days DTIC, 200 mg/m²/day i.v. × 5 days	93
	Oblimersen, 7.7 mg/kg/day CIV × 5 days DTIC, 1000 mg/m² day 6	93
Prostate	Oblimersen, 5 mg/kg/day CIV × 14 days Mitoxantrone, 12 mg/m² i.v. day 8	69
	Oblimersen, 7 mg/kg/day CIV × 5 days Docetaxel, 75 mg/m² i.v. day 6	89
Small-Cell Lung	[a]Oblimersen, 3 mg/kg/day CIV × 7 days Paclitaxel, 150 mg/m² i.v. day 6	90
Breast	[a]Oblimersen, 4 mg/kg/day CIV × 21 days Docetaxel, 35 mg/m² i.v. weekly	92
Colorectal	Oblimersen, 7 mg/kg/day CIV × 7 days Irinotecan, 280 mg/m² i.v. day 6	91
AML	[a]Oblimersen, 7 mg/kg/day CIV × 10 days Fludarabine, 15 mg/kg i.v. day 6–10 Cytarabine, 1000 mg/m² i.v. days 6–10	94

Abbreviations: CIV, continuous intravenous infusion; DTIC, dimethyltriazeno-imidazole carboxamide (dacarbazine); i.v., intravenously; AML, acute myelogenous leukemia.
[a]Maximum tolerated dose not defined.

factor that predicts earlier relapse and decreased survival.[86,87] In preclinical studies, oblimersen in combination with dacarbazine produced eradication of tumors and long-term cures in mice that bore xenotransplanted human melanoma tumor cell lines.[63] In the phase I evaluation of this combination, 14 metastatic patients were treated with the combination of oblimersen sodium at doses of 0.6 to 6.5 mg/kg/day by continuous intravenous infusion for 14 days, along with dacarbazine, 200 mg/m^2, administered starting on day 5 for 5 days and repeated every month (Table 1.2). An MTD was not specifically determined for this combination; however, the highest dose of oblimersen did reach an average steady-state concentration of 6.5 μg/mL, exceeding the concentrations necessary for Bcl-2 inhibition in vitro. The major toxicities of the combination were largely attributed to the dacarbazine, although fever attributed to oblimersen was observed at doses greater than 4.0 mg/kg/day. Melanoma metastases biopsy samples were assayed for Bcl-2 expression and demonstrated a 40% median reduction in Bcl-2 expression after 5 days of oblimersen therapy when compared with pretreatment values. In addition, the rate of apoptotic nuclei measured in these metastatic tumor biopsy specimens increased from a pretreatment mean value of 0.85% to 3.17% after 5 days of oblimersen therapy, and it further increased to 19.4% after dacarbazine administration. Although not the primary endpoint of this dose-escalation study, one complete response, two partial responses, and two minor responses were observed in 14 evaluable patients. This response rate compares favorably with the known single-agent activity of dacarbazine in metastatic melanoma.[88] The partial responses were also considered impressive because both patients had received prior immunotherapy and chemotherapy. To further address the effectiveness of this combination and the role of Bcl-2 inhibition in enhancing the anti-tumor activity of dacarbazine in malignant melanoma, a randomized study of dacarbazine with or without oblimersen was initiated.

Bcl-2 protein expression may have a role in mediating the transition from hormone-sensitive to hormone-refractory prostate cancer. On the basis of the frequency of Bcl-2 protein expression hormone-refractory prostate cancer specimens and also on the intrinsic chemoresistance of this disease, several phase I studies have examined oblimersen in combination with mitoxantrone or docetaxel (Table 1.2). The results of these studies indicate that oblimersen sodium at doses of 5–7 mg/kg/day can be combined safely with these cytotoxic agents at their full doses, and the toxicity associated with the combinations are predominantly those associated with the cytotoxic chemotherapeutic agent.[69,89] Furthermore, assays of peripheral blood mononuclear cells indicate that Bcl-2 protein expression is markedly reduced after 5 days of oblimersen therapy.

Disease-specific studies that combine oblimersen with a broad array of chemotherapeutic agents have been initiated or are completed (Table 1.2). The results indicate that oblimersen can be feasibly administered with full or near-full doses of the commonly indicated chemotherapeutic agents to patients with colorectal carcinoma (irinotecan), small-cell lung cancer (paclitaxel), acute myelogenous leukemia (cytarabine), and breast cancer (docetaxel).[90-92] In some of these studies, particularly the acute myelogenous leukemia and melanoma studies, responses have been observed after the reintroduction of previously used cytotoxic chemotherapeutic agents.[93,94] The results imply that Bcl-2 expression may be responsible for both intrinsic and acquired chemotherapy resistance, and reversal of clinical resistance may occur in some patients with oblimersen therapy.

There are several challenges for the successful clinical development of targeted agents whose mechanism of action is largely confined to the enhancement of currently available chemotherapy. Historically, the only successful regulatory approval of such an agent was folinic acid used in combination with 5-FU to enhance the activity of the latter agent for the treatment of colorectal carcinoma. Single-arm phase II studies have several limitations with regard to the true assessment of an agent such as oblimersen. The small sample size of these studies does not permit sufficient statistical confidence that the response rate observed is actually different from that observed with the single-agent chemotherapeutic agent alone. Therefore, randomized comparative studies are required to fully determine the therapeutic benefit, if any, of oblimersen added to a cytotoxic agent. Currently, several studies have been initiated over a broad spectrum of malignancies, including melanoma, non–small cell lung cancer (second line), small-cell lung cancer, CLL, acute myelogenous leukemia, and myeloma (Table 1.3). What is not currently available for most malignancies is an understanding of the predictive biomarkers that will identify which patient population will experience maximal therapeutic gain from Bcl-2 inhibition.

PATIENT SELECTION AND PREDICTIVE BIOMARKERS

Of the clinical and biologic questions that remain to be answered for Bcl-2–targeted therapy, none is more important than the identification of subpopulations that will derive maximal benefit from anti–Bcl-2 therapy. Resistance to chemotherapy, hormone therapy, and irradiation is a multifactorial process, with Bcl-2 being but one mechanism. Unfortunately, the degree of Bcl-2 expression, in isolation, may not be sufficient for predicting activity. Oblimersen has demonstrated enhanced anti-tumor activity of several apoptosis-inducing agents in both low and high Bcl-2–expressing cell lines.[95] Biomarkers other than Bcl-2 expression may be more useful and may identify populations that are destined to respond or may alternatively identify populations that will not respond (e.g., those

TABLE 1.3 Randomized Studies Planned or Initiated Examining the Efficacy of Oblimersen in Combination with Antineoplastic Agents

Tumor Site	Treatment Arms	Indication
Melanoma	DTIC (± oblimersen	1st line
CLL	Fludarabine/cyclophosphamide ± oblimersen	2nd line
Myeloma	Dexamethasone ± oblimersen	Relapsed Refractory
NSCLC	Docetaxel ± oblimersen	2nd line
Small-Cell Lung	Carboplatin/etoposide ± oblimersen (CALGB)	1st line
AML	Daunorubicin/cytarabine ± oblimersen	1st line
Prostate	Docetaxel ± oblimersen (NCIC/EROTC)	1st line (hormone refractory)

Abbreviations: DTIC, dimethyltriazeno-imidazole carboxamide (dacarbazine); AML, acute myelogenous leukemia; NSCLC, non–small cell lung carcinoma; CLL, chronic lymphocytic leukemia; CALGB, cancer and leukemia group B; EROTC, European Organization for Research and Treatment of Cancer; NCIC, National Cancer Institute of Canada.

with diminished Bax expression) to oblimersen-based therapy. Experience with the prototypic molecularly targeting agent trastuzumab indicates that identifying expression of the target alone (e.g., Her2 2+ or 3+) without discerning the subgroups in which tumor growth and biology are predictive of response (e.g., HER2 amplification) may reduce the likelihood of a successful outcome in randomized studies.[96,97] The identification of these subpopulations may be critical for targeted therapies, such as oblimersen, to successfully demonstrate an improvement in outcome in randomized studies.

CURRENT STATUS OF BCL-2 ANTISENSE STRATEGIES

The randomized studies of oblimersen combined with chemotherapy for the treatment of melanoma and CLL are approaching completion, with definitive results likely in 2003 and 2004. These two tumor sites represent good indications to test Bcl-2 inhibition by oblimersen. Both of these malignant diseases strongly express Bcl-2 in most patients. Furthermore, metastatic melanoma is an intrinsically chemoresistant disease with few therapeutic options, whereas CLL has a surfeit of active agents but is rarely curable. The results of these studies will not only define the importance of oblimersen in the treatment of these two indications but will also have significant implications for the validity of antisense oligonucleotide therapeutics and the value of Bcl-2 as a molecular target in the treatment of a broad spectrum of malignancies.

REFERENCES

1. Thornberry NA. Caspases: a decade of death research. Cell Death Differ 1999;6:1023–1027.
2. Thornberry NA, Lazebnik Y. Caspases: enemies within. Science 1998;281:1312–1316.
3. Keane MM, Rubinstein Y, Cuello M et al. Inhibition of NF-kappaB activity enhances TRAIL mediated apoptosis in breast cancer cell lines. Breast Cancer Res Treat 2000;64:211–219.
4. Sun SY, Yue P, Zhou JY et al. Overexpression of BCL2 blocks TNF-related apoptosis-inducing ligand (TRAIL)-induced apoptosis in human lung cancer cells. Biochem Biophys Res Commun 2001;280:788–797.
5. Tsujimoto Y, Finger LR, Yunis J et al. Cloning of the chromosome breakpoint of neoplastic B cells with the t(14;18) chromosome translocation. Science 1984;226:1097–1099.
6. Tsujimoto Y, Cossman J, Jaffe E et al. Involvement of the bcl-2 gene in human follicular lymphoma. Science 1985;228:1440–1443.
7. Tsujimoto Y, Ikegaki N, Croce CM. Characterization of the protein product of bcl-2, the gene involved in human follicular lymphoma. Oncogene 1987;2:3–7.
8. Zha H, Reed JC. Heterodimerization-independent functions of cell death regulatory proteins Bax and Bcl-2 in yeast and mammalian cells. J Biol Chem 1997;272: 31482–31488.
9. Zha H, Aime-Sempe C, Sato T et al. Proapoptotic protein Bax heterodimerizes with Bcl-2 and homodimerizes with Bax via a novel domain (BH3) distinct from BH1 and BH2. J Biol Chem 1996;271:7440–7444.
10. Tanaka S, Saito K, Reed JC. Structure-function analysis of the Bcl-2 oncoprotein: addition of a heterologous transmembrane domain to portions of the Bcl-2 beta protein restores function as a regulator of cell survival. J Biol Chem 1993;268:10920–10926.

11. Yang Korsmeyer SJ. Molecular thanatopsis: a discourse on the BCL2 family and cell death. Blood 1996;88:386–401.

12. Korsmeyer SJ. Regulators of cell death. Trends Genet 1995;11:101–105.

13. Schendel SL, Xie Z, Montal MO et al. Channel formation by antiapoptotic protein Bcl-2. Proc Natl Acad Sci USA 1997;94:5113–5118.

14. Minn AJ, Velez P, Schendel SL et al. Bcl-x(L) forms an ion channel in synthetic lipid membranes. Nature 1997;385:353–357.

15. Schlesinger, PH, Gross A, Yin XM et al. Comparison of the ion channel characteristics of proapoptotic BAX and antiapoptotic BCL-2. Proc Natl Acad Sci USA 1997;94:11357–11362.

16. Krajewski S, Bodrug S, Krajewska M et al. Immunohistochemical analysis of Mcl-1 protein in human tissues: differential regulation of Mcl-1 and Bcl-2 protein production suggests a unique role for Mcl-1 in control of programmed cell death in vivo. Am J Pathol 1995;146:1309–1319.

17. Krajewska M, Fenoglio-Preiser CM, Krajewski S et al. Immunohistochemical analysis of Bcl-2 family proteins in adenocarcinomas of the stomach. Am J Pathol 1996;149:1449–1457.

18. Krajewski S, Thor AD, Edgerton SM et al. Analysis of Bax and Bcl-2 expression in p53-immunopositive breast cancers. Clin Cancer Res 1997;3:199–208.

19. Graninger WB, Seto M, Boutain B et al. Expression of Bcl-2 and Bcl-2-Ig fusion transcripts in normal and neoplastic cells. J Clin Invest 1987;80:1512–1515.

20. McDonnell TJ, Deane N, Platt FM et al. bcl-2-immunoglobulin transgenic mice demonstrate extended B cell survival and follicular lymphoproliferation. Cell 1989;57:79–88.

21. Gil J, Yamamoto H, Zapata JM et al. Impairment of the proapoptotic activity of Bax by missense mutations found in gastrointestinal cancers. Cancer Res 1999;59:2034–2037.

22. Ionov Y, Yamamoto H, Krajewski S et al. Mutational inactivation of the proapoptotic gene BAX confers selective advantage during tumor clonal evolution. Proc Nat Acad Sci USA. 2000;97:10872–10877.

23. Tai YT, Lee S, Niloff E et al. BAX protein expression and clinical outcome in epithelial ovarian cancer. J Clin Oncol 1998;16:2583–2590.

24. Rampino N, Yamamoto H, Ionov Y et al. Somatic frameshift mutations in the BAX gene in colon cancers of the microsatellite mutator phenotype. Science 1997;275:967–969.

25. Krajewski S, Blomqvist C, Franssila K et al. Reduced expression of proapoptotic gene BAX is associated with poor response rates to combination chemotherapy and shorter survival in women with metastatic breast adenocarcinoma. Cancer Res 1995;55:4471–4478.

26. Krajewski S, Krajewska M, Ehrmann J et al. Immunohistochemical analysis of Bcl-2, Bcl-X, Mcl-1, and Bax in tumors of central and peripheral nervous system origin. Am J Pathol 1997;150:805–814.

27. Krajewski S, Bodrug S, Gascoyne R et al. Immunohistochemical analysis of Mcl-1 and Bcl-2 proteins in normal and neoplastic lymph nodes. Am J Pathol 1994;145:515–525.

28. Bauer JJ, Sesterhenn IA, Mostofi FK et al. Elevated levels of apoptosis regulator proteins p53 and bcl-2 are independent prognostic biomarkers in surgically treated clinically localized prostate cancer. J Urol 1996;156:1511–1516.

29. Bhatavdekar JM, Patel DD, Ghosh N et al. Coexpression of Bcl-2, c-Myc, and p53 oncoproteins as prognostic discriminants in patients with colorectal carcinoma. Dis Colon Rectum 1997;40:785–790.

30. Bubendorf L, Sauter G, Moch H et al. Prognostic significance of Bcl-2 in clinically localized prostate cancer. Am J Pathol 1996;148:1557–1565.

31. Gascoyne RD, Adomat SA, Krajewski S et al. Prognostic significance of Bcl-2 protein expression and Bcl-2 gene rearrangement in diffuse aggressive non-Hodgkin's lymphoma. Blood 1997;90:244–251.

32. Moul JW, Bettencourt MC, Sesterhenn IA et al. Protein expression of p53, bcl-2, and KI-67 (MIB-1) as prognostic biomarkers in patients with surgically treated, clinically localized prostate cancer. Surgery 1996;120:159-66; discussion 66–67.

33. Cox G, Louise Jones J, Andi A et al. Bcl-2 is an independent prognostic factor and adds to a biological model for predicting outcome in operable non-small cell lung cancer. Lung Cancer 2001;34:417–426.

34. Han H, Landreneau RJ, Santucci TS et al. Prognostic value of immunohistochemical expressions of p53, HER-2/neu, and bcl-2 in stage I non-small-cell lung cancer. Hum Pathol 2002;33:105–110.

35. Silvestrini R, Veneroni S, Daidone MG et al. The Bcl-2 protein: a prognostic indicator strongly related to p53 protein in lymph node-negative breast cancer patients. J Natl Cancer Inst 1994;86:499–504.

36. Miyashita T, Reed JC. Bcl-2 oncoprotein blocks chemotherapy-induced apoptosis in a human leukemia cell line. Blood 1993;81:151–157.

37. Ohmori T, Podack ER, Nishio K et al. Apoptosis of lung cancer cells caused by some anti-cancer agents (MMC, CPT-11, ADM) is inhibited by bcl-2. Biochem Biophys Res Commun 1993;192:30–36.

38. Walton MI, Whysong D, O'Connor PM et al. Constitutive expression of human Bcl-2 modulates nitrogen mustard and camptothecin induced apoptosis. Cancer Res 1993;53:1853–1861.

39. Teixeira C, Reed JC, Pratt MA. Estrogen promotes chemotherapeutic drug resistance by a mechanism involving Bcl-2 proto-oncogene expression in human breast cancer cells. Cancer Res 1995;55:3902–3907.

40. Violette S, Poulain L, Dussaulx E et al. Resistance of colon cancer cells to long-term 5-fluorouracil exposure is correlated to the relative level of Bcl-2 and Bcl-X(L) in addition to Bax and p53 status. Int J Cancer 2002;98:498–504.

41. Gleave M, Tolcher A, Miyake H et al. Progression to androgen independence is delayed by adjuvant treatment with antisense Bcl-2 oligodeoxynucleotides after castration in the LNCaP prostate tumor model. Clin Cancer Res 1999;5:2891–2898.

42. Raffo AJ, Perlman H, Chen MW et al. Overexpression of bcl-2 protects prostate cancer cells from apoptosis in vitro and confers resistance to androgen depletion in vivo. Cancer Res 1995;55:4438–4445.

43. Pratt MA, Krajewski S, Menard M et al. Estrogen withdrawal-induced human breast cancer tumour regression in nude mice is prevented by Bcl-2. FEBS Lett 1998; 440:403–408.

44. Huang ST, Cidlowski JA. Phosphorylation status modulates Bcl-2 function during glucocorticoid-induced apoptosis in T lymphocytes. FASEB J 2002;16:825–832.

45. Torcia M, De Chiara G, Nencioni L et al. Nerve growth factor inhibits apoptosis in memory B lymphocytes via inactivation of p38 MAPK, prevention of Bcl-2 phosphorylation, and cytochrome c release. J Biol Chem 2001;276:39027–39036.

46. Blagosklonny MV. Unwinding the loop of Bcl-2 phosphorylation. Leukemia 2001;15:869–874.

47. Park JW, Choi YJ, Jang MA et al. Arsenic trioxide induces G2/M growth arrest and apoptosis after caspase-3 activation and bcl-2 phosphorylation in promonocytic U937 cells. Biochem Biophys Res Commun 2001;286:726–734.

48. Calastretti A, Bevilacqua A, Ceriani C et al. Damaged microtubules can inactivate BCL-2 by means of the mTOR kinase. Oncogene 2001;20:6172–6180.

49. Furukawa Y, Iwase S, Kikuchi J et al. Phosphorylation of Bcl-2 protein by CDC2 kinase during G2/M phases and its role in cell cycle regulation. J Biol Chem 2000;275:21661–21667.

50. Shitashige M, Toi M, Yano T et al. Dissociation of Bax from a Bcl-2/Bax heterodimer triggered by phosphorylation of serine 70 of Bcl-2. J Biochem 2001;130:741–748.

51. Haldar S, Jena N, Croce CM. Inactivation of Bcl-2 by phosphorylation. Proc Natl Acad Sci USA 1995;92:4507–4511.

52. Haldar S, Chintapalli J, Croce CM. Taxol induces bcl-2 phosphorylation and death of prostate cancer cells. Cancer Res 1996;56:1253–1255.

53. Wang JL, Zhang ZJ, Choksi S et al. Cell permeable Bcl-2 binding peptides: a chemical approach to apoptosis induction in tumor cells. Cancer Res 2000;60:1498–1502.

54. Wang JL, Liu D, Zhang ZJ et al. Structure-based discovery of an organic compound that binds Bcl-2 protein and induces apoptosis of tumor cells. Proc Natl Acad Sci USA 2000;97:7124–7129.

55. Paterson BM, Roberts BE, Kuff EL. Structural gene identification and mapping by DNA-mRNA hybrid-arrested cell-free translation. Proc Natl Acad Sci USA 1977;74:4370–4374.

56. Zamecnik PC, Goodchild J, Taguchi Y et al. Inhibition of replication and expression of human T-cell lymphotropic virus type III in cultured cells by exogenous synthetic oligonucleotides complementary to viral RNA. Proc Natl Acad Sci USA 1986;83:4143–4146.

57. Stephenson ML, Zamecnik PC. Inhibition of Rous sarcoma viral RNA translation by a specific oligodeoxyribonucleotide. Proc Natl Acad Sci USA 1978;75:285–288.

58. Zamecnik PC, Stephenson ML. Inhibition of Rous sarcoma virus replication and cell transformation by a specific oligodeoxynucleotide. Proc Natl Acad Sci USA 1978;75:280–284.

59. Crooke ST. Molecular mechanisms of antisense drugs: RNase H. Antisense Nucleic Acid Drug Dev 1998;8:133–134.

60. Goodchild J, Agrawal S, Civeira MP et al. Inhibition of human immunodeficiency virus replication by antisense oligodeoxynucleotides. Proc Natl Acad Sci USA 1988;85:5507–5511.

61. Crooke ST. Molecular mechanisms of action of antisense drugs. Biochim Biophys Acta 1999;1489:31–44.

62. Ziegler A, Luedke GH, Fabbro D et al. Induction of apoptosis in small-cell lung cancer cells by an antisense oligodeoxynucleotide targeting the Bcl-2 coding sequence. J Natl Cancer Inst 1997;89:1027–1036.

63. Jansen B, Schlagbauer-Wadl H, Brown BD et al. bcl-2 antisense therapy chemosensitizes human melanoma in SCID mice. Nat Med 1998;4:232–234.

64. Gleave ME, Miayake H, Goldie J et al. Targeting bcl-2 gene to delay androgen-independent progression and enhance chemosensitivity in prostate cancer using antisense bcl-2 oligodeoxynucleotides. Urology 1999;54:36–46.

65. Benimetskaya L, Miller P, Benimetsky S et al. Inhibition of potentially anti-apoptotic proteins by antisense protein kinase C-alpha (Isis 3521) and antisense bcl-2 (G3139) phosphorothioate oligodeoxynucleotides: relationship to the decreased viability of T24 bladder and PC3 prostate cancer cells. Mol Pharmacol 2001;60:1296–1307.

66. Wacheck V, Heere-Ress E, Halaschek-Wiener J et al. Bcl-2 antisense oligonucleotides chemosensitize human gastric cancer in a SCID mouse xenotransplantation model. J Mol Med 2001;79:587–593.

67. Campos L, Sabido O, Rouault JP et al. Effects of BCL-2 antisense oligodeoxynucleotides on in vitro proliferation and survival of normal marrow progenitors and leukemic cells. Blood 1994;84:595–600.

68. Klasa RJ, Bally MB, Ng R et al. Eradication of human non-Hodgkin's lymphoma in SCID mice by BCL-2 antisense oligonucleotides combined with low-dose cyclophosphamide. Clin Cancer Res 2000;6:2492–2500.

69. Chi KN, Gleave ME, Klasa R et al. A phase I dose-finding study of combined treatment with an antisense Bcl-2 oligonucleotide (Genasense) and mitoxantrone in patients with metastatic hormone-refractory prostate cancer. Clin Cancer Res 2001;7:3920–3927.

70. Miayake H, Tolcher A, Gleave ME. Chemosensitization and delayed androgen-independent recurrence of prostate cancer with the use of antisense Bcl-2 oligodeoxynucleotides. J Natl Cancer Inst 2000;92:34–41.

71. Koty PP, Zhang H, Levitt ML. Antisense bcl-2 treatment increases programmed cell death in non-small cell lung cancer cell lines. Lung Cancer 1999;23:115–127.

72. Lacy J, Loomis R. Bcl-2 antisense (G3139, oblimersen) enhances the in vitro and in vivo responses of EBV-associated lymphoproliferative disease to rituximab [abstract 2853]. Proc Am Assoc Cancer Res 2002;43:575.

73. Sanchez-Garcia I, Grutz G. Tumorigenic activity of the BCR-ABL oncogenes is mediated by BCL2. Proc Natl Acad Sci USA 1995;92:5287–5291.

74. Tauchi T, Nakajima A, Sumi M et al. G3139 (Bcl-2 antisense oligonucleotide) is active against Gleevec-resistant BCR-ABL-positive cells [abstract 4702]. Proc Am Assoc Cancer Res 2002;43:949.

75. Jahrsdorfer B, Jox R, Muhlenhoff L et al. Modulation of malignant B cell activation and apoptosis by bcl-2 antisense ODN and immunostimulatory CpG ODN. J Leukoc Biol 2002;72:83–92.

76. Leung S, Miyake H, Zellweger T et al. Synergistic chemosensitization and inhibition of progression to androgen independence by antisense Bcl-2 oligodeoxynucleotide and paclitaxel in the LNCaP prostate tumor model. Int J Cancer 2001;91:846–850.

77. Wacheck V, Krepler C, Thallinger C et al. Anti-tumor effect of G3139 Bcl-2 antisense oligonucleotide (Genasense) is not mediated by immune-stimulation of SCID mice [abstract 2861]. Proc Am Assoc Cancer Res 2002;43:577.

78. Raynaud FI, Orr RM, Goddard PM et al. Pharmacokinetics of G3139, a phosphorothioate oligodeoxynucleotide antisense to bcl-2, after intravenous administration or continuous subcutaneous infusion to mice. J Pharmacol Exp Ther 1997;281:420–427.

79. Lopes, Mayer LD. Pharmacokinetics of Bcl-2 antisense oligonucleotide (G3139) combined with doxorubicin in SCID mice bearing human breast cancer solid tumor xenografts. Cancer Chem Pharmacol 2002;49:57–68.

80. Webb A, Cunningham D, Cotter F et al. BCL-2 antisense therapy in patients with non-Hodgkin lymphoma. Lancet 1997;349:1137–1141.

81. Waters JS, Webb A, Cunningham D et al. Phase I clinical and pharmacokinetic study of bcl-2 antisense oligonucleotide therapy in patients with non-Hodgkin's lymphoma. J Clin Oncol 2000;18:1812–1823.

82. Morris MJ, Tong WP, Cordon-Cardo C et al. Phase I trial of BCL-2 antisense oligonucleotide (G3139) administered by continuous intravenous infusion in patients with advanced cancer. Clin Cancer Res 2002;8:679–683.

83. O'Brien S, Giles F, Rai K et al. Bcl-2 antisense (Genasense) as monotherapy for refractory chronic lymphocytic leukemia. Blood 2001;98:772a.

84. Pepper C, Thomas A, Hoy T et al. Antisense-mediated suppression of Bcl-2 highlights its pivotal role in failed apoptosis in B-cell chronic lymphocytic leukaemia. Br J Haematol 1999;107:611–615.

85. Yamamura K, Kamada S, Ito S et al. Accelerated disappearance of melanocytes in bcl-2-deficient mice. Cancer Res 1996;56:3546–3550.

86. Selzer E, Schlagbauer-Wadl H, Okamoto I et al. Expression of Bcl-2 family members in human melanocytes, in melanoma metastases and in melanoma cell lines. Melanoma Res 1998;8:197–203.

87. Grover R, Wilson GD. Bcl-2 expression in malignant melanoma and its prognostic significance. Eur J Surg Oncol 1996;22:347–349.

88. Chapman PB, Einhorn LH, Meyers ML et al. Phase III multicenter randomized trial of the Dartmouth regimen versus dacarbazine in patients with metastatic melanoma. J Clin Oncol 1999;17:2745–2751.

89. Tolcher AW. Preliminary phase I results of G3139 (bcl-2 antisense oligonucleotide) therapy in combination with docetaxel in hormone-refractory prostate cancer. Semin Oncol 2001;28:67–70.

90. Rudin CM, Otterson GA, Mauer AM et al. A pilot trial of G3139, a bcl-2 antisense oligonucleotide, and paclitaxel in patients with chemorefractory small-cell lung cancer. Ann Oncol 2002;13:539–545.

91. Ochoa L, Kuhn J, Salinas R et al. A phase I pharmacokinetic and biologic correlative study of G3139 and irinotecan in patients with metastatic colorectal cancer. Proc Am Soc Clin Oncol 2001;20:75a.

92. Chen HX, Marshall JL, Trocky N et al. A phase I study of Bcl-2 antisense G3139 and weekly docetaxel in patients with advanced breast cancer and other solid tumors [abstract 692]. Proc Am Soc Clin Oncol 2000;19:178.

93. Jansen B, Wacheck V, Heere-Ress E et al. Chemosensitisation of malignant melanoma by BCL2 antisense therapy. Lancet 2000;356:1728–1733.

94. Marcucci G, Byrd JC, Catalano SR, et al. Phase 1 and pharmacodynamic studies of G3139, a Bcl-2 antisense oligonucleotide, in combination with chemotherapy in refractory or relapsed acute leukemia. Blood 2003;101:425–432.

95. Gazitt Y, Liu QY, Vesole D. Bcl-2 antisense oligonucleotides enhances apoptosis and cytotoxicity in drug-resistant myeloma cells [abstract 2688]. Blood 2001;98:641a.

96. Vogel CL, Cobleigh MA, Tripathy D et al. Efficacy and safety of trastuzumab as a single agent in first-line treatment of HER2-overexpressing metastatic breast cancer. J Clin Oncol. 2002;20:719–726.

97. Slamon DJ, Leyland-Jones B, Shak S et al. Use of chemotherapy plus a monoclonal antibody against HER2 for metastatic breast cancer that overexpresses HER2. N Engl J Med. 2001;344:783–792.

98. Campos L, Rouault JP, Sabido O et al. High expression of bcl-2 protein in acute myeloid leukemia cells is associated with poor response to chemotherapy. Blood. 1993;81:3091–3096.

99. Ravandi F, Kantarjian HM, Talpaz M et al. Expression of apoptosis proteins in chronic myelogenous leukemia: associations and significance. Cancer 2001;91:1964–1972.

100. Zutter M, Hockenbery D, Silverman GA et al. Immunolocalization of the Bcl-2 protein within hematopoietic neoplasms. Blood 1991;78:1062–1068.

101. Harada N, Hata H, Yoshida M et al. Expression of Bcl-2 family of proteins in fresh myeloma cells. Leukemia 1998;12:1817–1820.

102. Tang L, Tron VA, Reed JC et al. Expression of apoptosis regulators in cutaneous malignant melanoma. Clin Cancer Res 1998;4:1865–1871.

103. Apakama I, Robinson MC, Walter NM et al. bcl-2 overexpression combined with p53 protein accumulation correlates with hormone-refractory prostate cancer. Br J Cancer 1996;74:1258–1262.

104. McDonnell TJ, Navone NM, Troncoso P et al. Expression of bcl-2 oncoprotein and p53 protein accumulation in bone marrow metastases of androgen independent prostate cancer [see comments]. J Urol 1997;157:569–574.

105. Colombel M, Symmans F, Gil S et al. Detection of the apoptosis-suppressing oncoprotein bcl-2 in hormone-refractory human prostate cancers. Am J Pathol 1993;143:390–400.

106. Termuhlen PM, Sweeney-Gotsch BM, Berman RS et al. Increased apoptosis in metastatic human colonic adenocarcinomas. Cancer Biol Ther 2002;1:58–63.

107. Ofner D, Riehemann K, Maier H et al. Immunohistochemically detectable bcl-2 expression in colorectal carcinoma: correlation with tumour stage and patient survival. Br J Cancer 1995;72:981–985.

108. Carbognani P, Tincani G, Crafa P et al. Biological markers in non-small cell lung cancer. Retrospective study of 10 year follow-up after surgery: Immunohistochemical demonstration of apoptosis-regulated proteins, Bcl-2 and Bax, in resected non-small-cell lung cancers. J Cardiovasc Surg 2002;43:545–548.

109. Han H, Landreneau RJ, Santucci TS et al. Prognostic value of immunohistochemical expressions of p53, HER-2/neu, and bcl-2 in stage I non-small-cell lung cancer. Human Pathol 2002;33:105–110.

110. Higashiyama M, Doi O, Kodama K et al. Bcl-2 oncoprotein expression is increased especially in the portion of small cell carcinoma within the combined type of small cell lung cancer. Tumour Biol 1996;17:341–344.

111. Jiang SX, Kameya T, Sato Y et al. Bcl-2 protein expression in lung cancer and close correlation with neuroendocrine differentiation. Am J Pathol 1996;148:837–846.

Chapter 2

Translational Regulation of Thymidylate Synthase and the Cell Cycle: Insights for Clinical Drug Development

John C. Schmitz, Edward Chu

Thymidylate synthase (TS) is a folate-dependent enzyme that catalyzes the reductive methylation of 2′-deoxyuridine-5′-monophosphate (dUMP) by the reduced folate 5,10-methylenetetrahydrofolate (CH_2THF) to thymidylate (dTMP) and dihydrofolate (Fig. 2.1).[1,2] Once synthesized, dTMP is further metabolized within the cell to the dTTP triphosphate form, an essential precursor for DNA synthesis. While dTMP can be formed through the salvage pathway, a process that is catalyzed by thymidine kinase, the TS-catalyzed reaction provides for the sole intracellular de novo source of dTMP. This reaction plays a central role in DNA biosynthesis, and given that inhibition of this reaction results in immediate cessation of cellular proliferation and growth, TS represents an important target for cancer chemotherapy.[3,4]

Several lines of evidence provide further support to the concept that TS is an important chemotherapeutic target. The first comes from in vitro, in vivo, and clinical studies that show a strong association between the level of expression of

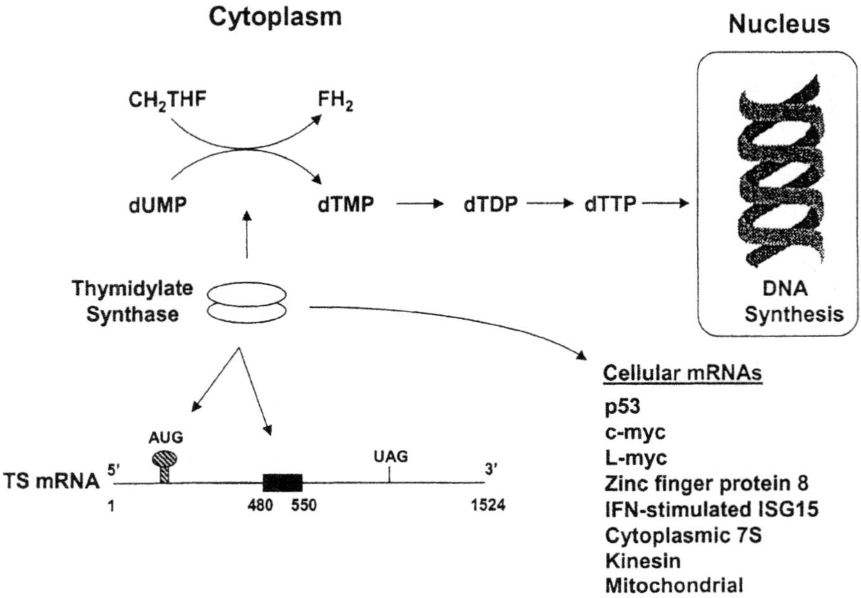

FIGURE 2.1 Enzymatic and RNA binding functions of thymidylate synthase.

TS enzyme activity and TS protein and fluoropyrimidine sensitivity.[5-7] It is well established that neoplastic cell lines and tumors expressing higher levels of TS are relatively more resistant to the cytotoxic and anti-tumor effects of the fluoropyrimidines and antifolate analogues that target TS. Second, a strong correlation exists between the level of inhibition of TS enzyme activity in patient tumor specimens after treatment with 5-FU and the eventual clinical response to 5-FU–based chemotherapy.[8,9] Third, the improved response rates observed when 5-FU is combined with the reduced folate leucovorin as compared with the response rates observed with single-agent 5-FU provide support to the cell-free studies that showed that TS enzyme inhibition was optimally maintained in the presence of increasing concentrations of the reduced folate CH_2THF.[10-15] Clinical trials with the antifolate analogue ZD1694, a specific inhibitor of TS, have shown promising activity against advanced colorectal cancer, with response rates ranging from 25% to 30%. These responses are comparable to those observed with the combination of 5-FU and leucovorin, and for this reason, ZD1694 has been approved for use as first-line therapy for metastatic colorectal cancer in several countries in Europe and Asia, as well as in Australia and Canada.[16-18] Finally, pemetrexed (LY231514, multitargeted antifolate) is an antifolate analogue that inhibits TS as well as other folate-dependent enzymes, including dihydrofolate reductase, aminoimidazole carboxamide ribonucleotide formyltransferase, and glycinamide ribonucleotide formyltransferase.[19] In several phase II studies, this agent has shown clinical activity against colorectal cancer as well as non–small cell lung cancer.[20] A recently completed phase III study revealed that treatment with this agent in combination with cisplatin significantly improved response rate and overall survival in patients with malignant pleural mesothelioma when compared with single-agent cisplatin.[21]

REGULATION OF TS EXPRESSION

Several groups have described rapid increases in TS enzyme levels in various in vitro, in vivo, and clinical model systems after short-term exposure to antifolates and fluoropyrimidines.[22-27] It was postulated that the drug-mediated induction of TS may represent a mechanism for the acute development of resistance to (5-FU) chemotherapy in a way that has direct biologic and clinical relevance. Although the molecular mechanisms mediating the 5-FU–induced expression of TS were not well characterized in these initial studies, several possibilities were proposed, including increased transcription of TS-specific sequences, enhanced stability of TS messenger RNA, increased efficiency of TS mRNA translation, and enhanced stability of TS protein. Intense research efforts subsequently focused on elucidating the critical biochemical and molecular events that control the 5-FU–mediated acute induction of TS. Keyomarsi et al[28] demonstrated that treatment of human breast cancer MCF-7 cells with the quinazoline antifolate analogue raltitrexed (ZD1694, Tomudex, TDX) gave rise to an acute 10- to 40-fold increase in levels of TS enzyme activity with no associated change in TS mRNA levels. The presence of the protein synthesis inhibitor cycloheximide effectively blocked the elevation in TS enzyme levels after exposure to ZD1694, providing suggestive evidence for a translational regulatory event.

Studies from our own laboratory using a human colon cancer H630 cell line as a model system revealed that the increase in TS enzyme activity and TS protein expression in response to short-term exposures to 5-FU was not associated with a corresponding change in the level of TS mRNA expression.[29,30] Although most of the induced protein was complexed with the 5-FU metabolite FdUMP, a nearly 50% increase in free levels of TS protein was also observed. Thus, the induction of TS protein in response to 5-FU exposure allowed free TS to remain at levels 50% greater than baseline, such that thymidylate and DNA biosynthesis could be maintained in the face of a cytotoxic stress, such as that posed by 5-FU. Further work revealed that the increase in TS protein expression resulted directly from new synthesis of TS protein and not from alterations in protein stability. In addition, repression of the 5-FU–mediated induction of TS by the cytokine interferon-γ at non–growth inhibitory drug concentrations was associated with a nearly 20-fold increase in the cytotoxic effects of 5-FU. Of note, the negative effect of interferon-γ on TS expression was also controlled at the translational level. This study provided the first direct evidence for the role of translational regulation in an intact biologic system and highlighted the biologic relevance of this regulatory process.

Recently, Welsh et al[31] investigated the induction of TS in a wide range of human cancer cell lines and nontransformed human fibroblasts after short-term exposure to the antifolate analogue ZD9331. Although a 6- to 10-fold induction of TS protein expression was observed in various human cancer cell lines, a significantly greater level of TS induction was noted in nontransformed human fibroblasts treated with equitoxic doses of drug. Additional in vivo experiments using the L5178Y/TK mouse lymphoma model implanted into DBA2 mice identified significantly higher levels of induction of TS protein in normal intestinal epithelial cells than in tumor cells.

Over the past few years, our laboratory has conducted an extensive series of studies to more carefully elucidate the regulation of TS mRNA translation in response to exposure to cytotoxic stress. The current working model for the translational autoregulatory control of TS and the interaction between TS protein and its own TS mRNA is presented in Figure 2.2. This regulatory process is well established as an important mechanism controlling the expression of various bacteriophage and prokaryotic systems.[32-36] However, TS represents the first eukaryotic gene whose expression is controlled in such a manner. The expression of three other eukaryotic proteins, namely dihydrofolate reductase,[37-39] p53,[40,41] and serine hydroxymethyltransferase,[42] is controlled by a similar autoregulatory feedback mechanism.

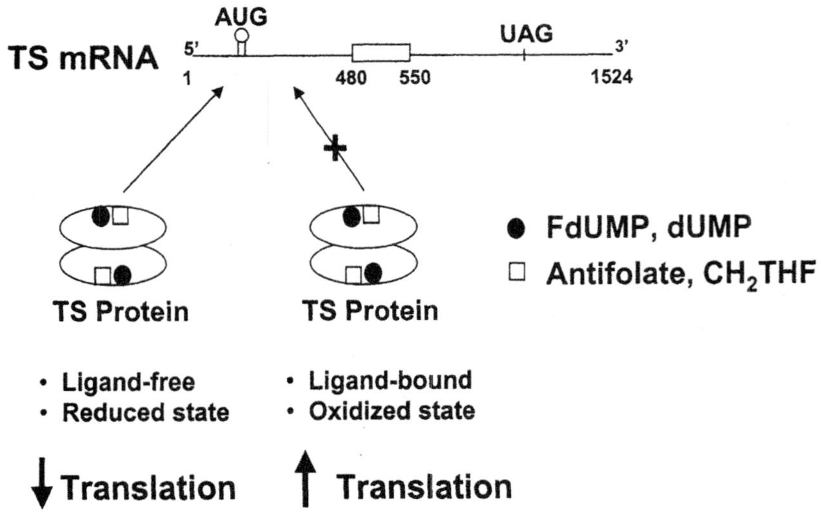

FIGURE 2.2 Model for translational autoregulation of thymidylate synthase.

Two different *cis*-acting sequences have been identified on human TS mRNA, and each element binds with high affinity, on the order of 1–3 nM, to TS.[43,44] The first site is a 30-nucleotide (nt) sequence corresponding to nt 80–109 and includes the translational start site within the loop aspect of a stable stem-loop structure. The second site is contained within a 70-nt sequence corresponding to nt 480–550 in the protein-coding region. This second *cis* element is sufficient to confer the property of translational regulation onto a heterologous luciferase reporter gene and requires the presence of an intact TS protein for its biologic effect.[45] Although this sequence is able to function independently of the 5′-upstream *cis* element in vivo, our studies suggest that both elements are required for complete translational autoregulatory activity.

Significant efforts have been placed on defining the essential molecular factors that mediate the interaction between TS protein and its own target TS mRNA. Our laboratory has shown that the RNA binding activity of human recombinant TS is exquisitely redox sensitive and requires the presence of at least one free sulfhydryl group.[46] In addition to the redox state, the state of occupancy of the TS protein represents another critical determinant of RNA binding. Specifically, when TS is ligand-free, maximal RNA binding activity is maintained, thereby resulting in complete translational repression of TS mRNA. In contrast, when TS is bound by either of its physiologic substrates dUMP or the reduced folate CH_2THF or is bound by the 5-FU nucleotide metabolite FdUMP, TS is unable to bind to its target mRNA (Fig. 2.2). In addition, incubation of TS with various antifolate analogues, including ZD1694 and LY231514, significantly impairs its ability to interact with TS mRNA. The end result of this disruption in RNA binding activity is abrogation of translational repression, thereby resulting in increased synthesis of new TS protein.[46] Such a condition would exist in cells exposed to direct inhibitor compounds of TS, whether it be nucleotide analogues, such as 5-FU, or antifolate analogues, such as ZD1694. Thus, this model provides rationale for the acute induction of TS that arises in direct response to exposure to the class of TS inhibitor compounds. Abrogation of this normal TS translational autoregulatory process may represent a biologically relevant mechanism to maintain normal cellular synthetic function in the setting of an acute cellular stress, such as exposure to an antineoplastic agent. Finally, it offers a novel mechanism for the development of acute drug resistance to compounds that specifically target TS.

TS AS A TRANSLATIONAL REGULATOR OF CELLULAR GENE EXPRESSION AND THE CELL CYCLE

There are growing examples in the literature documenting that a given RNA binding protein has the potential to interact with more than one cellular mRNA species.[47,48] The best-characterized example of such an RNA binding protein is the iron-responsive factor, which binds to its target iron-responsive element located within the 5′-untranslated regions (5′-UTR) of ferritin and erythroid 5-aminolevulinate synthase mRNAs and within the 3′-UTR of the transferrin receptor mRNA.[49,50] The ability of iron-responsive factor to coordinately regulate these different mRNAs allows for exquisite control of iron metabolism within the cell. With this in mind, studies were undertaken in our laboratory to determine whether TS, in its role as an RNA binding protein, might be able to interact with other cellular RNAs. For these studies, we developed a novel immunoprecipitation-RNA:random polymerase chain reaction method to isolate TS ribonucleoprotein (RNP) complexes from intact human colon cancer H630 cells.[51] This technique was based on the original immunoprecipitation procedure of Steitz[52] and was modified by incorporating an RNA:random polymerase chain reaction method developed by Froussard.[53] With this approach, eight different cellular RNAs that formed an RNP complex with TS were isolated (Fig. 2.1).[51] Although TS was one of the RNAs identified in this RNP complex, p53 and two members of the *myc* family of transcription factors, c- and L-*myc,* were also isolated. In addition, the mRNA encoding the 15-kd_a, interferon-stimulated protein (ISG15) was also identified. These mRNAs were of particular interest because they each play a critical role in cell cycle progression, DNA synthesis, and apoptosis. Careful analysis of the eight RNA sequences has, to date, failed to identify a consensus nucleotide sequence. However, one potential drawback of such an approach is that most of the RNA binding proteins characterized to date appear to recognize a sequence contained within the context of a stable secondary structure as opposed to a simple sequence. Future studies will focus on more precisely defining the consensus sequence(s) and/or secondary structure(s) required for both protein recognition and regulated expression of these various genes. In fact, there is emerging preliminary evidence to suggest the presence of such a consensus secondary structure among these different cellular mRNAs.

The critical role of p53 in tumor suppression, cell cycle regulation, cell cycle arrest, and the cellular response to DNA damage has been extensively reviewed.[54-56] The mechanisms controlling the expression of p53, in response to genotoxic and/or cytotoxic stress, are complex. Much of the work performed to date has shown that the induction of p53 after exposure to DNA-damaging agents is controlled at the posttranslational level, mainly through enhanced stability of the protein.[54,55,57] It is now well established that posttranslational modifications, including phosphorylation and acetylation at both the amino and the carboxy terminus, are critical for the activation of DNA binding activity.[58-60] However, there is growing evidence that translational control may play an important role in the induction and activation of p53 in response to exposure to cytotoxic agents.[61] For example, when murine fibroblast Swiss 3T3 cells were exposed to γ-irradiation, the expression of p53 protein increased significantly, whereas the corresponding p53 mRNA levels were unchanged.[40] Treatment with the transcriptional inhibitor actinomycin D did not alter the induced levels of p53 protein, in contrast to treatment with cycloheximide, which completely repressed the induced synthesis of p53. Subsequent investigations have confirmed that the expression of p53 is controlled, in part, at the translational level through an autoregulatory feedback loop that is identical to what has been previously described for TS and dihydrofolate reductase. One element in the 5′-UTR of murine p53 mRNA has been identified as a *cis*-acting target sequence for p53 protein, whereas the essential *cis*-acting element for human p53 mRNA has been localized to the 3′UTR.[62]

Given our observation that a TS RNP complex composed of TS protein and a sequence corresponding to human p53 mRNA was isolated from human colon cancer cells, further investigations were performed to confirm the interaction between TS protein and p53 mRNA and to elucidate the potential biologic consequences of such an interaction. Using a combination of RNA gel shift and in vitro translation assay systems, we demonstrated that TS binds with specificity and relatively high affinity to a sequence within the protein-coding region of p53 mRNA at the C-terminal region.[63,64] The functional consequence of this RNA–protein interaction is translational repression. These studies have been extended to the in vivo setting to document the biologic relevance of the TS protein–p53 mRNA interaction. As part of these studies, human colon cancer RKO cells were transfected with the human TS complementary DNA under the control of a tetracycline-inducible expression system. Treatment of TS-transfected RKO cells with doxycycline (1 μg/mL), a tetracycline analogue, resulted in a 15-fold induction of TS protein, which was accompanied by a dramatic decrease in the expression of p53 protein. Of note, no corresponding change in p53 mRNA levels was observed. Immunoprecipitation studies to isolate TS RNP complexes revealed a significantly greater level of p53 mRNA bound to TS protein in doxycycline-treated cells than occurred in uninduced cells.

As a second model system, TS-deficient, parent HCT-C18 cells expressing a functionally inactive TS were transfected with a human His-Tag TS complementary DNA under the control of a constitutive cytomegalovirus promoter. The expression of p53 in these TS-transfected cells (HCT-C18:His-TS+) was markedly decreased, and this decreased p53 expression was controlled at the translational level. These TS-overexpressing cells were significantly impaired in their ability to arrest at either the G_1/S or the G_2/M boundary, in response to γ-irradiation and/or treatment with various anticancer drugs, including doxorubicin and 5-FU, when compared with their corresponding parent HCT-C18 cells.[64] In addition, the apoptotic response to drug exposure was dramatically reduced in TS-overexpressing cells, as evidenced by decreased activation of caspase 3 after treatment with 5-FU. More recently, we have shown that TS-overexpressing, HCT-C18:His-TS+ cells are significantly more resistant to TS inhibitor compounds, such as 5-FU and ZD1694, as well as to non–TS-related anticancer agents, such as doxorubicin and cisplatin, by up to four- to sevenfold.[65] These observations lend support for the biologic relevance of the interaction between TS and p53 mRNA. In addition, they suggest that loss of p53 function through translational repression results in an altered cell cycle checkpoint, an altered apoptotic response, and the development of pleiotropic drug resistance.

Taken together, these studies show that TS, in its capacity as an RNA-binding protein, interacts with high affinity with its own mRNA as well as with the p53 mRNA and other cellular mRNAs. Thus, TS may be involved in the coordinate regulation of expression and/or function of other genes. Given the importance of p53 in the cell cycle and in the maintenance of the requirements for cellular growth and proliferation, it is conceivable that TS may play an essential role as a regulator of cell cycle–directed events. This effect may be especially relevant given the essential role of TS in providing the requisite nucleotide substrates for DNA biosynthesis. Studies in our laboratory are currently focused on more precisely defining the molecular elements that mediate the interaction between TS protein and p53 mRNA, with emphasis on defining the *cis*-acting elements of each of these mRNAs. In addition, studies are in progress to determine whether the same domain or domains are involved in the binding of TS to its own cognate TS mRNA as well as to other cellular mRNAs. Finally, extensive efforts are being directed at elucidating the downstream biologic consequences of TS-mediated suppression of p53 mRNA translation, with specific emphasis on cell cycle progression, cell cycle arrest, apoptosis, and chemosensitivity.

FUTURE PERSPECTIVES

There are several issues that remain to be addressed regarding the molecular basis for the interaction between TS and its own TS mRNA as well as with other cellular mRNAs. First, a more thorough understanding of the optimal nucleotide sequences and/or the secondary structures required for protein recognition is required. Second, further studies will need to focus on more precisely defining the critical amino acids and binding domain(s) on the TS protein that is needed for RNA recognition. Definitive characterization of both the critical RNA binding domain(s) as well as the essential nucleotide sequences and/or secondary structures awaits the results of x-ray crystallography and/or nuclear magnetic resonance analysis of the TS protein–TS mRNA complex. Although these structural studies have been limited, to date, by the availability of only small amounts of pure TS mRNA and human TS protein, these technical limitations should be resolved in the very near future.

A third important issue relates to the intracellular localization of the TS protein–TS mRNA complex as well as the cellular localization of the other TS RNP complexes. For this work, our laboratory is developing an in vivo fluorescence immunohistochemical approach. As a first step, we have generated a series of deletional TS complementary DNA constructs with a His-Tag placed at either the 5′ or the 3′ terminus, and these respective constructs have been transfected into human colon cancer RKO cells. The intracellular localization of these deletion proteins was compared with that of the wild-type, full-length human TS protein.[66] Our preliminary studies thus far have revealed that deletion of the first 10 amino acids at the amino terminus and deletion of nine amino acids at the carboxy terminus significantly altered cellular localization. Wild-type human TS protein was distributed uniformly throughout the cell in both the nucleus and the cytoplasm. In contrast, the deleted TS proteins localized exclusively to the cytoplasm with absolutely no nuclear localization. Studies are in progress to isolate the cellular location of TS mRNA by use of in situ hybridization. Once these initial series of experiments are performed, co-localization studies are planned to determine the actual cellular location of the TS RNP complex.

One issue raised by this work relates to how direct binding of TS to sequences in the protein-coding region of cellular mRNAs results in translational repression. Given the absence of truncated protein products for either c-Myc or p53, these findings would suggest that binding of TS interferes, in some manner, either with binding of the translational machinery, including ribosomes and translational initiation factors near or at the cap site, or with the process of ribosomal scanning. Clearly, for this to occur, some form of interactive "cross-talk" between the 5′ end of the mRNA and the protein-coding region must take place. Although much of the early work on translation identified the 5′-UTR as playing a major role in mediating translational initiation, these studies contribute to the growing body of evidence suggesting that sequences in both the protein-coding region and in the 3′-UTR may play critical roles in translational initiation. In addition, translational repression of TS, p53, or c-*myc* mRNA by TS protein does not lead to the generation of truncated protein products, a finding that implicates the direct inhibition of either translational initiation or ribosomal scanning rather than inhibition of protein elongation. Although the exact mechanism by which this occurs remains unclear, possible explanations include (1) binding of TS to the protein-coding region of each of these mRNA's results in stabilization of an RNA secondary structure, which in some manner impairs translational initiation and/or ribosomal scanning, or (2) an interaction that takes place between the TS RNP complex and the 5′-UTR to prevent the various translational initiation factors and/or ribosomes from initiating the process of translation.

Finally, what are the potential biologic consequences of translational repression of p53, c-*myc,* and other cellular RNAs by TS? Based on our current working model, TS-overexpressing cells exposed to exogenous DNA damage are impaired in their G_1 and/or G_2 checkpoint function. Moreover, these cells are unable to undergo apoptosis in response to a cytotoxic stress. These observations have direct and immediate relevance to the effective delivery of cancer chemotherapy and suggest a rational mechanism for the development of cellular drug resistance. Clearly, an enhanced understanding of the essential molecular elements underlying the translational repressive effects of TS on p53 and c-*myc* may provide insights into the design of novel treatment strategies that can help restore the normal cell cycle checkpoint function and chemosensitivity.

DEVELOPMENT OF NOVEL THERAPEUTIC APPROACHES TO INHIBIT THYMIDYLATE SYNTHASE

The molecular-based studies have expanded our current understanding of TS as an RNA binding protein and should provide fascinating new insights into the role of TS as an important regulator of certain critical aspects of cellular metabolism. However, such a detailed characterization of the interaction of TS with its own TS mRNA as well as with other cellular RNAs may also serve as the rational basis for the future development of novel therapeutic approaches. As we and other investigators have shown, one of the potential limitations of treatment with TS inhibitor compounds is that a paradoxical increase in TS protein expression can be observed that results in the development of acute cellular drug resistance. As outlined in Table 2.1, several potential strategies can be developed that are a direct result of our molecular-based studies. For example, identification of the specific RNA binding domain may result in the development of novel inhibitors of TS enzymatic activity that would still allow for formation of the TS mRNA–TS protein complex in vivo. A stable ternary complex composed of inhibitor, TS protein, and TS mRNA might then result in marked suppression of new TS protein synthesis. As an alternative approach, identification of the putative RNA binding domain may lead to the development of a small peptide that would then be used to target TS mRNA and repress new TS protein synthesis. The use of innovative modeling programs may identify small "designer" molecules that mimic the structural features of the binding peptide. Certainly, the potential advantage of such an approach would be that novel organic molecules with enhanced spatial and biophysical and biochemical properties could be designed. Currently, this strategy is being taken in anti-HIV drug development, in which small basic Rev and Tat peptides that mimic the function of their corresponding native proteins are being to tested for their ability to inhibit HIV viral replication.[67]

TABLE 2.1 Novel Therapeutic Approaches to Inhibit TS

- Identify lead compounds that inhibit TS enzyme activity and still allow for RNA binding.
- Identify small molecules that directly target cis-acting sequences on TS mRNA to inhibit translation.
- Design antisense, ribozyme, and/or siRNA molecules that target cis-acting sequences on TS mRNA.
- Design peptides and/or small designer molecules that target TS mRNA to inhibit translation.
- Design consensus RNA sequence with high-affinity binding to sequester and/or inhibit TS protein.

Identification of the consensus nucleotide sequence and/or secondary structure containing the high-affinity protein binding site may lead to the design of an RNA oligonucleotide that can be used to sequester and/or repress TS enzymatic function. An alternative strategy would be to identify a consensus nucleotide sequence/structure that might serve as the target for either antisense-, ribozyme-, or siRNA-based strategies with resultant inhibition of TS protein synthesis. However, one significant drawback of the use of nucleic acids, whether it be RNA or DNA, is the inherent difficulty in efficiently and specifically delivering them into their target cells. The use of molecular modeling programs to design small organic molecules that closely resemble the consensus RNA sequence and/or structure may help circumvent this problem. Such compounds could then be delivered with much greater efficiency and at relatively higher concentrations into malignant cells than their nucleic acid counterparts.

In an effort to circumvent the translational induction of TS, our laboratory and others have developed an antisense oligonucleotide strategy to inhibit the process of TS mRNA translation (Fig. 2.3). The initial focus was on developing antisense DNA oligos as therapeutic molecules. Ferguson et al[68,69] targeted the 3′UTR of human TS mRNA with phosphorothioate DNA oligodeoxynucleotides (ODNs) containing 6-nt methoxyethoxy ends. Treatment of human cervical cancer HeLa cells with these ODNs resulted in decreased expression of both TS

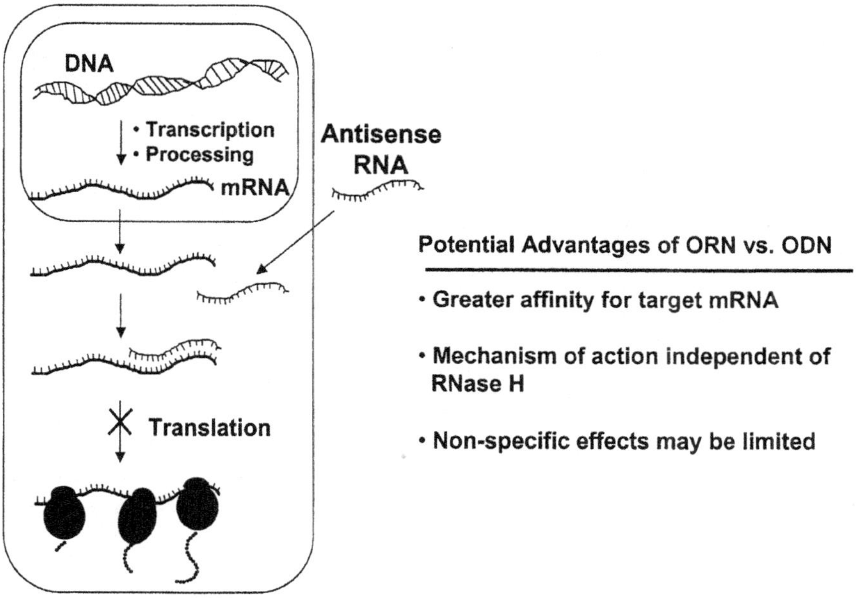

FIGURE 2.3 Antisense strategy to inhibit thymidylate synthase (TS) expression.

mRNA and TS protein levels, causing inhibition of cell proliferation. They also observed that antisense treatment sensitized parental and FUdR-resistant cell line to FUdR. Further studies from the same group demonstrated that TS-targeted ODN 83, but not a control ODN, exerted a G_2/M cell cycle block in HeLa cells, in contrast to classical TS inhibitors, which arrested cells in the G_1 or S phase.[70] Lin et al[71] targeted the protein coding region of TS mRNA (nt 201–217) with a phosphorothioate ODN, ATS-2. This ODN inhibited TS protein expression in human HEK cells by 90% after 24 hours. Effective inhibition of cell proliferation (98%) was observed at a concentration of 200 nM of ATS-2. In addition, they observed a block at the S phase of the cell cycle after ODN treatment. Although this finding is in direct contrast to the work previously reported by Ferguson et al,[68,69] this potential discrepancy may be related to the different cell lines and the specific cellular context being investigated. Thymidine supplementation was unable to rescue HEK cells from antisense treatment, whereas treatment of HeLa cells with thymidine effectively abrogated its effect. HEK cells incorporated 15 times less [^{3}H]thymidine than HeLa cells, suggesting that the TS-dependent pathway might be playing a role in determining the cell cycle response to TS-targeted ODNs. One major limitation of phosphorothioate ODNs is that their effects tend to be relatively nonspecific. It appears that only a five-base-pair recognition with the target mRNA is sufficient to induce RNase H-mediated degradation of the mRNA.[72] This fact could lead to a host of nonspecific interactions with unrelated cellular mRNAs and/or proteins.

Our own laboratory has attempted to circumvent the translational induction of TS by designing antisense RNA molecules that directly inhibit the process of TS mRNA translation. There are several advantages of oligoribonucleotides (ORNs) over their corresponding ODNs (Fig. 2.3). First, ORNs bind their target RNA sequence with markedly higher affinity, resulting in a more thermally stable ORN-RNA complex than the corresponding ODN-RNA. Second, RNA-RNA duplexes are not substrates for RNase H. As a result, the antisense ORN approach does not require an RNase H-dependent mechanism for its biologic effect. Finally, because ORNs do not activate degradation of their target RNA sequence, nonspecific effects may be limited because interaction of the ORNs with an unrelated cellular mRNA would result in only temporary inhibition of translation. In contrast, nonspecific binding of ODNs may result in irreversible degradation of certain critical cellular mRNAs. Thus, treatment with ODNs has a higher risk of activating undesirable nonspecific effects on cellular gene expression.

Using a rabbit reticulocyte in vitro translation system, we showed that a 30-nt native 2′-OH antisense ORN, targeted at the *cis*-acting element located at nt 80–109 of the 5′-upstream region of human TS mRNA, was able to potently repress TS mRNA translation.[73] This sequence was selected because our in vitro and in vivo work showed that it was an essential TS-response element and was critical for the process of TS translational autoregulation. We observed that the effect of this antisense TS ORN was specific in that it was unable to inhibit translation of control mRNAs, including *Escherichia coli* TS and p53. In order to make the ORN less susceptible to RNase degradation, we then designed ORNs with a modification on the ribose ring and observed that antisense 2′-*O*-methyl ORNs with either a phosphodiester or a phosphorothioate backbone were able to repress TS mRNA translation to an even greater extent than the native 2′-OH ORN. However, greater nonspecific effects on mRNA translation were observed with the 2′-O-methyl phosphorothioate ORN. These initial experiments revealed that antisense ORNs targeted at the 5′-*cis*-acting binding element of human TS mRNA could serve as potent inhibitors of TS mRNA translation.

We then extended these initial in vitro translation studies to an intact biologic system in which we showed that the 30-nt antisense 2′-*O*-methyl ORN effectively suppressed the expression of TS protein in a dose- and time-dependent manner in human colon cancer RKO cells.[74] With regard to the molecular level at which this ORN was exerting its effect, RNA Northern blot analysis revealed that the expression of TS mRNA remained unchanged with ORN treatment. These results suggested the role of a posttranscriptional mechanism. After antisense treatment, the half-life of TS protein was similar to that in untreated RKO cells. Taken together, these findings indicated that the antisense TS ORN exerts its suppressive effects at the level of translation, most likely through a process of translational arrest. Furthermore, control sense and mismatched ORNs had absolutely no effect on expression of TS protein. However, in cell proliferation assays, antisense and control ORNs inhibited cell growth to a similar extent, suggesting that the cytotoxic effects might be due to nonspecific interactions with cellular proteins and/or nonspecific effects caused by free 2′-O-methyl ribonucleotides that arise from ORN degradation. The nonspecific effects observed with these modified ORNs represent a significant limitation in their use as therapeutic agents.

As an alternative approach to using antisense oligos, we recently designed small interfering dsRNAs (siRNAs), which degrade target mRNAs through a process called RNA interference (RNAi). RNAi is an evolutionarily conserved process that maintains the genomic integrity of cellular organisms by silencing transposons and guarding against exogenous viral infection.[75-77] The molecular mechanism involves cleavage of the dsRNA by an RNase III–like endonuclease (Dicer) to small 21- to 25-nt dsRNAs (Fig. 2.4).[78-80] These siRNAs are bound in an endonuclease RNA–induced silencing complex, and the antisense strand is then used as a guide to target complementary mRNAs for degradation.[81] Although RNAi has gained rapid acceptance as a tool for studying gene function in *Caenorhabditis elegans* and *Drosophila,* its application in mammalian systems has been limited. Introduction of long dsRNA into mammalian cells results in a global shutdown of mRNA translation as well as nonspecific mRNA degradation.[82,83] However, 21-nt siRNA intermediates can function by themselves as potent activators of RNAi. Recent studies have shown that synthetic 21-nt siRNAs can function as potent activators of RNAi without inducing nonspecific effects on mRNA translation.[84,85]

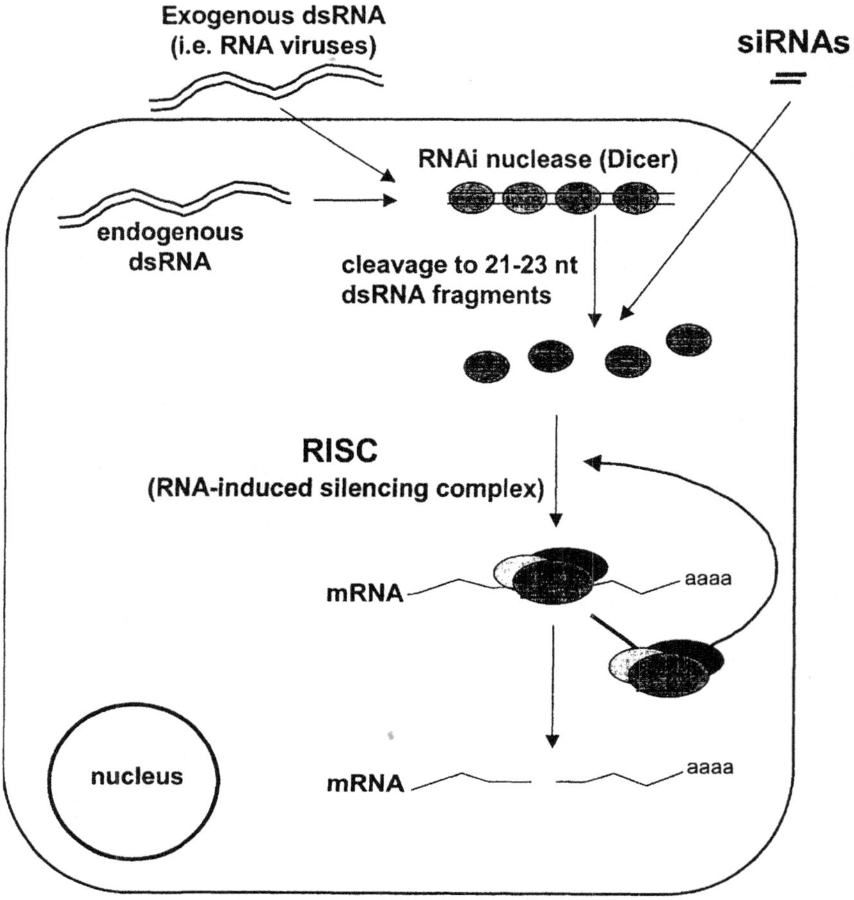

FIGURE 2.4 RNA interference strategy to inhibit thymidylate synthase (TS) expression.

With this in mind, we designed an siRNA that targeted the human TS mRNA at nucleotides 200–219. As seen in Figure 2.5A, levels of TS protein were significantly decreased after transfection of TS200 siRNA into human colon cancer RKO cells. Maximal suppression of TS protein was observed after 48 hours. Even after 5 days, the level of TS protein was 85% less than untreated cells. To confirm the molecular level at which the siRNA was exerting its biologic effect, TS mRNA levels were analyzed by Northern blot analysis. Figure 2.5B shows that TS mRNA is rapidly degraded, achieving maximal reduction by 12 hours, in contrast to control levels of 28S RNA, which remain completely unchanged. To demonstrate specificity of action, the expression of several other cellular proteins were determined by Western blot after siRNA transfection. As seen in Figure 2.5C, expression of topoisomerase I and α-tubulin remained unaffected by the

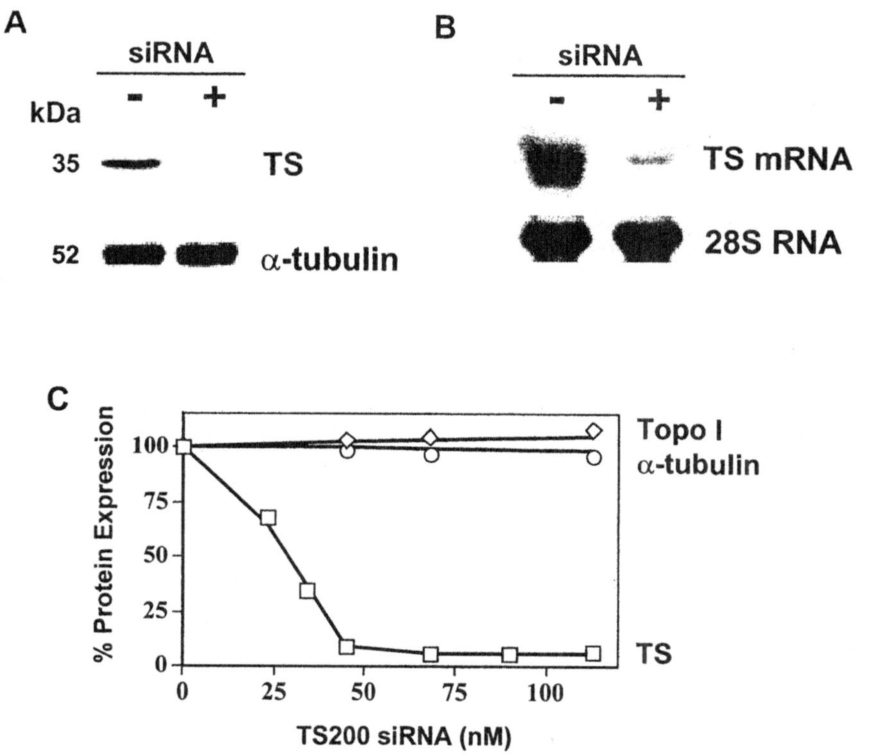

FIGURE 2.5 A, Effect of small interfering RNAs (siRNAs) on thymidylate synthase (TS) protein expression. B, Effect of siRNAs on TS messenger RNA (mRNA) expression. C, Effect of siRNAs on expression of unrelated cellular proteins, topoisomerase I, and α-tubulin.

TS200 siRNA. Additional control experiments were performed to document that each respective strand of the TS200 siRNA duplex had no effect on expression of TS protein. These studies provided strong evidence that an siRNA targeted at a sequence on the human TS mRNA can effectively and specifically down-regulate TS mRNA and TS protein expression.

We next investigated the effects of these TS-targeted siRNAs on cell growth and proliferation. RKO cells were transfected with increasing concentrations of TS200 siRNA for 5 hours and allowed to grow for an additional 72 hours; cell number was then determined. Under these conditions, we observed a marked dose-dependent effect of TS200 siRNA on RKO cell proliferation, with an inhibitory concentration of 50% (IC_{50}) of 80 nM. In contrast, a mismatched siRNA as well as an siRNA directed against a luciferase mRNA sequence had absolutely no growth-inhibitory effects.

To determine whether siRNAs would be effective against TS-overexpressing cancer cells, cell growth studies were performed with RKO-TDX cells. These cells are 2000 times more resistant to TDX than parental RKO cells and express approximately 20-fold higher levels of TS protein. Treatment of resistant RKO-TDX cells with TS200 siRNA resulted in IC_{50} values similar to those occurring with parental RKO cells (IC_{50}, 100 nM). Together, these studies suggest that siRNA targeting of TS mRNA is an effective approach to down-regulate TS expression in RKO and TS-overexpressing RKO-TDX cancer cells. In contrast to the antisense oligo approach, whether it be DNA or RNA, siRNAs are more specific and more potent inhibitors of TS expression, requiring 200-fold lower concentrations. These preliminary results suggest that siRNAs may have potential therapeutic use as anticancer agents, either by themselves or in combination with currently available TS inhibitor compounds.

However, several limitations remain for the RNAi strategy to be developed in the clinical setting. Given the negative charge of their backbone, siRNAs generally exhibit poor uptake into cultured cells and require the formation of a lipid complex for uptake into the cell. Another major obstacle is the potential susceptibility to nuclease degradation. To date, all reported studies using siRNAs suggest that modification of the backbone and/or ribose ring significantly impairs their ability to suppress cellular gene expression.[86,87] Finally, the issue of specificity of siRNAs is critical and is one that remains to be more carefully elucidated.

In addition to targeting TS mRNA with nucleic acid–based strategies, several investigators have designed small molecules to target specific sites on TS mRNA. Tok et al[88] demonstrated that a series of aminoglycoside antibiotic compounds were able to interact directly with the putative stem-loop structure in the 5′UTR of human TS mRNA (nt 80–109) in a specific and saturable fashion. When compared with the other aminoglycosides tested, neomycin B was found to interact with TS mRNA with the highest binding affinity, with a binding constant of approximately 0.9 μM. A detailed RNA footprinting analysis revealed that the "CC" bulge in the stem-loop structure was critical as a recognition site for aminoglycoside binding. However, when a hybrid RNA consisting of the CC bulge and a 16S rRNA loop region was constructed, the investigators observed that the aminoglycosides bound equally well to this fusion RNA, a finding that brought into question the specificity of binding of these compounds to the human TS mRNA. Given the relative lack of binding specificity, along with the relatively high binding constants (approximately 1 μM), these results suggest that aminoglycosides themselves would be ineffective in regulating the expression of TS. However, these studies identify the aminoglycoside structure as a potential lead molecule for the design and development of novel and more potent molecules that could target human TS mRNA and subsequently interfere with the translation and synthesis of new TS protein.

Cho and Rando[89] recently showed that the DNA intercalating agent Hoechst 33258 is able to bind to the same site on human TS mRNA, with a dissociation constant of 60 nM. A series of carefully performed RNA footprinting analyses confirmed that the bulge in the stem-loop structure was critical as an RNA recognition site for binding. These investigators also identified that the GC base pair adjacent to the CC bubble was critical for binding of Hoechst 33258. Although further studies are required to identify novel small molecules that specifically bind TS mRNA, these preliminary studies suggest that a small molecule approach that directly targets the process of TS mRNA translation may have therapeutic potential.

Finally, one of the potential limitations of TS inhibitor therapy is that treatment with anticancer agents, such as 5-FU and the antifolate analogue ZD1694, disrupts the normal interaction between TS protein and its target TS mRNA, resulting in new synthesis of TS protein. This process is highlighted in Figure 2.2. At the present time, the precise mechanism or mechanisms by which ligand binding disrupts RNA recognition remains to be defined. However, two main possibilities exist. First, molecular modeling studies have shown that *E. coli* and human TS undergo a marked conformational change on binding of inhibitor compounds such as FdUMP and the antifolate analogues CB3713 and ZD1694. It is conceivable then that binding by the inhibitor compound alters the conformation of TS in such a manner so as to make the critical domain or domains on TS no longer accessible for RNA binding. An alternative possibility is that the substrate and RNA binding domains of the protein may overlap with one another. Recent work from our laboratory has identified a 35-amino-acid sequence within the folate-binding domain that directly interacts with human TS mRNA, providing support for this second possibility. On the basis of these studies, one approach that could be taken therapeutically would be to identify compounds with potent inhibitory activity against the catalytic function of TS enzyme but would still allow for TS to interact with its target TS mRNA. Preliminary work from our laboratory has shown that incubation of TS with three antifolate analogs in current clinical practice (MTX, ZD1694, and LY2311514) significantly repress its RNA binding activity. In contrast, incubation of TS protein with the diglutamate form of the antifolate analogue 1843U89, another agent that is undergoing clinical testing, did not alter RNA binding, even at drug concentrations approaching 1 mM. This analogue is significantly more potent as an inhibitor of TS enzyme activity than ZD1694 or LY231514. Of note, x-ray crystal studies suggest that the binding of this compound to TS is distinct in the side chain and the third ring from that of other antifolate analogues. This compound has recently been reformulated through encapsulation in liposomes (GS7904L), and our recent studies suggest that this liposomal form of 1843U89 is also unable to abrogate the RNA binding activity of TS. Further investigations are now in progress to determine whether 1843U89, its liposomal counterpart, and other novel antifolate compounds may be able to inhibit TS enzyme activity, maintain RNA binding activity, and prevent the drug-mediated induction of TS expression, thereby preventing and/or overcoming the potential development of acute cellular drug resistance.

DISCUSSION

In this chapter, we review the critical role of translational regulation as a mechanism for regulating TS expression. For well over 40 years, this enzyme served a critical catalytic function by providing essential nucleotide precursors for DNA biosynthesis. However, it is now well established that TS also serves an important role as an RNA binding protein. Our laboratory has shown that TS binds with high affinity to its own mRNA, on the order of 1–3 nM, and directly regulates its own biosynthesis through a novel translational autoregulatory feedback mechanism. Through its role as an RNA binding protein, TS is also able to interact with several cellular mRNAs, including those corresponding to the p53 and the myc family of transcription factors. In each of these instances, TS functions as a translational repressor to coordinately regulate the expression and/or function of these important genes. Recent evidence from our group suggests that TS is an effective and potent translational regulator of cell cycle arrest, apoptosis, and chemosensitivity.

The molecular-based studies outlined herein should help expand our current understanding of TS as an RNA binding protein, and they provide new insights into the role of TS as a critical regulator of certain essential aspects of cellular metabolism and intracellular signaling. Moreover, such studies are the rational basis for the future development of novel therapeutic strategies that can be used either alone or in combination with other well-established anticancer agents. Several of these therapeutic approaches are currently under development in our laboratory as well as in others in order to translate more specific and effective therapies into the clinic for the treatment of human cancers.

ACKNOWLEDGMENTS

The authors wish to thank the members of our laboratory, both past and present, for their dedicated research efforts and contributions to this work. The authors would also like to express their thanks to the Yale Cancer Center, Yale University School of Medicine, and the VA CT Healthcare System for their continued support of this research. This work was supported by grants from the National Cancer Institute (CA16359 and CA75712 to E.C.) and from the Department of Veterans Affairs (VA Merit Review Award to E.C.).

REFERENCES

1. Santi DV, Danenberg PV. Folates in pyrimidine nucleotide biosynthesis. In: Blakely RL, Benkovic SJ, eds. Folate and Pteridines. New York: Wiley, 1984:345–398.
2. Carreras C, Santi DV. The catalytic mechanism and structure of thymidylate synthase. Annu Rev Biochem 1995;64:721–762.

3. Danenberg PV. Thymidylate synthase: a target enzyme in cancer chemotherapy. Biochem Biophys Acta 1977;473:73–79.
4. Hardy LW, Finer-Moore JS, Montfort WR et al. Atomic structure of thymidylate synthase: target for rational drug design. Science 1987;235:448–455.
5. Johnston PG, Liang CM, Henry S et al. Production and characterization of monoclonal antibodies that localize thymidylate synthase in the cytoplasm of human cells and tissue. Cancer Res 1991;51:6668–6676.
6. Leichman L, Danenberg K, Baranda J et al. Quantitation of intratumoral thymidylate synthase expression predicts for disseminated colorectal cancer response and resistance to protracted-infusion fluorouracil and weekly leucovorin. J Clin Oncol 1997;10:3223–3230.
7. Lenz HJ, Hayashi K, Salonga D et al. p53 mutations and thymidylate synthase messenger RNA levels in disseminated colorectal cancer: an analysis of response and survival. Clin Cancer Res 1998;4:1243–1250.
8. Swain SM, Lippman MC, Egan EF et al. 5-Fluorouracil and high-dose leucovorin in previously treated patients with metastatic breast cancer. J Clin Oncol 1989;7:890–899.
9. Van der Wilt CL, Pinedo HM et al. Elevation of thymidylate synthase following 5-fluorouracil treatment is prevented by the addition of leucovorin in murine colon tumors. J Clin Oncol 1994;12:2035–2042.
10. Santi DV, McHenry CS, Sommer H. Mechanism of interaction of thymidylate synthetase with 5-fluorodeoxyuridylate. Biochemistry 1974;13:471–480.
11. Keyomarsi K, Moran RG. Folinic acid augmentation of the effects of fluoropyrimidines on murine and human leukemic cells. Cancer Res 1988;46:5229–5235.
12. Erlichman C, Fine S, Wong A et al. A randomized trial of fluorouracil and folinic acid in patients with metastatic colorectal carcinoma. J Clin Oncol 1988;6:469–475.
13. Poon MA, O'Conell MJ, Moertel CG et al. Biochemical modulation of fluorouracil: evidence of a significant improvement of survival and quality of life in patients with advanced colorectal carcinoma. J Clin Oncol 1989;10:1407–1418.
14. Modulation of fluorouracil by leucovorin in patients with advanced colorectal cancer: evidence in terms of response rate. Advanced Colorectal Cancer Meta-Analysis Project. J Clin Oncol 1992;10:896–903.
15. Rustum YM, Harstrick A, Cao S et al. Thymidylate synthase inhibitors in cancer therapy: direct and indirect inhibitors. J Clin Oncol 1997;15:389–400.
16. Cunningham D, Zalcberg JR, Rath U et al. Tomudex Colorectal Cancer Study Group. Tomudex (ZD1694): results of a randomized trial in advanced colorectal cancer demonstrate efficacy and reduced mucositis and leucopenia. Eur J Cancer 1995;12:1945–1954.
17. Zalcberg JR, Cunningham D, van Cutsem E et al. ZD1694: a novel thymidylate synthase inhibitor with substantial activity in the treatment of patients with advanced colorectal cancer. J Clin Oncol 1996;14:716–721.
18. Cocconi G, Cunninghman D, van Cutsem E et al. Open, randomized, multicenter trial of raltitrexed versus fluorouracil plus high-dose leucovorin in patients with advanced colorectal cancer. J Clin Oncol 1998;16:2943–2952.
19. Schultz RM, Chen VJ, Bewley JR et al. Biological activity of the multitargeted antifolate, MTA (LY231514), in human cell lines with different resistance mechanisms to antifolate drugs. Semin Oncol 1999;26:68–73.
20. O'Dwyer PJ, Nelson K, Thornton DE. Overview of phase II trials of MTA in solid tumors. Semin Oncol 1999;26:99–104.

21. Vogelzang N, Rusthoven J, Paoletti P et al. Phase III single-blinded study of pemetrexed + cisplatin vs. cisplatin alone in chemonaive patients with malignant pleural mesothelioma [abstract 5]. Proc Am Soc Clin Oncol 2002;21, abstract 2.
22. Labow R, Maley GF, Maley F. The effect of methotrexate on enzyme induced following partial hepatectomy. Cancer Res 1969;29:366–372.
23. Bonney RJ, Maley F. Effect of methotrexate on thymidylate synthetase in cultured parenchymal cells isolated from regenerating rat liver. Cancer Res 1975;35:1950–1956.
24. Spears CP, Shahinian AH, Moran RG et al. In vivo kinetics of thymidylate synthase inhibition in 5-fluorouracil-sensitive and-resistant murine colon adenocarcinoma. Cancer Res 1982;42:450–456.
25. Washtein WL. Increased levels of thymidylate synthetase in cells exposed to 5-fluorouracil. Mol Pharmacol 1984;25:171–177.
26. Swain SM, Lippman MC, Egan EF et al. 5-Fluorouracil and high-dose leucovorin in previously treated patients with metastatic breast cancer. J Clin Oncol 1989;7:890–899.
27. Van der Wilt CL, Pinedo HM et al. Elevation of thymidylate synthase following 5-fluorouracil treatment is prevented by the addition of leucovorin in murine colon tumors. J Clin Oncol 1994;12:2035–2042.
28. Keyomarsi K, Samet J, Molnar G et al. The thymidylate synthase inhibitor, ICI D1694, overcomes translational detainment of the enzyme. J Biol Chem 1993;268:15142–15149.
29. Chu E, Zinn S, Boarman D et al. Interaction of gamma interferon and 5-fluorouracil in the H630 human colon carcinoma cell line. Cancer Res 1990;50: 5834–5840.
30. Chu E, Koeller DM, Johnston PG et al. Regulation of thymidylate synthase in human colon cancer cells treated with 5-fluorouracil and interferon-gamma. Mol Pharmacol 1993;43:527–533.
31. Welsh SJ, Titley J, Brunton L et al. Comparison of thymidylate synthase (TS) protein upregulation after exposure to TS inhibitors in normal and tumor cell lines and tissues. Clin Cancer Res 2000;6:2538–2546.
32. Carey J, Cameron V, de Haseth PL et al. Sequence-specific interaction of R17 coat protein with its ribonucleic acid binding site. Biochemistry 1983;22:2601–2610.
33. Bernardi A, Spahr PF. Nucleotide sequence at the binding site for coat protein on RNA of bacteriophage R17. Proc Natl Acad Sci USA 1972;69:3033–3037.
34. Winter RB, Morrissey L, Gauss P et al. Bacteriophage T4 regA protein binds to mRNAs and prevents translation initiation. Proc Natl Acad Sci USA 1987;94:7822–7826.
35. Andrake M, Guild N, Hsu T et al. DNA polymerase of bacteriophage T4 is an autogenous translational repressor. Proc Natl Acad Sci USA 1988;85:7942–7946.
36. Gold L. Posttranscriptional regulatory mechanisms in Escherichia coli. Ann Rev Biochem 1988;57:199–233.
37. Chu E, Takimoto CH, Voeller D et al. Specific binding of human dihydrofolate reductase protein to dihydrofolate reductase messenger RNA in vitro. Biochemistry 1993;32:4756–4760.
38. Ercikan E, Banerjee D, Waltham M et al. Translational regulation of the synthesis of dihydrofolate reductase. Adv Exp Med Biol 1993;338:537–540.
39. Ercikan-Abali EA, Banerjee D, Waltham MC et al. Dihydrofolate reductase protein inhibits its own translation by binding to dihydrofolate reductase mRNA sequences within the coding region. Biochemistry 1997;36:12317–12322.
40. Mosner JT, Mummenbrauer C, Bauer G et al. Negative feedback regulation of wild-type p53 synthesis. EMBO J 1995;14:4442–4449.

41. Fu L, Minden D, Benchimol S. Translational regulation of human p53 expression. EMBO J 1996;15:4392–4401.

42. Liu X, Reig B, Nasrallah IM et al. Human cytoplasmic serine hydroxymethyltransferase is an mRNA binding protein. Biochemistry 2000;39:11523–11531.

43. Chu E, Koeller DM, Casey JL et al. Autoregulation of human thymidylate synthase messenger RNA translation by thymidylate synthase. Proc Natl Acad Sci USA 1991;88:8977–8981.

44. Chu E, Voeller DM, Koeller DM et al. Identification of an RNA binding site for human thymidylate synthase. Proc Natl Acad Sci USA 1993;90:517–521.

45. Lin X, Parsels LA, Voller DM et al. Characterization of a cis-acting regulatory element in the protein coding region of thymidylate synthase mRNA. Nucleic Acids Res 2000;28:1381–1389.

46. Chu E, Voeller DM, Morrison PF. The effect of reducing reagents on binding of thymidylate synthase protein to thymidylate synthase messenger RNA. J Biol Chem 1994;269:20289–20293.

47. Steitz TA. RNA recognition by proteins. In: Gesteland RF, Cech TR, Atkins JF, eds. The RNA world. Cold Spring Harbor: Cold Spring Harbor Press, 1999: 427–450.

48. Melefors O, Hentze MW. Translational regulation by mRNA/protein interactions in eukaryotic cells: ferritin and beyond. Bioessays 1993;15:85–90.

49. Klausner RD, Rouault TA, Harford JB. Regulating the fate of mRNA: the control of cellular iron metabolism. Cell 1993;72:19–28.

50. Henderson BR, Menotti E, Bonnard C et al. Optimal sequence and structure of iron-responsive element. J Biol Chem 1994;269:17481–17489.

51. Chu E, Cogliati T, Copur SM et al. Identification of in vivo target RNA sequences bound by thymidylate synthase. Nucleic Acids Res 1996;24:3222–3228.

52. Steitz J. Immunoprecipitation of ribonucleoproteins using autoantibodies. Methods Enzymol 1989;180:468–481.

53. Froussard P. rPCR: a powerful tool for random amplification of whole RNA sequences. PCR Methods Appl 1992;2:185–190.

54. Ko LJ, Prives C. p53: puzzle and paradigm. Genes Dev 1996;10:1054–1072.

55. Levine AJ. p53, the cellular gatekeeper for growth and division. Cell 1997;88:323–331.

56. Mowat MRA. p53 in tumor progression: life, death and everything. Adv Cancer Res 1998;74:25–48.

57. Maltzman W, Czyzyk L. UV irradiation stimulates levels of p53 cellular tumor antigen in nontransformed mouse cells. Mol Cell Biol 1984;4:1689–1694.

58. Shieh SY, Ikeda M, Taya Y et al. DNA damage-induced phosphorylation of p53 alleviates inhibition by MDM2. Cell 1997;91:325–334.

59. Gu W, Roeder RG. Activation of p53 sequence-specific DNA binding by acetylation of the p53 C-terminal domain. Cell 1997;90:595–606.

60. Sakaguchi K, Herrera JE, Saito W et al. DNA damage activates p53 through a phosphorylation-acetylation cascade. Genes Dev 1998;12:2831–2841.

61. Kastan MB, Onyekwere O, Sidransky D et al. Participation of p53 protein in the cellular response to DNA damage. Cancer Res 1991;51:6304–6311.

62. Fu L, Benchimol S. Participation of the human p53 3′-UTR in translational repression and activation following gamma-irradiation. EMBO J 1997;16:4117–4125.

63. Chu E, Copur SM, Ju J et al. Thymidylate synthase protein and p53 mRNA form an in vivo ribonucleoprotein complex. Mol Cell Biol 1999;19:1582–1594.

64. Ju J, Pederson-Lane J, Maley F et al. Regulation of p53 expression by thymidylate synthase. Proc Natl Acad Sci USA 1999;96:3769–3774.

65. Ju J, Chu E. Translational regulation of 5-FU-induced p53 expression in human cancer RKO cell. Proc Am Assoc Cancer Res 2000; 41:854, 5422a.

66. Liu J, Maley F, Chu E. Intracellular localization of human thymidylate synthase. Proc Am Assoc Cancer Res 2000;41:149, 954a.

67. Green M, Ishino M, Loewenstein PM. Mutational analysis of HIV-1 Tat minimal domain peptides: identification of trans-dominant mutants that suppress HIV-LTR-driven gene expression. Cell 1989;58:215–223.

68. Ferguson PJ, Collins O, Dean, NM et al. Antisense down-regulation of thymidylate synthase to suppress growth and enhance cytotoxicity of 5-FUdR, 5-FU and Tomudex in HeLa cells. Br J Pharmacol 1999;127:1777–1786.

69. Ferguson PJ, DeMoor JM, Vincent MD et al. Antisense-induced down-regulation of thymidylate synthase and enhanced cytotoxicity of 5-FUdR in 5-FUdR-resistant HeLa cells. Br J Pharmacol 2001;134:1437–1446.

70. Berg RW, Werner M, Ferguson PJ et al. Tumor growth inhibition in vivo and G2/M cell cycle arrest induced by antisense oligodeoxynucleotide targeting thymidylate synthase. J Pharmacol Exp Ther 2001;298:477–484.

71. Lin S, Ts'O P, Sun S et al. Inhibition of thymidylate synthase activity by antisense oligodeoxynucleotide and possible role in thymineless treatment. Mol Pharmacol 2001;60:474–479.

72. Stein CA. Is irrelevant cleavage the price of antisense efficacy? Pharmacol Ther 2000;85:231–236.

73. Schmitz JC, Agrawal S, Chu E. Repression of human thymidylate synthase mRNA translation by antisense 2′-O-methyl oligoribonucleotides. Antisense Nucleic Acid Drug Dev 1998;8:371–378.

74. Schmitz JC, Yu D, Agrawal S et al. Effect of 2'-O-methyl antisense ORNs on expression of thymidylate synthase in human colon cancer RKO cells. Nucleic Acids Res 2000;29: 415–422.

75. Bernstein E, Denli AM, Hannon GJ. The rest is silence. RNA 2001;7:1509–1521.

76. Sharp PA. RNA interference-2001. Genes Dev 2001;15:485–490.

77. Zamore PD. RNA interference: listening to the sound of silence. Nat Struct Biol 2001;8:746–750.

78. Hamilton AJ, Baulcombe DC. A species of small antisense RNA in posttranscriptional gene silencing in plants. Science 1999;286:950–952.

79. Elbashir SM, Lendeckel W, Tuschl T. RNA interference is mediated by 21- and 22-nucleotides RNAs. Genes Dev 2001;15:188–200.

80. Zamore PD, Tuschl T, Sharp PA et al. RNAi: double-stranded RNA directs the ATP-dependent cleavage of mRNA at 21 to 23 nucleotide intervals. Cell 2000;101:25–33.

81. Hammond SM, Berstein E, Beach D et al. An RNA-directed nuclease mediates post-transcriptional gene silencing in Drosophila cells. Nature 2000;404:293–296.

82. Williams BR. Role of the double-stranded RNA-activated protein kinase (PKR) in cell regulation. Biochem Soc Trans 1997;25:509–513.

83. Player MR, Torrence PF. The 2-5A system: modulation of viral and cellular processes through acceleration of RNA degradation. Pharmacol Ther 1998;78:55–113.

84. Caplen NJ, Parrish S, Imani F et al. Specific inhibition of gene expression by small double-stranded RNAs in invertebrate and vertebrate systems. Proc Natl Acad Sci USA 2001;98:9742–9747.

85. Elbashir SM, Harborth J, Lendeckel W et al. Duplexes of 21-nucleotide RNAs mediate RNA interference in cultured mammalian cells. Nature 2001;411:494–498.

86. Elbashir SM, Martinez J, Patkaniowsha A et al. Functional anatomy of siRNAs for mediating efficient RNAi in Drosophila melanogaster embryo lysate. EMBO J 2001;20:6877–6888.

87. Parrish S, Fleenor J, Xu S et al. Functional anatomy of a dsRNA trigger: differential requirement for the two trigger strands in RNA interference. Mol Cell 2000;6:1077–1087.

88. Tok JB, Cho J, Rando RR. Aminoglycoside antibiotics are able to specifically bind the 5′-untranslated region of thymidylate synthase messenger RNA. Biochemistry 1999;38:199–206.

89. Cho J, Rando RR. Specific binding of Hoechst 33258 to site 1 thymidylate synthase mRNA. Nucleic Acids Res 2000;28:2158–2163.

Chapter 3

Radioimmunotherapy for Non-Hodgkin's Lymphoma

Susan Tinsley Schumer, MD

Robin M. Joyce, MD

In March 2002, the US Food and Drug Administration licensed the first radioimmunotherapeutic for human use. Yttrium-90 ibitromomab tiuxetan (Zevalin; IDEC Pharmaceuticals, San Diego, CA) is the first in a series of radioimmunotherapeutics to become available for the treatment of non-Hodgkin's lymphoma (NHL). This review discusses the general principles of radioimmunotherapy and some of the clinical data on several radioimmunoconjugates in development for the treatment of NHL. Clinical data from published trials is reviewed; data that are available only in abstract form is not included. The reader is referred to several excellent reviews for a more detailed discussion of the preclinical work, other targeting moieties, and radioimmunotherapy in other malignancies.[1-4]

The NHLs represent a heterogeneous collection of lymphoid neoplasms whose incidence is rising dramatically in all age groups. An estimated 56,000 new cases will be diagnosed in the United States this year.[5] More than 80% of these cases are of B-cell origin. The incidence of indolent (World Health Organization classification) lymphomas as a subgroup is approximately 40%; however, given their longer natural history, their prevalence in North America accounts for about 65% of NHLs.[6] These lymphomas are often disseminated at presentation, and although they are initially responsive to chemotherapy, relapse is virtually inevitable. Multiple chemotherapy agents are active against these indolent lymphoid neoplasms; these agents include alkylating agents (chlorambucil, cyclophosphamide), anthracyclines, and purine analogues (fludarabine, cladribine). The reported response rate (RR) for purine analogues is between 30% and 66%.[7-9] Unfortunately, none of these therapies have demonstrated a survival benefit,[10] and remission durations appear to be progressively shorter when patients are treated with alkylator-based therapy. In patients with minimal disease burden and an excellent performance status, myeloablative therapy has been pursued.[11-13] This approach is limited by the requirement of a minimal disease state as well as by the high frequency of overt bone marrow involvement. More aggressive, but still subablative, chemotherapy combinations, such as fludarabine, mitoxantrone and dexamethasone (FND) or fludarabine and cyclophosphamide (FC), have demonstrated significant activity against this disease but are frequently complicated by opportunistic infections.[14,15] Moreover, these approaches have failed to produce durable remissions. Recently, the introduction of immunotherapeutic agents has further advanced the treatment of NHL. Rituximab is a chimeric anti-CD20 monoclonal antibody that was approved by the US Food and Drug Administration in 1997 for the treatment of relapsed or refractory low-grade or follicular NHL. In the pivotal trial, rituximab demonstrated an overall response (OR) rate of 48%, with a complete response (CR) rate of 6% and a time to progression of 13 months.[16]

Aggressive lymphomas constitute 40% of NHLs in the World Health Organization classification. They are characterized by rapid progression and death within a matter of months. A proportion of patients can be cured with combination anthracycline-based chemotherapy. Of patients who do not obtain a durable remission, a small proportion can be cured with high-dose chemotherapy and autologous stem cell rescue.[17]

Lymphoma is inherently radiosensitive and has a steep dose-response curve.[18-21] External-beam radiation is often used to palliate focal areas of disease, and approximately half of stage I follicular lymphomas can be cured with involved-field radiation therapy. Unfortunately, most patients with indolent NHL present with disseminated disease, posing a practical obstacle to the use of external-beam radiation therapy. The ability to target multiple sites of disease, while sparing normal tissue, would therefore be a great therapeutic advance. Radioimmunotherapy (RIT) delivers systemic radiation through targeted radiolabeled monoclonal antibodies. Along with targeting multiple disease sites, RIT may have a benefit over external-beam radiation therapy by delivering a continuous low dose rate of radiation. Radioimmunotherapy also has advantages over treatment with unlabeled monoclonal antibodies.[22] Radioimmunoconjugates do not rely on the immune system for their antitumor effect. This may be relevant in a disease where the immune system of the patient is impaired. In addition, through therapeutic beta emissions, radiolabeled antibodies exert their effect over several cell diameters and kill neighboring cells through "cross-fire." This helps to overcome some of the barriers to uniform antibody distribution: nonuniform blood flow, elevated interstitial pressures, and absent antigenic targets. This may be especially important in bulky tumors in which the efficacy of immunotherapy is limited.

There are three general components of successful radioimmunotherapy (Table 3.1): (1) a suitable target, (2) a targeting moiety, (3) and an effector mechanism or isotope. To be effective, RIT targets should be selective for neoplastic cells. This selectivity can be the result of overexpression (e.g., carcinoembryonic antigen in epithelial malignancies) or abnormal expression (e.g., MUC-1) of the antigen. The targets should be continually expressed on tumor cells with little modulation or shedding into the circulation. If the antigen is not tumor specific, but rather tumor associated and tissue specific, it also should not be expressed on the tissue's stem cell.

The idiotype of B cells represents a tumor-specific target for lymphoid malignancies. At present, CD20 is the most well-studied tissue specific B-cell antigen. It is a 32-kd phosphoprotein that is integral to the B-cell membrane. It is expressed by more than 95% of B-cell neoplasms and early pre–B cells and is not present on hematopoietic stem cells or mature plasma cells.[23,24] On antibody binding, the antigen is not shed, modulated, or internalized. CD22 is another B lymphocyte membrane protein; it translocates to the cytoplasm when it is bound by antibody and is later reexpressed on the plasma membrane. Certain HLA-DR epitopes on B-cell surfaces have been used as targets for antibody-directed therapy.

The targeting moiety, or antibody, is another important element of radioimmunotherapy. The antibody should have high affinity to the selected antigen, low immunogenicity, optimal tumor penetration, and rapid clearance from normal tissues. Various immunoglobulin molecules have been studied in RIT, including antibody fragments and subfragments, such as bivalent $F(ab')_2$ and monovalent Fab′ fragments; monoclonal murine antibodies; and reengineered chimeric and humanized antibodies. Chimeric antibodies contain a human antibody Fc component grafted onto a murine antigen-binding domain. In contrast, the humanized antibodies are engineered to contain only a few murine molecules in the $F(ab')_2$ segment. These manipulations may lead to better engagement of human effector molecules, activation of the complement cascade, and less immunogenicity. The shorter half-life of the murine antibodies may be advantageous when radioisotopes are used. The biologic half-life of these antibodies and the physical half-life of the isotope are optimal in this situation and may minimize toxicity to nontarget organs. However, the immunogenicity of the murine proteins can result in the formation of neutralizing human anti-mouse antibodies (HAMA) and human anti-chimeric antibodies (HACA). This occurs most frequently with repeated antibody dosing and may limit the utility of these molecules.[25,26]

TABLE 3.1 Characteristics of Selected Radioimmunotherapeutic Agents

RIT Agent	Labeled Antibody	"Cold" Pretherapy Antibody	Target Antigen	Isotope	Chelating Agent
^{90}Y ibritumomab tiuxetan	Ibritumomab (murine IgG1 K)	Rituximab	CD20	^{90}Y	Tiuxetan (DTPA derivative)
^{131}I tositumomab	Tositumomab (murine IgG2a)	Tositumomab	CD20	^{131}I	—
^{131}I or ^{67}Cu Lym-1	Lym-1 (murine IgG2a)	Lym-1	HLA-DR 10	^{131}I ^{67}Cu	— TETA
^{131}I or ^{90}Y epratuzumab	Epratuzumab (humanized IgG)	Epratuzumab	CD22	^{131}I ^{90}Y	— DTPA derivative

Abbreviations: DTPA, diethylenetriamine penta-acetic acid; IgG, immunoglobulin G; RIT, radioimmunotherapy.

The radioisotope is the third component of radioimmunotherapy (Table 3.2). To date, two isotopes have been extensively studied for clinical use: iodine-131 (^{131}I) and yttrium-90 (^{90}Y). The early studies were performed with iodine 131 (^{131}I), which is easily generated and emits both beta and gamma energies. The mean beta energy is 0.6 MeV, most of which is deposited over a 50-cell radius. Its half-life is 193 hours. This is longer than most antibodies, thereby creating the potential for prolonged radiation exposure if free isotope is available to the patient. Significant dehalogenation occurs via a native dehalogenase, yielding circulating free ^{131}I. This free ^{131}I is either rapidly excreted or accumulated in the thyroid, necessitating the prophylactic use of iodine. ^{131}I also emits gamma irradiation. This is useful for tumor imaging but exposes the patient's distant tissues to excess radiation and potentially exposes clinical personnel and household members to radiation as well. Many states require protective hospitalization and shielding when this radionuclide is used.[27,28]

Radioactive metals are the other source of isotope. Yttrium 90 (^{90}Y) is the best studied and most readily available radioactive metal. This isotope has a pure high-energy beta emission (2.3 MeV) and has no need for special isolation or protective measures. The higher-energy beta emission produces an increase in the cell-killing radius to approximately 250 cells (5 mm). This may be advantageous in bulky tumors. The half-life of ^{90}Y is 64 hours, approximating the biologic half-life of the targeting antibody. Preclinical trials demonstrate that tumor uptake might be faster for ^{90}Y-labeled antibodies than for ^{131}I-labeled antibodies.[29] Because ^{90}Y is a pure beta emitter, it is not suitable for imaging or dosimetry. Indium 111 (^{111}In) is a gamma-emitting isotope with a biodistribution and a half-life similar to those of ^{90}Y but without therapeutic beta emissions. It is commonly used for dosimetry and imaging in clinical trials involving ^{90}Y-radiolabeled antibodies. Because yttrium is naturally deposited in bone, it must be administered with an extremely avid chelating molecule.

Copper 67 (^{67}Cu) is a second radiometal being investigated in RIT. It emits therapeutically useful beta particles of moderate energy (0.14 MeV) as well as

TABLE 3.2 Properties of Commonly Used Isotopes in Radioimmunotherapy

Isotopes	Mean Energy[a] (MeV)	Energy Emitted	Half-Life (hours)	Path Length[a] (mm)	Comments
^{131}I	0.6	β, γ	193	0.8 mm	Requires prophylactic iodine to protect thyroid
^{90}Y	2.3	β	64	5.3 mm	No gamma emission so unable to use for imaging
^{67}Cu	0.14	β, γ	62	0.6 mm	Rare isotope

[a]Refers to energy for the β component.

gamma photons that permit imaging studies but still allow for outpatient therapy. It has a long half-life (62 hours), similar to the residence time of monoclonal antibodies in tumors,[30,31] and is not deposited in the skeleton or bone marrow. This leads to delivery of a greater radiation dose to tumors and achieves a higher therapeutic index. In addition, ^{67}Cu has microdosimetry properties similar to those of ^{131}I but appears to provide better tumor imaging.[31] In small comparative studies with ^{131}I, ^{67}Cu achieved higher peak and mean tumor concentrations, had a longer biologic half-life, and delivered a lower radiation dose to the bone marrow.[32] Both nuclides delivered similar radiation doses to all other organs except the liver, which received a greater radiation dose from ^{67}Cu because of recycling by ceruloplasmin in the liver. However, hepatotoxicity was not observed in early clinical trials.[31,33,34]

A significant obstacle to the optimal use of radiometals in RIT has been the development of high-affinity chelators that can form a stable bond to the targeting antibodies without altering their binding characteristics. The yttrium chelator tiuxetan is a derivative of diethylenetriamine penta-acetic acid (DTPA) that maintains affinity with enhanced stability. TETA (1,4,7,11 tetraazacyclotetradecane-N,N′,N″,N‴-tetra-acetic acid) is the copper chelator that selectively binds ^{67}Cu and joins it to the Lym-1 antibody, forming the radioimmunoconjugate ^{67}Cu 2IT-BAT-Lym-1. This complex has demonstrated exceptional structural stability and functional integrity.[31,35]

The general treatment schema and trial enrollment criteria are similar for most of the RIT agents and their studies. Patients receive an initial dose of unlabeled ("cold") antibody before the radiolabeled antibodies are infused. This pretreatment cold antibody blocks nonspecific antigen-binding sites in the blood and reticuloendothelial system, thereby improving tumor targeting and providing more favorable biodistribution and pharmacokinetics.[36,37] Before the therapeutic RIT dose, a small tracer dose of radiolabeled antibody is injected (after a dose of cold antibody). Serial imaging is then performed to evaluate tumor uptake and dosimetry. The therapeutic radioimmunoconjugte is then administered 1–2 weeks later. When iodinated radiolabeled antibodies are used, standard pharmaceutical thyroid protection (potassium perchlorate and saturated solution of potassium iodide) is incorporated. In general, most RIT studies require evidence of adequate hematopoieses (absolute neutrophil count [ANC] > 1500 cells/mm^3 and platelet count > 100,000 cells/mm^3), minimal bone marrow involvement by NHL (< 25%), no HAMA or HACA, and adequate organ function.

^{90}Y-IBRITUMOMAB TIUXETAN

^{90}Y ibritumomab tiuxetan is a radiolabeled molecule composed of a murine immunoglobulin G1 (IgG1) K monoclonal antibody and the isotope ^{90}Y, bound by the chelator tiuxetan. The monoclonal antibody is the parent murine antibody used in the development of rituximab. It recognizes the CD20 antigen with high affinity and high specificity.

The initial clinical studies with ^{90}Y ibritumomab tiuxetan aimed to determine the biodistribution and radiation dose delivered to both the tumor and to normal tissues. The first phase I/II dose escalation trial demonstrated activity of ^{90}Y ibritumomab tiuxetan and determined the maximal tolerated dose of this agent.[38] In this trial, 14 patients with relapsed or refractory low- or intermediate-grade B cell NHL were treated with escalating doses of ^{90}Y ibritumomab tiuxetan until they reached a myelosuppressive dose requiring peripheral blood stem cell reinfusion. All but one patient had stage III or IV disease, and more than half had extranodal involvement. Many patients were heavily pretreated, progressing after a mean of 2.9 regimens (range, 1–5).

Early in the trial, biodistribution studies using ^{111}In ibritumomab tiuxetan were performed in patients receiving $\leq$ 30 mCi of ^{90}Y ibritumomab tiuxetan. These studies evaluated the impact of the pretreatment unlabeled antibody on the biodistribution of ^{111}In ibritumomab tiuxetan and demonstrated that the unlabeled antibody improved biodistribution of the radiolabel and increased visualization of known disease sites. Detection was further enhanced with higher doses of unlabeled antibody. Eighteen percent of known disease sites were visualized when ^{111}In ibritumomab tiuxetan was given alone; however, 56% were seen after pretreatment with 1 mg/kg of unlabeled antibody, and 92% were visualized after 2.5 mg/kg of antibody. Occult sites of disease and splenomegaly were also detected. Based on these results, all patients in this and subsequent trials received unlabeled antibody injections before all ^{111}In- and ^{90}Y-labeled ibritumomab tiuxetan infusions.

Biodistribution studies were performed in a standard fashion immediately after administration of ^{111}In ibritumomab tiuxetan (5 mCi).[38] Whole-body anterior and posterior images were obtained immediately after infusion and at 14, 18, 24, 48, and 72 hours after injection. Whole-body average retention times were estimated by use of an existing algorithm based on a single exponential analysis. Regions of interest were marked for recognizable organs and tumor lesions. Tumor dosimetry was compared with organ dosimetry. Treatment with ^{90}Y ibritumomab tiuxetan was performed if the estimated cumulative dose of ^{90}Y ibritumomab tiuxetan was less than 10 times the whole-body dose and if the estimated liver dose was < 1500 cGy. After demonstrating adequate dosimetry, patients in this trial were treated with escalating ^{90}Y ibritumomab tiuxetan ranging from 13.5 to 50 mCi. An impressive RR of 72% occurred in this study, and the CR rate was 33%. At the time of publication, the longest CR was greater than 29 months.

Nonhematologic toxicity was generally mild and included grade 1 and 2 fever and a rash (10 patients) that was immediately reversible with antihistamines. Several grade 2 and 3 infections, which responded to antibiotic therapy, also occurred. Three months after treatment, there was no change in immunoglobulin levels; however, four patients developed HAMA during the first year.

Hematologic toxicity was the dose-limiting factor. Peripheral blood stem cells were uniformly required at the 50-mCi dose but never at the 30-mCi dose.

A second phase I/II study was performed to compare two pretreatment doses of unlabeled antibody (rituximab, 100 mg/m^2 or 250 mg/m^2) and to determine the maximum tolerated dose (MTD) of ^{90}Y ibritumomab tiuxetan when it was used as a single dose without peripheral blood stem cell support.[39] The patient population was similar to that of the previous study. Both doses of rituximab showed similar imaging and dosimetric characteristics. The 250-mg/m^2 dose was chosen for future studies. Patients received escalating ^{90}Y ibritumomab tiuxetan doses of 0.2, 0.3, and 0.4 mCi/Kg. The 0.4-mCi/kg dose was found to be the MTD, and the 0.3-mCi/kg dose was selected for patients with a baseline platelet count of 100 to 149,000/μL. In both cases, the maximum infused dose was set at 32 mCi.

Fifty-one patients were evaluated in an intent-to-treat analysis. The OR rate for the study was 67% (26% CRs and 41% PRs), and the median duration of response was estimated at 11.7 months. When stratified by histology, the RR was 82% for low-grade NHLs and 43% for intermediate-grade disease. Independent predictors of response included low-grade follicular histology, absence of bone marrow involvement, and nonbulky disease. The adverse events were mainly hematologic and seemed to correlate with the degree of lymphomatous bone marrow involvement.

A randomized phase III trial comparing ^{90}Y ibritumomab tiuxetan with a standard course of rituximab was then performed (Table 3.3).[40] This was the first trial to compare the safety and efficacy of an unlabeled monoclonal antibody with those of a radiolabeled one. One hundred forty-three patients from 27 institutions with CD20+ B-cell NHL were enrolled. Patients were required to meet standard entrance criteria for RIT, including lack of HAMA or HACA and minimal bone marrow involvement. The primary study objective was OR rate, as determined by an independent third-party panel of radiologists and oncologists who were expert in lymphoma. The ^{90}Y ibritumomab tiuxetan regimen (73 patients) consisted of day 1 rituximab (250 mg/m^2) followed by ^{111}In-labeled ibritumomab (5 mCi) and day 8 rituximab (250 mg/m^2) and 0.4 mCi/kg (maximum 32 mCi) ^{90}Y conjugated ibritumomab tiuxetan (hereafter referred to as standard ^{90}Y ibritumomab tiuxetan treatment course). The control arm (70 patients) received 4 weekly rituximab doses (375 mg/m^2). Patients were stratified by histology type (International Working Formulation [IWF] type A, follicular or transformed) before randomization. Baseline characteristics in both arms were well balanced. There were no statistical differences between the ^{90}Y ibritumomab tiuxetan and rituximab groups in regard to median number of prior therapies (2), age, bone marrow involvement (42% vs 34%), splenomegaly (10% vs 4%), bulky disease > 5 cm (45% vs 44%), elevated LDH (19% vs 14%), chemotherapy resistance (49% vs 47%), performance status, International Prognostic Index (IPI), and extranodal disease.

TABLE 3.3 Important Trials for ^{90}Y Ibritumomab Tiuxetan

Study	Type of Trial	*N*	Patient Characteristics	^{90}Y Ibritumomab tiuxetan Dose[a,b] (mCi)	R	CR	Median DR (months)	Comments
Witzig et al (2002)[40]	Phase III randomized trial Total $N = 143$	^{90}Y ibritumoma b tiuxetan arm, 73	Relapsed or refractory low-grade, follicular, or transformed NHL	0.4 mCi/kg as single dose	80%	30%	14.2	OR rate and CR for ^{90}Y ibritumomab tiuxetan statistically superior to rituximab. Demonstrated improvement in QOL.
		Rituximab control arm, 70		Rituximab, 375 mg/m^2 weekly × 4 doses	56%	16%	12.1	
Witzig et al (2002)[43]	Phase II trial	57 (3 with nonfollicular NHL);	Relapsed or refractory follicular NHL; Rituximab refractory	0.4 mCi/kg as single dose	74%[c]	15%[c]	6.4	<2% HAMA. Demonstrated improvement in QOL.
Wiseman et al (2002)[42]	Phase II trial	30	Relapsed or refractory low-grade, follicular, or transformed NHL. Mild thrombocytopenia	0.3 mCi/kg as single dose	83%	37%	11.7	Reduced dose ^{90}Y ibritumomab tiuxetan determined to be safe in patients with mild thrombocytopenia.

Abbreviations: OR, overall response; CR, complete response; DR, duration of response; RIT, radioimmunotherapy; R, response; NHL, non-Hodgkin's lymphoma; QOL, quality of life; HAMA, human anti-mouse antibodies.

[a]Standard ^{90}Y ibritumomab tiuxetan treatment course: unlabeled antibody (rituximab, 250 mg/m^2) infused on day 1, followed by ^{111}In ibritumomab tiuxetan (5 mCi) for imaging. On day 8, unlabeled antibody (rituximab, 250 mg/m^2) was again infused, followed by therapeutic dose of ^{90}Y ibritumomab tiuxetan.

[b]Maximum infused dose was 32 mCi.

[c]RR and CR calculated for the 54 patients with follicular NHL.

The ^{90}Y ibritumomab tiuxetan group demonstrated a statistically significant improvement in OR rate (80% vs 56%, $P = 0.002$). This group had a complete remission rate of 30%, compared with a 16% complete remission rate in the rituximab control group ($P = 0.04$). Patients with follicular histology responded most often with an OR rate of 86%, compared with OR rates of 67% and 56% in the IWF A (small lymphocytic) and transformed groups, respectively. The duration of remission in the ^{90}Y ibritumomab tiuxetan group was 14.2 months, versus 12.1 months in the rituximab group. This difference was not statistically significant; however, this study was not powered to detect differences in this endpoint. The median time to next therapy for the ^{90}Y ibritumomab tiuxetan group had not been reached at the time of publication. When analyzed by prognostic variables, patients considered to be chemotherapy resistant (no response to the most recent chemotherapy or a response with progression in < 6 months) showed a higher RR (63%) to ^{90}Y ibritumomab tiuxetan than to rituximab (RR, 43%; $P = 0.078$). Quality of life, as measured by the Functional Assessment of Cancer Therapy-General (FACT-G) score showed a statistically significant improvement in the ^{90}Y ibritumomab tiuxetan group at 3 months. This improvement in self-assessed quality of life is especially meaningful given the palliative nature of treatment for this population.

The overall incidence of nonhematologic adverse events was low and was similar in both treatment arms. During the treatment period, the most frequent treatment-related adverse events for the ^{90}Y ibritumomab tiuxetan and rituximab arms, respectively, included asthenia (40%, 33%), nausea (33%, 14%), chills (18%, 29%), throat irritation (18%, 14%), fever (14%, 16%), headache (12%, 16%), and vomiting (14%, 6%).

In the ^{90}Y ibritumomab tiuxetan group, transient hematologic toxicity was observed. The median ANC nadir was 900 cells/mm^3, and the median time to recovery (ANC to >1000 cells/mm^3) was 8 days for the 57 patients with grade 3 or 4 toxicity. Seven patients received granulocyte colony stimulating factor treatments, and five patients received prophylactic antibiotics. Flow cytometry analysis of a subset of 72 patients demonstrated prompt depletion of circulating B cells to below the detectable range, with recovery beginning 6 months after therapy. However, plasma immunoglobulin levels remained in the normal range. The overall incidence of serious clinical infections in this trial was low (7%). Thus, despite neutropenia and a transient depletion of normal peripheral blood B cells, ^{90}Y ibritumomab tiuxetan therapy did not result in significant hypogammaglobulinemia, and more importantly, it did not result in an excessive infectious risk. Significant thrombocytopenia and anemia also occurred with ^{90}Y ibritumomab tiuxetan treatment but were much less common. The median nadir platelet count was 41,000 cells/mm^3 and developed 54 days after treatment. Four patients (5.5%) experienced grade 4 thrombocytopenia, but there were no hospitalizations for bleeding. Thirteen patients received platelet transfusions. The nadir hemoglobin value was 10.8 g/dL, occurring on day

70. Nine patients received red blood cell transfusions, and four patients received erythropoietin.

Dosimetry results for 72 of the patients treated with ^{90}Y ibritumomab tiuxetan demonstrated that ^{90}Y ibritumomab tiuxetan infused at 0.4 mCi/kg delivered an acceptable radiation dose to normal organs and red marrow by never exceeding the protocol-defined acceptable doses for normal organs (<2000 cGy) or bone marrow (300 cGy). The median estimated radiation doses for critical organs were as follows: 779 cGy to spleen, 532 cGy to liver, 215 cGy to lungs, 15 cGy to kidneys, and 71 cGy to red marrow.[41]

A phase II study was designed to evaluate the safety and efficacy of reduced-dose ^{90}Y ibritumomab tiuxetan in patients with mild thrombocytopenia (100,000 to 149,000 platelets/mm3).[42] The trial also evaluated the ability of the baseline platelet count to select a safe and effective ^{90}Y ibritumomab tiuxetan dose and thereby eliminate the need for dosimetry. The study involved 30 patients with advanced, relapsed or refractory, low-grade, follicular or transformed B-cell NHL who had failed to respond to conventional chemotherapy. Ninety percent of patients had stage III/IV disease, and 67% had bone marrow involvement. Patients were treated according to the standard ^{90}Y ibritumomab tiuxetan treatment protocol using a lower dose of ^{90}Y ibritumomab tiuxetan (0.3 mCi/kg; maximum 32 mCi). The OR rate was 83% (25/30 patients), with a 37% CR rate (11 patients), a 6.7% (unconfirmed complete response CRu) rate (2 patients), and a 40% PR rate (12 patients). Kaplan-Meier–estimated median (time to progression TTP) for responders was 12.6 months. Hematologic toxicity was transient and reversible. Blood count nadirs included an ANC of 600 cells/mm^3, a platelet count of 26,000 cells/mm^3, and a hemoglobin level of 10.1 gm/dL. Grade 4 neutropenia and thrombocytopenia occurred in 33% and 13% of patients, respectively, with a median time to recovery of 14 days. The incidence of grade 4 thrombocytopenia was significantly associated with increased bone marrow involvement (P = 0.049). Thus, reduced-dose ^{90}Y ibritumomab tiuxetan was determined to be safe and effective in this patient population. In addition, the clinical variables of baseline platelet count, the percent of NHL bone marrow involvement, and the patient weight predicted for toxicity and allowed dosing without dosimetry.

A second, nonrandomized, multicenter study was designed to evaluate the efficacy and safety of a single course of ^{90}Y ibritumomab tiuxetan radioimmunotherapy in patients with rituximab-refractory follicular B-cell NHL.[43] Patients were considered to be refractory to rituximab if they had failed to respond or had responded and progressed in less than 6 months after a standard 4-week course of rituximab. Fifty-seven patients with relapsed or refractory NHL (54 follicular, 3 nonfollicular) were enrolled. Patients were heavily pretreated (median of four prior therapies) and displayed numerous poor prognostic features: bulky disease (> 5 cm) in 76%, splenomegaly in 12%, and resistance to last chemotherapy regimen in 67%. All patients received a standard ^{90}Y ibritumomab tiuxetan treatment course with a ^{90}Y ibritumomab tiuxetan dose of 0.4 mCi/kg (maximum dose, 32 mCi). The study's primary endpoint was OR rate. This and duration of response were also compared with the same values for the patients' most recent rituximab and chemotherapy treatments. In the 54 patients with follicular NHL, the OR rate was 74% (32/54) and the CR was 15%. This OR rate was significantly higher than that of the last rituximab therapy (59% vs 32%; $P = 0.002$) but was not significantly different from the response to the last chemotherapy. Fifty-one percent (19/37) of patients who had not responded to their last rituximab treatment derived a response to ^{90}Y ibritumomab tiuxetan. Kaplan-Meier–estimated median TTP was 8.7 months (range, 1.7 to ≥25.9 months) for responders, and the estimated median duration of response was 6.4 months (range, 0.5 to ≥24.9 months). Although retreatment with a monoclonal antibody–based regimen raised the concern for HAMA or HACA formation, only one patient (< 2%) experienced HAMA in this study.

A review of integrated safety evaluations from 211 patients treated on these four trials showed ^{90}Y ibritumomab tiuxetan to be safe and well tolerated.[39,40,42,43] Adverse events were primarily hematologic, transient, and reversible, with severity being related to baseline platelet count and degree of bone marrow involvement. Most nonhematologic adverse events were grade 1 and 2 and were related to rituximab infusions. No major organ dysfunction was observed. Despite myelosuppression, the infection risk was not high, and only 7.6% of patients required hospitalization for infection.[40,43] The incidences of HAMA and HACA were 1.4% (three patients) and 0.5% (one patient), respectively. There were rare cases of myelodysplasia or acute myelogenous leukemia AML/ (four patients, 1.9%), which is well beneath the anticipated rate of 4%–8% in this heavily pretreated population.[44]

Based on these trials, ^{90}Y ibritumomab tiuxetan was approved by the food and Drug Administration for the treatment of relapsed or refactory low-grade follicular or transformed NHL.Further development with this agent is ongoing. Investigators are studying a broader patient population and the efficacy of new dosing protocols and combination therapy. Current trials are enrolling patients with mantle cell NHL and patients who have undergone prior bone marrow transplant. Other studies are looking at the efficacy and toxicity of multidose ^{90}Y ibritumomab tiuxetan treatment, the use of myeloablative doses with hematopoietic stem cell support, and the combination of RIT with chemotherapy.

^{131}I TOSITUMOMAB

^{131}I tositumomab (Bexxar; Corixa Corporation, Seattle, WA) is a murine IgG2a anti-CD20 molecule that is covalently linked to an iodine isotope via a tyrosine residue (Table 3.1). This linkage is stable; however, there is native dehalogenase in human tissue that can release free iodine at varying rates. The immunoglobulin molecule itself can also be degraded. The free iodine-tyrosine molecules can deposit in the thyroid and stomach and are cleared by the kidney. In order to properly dose individual patients and optimize radiation doses absorbed by both normal and tumor tissues, individual patient doses need to be calculated. This individual dosimetry can address interpatient variability that cannot be accounted for by weight-based dosing alone. This internal individual dosimetry can be performed with the ^{131}I radionuclide itself, which is an advantage of the ^{131}I conjugate. This isotope emits both intermediate-energy beta particles (0.606 mEV with a path length of 0.8 mm) and gamma photons suitable for imaging.

In the phase I ^{131}I-anti B1 (tositumomab) dose-escalation study, therapeutic doses of ^{131}I were determined following imaging and dosimetry calculations to allow delivery of a specified total-body radiation dose (TBD).[45] Total-body doses were escalated from 25–85 cGy in sequential groups of patients with relapsed NHL. The maximal tolerated total body dose was 75 cGy. Twenty-eight patients were treated with doses ranging from 34–161 mCi, resulting in 14 complete remissions. Responses were seen in all patients with low-grade lymphoma. The median duration of response for all patients was 16.5 months. Two forms of toxicity were generally observed. The first related to infusional toxicities commonly seen with monoclonal antibody therapy; the second, and dose-limiting toxicity, was hematologic.

Kaminski et al[46] reported the long-term results of a phase I/II study of ^{131}I tositumomab in 59 patients treated at the University of Michigan (Table 3.4). Patients met the standard entrance requirements for RIT. The first 25 patients in this cohort received varying doses of unlabeled tositumomab to determine optimal targeting. The remaining 34 patients were treated with the chosen cold antibody dose of 450 mg. Patients received standard pharmacologic thyroid protection. Data from the previously discussed phase I study were also included in this long-term follow-up. Patients were eligible for retreatment if they had not responded to prior therapy or had relapsed and were HAMA negative. Seventy-one percent had low-grade or low-grade–transformed NHL histologies. Patients had received a median of three prior regimens and had refractory disease, although some did receive ^{131}I tositumomab as their first therapy. Twenty patients were treated at the MTD of 75 cGy TBD, but there was a wide range of administrated doses (56.8–153 mCi). Six patients did not receive a therapeutic dose, because of either rapid disease progression or early development of HAMA. In an intent-to-treat analysis the OR rate was 71%. In the 42 patients with low-grade histologies, the RR was 83%, compared with 41% in those with intermediate- or high-grade NHL. Patients with transformed lymphomas responded similarly to those with low-grade histologies. In patients with prior remissions of more than 6 months duration, the RR was 100%, and the progression-free survival was 17 months. In general, RR was observed to directly correlate with total body dose. Patients who received less than 65 cGy of radiation had a RR of 57%, compared with a RR of 86% in those receiving more than 65 cGy. All of the patients who had a duration of response greater than 1.5 years received a TBD of more than 55 cGy.

Of the 14 patients treated after autologous stem cell transplantation, the OR rate was 50%. The median progression-free survival in responders had not been reached at 4.7 years follow-up, and four patients remained disease free more than 3 years after treatment. Seven patients received a second dose of ^{131}I tositumomab

TABLE 3.4 Important Trials for ^{131}I Tositumomab

Study	Type Of Trial	*N*	Patient Characteristics	^{131}I Tositumomab TBD (cGy)[a,b]	R	CR	Duration[c] (months)	Comments
Kaminski et al (2000)[46]	Phase I/II	59	Relapsed or refractory NHL (14 post-ASCT)	Escalating single dose given to establish MTD. 7 patients received a second dose.	71%	34%	12 (PFS at 3 years)[c]	Established MTD: 75 cGy in non ASCT patients, 45 cGy in post-ASCT patients. 5 developed MDS (long term follow-up).
Vose et al (2000)[47]	Phase II	47	Relapsed or refractory low-grade or low-grade transformed NHL. All had received prior anthracycline-based chemotherapy. Relapse < 12 months	Single dose of 75 cGy or 65 cGy (if platelet count <1500,000).	57%	32%	9.9 (median DR)	Response rate similar in low-grade and transformed low-grade NHL.
Kaminski et al(2001)[48]	Non randomized phase III	60	Chemotherapy refractory low-grade or low-grade transformed NHL. Relapse < 6 months	Single dose of 75 cGy	65%	20%	6.5 (median DR)	Trial designed to compare efficacy of ^{131}I tositumomab with that of a patient's LQC. ^{131}I tositumomab found to be significantly more efficacious that the LQC
Press et al (1993)[49] Liu et al (1998)[51]	Phase I/II	29	Relapsed low- and intermediate-grade NHL.	Myeloablative dose followed by ASCT. Dose based on estimated absorbed radiation dose to critical organs.	86%	79%	42% (PFS rate at 4 years)[c]	Cardiopulmonary toxicity was dose limiting. 13 patients remained in CR greater than 3 years. No MDS seen

N, number of patients in trial; TBD, total body dose; RR, overall response rate; CR, complete response; DR, duration of response; PFS, progression free survival; LQC, last qualifying chemotherapy; autologous stem cell transplant (ASCT)

[a]Goal total body dose (TBD) absorbed. Administered dose of ^{131}I tositumomab (mCi) calculated based on individual dosimetry.

[b]Standard course of ^{131}I tositumomab: unlabeled antibody infusion (450 mg) followed by tracer dose of ^{131} I tositumomab (5 mCi) for dosimetry given on day 0. Therapeutic dose delivered between day 7 and 15 after an infusion of unlabeled antibody (450 mg). All patients receive standard pharmacologic thyroid protection.

[c]Outcome measurements of duration varied in different trials. PFS, median DR, and PFS rate all used in above.

because they had an incomplete response to the initial therapy dose. In only one of these patients did stable disease convert to PR. Sixteen patients were retreated because of relapse after an initial response. Fifty-six percent of these patients had a second response, and the median progression-free survival was 11.4 months. Three patients remained in a continued CR 37 months after retreatment.

Early adverse events associated with ^{131}I tositumomab therapy consisted of grade I and II infusion-related toxicities. The dose-limiting toxicity was hematologic. The median times to platelet and neutrophil nadir from the time of treatment were 35 and 43 days, respectively, and the median times to recovery were 51 and 64 days, respectively. Three of twenty patients received either platelet or red cell transfusions. Hematologic toxicity was similar in retreated patients. Based on hematologic toxicity, the MTD was established as a TBD of 75 cGy in patients who had not undergone prior stem cell transplantation and 45 cGy in those who had received prior myeloablative therapy. As expected, there was a substantial drop in circulating B cells, but they were back to the normal range by 3.6 months. There was no change in T-cell number.

Kaminski was also able to report on the late effects of ^{131}I tositumomab use. An elevation of thyroid-stimulating hormone was noted in five patients 3 to 29 months after treatment.[46] Five patients were also diagnosed with myelodysplasia 1.2 to 7.5 years after ^{131}I treatment. These patients had been heavily treated with a median of four prior chemotherapies, including alkylating agents. Bone marrow cytogenetics were available on four cases, and all showed clonal abnormalities involving chromosome 5, chromosome 7, or both. Three patients were diagnosed with solid tumors after RIT (two transitional cell carcinoma of the bladder, one squamous cancer of rectum). Seventeen percent of patients experienced HAMA after therapeutic RIT doses, but no patient who received only one dosimetric dose of ^{131}I tositumomab was prevented from receiving a therapeutic treatment as a result of HAMA.

This cohort of patients represents the longest follow-up of patients treated with RIT. Both early and late toxicities were acceptable, and a significant proportion of patients with low-grade lymphomas appeared to benefit from this treatment. Many patients who responded to RIT experienced a longer remission than that achieved with the most recent chemotherapy.

A phase II study of 47 patients treated with the standard ^{131}I tositumomab treatment schema was conducted at seven sites throughout the United States and England.[47] Patients were required to have relapsed or refractory low-grade or transformed CD20+ NHL, including prior treatment with a regimen containing an anthracycline or anthracenedione. Patients who had experienced a relapse needed to demonstrate disease progression within 1 year of the last chemotherapy. After the therapeutic dose of ^{131}I tositumomab was administered, patients were kept in isolation until they emitted $\leq$5 mrem/h at one meter (usually 3–4 days). Seventy-seven percent of the patients were able to receive a full therapeutic dose of 75 cGy. The average tumor dose was 10 times the total body dose, and all normal tissues received doses well below the tolerances calculated for external-beam radiation therapy. The OR rate was 57%, and the CR rate was 32%. The median duration of response for all patients was 9.9 months; however, for those achieving a CR, the median duration for response was 19.9 months. Six patients were reported to have ongoing CRs lasting 26.9+ to 33.8+ months. Similar results were observed for both low-grade and transformed NHL. There were no infusion-related toxicities in 83% of infusions. In the remainder, there were mild, grade 1 or 2, toxicities that mainly occurred during the first exposure to tositumomab with the dosimetric dose. Fatigue, mild nausea, and fever were the most common nonhematologic toxicities. Hematologic toxicity was similar to that in other studies, with 26% of patients receiving platelet transfusions and 21% receiving red blood cell transfusions. There was no HAMA formation in the 45 patients who received a single dosimetric dose of ^{131}I tositumomab.

A nonrandomized phase III trial was subsequently designed as the pivotal trial for ^{131}I tositumomab in patients with refractory low-grade or transformed NHL.[48] The study targeted an especially poor prognostic group of patients with chemotherapy-refractory disease, defined as no response or initial response followed by relapse and disease progression less than 6 months after the last qualifying chemotherapy (LQC). All patients were required to have received at least two qualifying chemotherapy regimens, and only certain prospectively determined regimens were used to determine the chemotherapy refractory status. The goal of the study was to compare the efficacy ^{131}I tositumomab treatment with that of a patient's LQC by comparing response and duration of response in each group. Patients therefore served as at their own control. An independent review panel of physicians was used to assess response.

Sixty patients were enrolled and 58 treated with a therapeutic dose of 75 cGy TBD (65 cGy in patients with a platelet count of < 150,000 cells/mm^3) administered according to the previously described ^{131}I tositumomab treatment program. Nearly all patients had stage III/IV disease, and 38% had biopsy-confirmed, transformed, low-grade NHL. Patients had received an average of four prior chemotherapies, including a doxorubicin-containing regimen in 78% of cases. The median time from LQC to the administration of ^{131}I tositumomab was 4.4 months. In an intent-to-treat analysis, the RR for the LQC was 28% (17/60), compared with the RR of 65% (39/60) for ^{131}I tositumomab ($P < 0.001$). The median duration of response for the ^{131}I tositumomab–treated group was 6.5 months, compared with 3.4 months for the LQC. A CR was achieved in three patients receiving the LQC versus 12 patients receiving the ^{131}I tositumomab therapy. For those who achieved a CR, the median response duration was 6.1 months for the LQC and had not been reached for ^{131}I tositumomab, with over 47 months of follow-up. An independent review panel verified that of the 43 patients with nonequivalent durations of response (> 30 days difference), 32 (74%) had a longer duration of response after ^{131}I tositumomab ($P < 0.001$). Hematologic toxicity was the most significant and was similar to the previously reported studies. The most common nonhematologic toxicities were usually transient and included mild-to-moderate asthenia, fever, and nausea. With long-term follow-up, four patients were diagnosed with myelodysplasia at a median of 35.5 months (range, 20.6–40.9 months) after ^{131}I tositumomab treatment. Based on the data of this and prior studies, ^{131}I tositumomab is currently before the Food and Drug Administration for consideration in the treatment of NHL.

The safety and efficacy of myeloablative ^{131}I tositumomab therapy with autologous bone marrow support has also been investigated. Press et al[49] were the first to report on the use of myeloablative RIT in NHL in their phase I dose-escalation trial of ^{131}I-labeled anti-CD20 (B1 and IF-5) and anti-CD37 (MB-1) antibodies. They enrolled 43 patients with advanced-stage, heavily pretreated, relapsed low- and intermediate-grade B cell NHL. Biodistribution studies demonstrated favorable antibody distribution in 24 patients, and 19 were subsequently treated with a single therapeutic dose of ^{131}I-labeled antibody followed by autologous marrow reinfusion. Twelve of these patients received ^{131}I B1 (now referred to as ^{131}I tositumomab) therapy. RIT doses were individualized (range, 234–777 mCi) on the basis of antibody biodistribution and a targeted ^{131}I dose to the normal organ receiving the most radiation. Escalating doses were given, and the ^{131}I tositumomab dose of 27 Gy was established to be the MTD for normal organs. Cardiopulmonary complications were the dose-limiting nonhematologic toxicity. The OR rate in this trial was 95%, and 85% of patients achieved a CR. The median duration of response for patients treated with ^{131}I tositumomab was greater than 11 months.

Based on these promising results, these investigators conducted a phase II trial with ^{131}I tositumomab given at maximally tolerated myeloablative doses followed by marrow/stem cell rescue.[50] The trial involved 25 patients (including four from the phase I study) with advanced stage, relapsed, B-cell NHL, most of who had low-grade follicular lymphoma. Twenty-two patients demonstrated favorable antibody biodistribution, and 21 received therapeutic ^{131}I tositumomab infusions calculated to deliver 25–31 cGy of radiation to critical organs. The lung was the dose-limiting organ in 20 of 21 cases. Analysis of long-term follow-up for the 29 patients treated with myeloablative ^{131}I tositumomab doses on these phase I and II trials revealed major responses in 25 (86%) patients, with 79% achieving a CR.[51] At a median follow-up of 42 months, 68% of patients remained alive, and the progression-free survival rate was 42%. Thirteen of 29 patients were in continued CR for more than 3 years. Serious early toxicities included severe myelosuppression, two cases of grade III cardiopulmonary toxicity, and three episodes of severe infection, one of which was fatal. Thyroid dysfunction was the most common long-term toxicity, with 62% of patients developing hypothyroidism. There were no cases of myelodysplasia, and the cumulative incidence of HAMA development was 35%.

In an attempt to further increase the efficacy of RIT in NHL, the combination of radioimmunotherapy and high-dose chemotherapy with autologous stem cell rescue has been evaluated. In a phase I/II study combining high-dose etoposide and cyclophosphamide chemotherapy with ^{131}I tositumomab, the feasibility and MTD of ^{131}I tositumomab therapy in this setting were determined.[52] Efficacy endpoints were also evaluated, and they demonstrated an overall survival of 83% and a progression-free survival of 68% at 2 years. Combination RIT and high-dose chemotherapy with autologous stem cell transplantation has also been evaluated in patients with relapsed or refractory mantle cell NHL.[53] In a small trial involving 16 patients treated with a regimen similar to that of the previous study, an OR rate of 100% and a CR rate of 91% were observed in 11 patients with measurable disease. Overall survival at 3 years from transplantation was estimated to be 93%, and the progression-free survival was 61%.

^{131}I AND ^{67}CU RADIOLABELED LYM-1

Lym-1 is a third radiolabeled antibody under investigation for the treatment of NHL. It targets a discontinuous epitope on the human leukocyte antigen (HLA)-DR 10-β subunit located on the surface membrane of most malignant B cells.[54,55] This antigen has several unique properties that make it an attractive target for RIT.[55,56] It is highly expressed on most B cell lymphomas but is expressed to a lesser extent on normal B cells. It is not shed, modulated, or internalized on antibody binding, nor is it found free in the serum.

The Lym-1 antibody is a murine IgG2a MAb produced by fusion with splenic lymphocytes of mice that have been hyperimmunized with nuclei from Raji Burkitt's lymphoma. It selectively binds to B-cell lymphomas and leukemias and demonstrates a greater avidity for malignant B cells than normal B lymphocytes. Early studies demonstrated that 80% of B-cell NHL and 40% of chronic lymphocytic leukemia (CLL) cases reacted with Lym-1, whereas only 8% of normal circulating B lymphocytes reacted with this antibody.[55,56] Further, Lym-1 does not react with other hematopoietic cells or normal tissues.[55]

The antitumor effect of the Lym-1–radiolabeled antibody comes from the activity of the attached radioisotope. Although the unlabeled Lym-1 antibody can trigger antibody-dependent cellular cytotoxicity and complement-dependent cytotoxicity in vitro, it has little therapeutic effect in vivo.[57] When Lym-1 is conjugated to a radionuclide, such as ^{131}I and ^{67}Cu, however, it has shown impressive activity.

DeNardo and associates[37] have performed most of the work with this radiolabeled antibody, initially looking at ^{131}I Lym-1 and more recently exploring the possible advantages of ^{67}Cu Lym-1. They have also explored the role of dose fractionation in RIT as a way to increase the tumor dose and reduce the toxicity to normal tissue. Support for this approach comes, in part, from work with a colon cancer xenograft mouse model that demonstrated that dividing a lethal dose of radiation into two doses could achieve tumor growth arrest in 90% of tumors and reduce mortality to only 10%. Dividing the dose into three fractions allowed an additional 50% increase in the tolerated dose.[58]

^{131}I LYM-1

DeNardo et al[59] published the first account of ^{131}I Lym-1 therapy when they treated a patient with Richter's transformation of CLL. Since then, this group has treated more than 50 patients with ^{131}I Lym-1, attempting to define the optimal dose, schedule, and toxicity for this radioimmunoconjugate. In these studies, all patients were required to have tumors with Lym-1 reactivity and no HAMAs.

In an early pilot study involving five patients with refractory CLL, ^{131}I Lym-1 was administered every 2 to 6 weeks in doses ranging from 20–65 mCi.[60] All patients were heavily pretreated and had experienced disease progression after intensive multiple drug chemotherapies. They had advanced-stage disease (Rai stage III or IV) with diffuse marrow involvement, and most had some degree of thrombocytopenia. The authors observed a dramatic regression in the lymphadenopathy of all patients; four patients achieved a PR and one patient attained a CR. Two patients were also noted to have normalization of their leukocyte count. Although the partial responses were short lived, the patient achieving a CR was alive 24 months after treatment although this patient had restarted on chemotherapy.

In a "low-dose" trial involving 30 patients (25 with NHL and five with CLL), subjects were treated with fractionated low doses of ^{131}I Lym-1 (30 or 60 mCi at 2- to 6-week intervals) toward a cumulative dose of 300 mCi.[61] Early data for some of these patients was included in the previous report. All cases were refractory to standard chemotherapy, and most had stage IV disease along with other poor prognostic factors. The majority of NHL cases were intermediate or high grade, and many patients had diffuse lymphomatous bone marrow involvement. Eleven of the 30 patients completed the intended 300-mCi dose, and the mean follow-up time was 10.4 years. Twenty-five of 30 patients (83%) showed tumor regression, with 47% meeting criteria for a PR and 10% achieving a CR. Fifty-seven percent (17/25) had durable responses, including the three patients with a CR. Further analysis of those who had received higher dose of ^{131}I Lym-1 (> 180 mCi) showed a 94% (17/18) RR. Responses occurred both in patients with NHL and in those with CLL.

A follow-up trial was then designed to define the MTD of the first two doses (of a maximum of four doses) of ^{131}I Lym-1 therapy.[62] Twenty patients with refractory NHL were enrolled (21 times), and all but one had stage IV disease. Later in the trial, patients with extensive NHL bone marrow involvement were excluded. Nearly two thirds of patients had diffuse large-cell NHL. Patients were heavily pretreated, and most had bulky tumors (≥ 7 cm). Fourteen of 21 (67%) patients received two doses of ^{131}I Lym-1 therapy, and six received all four doses. Complications of NHL were the reason most patients did not receive a second dose. The OR rate was 52%. Seven patients achieved a CR lasting a mean of 14 months. Of the 14 patients who received at least two doses of ^{131}I Lym-1, 71% responded. All three of the subjects who received the highest dose (100 mCi) of

^{131}I Lym-1 achieved a CR, with responses lasting from 8.8 months to 24 months. Responses were seen in all histologic grades, including four of the eight transformed NHLs and 46% of the diffuse large-cell lymphomas. The median survival for responders was 19.5 months.

There were no treatment-related deaths or episodes of significant bleeding in any of the trials. The side effects related to the Lym-1 antibody were mild and typical for immunotherapy treatment. Hematologic toxicity was the most significant, with 88% of patients experiencing grade 3 or 4 toxicity when they were treated in the MTD trial.[62] Thrombocytopenia was the most severe and dose limiting toxicity. The development of HAMA occurred in seven (30%) of those in the MTD trial.

^{67}CU 2IT-BAT-LYM-1

More recently, the radiometal ^{67}Cu has been conjugated to Lym-1 because of its promising physical and chemical properties.[31] ^{67}Cu emits therapeutically useful beta particles as well as gamma photons for imaging. It achieves a greater mean tumor concentration than ^{131}I and has a more favorable therapeutic index.[32] The drawback of using ^{67}Cu relates to its greater expense, its potential to accumulate in the liver, and the fact that it is less readily available.[33,34] To provide a stable complex for clinical use, ^{67}Cu is joined to the Lym-1 antibody by the macrocyclic chelator TETA.[34,35] This yields the radiopharmaceutical ^{67}Cu 2IT-BAT-Lym-1.

Three small clinical trials have been published looking at ^{67}Cu 2IT-BAT-Lym-1 therapy in NHL. An early study evaluated the pharmacokinetics and dosimetry of this agent given at imaging doses.[63] Radiation doses were found to be higher in tumors compared with normal organs. The next study attempted to define the MTD of the first two doses (of a maximum of four) of ^{67}Cu 2IT-BAT-Lym-1 given 4 weeks apart.[34] The starting dose of 60 mCi/m2 was based on the MTD and the comparative dosimetry for ^{131}I Lym-1. This starting dose proved to be the MTD; three of three patients experienced grade 3 or 4 hematologic toxicity and required platelet transfusions. Tumor regression was seen in all patients, and the maximum effect was observed at 1 week. The radiation dose to the liver was higher than that to other normal tissues, but there was no evidence of hepatotoxicity. Encouraged by these prior studies, a phase I/II trial was conducted in 12 patients with relapsed or refractory NHL.[31,33] Eleven patients had intermediate- or high-grade disease (IWF classification), and all patients had stage III/IV disease, including half with bone marrow involvement (making up $< 25\%$ of the marrow). The first three patients (phase I) received a ^{67}Cu 2IT-BAT-Lym-1 dose of 60 mCi/m^2, and the next nine (phase II) received either 50 or 25 mCi/m^2, with the lower dose being given to patients with bone marrow involvement. Patients could receive a maximum of four doses, but only one patient received all four doses. The OR rate was 58%, and there was one CR (median response duration, 12 months) and six PRs (median response duration, 3 months). Hematologic toxicity was significant. Eighty-eight percent (7/8) of patients receiving a dose of 50 mCi/m^2 or more had grade III/IV thrombocytopenia, and 62% experienced grade III/IV neutropenia. Five of 12 patients (42%) experienced HAMA.

^{131}I AND ^{90}Y EPRATUZUMAB

LL2 is a fourth antibody used for RIT in lymphoma. It is directed against the B-cell antigen CD22, which is expressed on the surface of mature B cells and most NHL cells. This antigen is not present on stem cells and is lost during terminal differentiation before plasma cell development. On antibody binding, the CD22 antigen is rapidly internalized, only to be resynthesized and re-expressed on the cell surface for further binding. The process occurs quickly, with 50% of the internalized CD22 being re-expressed within 5 hours.[64] The LL2 antibody is highly selective. It reacts with mature B cells and virtually all NHLs, but it shows no affinity for megakaryocyte, myeloid, or erythroid cells.[65,66] It was first developed as a murine antibody (mLL2) but was later humanized (hLL2 or epratuzumab).[36]

Studies were initially conducted with ^{131}I-labeled mLL2 and F(ab')2 to assess the biodistribution, dosimetry, and efficacy of repeated low doses (< 30 mCi) of this radioimmunoconjugate. In the first study, 16 patients with NHL were initially infused with small "diagnostic" doses of ^{131}I mLL2 or F(ab') for pharmacokinetic and dosimetry evaluations.[67] Seven patients also received therapeutic doses of this agent, and five were assessable for response. Two patients demonstrated a PR, and two had a mixed response. In addition, one patient who received only the diagnostic dose of ^{131}I mLL2 attained a CR. With these promising results, a phase I/II trial was conducted involving 21 patients with B-cell NHL (including seven from the prior study) who had not responded to conventional chemotherapy.[36] Patients were given two low doses (< 30 mCi) of ^{131}I-labeled mLL2 or F(ab′)$_2$ per cycle, along with varying doses (2–20 mg) of unlabeled antibody administered simultaneously. Seventeen of 21 patients were assessable for response, 12 of whom had received at east one cycle of mLL2 therapy (~50 mCi). There were five responses (RR of 30%), including one CR lasting 5 months. Myelotoxicity was dose limiting, and HAMA responses occurred in four of 10 patients who received two radiolabeled mLL2 injections.

To evaluate the efficacy and toxicity of a multiple-dose regimen, Vose and colleagues[68] conducted a phase I/II trial involving four dose levels. Twenty-one patients received 2, 4, 6, or 8 doses of ^{131}I mLL2. Patients with indolent (11) and aggressive (10) NHLs were included, and 55% had bulky disease (>5 cm). Thirty-eight percent had received prior high-dose chemotherapy and hematopoietic stem cell support. Retreatment was permitted if patients continued to meet eligibility criteria, and eight patients did receive a second course. Fifteen patients were assessable for response, and seven responses occurred, including five CRs and two PRs. The OR rate was 33%, and responses were observed in both indolent and aggressive histologies. The median follow-up was 25 months, and the longest response was seen in a patient with large-cell NHL who attained a CR and remained failure-free at 43+ months. Three patients did become hypothyroid, and HAMA antibodies developed in four patients. As expected, hematologic toxicity was the most severe, with five patients requiring hematopoietic stem cell support (two after the first course of treatment). There were two cases of febrile neutropenia.

Juweid and colleagues[69] studied the pharmacokinetics, dosimetry, and immunogenicity of the radiolabeled humanized LL2 (epratuzumab) and compared the dosimetric attributes of ^{131}I and ^{90}Y. Twenty-two patients were involved in this pilot study: 14 received ^{131}I epratuzumab and eight received ^{90}Y epratuzumab. Patients had indolent, intermediate-grade, and aggressive B cell lymphomas, and all but one had stage III or IV disease. All patients had experienced disease progression after multiple-agent chemotherapy, and 12 had received high-dose chemotherapy with hematopoietic stem cell support. Patients received infusions of either ^{131}I- or ^{90}Y-labeled epratuzumab. The therapeutic radioactive antibody dose was based on an intended bone marrow dose of 50–100 cGy with the lower dose being given to patients who had undergone prior stem cell transplantation. Investigators found more favorable dosimetry with the ^{90}Y-labeled epratuzumab than with the ^{131}I epratuzumab. The estimated average tumor radiation dose for ^{90}Y epratuzumab was 21.5 cGy, which was 3.7-, 2.5-, 1.8-, and 2.5-fold that of the bone marrow, lungs, liver and kidney, respectively. Objective tumor responses occurred in two of 13 patients treated with ^{131}I epratuzumab and in two of seven patients treated with ^{90}Y epratuzumab.

CONCLUSION

The Food and Drug Administration approval of ^{90}Y ibritumomab tiuxetan for the treatment of relapsed and refractory NHL brings a distinctly new weapon to the oncologists' armamentarium. It is not a coincidence that NHL is the first malignancy to show success with this treatment. Lymphoma has a steep radiation dose response curve, and it has demonstrated response to antibody therapy in general. In addition, patients with lymphoma often have a sufficiently impaired immune system to make the rapid development of neutralizing antibodies less of a problem. There are several notable advantages of this new agent. ^{90}Y ibritumomab tiuxetan has shown significant activity in patients who are heavily pretreated, have bulky disease, and have diseases that are refractory to unlabeled antibody therapy (rituximab). Oncologists must always keep in mind, however, that these agents deliver ionizing radiation throughout the body.

Hematologic side effects are significant, yet because of limited extramedullary toxicity, the rate of infection is low. To avoid severe hematologic toxicity, patients in these clinical trials were carefully screened and required to demonstrate adequate hematopoiesis and minimal lymphomatous bone marrow involvement on bilateral core biopsies before enrollment. These trials revealed that the hematologic toxicity associated with ^{90}Y Ibritumomab tiuxetan is mainly related to the degree of lymphomatous bone marrow involvement and the baseline platelet count. Other predictors of prolonged myelotoxicity include prior history of failed stem cell collection, multiple cycles of fludarabine chemotherapy, and hypocellular marrow. Sophisticated dosimetry based on indium imaging and pharmacokinetic measurements of yttrium blood levels did not predict toxicity.

Oncologists must also be mindful of the unique time course associated with these toxicities. The myelosuppression occurring with RIT develops later and lasts longer than that experienced with chemotherapy. The onset of hematologic nadirs develops 4 weeks after ^{90}Y ibritumomab tiuxetan therapy and persists for 1 to 2 weeks. The use of neutrophil growth factor does not appear to be routinely necessary, but about 20%–25% of patients do require red cell transfusions during the course of therapy. The use of erythropoietin in this population of heavily pretreated patients may be beneficial. Finally, the radiation safety requirements for ^{90}Y ibritumomab tiuxetan are minimal. Only minute quantities of ^{90}Y are excreted in the urine, and studies evaluating radiation exposure to family members in intimate contact with the treated patient have failed to demonstrate significant radiation exposure.

^{90}Y ibritumomab tiuxetan is the first of what will likely be several agents in this entirely new class of therapeutics now available to the oncologist. Currently, the most important issue is appropriate patient selection. The sequence in which this therapy is integrated into a patient's overall treatment plan must also be addressed. Finally, as more agents become available, the oncologist will need to be able to judge the merits of each agent, including the type of pretreatment unlabeled antibody used, the risk of immunization, and the unique characteristics of each target and isotope. The next few years promise to bring answers to these questions through ongoing clinical research.

REFERENCES

1. Goldenberg DM. The role of radiolabeled antibodies in the treatment of non-Hodgkin's lymphoma: the coming of age of radioimmunotherapy. Crit Rev Oncol Hematol 2001;39:195–201.
2. Goldenberg D. Cancer Therapy with Radiolabelled Antibodies. Boca Raton: CRC Press, 1995.
3. Goldenberg DM. Targeted therapy of cancer with radiolabeled antibodies. J Nucl Med 2002;43:693–713.
4. Meredith RF, LoBuglio AF, Spencer EB. Recent progress in radioimmunotherapy for cancer. Oncology (Huntingt) 1997;11:979–984, 987; discussion 987–988.
5. Greenlee R, Murray T, Bolden S et al. Cancer statistics. CA Cancer J Clin 2000; 50:7–33.
6. Harris N, Jaffe E, Armitage J et al. Lymphoma classification: from R.E.A.L. to W.H.O. and beyond. Princ Prac Oncol 1999;13:1–14.
7. Whelan J, Davis C, Rule S et al. Fludarabine phosphate for the treatment of low grade lymphoid malignancy. Br J Cancer 1991;64:120–123.

8. Hochster HS, Kim KM, Green MD et al. Activity of fludarabine in previously treated non-Hodgkin's low-grade lymphoma: results of an Eastern Cooperative Oncology Group study. J Clin Oncol 1992;10:28–32.

9. Redman JR, Cabanillas F, Velasquez WS et al. Phase II trial of fludarabine phosphate in lymphoma: an effective new agent in low-grade lymphoma. J Clin Oncol 1992;10:790–794.

10. Longo D, DeVita VT Jr, Jaffe E, et al. Lymphocytic Lymphomas. In: DeVita VT Jr, Hellman S, Rosenberg SA, eds. Cancer: Principles & Practice of Oncology. Philadelphia: Lippincott, 1993:1859–1927.

11. Freedman A, Ritz J, Neuberg D et al. Autologous bone marrow transplantation in 69 patients with a history of low-grade B-cell non-Hodgkin's lymphoma. Blood 1991;77:2524–2529.

12. Fouillard L, Gorin N et al. Feasibility of autologous bone marrow transplantation for early consolidation of follicular non-Hodgkin's lymphoma. Eur J Haematol 1991;46:279–284.

13. Bastion Y, Brice P, Haioun C et al. Intensive therapy with peripheral blood progenitor cell transplantation in 60 patients with poor-prognosis follicular lymphoma. Blood 1995;86:3257–3262.

14. Zinzani PL, Magagnoli M, Moretti L et al. Fludarabine-based chemotherapy in untreated mantle cell lymphomas: an encouraging experience in 29 patients. Haematologica 1999;84:1002–1006.

15. Flinn IW, Byrd JC, Morrison C et al. Fludarabine and cyclophosphamide with filgrastim support in patients with previously untreated indolent lymphoid malignancies. Blood 2000;96:71–75.

16. McLaughlin P, Grillo-Lopez AJ, Link BK et al. Rituximab chimeric anti-CD20 monoclonal antibody therapy for relapsed indolent lymphoma: half of patients respond to a four-dose treatment program. J Clin Oncol 1998;16:2825–2833.

17. Philip T, Guglielmi C, Hagenbeek A et al. Autologous bone marrow transplantation as compared with salvage chemotherapy in relapses of chemotherapy-sensitive non-Hodgkin's lymphoma. N Engl J Med 1995;333:1540–1545.

18. Press O, Early J, Badger C et al. Treatment of refractory non-Hodgkin's lymphoma with radiolabeled MB-1 (anti-CD37) antibody. J Clin Oncol 1989;7:1027–1038.

19. Rubin P. Law and order of radiation sensitivity: absolute versus relative. Front Radiat Ther Oncol 1989;23:7–40.

20. Parker B, Vassos A, Halpern S et al. Radioimmunotherapy of human B-cell lymphoma with Y-conjugated anti-idiotype monoclonal antibody. Cancer Res 1990;50:1022s–1028s.

21. Fuks Z, Kaplan H. Recurrence rate following radiation therapy of nodular and diffuse malignant lymphomas. Radiology 1973;108:675–684.

22. DeNardo G, O'Donnell R, DeNardo S. Radiolabeled anti-lymphoma antibodies. In: G. Giaccone RS, P. Sondel, ed. Cancer Chemotherapy and Biological Response Modifiers, vol 19. New York: Elsevier Science, 2001:297–307.

23. Anderson KC, Bates MP, Slaughenhoupt BL et al. Expression of human B cell-associated antigens on leukemias and lymphomas: a model of human B cell differentiation. Blood 1984;63:1424–1433.

24. Press OW, Appelbaum F, Ledbetter JA et al. Monoclonal antibody 1F5 (anti-CD20) serotherapy of human B cell lymphomas. Blood 1987;69:584–591.

25. Meeker TC, Lowder J, Maloney DG et al. A clinical trial of anti-idiotype therapy for B cell malignancy. Blood 1985;65:1349–1363.

26. Khazaeli MB, Saleh MN, Wheeler RH et al. Phase I trial of multiple large doses of murine monoclonal antibody CO17-1A. II. Pharmacokinetics and immune response. J Natl Cancer Inst 1988;80:937–942.

27. Kaminski M, Zasadny K, Francis I et al. Radioimmunotherapy of B-cell lymphoma with ^{131}I: antiB1 (anti-CD20) antibody. N Engl J Med 1993;329:459–465.

28. Gates VL, Carey JE, Siegel JA et al. Nonmyeloablative iodine-131 anti-B1 radioimmunotherapy as outpatient therapy. J Nucl Med 1998;39:1230–1236.

29. Casey JL, King DJ, Chaplin LC et al. Preparation, characterisation and tumour targeting of cross-linked divalent and trivalent anti-tumour Fab' fragments. Br J Cancer 1996;74:1397–1405.

30. Smith A, Alberto R, Blaeuenstein P et al. Preclinical evaluation of 67Cu-labeled intact and fragmented anti-colon carcinoma monoclonal antibody MAb35. Cancer Res 1993;53:5727–5733.

31. O'Donnell RT, DeNardo GL, Kukis DL et al. 67Copper-2-iminothiolane-6-[p-(bromoacetamido)benzyl-TETA-Lym-1 for radioimmunotherapy of non-Hodgkin's lymphoma. Clin Cancer Res 1999;5:3330s–3336s.

32. DeNardo GL, Kukis DL, Shen S et al. 67Cu-versus 131I-labeled Lym-1 antibody: comparative pharmacokinetics and dosimetry in patients with non-Hodgkin's lymphoma. Clin Cancer Res 1999;5:533–541.

33. O'Donnell RT, DeNardo GL, Kukis DL et al. A clinical trial of radioimmunotherapy with 67Cu-2IT-BAT-Lym-1 for non-Hodgkin's lymphoma. J Nucl Med 1999;40:2014–2020.

34. Denardo GL, Denardo SJ, Kukis DL et al. Maximum tolerated dose of 67Cu-2IT-BAT-LYM-1 for fractionated radioimmunotherapy of non-Hodgkin's lymphoma: a pilot study. Anticancer Res 1998;18:2779–2788.

35. Kukis DL, DeNardo GL, DeNardo SJ et al. Effect of the extent of chelate substitution on the immunoreactivity and biodistribution of 2IT-BAT-Lym-1 immunoconjugates. Cancer Res 1995;55:878–884.

36. Juweid M, Sharkey RM, Markowitz A et al. Treatment of non-Hodgkin's lymphoma with radiolabeled murine, chimeric, or humanized LL2, an anti-CD22 monoclonal antibody. Cancer Res 1995;55:5899s–5907s.

37. DeNardo GL, DeNardo SJ, O'Grady LF et al. Fractionated radioimmunotherapy of B-cell malignancies with 131I-Lym-1. Cancer Res 1990;50:1014s–1016s.

38. Knox S, Goris M, Trisler K et al. Yttrium-90-labeled anti-CD20 monoclonal antibody therapy of recurrent B-cell lymphoma. Clin Cancer Res 1996;2:457–470.

39. Witzig T, White C, Wiseman G et al. Phase I/II trial of IDEC-Y2B8 radioimmunotherapy for treatment of relapsed or refractory CD20+ B-cell non-Hodgkin's lymphoma. J Clin Oncol 1999;17:3793–3803.

40. Witzig TE, Gordon LI, Cabanillas F et al. Randomized controlled trial of yttrium-90-labeled ibritumomab tiuxetan radioimmunotherapy versus rituximab immunotherapy for patients with relapsed or refractory low-grade, follicular, or transformed B-cell non-Hodgkin's lymphoma. J Clin Oncol 2002;20:2453–2463.

41. Wiseman GA, White CA, Sparks RB et al. Biodistribution and dosimetry results from a phase III prospectively randomized controlled trial of Zevalin radioimmunotherapy for low-grade, follicular, or transformed B-cell non-Hodgkin's lymphoma. Crit Rev Oncol Hematol 2001;39:181–194.

42. Wiseman GA, Gordon LI, Multani PS et al. Ibritumomab tiuxetan radioimmunotherapy for patients with relapsed or refractory non-Hodgkin lymphoma and mild thrombocytopenia: a phase II multicenter trial. Blood 2002;99:4336–4342.

43. Witzig TE, Flinn IW, Gordon LI et al. Treatment With ibritumomab tiuxetan radioimmunotherapy in patients with rituximab-refractory follicular non-Hodgkin's lymphoma. J Clin Oncol 2002;20:3262–3269.

44. Witzig T, White C, Flinn I et al. Zevalin radioimmunotherapy of rituximab-refractory follicular non-Hodgkin's lymphoma. Blood 2000;16:2183a.

45. Kaminski MS, Zasadny KR, Francis IR et al. Iodine-131-anti-B1 radioimmunotherapy for B-cell lymphoma. J Clin Oncol 1996;14:1974–1981.

46. Kaminski MS, Estes J, Zasadny KR et al. Radioimmunotherapy with iodine (131)I tositumomab for relapsed or refractory B-cell non-Hodgkin lymphoma: updated results and long-term follow-up of the University of Michigan experience. Blood 2000;96:1259–1266.

47. Vose JM, Wahl RL, Saleh M et al. Multicenter phase II study of iodine-131 tositumomab for chemotherapy-relapsed/refractory low-grade and transformed low-grade B-cell non-Hodgkin's lymphomas. J Clin Oncol 2000;18:1316–1323.

48. Kaminski MS, Zelenetz AD, Press OW et al. Pivotal study of iodine I 131 tositumomab for chemotherapy-refractory low-grade or transformed low-grade B-cell non-Hodgkin's lymphomas. J Clin Oncol 2001;19:3918–3928.

49. Press OW, Eary JF, Appelbaum FR et al. Radiolabeled-antibody therapy of B-cell lymphoma with autologous bone marrow support [see comments]. N Engl J Med 1993;329:1219–1224.

50. Press OW, Eary JF, Appelbaum FR et al. Phase II trial of 131I-B1 (anti-CD20) antibody therapy with autologous stem cell transplantation for relapsed B cell lymphomas. Lancet 1995;346:336–340.

51. Liu SY, Eary JF, Petersdorf SH et al. Follow-up of relapsed B-cell lymphoma patients treated with iodine-131-labeled anti-CD20 antibody and autologous stem-cell rescue. J Clin Oncol 1998;16:3270–3278.

52. Press OW, Eary JF, Gooley T et al. A phase I/II trial of iodine-131-tositumomab (anti-CD20), etoposide, cyclophosphamide, and autologous stem cell transplantation for relapsed B-cell lymphomas. Blood 2000;96:2934–2942.

53. Gopal AK, Rajendran JG, Petersdorf SH et al. High-dose chemo-radioimmunotherapy with autologous stem cell support for relapsed mantle cell lymphoma. Blood 2002;99:3158–3162.

54. Rose LM, Gunasekera AH, DeNardo SJ et al. Lymphoma-selective antibody Lym-1 recognizes a discontinuous epitope on the light chain of HLA-DR10. Cancer Immunol Immunother 1996;43:26–30.

55. Epstein AL, Marder RJ, Winter JN et al. Two new monoclonal antibodies, Lym-1 and Lym-2, reactive with human B-lymphocytes and derived tumors, with immunodiagnostic and immunotherapeutic potential. Cancer Res 1987;47:830–840.

56. DeNardo GL, O'Donnell RT, Rose LM et al. Milestones in the development of Lym-1 therapy. Hybridoma 1999;18:1–11.

57. Hu E, Epstein AL, Naeve GS et al. A phase 1a clinical trial of LYM-1 monoclonal antibody serotherapy in patients with refractory B cell malignancies. Hematol Oncol 1989;7:155–166.

58. Schlom J, Molinolo A, Simpson JF et al. Advantage of dose fractionation in monoclonal antibody-targeted radioimmunotherapy. J Natl Cancer Inst 1990;82:763–771.

59. DeNardo SJ, DeNardo GL, O'Grady LF et al. Treatment of a patient with B cell lymphoma by I-131 LYM-1 monoclonal antibodies. Int J Biol Markers 1987;2:49–53.

60. DeNardo GL, Lewis JP, DeNardo SJ, O'Grady LF. Effect of Lym-1 radioimmunoconjugate on refractory chronic lymphocytic leukemia. Cancer 1994;73:1425–1432.

61. DeNardo GL, DeNardo SJ, Lamborn KR et al. Low-dose, fractionated radioimmunotherapy for B-cell malignancies using 131I-Lym-1 antibody. Cancer Biother Radiopharm 1998;13:239–254.

62. DeNardo GL, DeNardo SJ, Goldstein DS et al. Maximum-tolerated dose, toxicity, and efficacy of (131)I-Lym-1 antibody for fractionated radioimmunotherapy of non-Hodgkin's lymphoma. J Clin Oncol 1998;16:3246–3256.

63. DeNardo SJ, DeNardo GL, Kukis DL et al. 67Cu-2IT-BAT-Lym-1 pharmacokinetics, radiation dosimetry, toxicity and tumor regression in patients with lymphoma. J Nucl Med 1999;40:302–310.

64. Shih LB, Lu HH, Xuan H et al. Internalization and intracellular processing of an anti-B-cell lymphoma monoclonal antibody, LL2. Int J Cancer 1994;56:538–545.

65. Pawlak-Byczkowska EJ, Hansen HJ, Dion AS et al. Two new monoclonal antibodies, EPB-1 and EPB-2, reactive with human lymphoma. Cancer Res 1989;49:4568–4577.

66. Stein R, Belisle E, Hansen HJ et al. Epitope specificity of the anti-(B cell lymphoma) monoclonal antibody, LL2. Cancer Immunol Immunother 1993;37:293–298.

67. Goldenberg DM, Horowitz JA, Sharkey RM et al. Targeting, dosimetry, and radioimmunotherapy of B-cell lymphomas with iodine-131-labeled LL2 monoclonal antibody. J Clin Oncol 1991;9:548–564.

68. Vose JM, Colcher D, Gobar L et al. Phase I/II trial of multiple dose 131iodine-MAb LL2 (CD22) in patients with recurrent non-Hodgkin's lymphoma. Leuk Lymphoma 2000;38:91–101.

69. Juweid ME, Stadtmauer E, Hajjar G et al. Pharmacokinetics, dosimetry, and initial therapeutic results with 131I- and (111)In-/90Y-labeled humanized LL2 anti-CD22 monoclonal antibody in patients with relapsed, refractory non-Hodgkin's lymphoma. Clin Cancer Res 1999;5:3292s–3303s.

Chapter 4

Molecular Markers in Acute Myeloid Leukemia

Michal Rose, MD

Nancy Berliner, MD

Molecular studies are becoming an integral part of the evaluation of acute myelogenous leukemia (AML). Using molecular techniques, genetic abnormalities are detectable in an ever-growing number of AML patients, thus adding critical information to routine clinical, morphologic, and cytogenetic data. These molecular studies are increasingly important in refining the diagnosis of AML and its subtypes, in determining prognosis, selecting therapy, and detecting minimal residual disease. The purpose of this review is to provide an update on the clinical applications of molecular studies in AML.

CLINICAL DECISIONS BASED ON CYTOGENETICS

The identification of recurring cytogenetic abnormalities in AML has contributed both to our understanding of the pathogenesis of AML and to the recognition of the heterogeneity in its prognosis and response to treatment. Cytogenetic information is the strongest predictor of the likelihood that a patient with AML will obtain a remission and be cured by current therapies.[1-4] Favorable-risk patients [t(8;21), inv(16) and t(15;17)] have a 5-year survival ranging from 56% to 65%, intermediate-risk patients [normal cytogenetics, –y, +8, +6 or del(12p)] have a 5-year survival ranging from 35% to 41%, and unfavorable-risk patients (abnormalities of 5, 7, 3q, or complex karyotypes with ≥ 3 abnormalities) have a 5-year survival of only 12-26%.[1,2,5]

Cytogenetic analysis now plays a critical role in the selection of therapy for AML. The most striking example is acute promyelocytic leukemia (APL) and its response to all-*trans* retinoic acid (ATRA). Randomized studies have demonstrated that overall survival is significantly prolonged when patients with the t(15;17) translocation are treated with ATRA in combination with chemotherapy during induction and consolidation.[6,7] Another compelling demonstration of the link between cytogenetics and therapy was provided by a Cancer and Leukemia Group B study that examined three dose schedules of cytarabine during consolidation. That study demonstrated that patients with cytogenetics that conferred a good prognosis [t(8;21) and inv(16)] had better survival rates when they were treated with high-dose cytarabine.[8] Patients with intermediate-risk cytogenetics did the same whether they received the high- or intermediate-dose cytarabine, and patients with poor-risk cytogenetics did poorly regardless of the dose of cytarabine used in consolidation.[8]

Despite the increasing awareness of the importance of cytogenetic data in prognosis and in therapeutic decision making, abnormalities are detected in only 40%–50% of patients with AML.[1] Although the accuracy of chromosome analysis has improved over the past 20 years, it is still suboptimal. In 2%–10% of patients, no cytogenetic information is obtained because of inadequate metaphases.[1] More significantly, the introduction of fluorescence in situ hybridization (FISH) and polymerase chain reaction (PCR) has demonstrated that molecular evidence of chromosomal translocations and deletions can be present despite normal cytogenetics as determined by conventional banding techniques. Recent studies have focused on the utility of these potentially more sensitive screening techniques for the detection of clinically important cytogenetic abnormalities.

Good-Prognosis Cytogenetic Abnormalities

Core Binding Factor Abnormalities: t(8;21) and inv(16) Core binding factor (CBF) is a transcription factor composed of two subunits, CBFα (also known as AML1), located on chromosome 21q22, and CBFβ, located on chromosome 16q22.[3,9,10] CBF regulates the expression of multiple genes that are important in normal hematopoiesis, including interleukin-3 (IL-3), granulocyte macrophage colony stimulating factor, macrophage colony stimulating factor, and genes involved in B- and T-cell maturation.[10] The t(8;21) translocation results in the fusion of the CBFα gene to ETO (*e*ight-*t*wenty-*o*ne). It is found in 5%–10% of de novo AML and is strongly associated with the FAB-M2 morphology.[3,9,10] The inv(16) abnormality, and less frequently the t(16;16) translocation, produces the CBFβ/smooth muscle myosin heavy chain (SMMHC, also known as MYH11) fusion protein and is found in 10%–20% of AML. These chromosome 16 abnormalities are most commonly found in the FAB-M4Eo subtype, but they may also be present in patients with M2 and M5 morphologies.[3,9,10]

Chimeric proteins produced by both the t(8;21) translocation and inv(16)/t(16;16) serve as dominant negative inhibitors of the normal CBF heterodimer.[10] The reliable identification of CBF AML patients is important both for determining prognosis and for choosing therapy because these patients have a better prognosis, especially when they receive intensive postremission therapy with high-dose cytarabine.[8]

Several studies have correlated the identification of the t(8;21) and inv(16) cytogenetic abnormalities with the detection by PCR of CBFα/ETO and CBFβ/MYH11 transcripts, respectively. On behalf of the Medical Research Council, Langabeer et al[11] reported on 396 patients with newly diagnosed AML who were screened for the presence of the t(8;21) translocation by conventional cytogenetics and for CBFα/ETO fusion transcripts by reverse transcriptase PCR (RT-PCR). Thirty-two cases of t(8;21) were detected by conventional cytogenetics, all of which were also PCR positive, but an additional 19 cases were detected by RT-PCR alone. Thus, in this study, 37% of patients with the CBFα/ETO transcript were not identified by conventional cytogenetics.[11] Similar results were reported by Andrieu et al[12] in a study of 64 patients with M1 or M2 AML: RT-PCR increased the detection rate of CBFα/ETO transcripts from 8% to 14%.

In three other studies, however, the difference between conventional cytogenetics and RT-PCR was not as pronounced. Rowe et al[13] found 31/412 (7.5%) patients with a cytogenetic t(8;21) and only two additional patients with the CBFα/ETO (determined by RT-PCR) in the absence of the t(8;21) translocation. Mitterbauer et al[14] screened 204 patients with AML, observing that 15 had a t(8;21) translocation and only two additional patients had a cryptic CBFα/ETO transcript. In the only prospective study specifically addressing this issue, Mrozek et al[15] studied 284 adult AML patients enrolled in the CALBG 9621 trial. Initial cytogenetic and RT-PCR analyses correctly classified 95.7% and 96.1% of patients, respectively. Cytogenetics were falsely negative in three CBFα/ETO patients who had unique variants of t(8;21). RT-PCR was presumed to be falsely positive for CBFα/ETO in two patients in whom multiple subsequent results were negative.[15]

Compared with the t(8;21) translocation, inv(16) is more difficult to detect by conventional cytogenetics, especially in suboptimal samples, and may be missed or misinterpreted as del(16).[16,17] Although the breakpoints within both the MYH11 and the CBFβ genes are more variable, RT-PCR detects most of the patients with CBFβ/MYH11 fusions.[16-18] Five studies have correlated cytogenetic analysis and RT-PCR for the detection of CBFβ/MYH11 fusion,[13,15,16,18,19] and here too, results are conflicting. In the 321 patients studied by Langabeer et al,[19] 21 had inv(16) determined by cytogenetics, all of which were positive by RT-PCR; however, CBFβ/MYH11 was detected by RT-PCR in 12 additional patients who did not have inv(16). In the study by Ritter et al,[16] among 121 patients with AML, five cases of CBFβ/MYH11 were detected by cytogenetics, and an additional two were detected by RT-PCR alone.

However, Rowe et al[13] and Mitterbauer et al[18] found a closer correlation between the two methods. In the former study, inv(16) was detected in 27/412 cases (6.6%) by cytogenetics, and no cryptic cases were detected by RT-PCR. In the second study, inv(16) was detected by cytogenetics in 18/241 (7.5%) patients, and an additional two cases were detected only by RT-PCR. A recent report by Mrozek et al[15] on behalf of the Cancer and Leukemia Group B demonstrated that both methods had their pitfalls. In this carefully conducted study of 284 patients, 27 were eventually determined to have the CBFb/MYH11 fusion; however, only 22 of these were initially detected by both methods. In one patient with positive RT-PCR, cytogenetics failed to yield metaphase cells. In two patients, reanalysis of their cytogenetic study after CBFβ/MYH11 had been detected by RT-PCR resulted in the detection of inv(16) in one case and t(16;16) in the other. One patient with typical inv(16) was negative by initial RT-PCR, but results of metaphase FISH and repeat RT-PCR of a sample in another vial were both positive for CBFb/MYH11. There was also one patient with the M4Eo subtype who had no evidence of either inv(16)/t(16;16) or the CBFβ/MYH11 product on RT-PCR, but both methods were found to be positive after reanalysis. In two patients, RT-PCR was believed to be falsely positive because the initial finding of a CBFβ/MYH11 transcript was not confirmed by subsequent analyses.[15]

The reasons for discordant results between different studies are not clearly evident. Most of the published data are retrospective and may be affected by RNA degradation in storage. The quality of cytogenetics varies by laboratory and by the freshness of the samples. At present, molecular analysis cannot replace cytogenetics, because it cannot cover the wide range of possible karyotypic abnormalities. Most investigators therefore conclude that molecular analysis and standard cytogenetics must be combined to maximize the likelihood of detecting these good prognosis abnormalities.

Acute Promyelocytic Leukemia Most AML cases with the morphologic and clinical features of APL have the t(15;17)(q12;q11) translocation, which results in the fusion of the promyelocytic leukemia (PML) gene on chromosome 15 with the retinoic acid receptor-α (RARα) gene on chromosome 17.[3,9] This balanced translocation results in the PML/RARα fusion protein in all patients and in the RARα/PML transcript in approximately 65% of patients. The PML/RARα fusion acts as a dominant negative inhibitor of the native proteins PML and RARα. This results in inhibition of apoptotic pathways, inhibition of retinoic acid–dependent transcription, and induction of a maturation arrest of neutrophil development at the promyelocyte stage. The role of the reciprocal, PML/RARα in the pathogenesis of APL is less clear, and current evidence suggests that RARα/PML is not required for the pathogenesis of APL but may contribute to the disease process.[20] Pharmacologic doses of ATRA can override the dominant inhibitory activity of PML/RARα and restore transcriptional activity of repressed genes.[10,20] ATRA induces maturation of blasts in patients with APL, and its use in combination with chemotherapy has led to a significant improvement in the cure of the disease.[6]

The breakpoint on chromosome 15 occurs at two major sites in the PML gene, intron 3 and intron 6, producing a short- and long-fusion messenger RNA product, respectively. Most studies have suggested that patients with the short isoform have an higher relapse rate and a shorter survival time.[21,22]

A series of alternative chromosomal translocations, involving the RARα gene fused to other partners, has been discovered (Table 4.1). These include t(11;17), involving the *PLZF* gene; t(5;17), involving the *NPM* gene; t(11;17), involving the *NuMA* gene; and der (17), involving the *STAT5b* gene.[20] APL blasts with fusion genes involving *NPM* and *NuMA* undergo differentiation when they are exposed to ATRA. However, the data are conflicting regarding the ATRA sensitivity of APL blasts harboring t(11;17), with most studies suggesting a lack of response.[10,23] However, a recent report by Petti et al[24] described a patient with PLZF/RARα APL who was treated at relapse with ATRA and low-dose hydroxyurea; the patient experienced a complete hematologic remission.

The optimal management of APL depends on a prompt diagnosis to enable the early introduction of ATRA therapy, along with induction chemotherapy. In most cases, the diagnosis of APL can be made by morphology because most APL blasts have distinct, heavy azurophilic granules, bundles of Auer rods, and bilobed nuclei. Diagnosis of the microgranular variant, which occurs in 15%–20% of cases, can be more challenging because the blasts have few if any granules.[25] Flow cytometry[26] and immunochemistry using antibodies against the PML protein[27,28] may aid in the rapid identification of these patients.

In approximately 10% of patients with a morphologic diagnosis of APL, t(15;17) is not detected, either because cytogenetic analysis is not successful or because of unusual rearrangements resulting in a fusion between RARα and a partner gene.[23,25] In a multicenter study by Grimwade et al,[23] of 611 patients with newly diagnosed APL by morphologic criteria, 9% lacked the t(15;17) translocation, despite a successful cytogenetic analysis. Diagnostic material from 60 pa-

TABLE 4.1 Translocations Involving RARα in APL

Chromosomal Abnormality	Partner Gene	Response to ATRA
t(15;17)(q22;q21)	*PML*	Yes
t(11;17)(q23;q21)	*PLZF*	No
t(5;17)(q35;q21)	*NPM*	Yes
t(11;17)(q13;q21)	*NuMa*	Yes
der(17)	*STAT5b*	No

Abbreviations: APL, acute promyelocytic leukemia; ATRA, all-*trans* retinoic acid.

tients with morphologic evidence of APL in the absence of t(15;17) were studied by FISH, RT-PCR, and/or Southern blotting techniques in a central workshop. In 42 of these patients, there was molecular evidence of PML/RARα fusion, due to either insertions (28/42) or more complex mechanisms, such as three-way translocations. In 11/60 patients, there was molecular evidence of PLZF/RARα rearrangements, and two patients had a t(5;17). In five of these 60 patients, no RARα rearrangements could be identified.

The yield of using molecular techniques to screen AML subtypes other than M3 for evidence of RARα rearrangements is low. In a study by Allford et al,[29] RT-PCR for PML/RARα and RARα/PML fusion transcripts was performed in diagnostic material from 530 patients who had AML subtypes other than M3, and only one case was detected.

In summary, the diagnosis of APL is usually evident by clinical and morphologic data, and it is confirmed in approximately 90% of patients by cytogenetic studies. However, RT-PCR or FISH analysis should be performed in all patients with newly diagnosed APL because these molecular studies can identify the specific RARα rearrangement and predict the likelihood of response to ATRA therapy. In patients with the PML/RARα translocation, the transcript size may yield prognostic information. Furthermore, the identification of the specific RARα rearrangement is essential to minimal residual disease monitoring, which is playing an increasing role in the treatment of these patients.

Summary: Role of RT-PCR for Good Prognosis Translocations in Newly Diagnosed AML Although RT-PCR is clearly more sensitive than cytogenetics in diagnosing well-defined gene rearrangements, currently available data regarding its ability to influence clinical decision making remain somewhat controversial. Most patients with good-prognosis rearrangements are probably detected by routine cytogenetics. However, given the significant impact of detecting the CBF- and PML/RAR-containing translocations on both prognosis and therapy, it seems likely that as these assays become more readily and routinely available, RT-PCR evaluation for these rearrangements will become a routine part of clinical practice.

Poor-Prognosis Cytogenetic Abnormalities

MLL (11q23 Abnormalities) Translocations involving the mixed-lineage leukemia (MLL, also known as ALL1, HTRX-1, and HRX) gene on chromosome 11q23 have been observed in both AML and acute lymphoid leukemia (ALL).[3,9,10] Rearrangements involving MLL are the most common cytogenetic abnormalities in acute leukemia in infants and young children.[3,9] In adult AML, translocations involving 11q23 are detected in 5%–10% of patients and are typically associated with acute myelomonocytic or acute monoblastic leukemia.[3,9] MLL leukemias often have biphenotypic antigen expression.[9] MLL abnormalities are found in 80% of secondary leukemia that arises after exposure to topoisomerase II inhibitors, such as epipodophyllotoxins and anthracyclines.[30] Typically, adult and pediatric patients with 11q23 rearrangements have a poor prognosis,[1] although t(9;11) in children may be associated with a more favorable prognosis.[31]

MLL is a highly conserved gene, which, through its regulation of the homeobox genes, is crucial for both embryonic development and normal hematopoiesis.[3,10] The MLL protein is thought to bind to the minor groove of DNA, alter chromatin structure, and facilitate binding of transcription factors at enhancer sites.[10] Translocations involving the MLL gene at 11q23 have been described with more than 40 different partners.[30] The most common of these in AML are 6q27 (AF6 gene), 9p22 (AF9 gene), 10p12 (AF10 gene), 17q21 (AF17 gene), and 19p13.1 (ELL or MEN gene).[9] All breakpoints of MLL are clustered in an 8.3-kb fragment between exons 8 and 14, an area rich in ALU repeats and harboring a topoisomerase II cleavage site.[30] The function of the many MLL fusion genes is poorly understood; however, the fusion proteins appear to cause leukemia by disrupting the ability of MLL to regulate homeobox gene expression.[10,30]

The multiple breakpoints in the MLL gene, and the large array of MLL fusion genes, have made the development of simple molecular assays for the screening for 11q23 rearrangements difficult. Poirel et al[32] screened 41 patients with M1 or M5 AML by Southern blotting with two MLL genomic probes, by RT-PCR, and by FISH. Twelve MLL-rearranged cases were found by Southern blotting, and of the 10 that had undergone cytogenetic analysis, only five were shown to have an 11q23 abnormality. Further characterization of 11 cases showed MLL self-fusions in four, MLL-AF6 in four, MLL-AF9 in two, and uncharacterized t(11;19) in one. Ibrahim et al[33] compared the occurrence of 11q23 abnormalities by karyotyping and MLL gene rearrangement assessed by Southern blotting in 311 adult patients with AML or myelodysplasia (MDS). Abnormal 11q23 by karyotype was found in 18 patients (5.8%), seven of whom did not have detectable MLL gene rearrangement by Southern blotting. Of the 35 patients with abnormal MLL by Southern blotting, only 11 had cytogenetic evidence of 11q23 abnormalities.[33] FISH[34] and "panhandle PCR"[35] may hold promise for clarifying the occurrence of 11q23 abnormalities, but these need to be tested in a larger number of patients.

Internal Tandem Duplications of the MLL Gene In addition to translocations involving a large array of genes, a significant number of adult AML patients harbor in-frame, internal tandem duplications (ITDs) of the MLL gene.[32,36,37] These partial tandem duplications are thought to be generated by homologous ALU recombination[38] and are found at low levels in the peripheral blood and bone marrow of nearly all healthy donors.[39] They are especially common in AML patients with trisomy 11, but they are also found in 5%–11% of patients with normal cytogenetics.[36] These ITDs are easier than 11q23 translocations to detect using RT-PCR, and several cohorts of AML patients have been studied for the frequency and clinical significance of their presence. Most researchers have found these ITDs to be associated with a higher relapse rate and/or decreased survival.[36,40,41] Dohner et al[40] performed Southern blot analysis for MLL ITDs in 525 adult patients with AML (age < 60 years). None of the patients with favorable karyotypes had MLL ITDs, but 7.7% of patients with normal karyotype and 8.5% of patients with abnormal karyotypes [excluding the 30 cases of t(11q23)] had MLL ITDs. Although presenting clinical features were not different between patients with and those without ITDs, relapse rate and median remission duration of the ITD-positive patients were shorter.[40]

Similar results were reported by Schnittger et al[42] using a RT-PCR assay in 387 cases of AML. A total of 13 (3.4%) cases were found to have an ITD, and 10 of these had a normal karyotype. Again, ITDs were not present in the patients with favorable karyotypes. Among 217 patients in this study on whom complete clinical data were available, 105 had a normal karyotype, and six of these had the MLL ITD (5.7%). Patients with MLL abnormalities had an inferior overall survival in this study.[42] Caligiuri et al[36] performed Southern blot analysis of the MLL gene in pretreatment samples from 98 adults with AML and normal cytogenetics. Eleven patients (11%) had evidence of a rearranged MLL gene, and sequencing, which was available in nine of these patients, demonstrated that all had tandem duplications. In this study, too, patients with a rearranged MLL gene had a shorter duration of complete remission than patients without MLL abnormalities.[36]

MLL Amplification A third mechanism by which the MLL gene may be involved in AML is gene amplification, which is most easily detected by FISH analysis. The MLL copy number ranges in reported cases from three to 90 copies. Patients with this abnormality tend to be older and to have other, complex cytogenetic abnormalities. They have a poor response to chemotherapy and a shortened survival.[43]

FLT3 Mutations in AML FLT3 (FMS-like tyrosine kinase 3, also called stem cell kinase 1 [STK1] and fetal liver kinase 2), belongs to the class III receptor tyrosine kinase family, which also includes c-KIT, platelet-derived growth factor receptor, and FMS. Like the other members of this family, its structure includes an extracellular region of five immunoglobulin-like domains, a transmembrane region, a juxtamembrane domain, and two tyrosine kinase domains (Fig. 4.1).[44,45] FLT3 protein is preferentially expressed on early hematopoietic and lymphoid progenitors. Several lines of evidence demonstrate that it plays an important role in early stem cell survival and myeloid differentiation. Stimulation with an agonist antibody against FLT3 expands myeloid and lymphoid cells, and antisense oligonucleotides against FLT3 block the formation of mature myeloid progenitor cells. Mice with disruption of FLT3 have deficiencies in B-lymphoid progenitors and stem cells and a reduced ability to reconstitute bone marrow in irradiated recipients.[45]

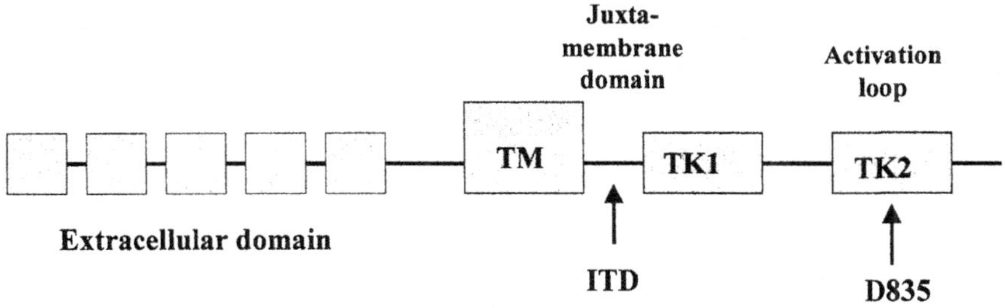

FIGURE 4.1 The structure of the FLT3 receptor. *Arrows* denote the sites of the common mutations. TM, transmembrane; TK, tyrosine kinase; ITD, internal tandem duplication.

The ligand of FLT3, FL, is expressed by bone marrow stromal cells and induces dimerization of FLT3 and phosphorylation of its intracellular tyrosine residues. This activates signal transduction pathways, including STAT5, mitogen-activated protein kinase, RAS, and phosphatidylinositol 3′ kinase.[45-47]

FLT3 is expressed at high levels in most cases of AML and pre-B-cell acute lymphoblastic leukemia and in some cases of myelodysplasia and T-cell ALL. It is expressed at high levels in many leukemia and lymphoma cell lines.[45] A serendipitous finding by Japanese researchers of unexpected longer transcripts of FLT3 in five patients with AML[44] led to the identification of the most commonly mutated gene in this disease, and it has had a significant impact on our understanding of the pathogenesis of AML.

FLT3 Internal Tandem Duplications (ITD) In 1996, Japanese researchers reported on five patients with AML and ITDs of sequences in the juxtamembrane domain of the FLT3 gene (exon 11, intron 11, and exon 12).[44] Strikingly, these duplications were all in-frame. In three of these patients who were also studied in remission, the abnormally long PCR products were absent. Subsequent studies have shown FLT3 ITD of various lengths and positions to be the most common gene mutation in AML, present in 20%–30% of patients.[48-53] FLT3 ITD are found most frequently in the M3 subtype of AML and have a lower incidence in secondary AML, MDS, and pediatric AML. FLT3 ITDs have not been reported in chronic myelogenous leukemia, lymphomas, T-cell ALL, myeloma, or chronic lymphocytic leukemia.[54]

In vitro studies have demonstrated that these ITDs result in constitutive activation of the FLT3 kinase and its signal transduction pathways.[46,47,55,56] FLT3-containing ITD mutations induced IL-3 and ligand-independent growth in IL-3–dependent cell lines such as BA/F3 and 32D cells.[46,47] Cells transfected with mutant FLT3 showed constitutive activation of STAT5, MAP kinase, and SHC.[46,47] Furthermore, murine bone marrow cells containing FLT3 ITD mutations caused a myeloproliferative disease in mice.[57]

These ITD are always in-frame and cluster in the juxtamembrane domain of the receptor. Kiyoi et al[55] postulated that because the DNA corresponding to this domain contains palindromic sequences, it is prone to forming single-strand secondary structures, such as hairpins, during DNA replication. The formation of these structures predisposes the cell to duplication errors. Cells that acquire an in-frame duplication in the juxtamembrane domain have a growth advantage and expand selectively.

Activating Mutation of D835 of FLT3 A second mutation of the intracellular domain of FLT3 has recently been described in AML in an intracellular portion of the receptor called the activation loop.[58] These patients have a substitution mutation of the highly conserved aspartic acid residue 835 of the activation loop. D835Y is the most commonly found mutation, but others have been described, including D835V, D835H, D835E, and D835N.[59] Homologous mutations in aspartic acid residues in the related receptor, c-kit, have been found in mastocytosis and gastrointestinal stromal tumors and cause constitutive activation of the receptor. Structural analysis studies of EphR2, another related receptor tyrosine kinase, have shown that the activation loop normally prevents activation of the receptor by blocking the binding of adenosine triphosphate to the active site of the enzyme.[60] Mutations of critical residues at this site cause the loop to fold out, exposing the active site and enabling activation of the receptor. When D835 mutant FLT3 complementary DNA was introduced into 32D cells, they proliferated without IL-3 or FL ligand.[59]

The Clinical Significance of FLT3 Mutations Four large clinical studies[51-53,59] and several smaller studies[48-50,54,61,62] have addressed the incidence and prognostic significance of FLT3 mutations in AML. The German AML Cooperative Group screened 1003 cases of AML for FLT3 ITDs and found them to be present in 23.5% of patients. The mutation was more common in patients with a normal karyotype, with the exception of patients with the t(15;17) translocation, in which 35.3% had FLT3 ITD. ITDs were more common in women, and the median age of patients with the mutation was lower than the median age of patients without FLT3 ITDs (54.9 vs 57.6 years). With a median follow-up of only 11.1 months, the complete remission rate and the overall survival were the same among patients with the mutation as it was in those without the mutation. However, patients with FLT3 ITDs had higher white blood cell counts at presentation and a higher relapse rate.[52]

A second German study of 979 patients with AML found similar results, with 20.4% of cases harboring FLT3 ITD mutations. Point mutations of codon 835 were also evaluated in this study, and 7.7% of patients had substitutions at this aspartic acid residue.[53] Seventeen patients (1.7%) had both activating mutations in FLT3. Thus, 26.4% of AML patients in this study had an activating mutation of FLT3. As in the previous study, FLT3 mutations were more prevalent in patients with normal karyotypes (32% vs 9.9%, $P < 0.001$), although 31% of patients with t(15;17) had FLT3 ITDs, and 90% (9/10) patients with the t(6;9) translocation had FLT3 ITDs. Both FLT3 mutations were associated with higher white blood cell count and a higher percentage of bone marrow blasts at presentation. In this study, there was no association between patient age and presence of FLT3 mutations. However, there was an association with French-American-British (FAB) subtype, with a low frequency of mutations in the M2 and M6 subtypes, and a high frequency in the M3 and M5 subtypes.

The median follow-up time in this study was only 12.2 months, and again, this short-term study did not find a clear impact of the presence of FLT3 mutations on overall survival. However, the ratio between mutant FLT3 and wild-type FLT3 proved to be of prognostic significance. This ratio ranged from 0.03 to 32.56, with a median of 0.78. Patients younger than 60 years with intermediate-risk cytogenetics had highly significant shorter overall survival when their ratio was above the median, compared with patients with a ratio below the median or patients without FLT3 ITD. Multivariate analysis confirmed that the mutant/wild-type ratio was an independent prognostic factor.

The third large clinical study to address these issues was the United Kingdom Medical Research Council AML study, in which 854 patients were screened for the presence of FLT3 ITDs.[51] The median follow-up of patients was 52 months, but some patients were followed up for more than 10 years. Only four patients in this series were older than 60 years. A FLT3 ITD mutation was found in 27% of the patients, and, as in previous studies, it was associated with a high white blood cell count at presentation, a high percentage of bone marrow blasts, the t(15;17) translocation (37%), and normal karyotypes (34%). The presence of FLT3 ITDs in this study was clearly associated with an increased relapse risk and worse overall survival, with 44% of patients without FLT3 ITDs being alive at 5 years, compared with 32% of patients with the FLT3 mutations.

Yamamoto et al[59] studied 429 patients with AML and found 7% D835 mutations and 18.9% ITD mutations. Clinical outcome was studied in a subgroup of 201 of these patients, none of whom had M3 leukemias. In this group, 22.9% had an ITD mutation, and 4% had a D835 mutation. As in previous studies, white blood cell counts at presentation were significantly higher in the ITD group compared with patients who did not have ITD but not in the D835 mutation group. At a median follow-up time of 50 months, patients with ITDs had significantly worse disease-free and overall survival, with 13.1% of patients with ITD being alive at 50 months, versus 37.1% of patients with wild-type FLT3.

In five smaller studies,[48-50,54,61,62] a combined total of 678 patients with AML were screened for FLT3 ITDs, and the prevalence of the mutations ranged from 13.2% to 28%. In the two largest of these studies that assessed clinical outcome,[49,62] the presence of FLT3 was a poor prognostic factor. In another of these studies,[48] 82 adults younger than 60 years of age with primary AML and normal cytogenetics were studied for FLT3 ITDs, and 23 (28%) were found to carry the mutation. Of these 23 patients, eight (35%) also lacked an FLT3 wild-type allele, and disease-free and overall survival were significantly inferior in this group, compared with patients who did not have ITDs and with patients who had both wild-type FLT3 and FLT3 ITDs.[48]

FLT3 ITDs were found in 34% of 140 older patients with AML (age > 55 years) and were not associated with an inferior outcome.[63] They appear to be less common in MDS and in therapy-related AML; they were found only in four (2.2%) of a combined total of 180 patients with MDS studied in four published reports[54,59,64,65] and in eight of 60 patients (13.3%) with therapy-related AML.[64,65]

In the six studies that have evaluated the incidence and significance of FLT3 ITDs in pediatric and infant AML, the mutation was found less frequently than in adults, with an incidence ranging between 5.3% and 16.5%. All studies found that it was associated with a poor prognosis.[66-71]

FLT3 as a Therapeutic Target in AML Because mutated FLT3 has been shown to cause constitutive activation of the receptor, to be leukemogenic in experimental systems, and to be a poor prognostic indicator in clinical studies of AML, it represents a rational therapeutic target in AML. Two inhibitors of FLT3, AG 1295 and CEP-701, are showing promising in vitro results.[72,73] Both inhibitors show specific toxicity to AML blasts harboring FLT3 ITD mutations. CEP-701 prolonged survival in a mouse model of FLT3 ITD leukemia.[73] A phase I study of oral CEP-701 has been completed, and the drug was well tolerated without serious toxicities.[73]

FLT3 Summary Activating mutations of the receptor tyrosine kinase FLT3 are found in approximately one third of patients with de novo AML, making this gene the most commonly mutated one in this disease. These mutations are more prevalent in patients with normal cytogenetics, t(15;17) AML, and t(6;9) AML, and are rarer in patients with t(8;21), inv(16), 11q23 rearrangements, and complex karyotypes. Most studies with sufficient follow-up have shown FLT3 mutations to be associated with decreased overall survival. There is evidence to suggest that these activating mutations are leukemogenic and may be appropriate therapeutic targets in AML. Clinical studies with FLT3 inhibitors in AML patients are underway.

MINIMAL RESIDUAL DISEASE (MRD)

Although most patients with AML achieve a remission with conventional chemotherapy, fewer than 50% are cured, indicating that morphology and cytogenetics are not sensitive enough to detect a small tumor burden. Furthermore, most studies that have evaluated prognostic factors in acute leukemia have demonstrated that the chance of cure is higher when the tumor burden is low. These facts point to the potential benefit of detecting minimal residual disease in AML. However, in contrast to ALL and CML, AML is a heterogeneous disease that cannot be monitored by a single translocation or gene rearrangement. Furthermore, studies of MRD in AML have shown that the significance of detection of disease differs between distinct subtypes of AML and that each subgroup needs to be studied separately (Table 4.2).

PCR of a leukemia-specific marker, which can detect one leukemic cell in 10^3 to 10^5 normal cells, is the most sensitive method for the detection of MRD. Other methods that have been utilized in MRD studies include FISH, Southern blotting, and flow cytometry; however, they have proved to be less sensitive than PCR. FISH is valuable for the detection of chromosomal deletions and duplications, which cannot be detected by PCR. Southern blotting requires relatively large amounts of DNA, is time consuming, and is not as sensitive as the other methods and thus is not used routinely for MRD detection.

Minimal Residual Disease in APL

The most extensive and informative studies of MRD in AML have been conducted in APL, capitalizing on the unique translocation that characterizes this leukemia. In the largest of these studies, Deverio et al[74] performed RT-PCR for the PML/RARα transcript in bone marrow samples of 163 patients with APL who were enrolled in an Italian, multicenter trial. All patients were treated uniformly with ATRA and idarubicin induction, followed by three courses of consolidation chemotherapy, and bone marrow samples were collected prospectively at predetermined intervals. The sensitivity of the PCR assay used in this study was 10^{-4}. All patients had a negative PCR result at the end of consolidation. In 21 patients, follow-up PCR converted to a positive result, and 20 of these patients experi-

TABLE 4.2 Significance of Minimal Residual Disease in AML Subtypes

Chromosome Abnormality	Significance of RT-PCR–Detectable MRD
t(15;17)	High risk of relapse if marrow (+) after consolidation or converts from (–) to (+). Treatment recommended in molecular relapse.
T(8;21)	May remain (+) in long-term remission. MRD detected by RT-PCR does not necessarily herald relapse and should not be treated. Role of quantitative PCR still being investigated.
inv(16)	Residual PCR (+) after therapy may decline over time. May remain (+) in long-term remission. MRD detected by RT-PCR does not necessarily herald relapse and should not be treated. Role of quantitative PCR still being investigated.

Abbreviations: MRD, minimal residual disease; RT-PCR, reverse transcriptase-polymerase chain reaction.

enced relapse at a median of 3 months after the first positive PCR result. Of the 142 patients who remained PCR negative, only eight had a hematologic relapse.[74]

In a follow-up study, Lo Coco et al[75] treated 14 patients with APL who experienced a *molecular* relapse (defined as the reappearance of the PML/RARα transcripts in two successive marrow samples) with ATRA followed by cytarabine/mitoxantrone chemotherapy, autologous transplantation, and/or ATRA maintenance. The 2-year survival estimate from time of relapse was 92% in this group, compared with only 37% in a previous series of patients who received the same treatment, but at the time of *hematologic* recurrence.

In a similar study, Jurcic et al[22] reported that among 47 patients with APL who underwent successful induction with ATRA followed by chemotherapy, only 3/41 with two or more negative PCR results had a relapse, compared with all four patients who had residual disease by PCR after consolidation.

These studies and others[76] have demonstrated that almost all patients who have a PCR result that is either persistently positive after consolidation or converts from negative to positive experience relapse. However, 5%–25% of patients with negative PCR results also experience relapse, indicating that the sensitivity of the PCR test used is not sufficient to detect all patients who may benefit from additional therapy. More sensitive PCR methods, which can detect one leukemic cell in 10^{-5} to 10^{-6} normal cells and can quantify the number of PML/RARα transcripts, are becoming increasingly available and automated,[3,77-80] although their clinical utility has yet to be evaluated in significant numbers of patients.

Based on available data, a reasonable approach to the monitoring of MRD in patients with APL who have achieved a molecular remission includes surveillance bone marrow evaluations every 3 months for the first 2 years after therapy, when the risk of relapse is the highest. All remission samples should be studied by RT-PCR for the PML/RARα transcript. Salvage therapy should be administered if two or more PCR results are positive in a patient who had achieved a prior molecular remission.

MRD in t(8;21) AML

The significance of MRD in patients with the t(8;21) translocation has not been studied as extensively as it has in APL. However, available data suggest that the CBFα/ETO fusion gene may be present at low levels in patients in long-term remission from their leukemia and does not necessarily identify patients who are at increased risk for relapse.[81-83] For example, Miyamoto et al[81] detected the CBFα/ETO transcript in all 18 patients who had been in complete remission for 12–150 months. There has been increasing interest in using quantitative PCR methods to try to identify which patients with evidence of persistence of the CBFα/ETO are at risk for recurrent disease. Tobal et al[80] studied 25 patients with t(8;21) AML by use of a competitive, quantitative RT-PCR assay and found that levels of CBFα/ETO transcript of up to 10^3 molecules per microgram of RNA in bone marrow were compatible with durable remission. The five patients with

0.71×10^5 to 2.27×10^5 molecules/μg of RNA had a hematologic relapse within 3–6 months of completing therapy. A small-scale study using quantitative real-time RT-PCR for the CBFα/ETO transcript and using fluorescently labeled hybridization probes showed this method to be reliable and sensitive.[84] This method, applied in large prospective trials, may help elucidate the prognostic implications of MRD detection in t(8;21) leukemia. At present, however, we lack sufficient data to make specific therapeutic decisions based on the detection of MRD in this subset of AML patients.

MRD in inv(16) AML

Data are similarly conflicting regarding the significance of the detection of the CBFβ/smooth muscle myosin heavy chain transcript in patients with M4Eo/inv(16) AML in remission, and there is an emerging role for quantitative, and especially real-time, PCR for detection of MRD in this leukemia.[85-87] Guerrasio et al[85] studied 36 patients with inv(16) leukemia by use of qualitative nested RT-PCR and quantitative real-time PCR. All patients in complete remission after consolidation therapy were still PCR positive; however, all patients who remained in remission for more than 12 months became PCR negative. In 16 of these patients, a quantitative real-time PCR was used, in which the CBFβ/smooth muscle myosin heavy chain transcript copy number was normalized for expression of the house-keeping gene ABL and expressed as fusion gene copy number per 10^4 copies of ABL. In the patients in complete remission, the mean copy number was significantly higher in the seven patients destined to relapse, compared with the patients who remained in complete remission. Using similar methods, Buonamici et al[86] studied 21 patients with inv(16) AML and showed that in those who were in remission, the presence of transcript ratios greater than 0.25% corresponded to a high risk of relapse, and ratios less than 0.12% were found in the patients who remained in remission. Results of large-scale studies using quantitative PCR methods are needed before clinical decisions can be based on the detection of MRD in inv(16) AML.

MRD in AML with Other Cytogenetic Abnormalities

The MLL gene may be fused with more than 40 partner genes in AML, making the development of PCR assays to detect MRD in these patients a formidable task. However, a small study by Mitterbauer et al[88] in six patients with the MLL-AF6 translocation demonstrated a good correlation between the detection of the abnormal transcript by RT-PCR and the subsequent recurrence of disease. A recent study evaluating the potential value of FLT3 mutations as markers for MRD has demonstrated that these mutations are unstable and may not be useful for the monitoring of patients in remission because different mutations may be acquired during relapse.[89]

DNA MICROARRAYS

DNA microarrays are powerful tools that can provide information on the expression profile of thousands of genes in a tumor sample. The technique involves the application of RNA from clinical samples to nucleic acid sequences immobilized on a solid surface. The hybridization patterns create enormous data sets, which then need to be analyzed to create clinically meaningful information.[90] The use of DNA microarrays in AML is only now emerging, but early studies suggest that this technique may prove powerful in the molecular characterization of this disease.

In the first published microarray analysis of acute leukemia, 72 samples were studied by use of an array of 6817 genes. The samples were easily sorted into AML and ALL on the basis of their gene expression pattern.[91] Armstrong et al[92] studied ALL carrying a 11q23 translocation and found a highly distinct gene expression profile that was easily separated from ALL without the MLL translocation and from AML. Two studies have compared expression profiles within AML subtypes and found distinct differences between them. Schoch et al[93] performed microarray analyses on bone marrow samples of 37 AML patients with t(8;21), t(15;17), or inv(16). They found a strong correlation between the specific cytogenetic abnormalities and three distinct, homogenous patterns of gene expression. Virtaneva et al[94] compared expression patterns of AML with trisomy 8 to AML with normal cytogenetics and found that trisomy 8 AML was associated with overexpression of genes on chromosome 8 and with down-regulation of genes involved on apoptosis. Thus, these preliminary studies suggest that DNA microarrays may have an increasing role in the characterization of AML subgroups and may contribute to our understanding of the disease, the identification of molecular therapeutic targets, and our ability to tailor therapy to the individual AML patient.

REFERENCES

1. Grimwade D, Walker H, Oliver F et al. The importance of diagnostic cytogenetics on outcome in AML: analysis of 1,612 patients entered into the MRC AML 10 Trial. Blood 1998;92:2322–2333.
2. Slovak M, Kopecky K, Cassileth P et al. Karyotypic analysis predicts outcome of preremission and postremission therapy in adult acute myeloid leukemia: a Southwest Oncology Group/Eastern Cooperative Oncology Group study. Blood 2000;96:4075–4083.
3. Willman C. Molecular evaluation of acute myeloid leukemias. Semin Hematol 1999;36:390–400.
4. Leith C, Kopecky K, Godwin J et al. Acute myeloid leukemia in the elderly: assessment of multidrug resistance (MDR1) and cytogenetics distinguishes biologic subgroups with remarkably distinct responses to standard chemotherapy: a Southwest Oncology Group study. Blood 1997;89: 3323–3329.
5. Appelbaum F. Molecular diagnosis and clinical decisions in adult acute leukemia. Semin Hematol 1999;36:401-410.
6. Dombret H, Fenaux P, Soignet S et al. Established practice in the treatment of patients with acute promyelocytic leukemia and the introduction of arsenic trioxide as a novel therapy. Semin Hematol 2002;39:8–13.

7. Tallman M, Nabhan C. Management of acute promyelocytic leukemia. Curr Oncol Rep 2002;4:381–389.
8. Bloomfield C, Lawrence D, Byrd J et al. Frequency of prolonged remission duration after high-dose cytarabine intensification in acute myeloid leukemia varies by cytogenetic subtype. Cancer Res 1998;58:4173–4179.
9. Hayashi Y. The molecular genetics of recurring chromosome abnormalities in acute myeloid leukemia. Semin Hematol 2000;37:368–380.
10. Dash A, Gilliland D. Molecular genetics of acute myeloid leukaemia. Best Pract Res Clin Haematol 2001;14:49–64.
11. Langabeer S, Walker H, Rogers J et al. Incidence of AML1/ETO fusion transcripts in patients entered into the MRC AML trials. Br J Haematol 1997;99:925–928.
12. Andrieu V, Radford-Weiss I, Troussard X et al. Molecular detection of t(8;21)/AML1-ETO in AML M1/M2: correlation with cytogenetics, morphology and immunophenotype. Br J Haematol 1996;92:855–865.
13. Rowe D, Cotterill S, Ross F et al. Cytogenetically cryptic AML1-ETO and CBF beta-MYH11 gene rearrangements: incidence in 412 cases of acute myeloid leukaemia. Br J Haematol 2000;111:1051–1056.
14. Mitterbauer M, Kusec R, Schwarzinger I et al. Comparison of karyotype analysis and RT-PCR for AML1/ETO in 204 unselected patients with AML. Ann Hematol 1998;76:139–143.
15. Mrozek K, Prior T, Edwards C et al. Comparison of cytogenetic and molecular genetic detection of t(8;21) and inv(16) in a prospective series of adults with de novo acute myeloid leukemia: a Cancer and Leukemia Group B study. J Clin Oncol 2001;19:2482–2492.
16. Ritter M, Thiede C, Schakel U et al. Underestimation of inversion (16) in acute myeloid leukaemia using standard cytogenetics as compared with polymerase chain reaction: results of a prospective investigation. Br J Haematol 1997;98:969–972.
17. Tobal K, Johnson P, Saunders M et al. Detection of CBFb/MYH11 transcripts in patients with inversion and other abnormalities of chromosome 16 at presentation and remission. Br J Haematol 1995;91:104–108.
18. Mitterbauer M, Laczika K, Novak M et al. High concordance of karyotype analysis and RT-PCR for CBF beta/MYH11 in unselected patients with acute myeloid leukemia. Am J Clin Pathol 2000;113:406–410.
19. Langabeer S, Walker H, Gale R et al. Frequency of CBFβ/MYH11 fusion transcripts in patients entered into the U.K. MRC AML trials. Br J Haematol 1997;96:736–739.
20. Melnick A, Licht J. Deconstructing a disease: RARα, its fusion partners, and their roles in the pathogenesis of acute promyelocytic leukemia. Blood 1999;93:3167–3215.
21. Slack J, Arthur D, Lawrence D et al. Secondary cytogenetic changes in acute promyelocytic leukemia: prognostic importance in patients treated with chemotherapy alone and association with the intron 3 breakpoint of the PML gene: a Cancer and Leukemia Group B study. J Clin Oncol 1997;15:1786–1795.
22. Jurcic J, Nimer S, Scheinberg D et al. Prognostic significance of minimal residual disease detection and PML/RAR-α isoform type: long-term follow-up in acute promyelocytic leukemia. Blood 2001;98:2651–2656.
23. Grimwade D, Biondi A, Mozziconacci M et al. Characterization of acute promyelocytic leukemia cases lacking the classic t(15;17): results of the European Working Party. Blood 2000;96:1297–1308.
24. Petti M, Fazi F, Gentile M et al. Complete remission through blast cell differentiation in PLZF/RARalpha-positive acute promyelocytic leukemia: in vitro and in vivo studies. Blood 2002;100:1065–1067.

25. Sainty D, Liso V, Cantu-Rajnoldi A et al. A new morphologic classification system for acute promyelocytic leukemia distinguishes cases with underlying PLZF/RARA gene rearrangements. Blood 2000;96:1287–1296.

26. Orfao A, Chillon M, Bortoluci A et al. The flow cytometric pattern of CD34, CD15 and CD13 expression in acute myeloblastic leukemia is highly characteristic of the presence of PML-RARalpha gene rearrangements. Haematologica 1999;84:405–412.

27. Villamor N, Costa D, Aymerich M et al. Rapid diagnosis of acute promyelocytic leukemia by analyzing the immunocytochemical pattern of the PML protein with the monoclonal antibody PG-M3. Am J Clin Pathol 2000;114:786–792.

28. Falini B, Flenghi L, Fagioli M et al. Immunocytochemical diagnosis of acute promyelocytic leukemia (M3) with the monoclonal antibody PG-M3 (anti-PML). Blood 1997;90:4046–4053.

29. Allford S, Grimwade D, Langabeer S et al. Identification of the t(15;17) in AML FAB types other than M3: evaluation of the role of molecular screening for the PML/RARα rearrangement in newly diagnosed AML. Br J Haematol 1999;105:198–207.

30. Bernasconi P, Boni M, Cavigliano P et al. Molecular genetics of acute myeloid leukemia. Ann NY Acad Sci 2002;963:297–305.

31. Rubnitz J, Raimondi S, Tong X et al. Favorable impact of the t(9;11) in childhood acute myeloid leukemia. J Clin Oncol 2002;20:2302–2309.

32. Poirel H, Rack K, Delabesse E et al. Incidence and characterization of MLL gene (11q23) rearrangements in acute myeloid leukemia M1 and M5. Blood 1996;87:2496–2505.

33. Ibrahim S, Estey E, Pierce S et al. 11q23 abnormalities in patients with acute myelogenous leukemia and myelodysplastic syndrome as detected by molecular and cytogenetic analyses. Am J Clin Pathol 2000;114.

34. Burg MVD, Beverloo H, Langerak A et al. Rapid and sensitive detection of all types of MLL gene translocations with a single FISH probe set. Leukemia 1999;13:2107–2113.

35. Megonigal M, Rappaport E, Wilson R et al. Panhandle PCR for cDNA: a rapid method for isolation of MLL fusion transcripts involving unknown partner genes. Proc Natl Acad Sci USA 2000;97:9597–9602.

36. Caligiuri M, Strout M, Lawrence D et al. Rearrangement of ALL1 (MLL) in acute myeloid leukemia with normal cytogenetics. Cancer Res 1998;58:55–59.

37. Yu M, Honoki K, Andersen J et al. MLL tandem duplication and multiple splicing in adult acute myeloid leukemia with normal karyotype. Leukemia 1996;10:774–780.

38. Strout M, Marcucci G, Bloomfield C et al. The partial tandem duplication of ALL1 (MLL) is consistently generated by Alu-mediated homologous recombination in acute myeloid leukemia. Proc Natl Acad Sci USA 1998;95:2390–2395.

39. Schnittger S, Wormann B, Hiddemann W et al. Partial tandem duplications of the MLL gene are detectable in peripheral blood and bone marrow of nearly all healthy donors. Blood 1998;92:1728–1734.

40. Dohner K, Tobis K, Ulrich R et al. Prognostic significance of partial tandem duplications of the MLL gene in adult patients 16 to 60 years old with acute myeloid leukemia and normal cytogenetics: a study of the Acute Myeloid Leukemia Study Group Ulm. J Clin Oncol 2002;20:3254–3261.

41. Shiah H, Kuo Y, Tang J et al. Clinical and biological implications of partial tandem duplication of the MLL gene in acute myeloid leukemia without chromosomal abnormalities at 11q23. Leukemia 2002;16:196–202.

42. Schnittger S, Kinkelin U, Schoch C et al. Screening for MLL tandem duplication in 387 unselected patients with AML identify a prognostically unfavorable subset of AML. Leukemia 2000;14:796–804.

43. Dolan M, McGlennen R, Hirsch B. MLL amplification in myeloid malignancies: clinical, molecular, and cytogenetic findings. Cancer Genet Cytogenet 2002;134:93–101.

44. Nakao M, Yokota S, Iwai T et al. Internal tandem duplication of the flt3 gene found in acute myeloid leukemia. Leukemia 1996;10:1911–1918.

45. Gilliland D, Griffin J. The roles of FLT3 in hematopoiesis and leukemia. Blood 2002;100:1532–1542.

46. Kiyoi H, Ohno R, Ueda R et al. Mechanism of constitutive activation of FLT3 with internal tandem duplication in the juxtamembrane domain. Oncogene 2002;21:2555–2563.

47. Hayakawa F, Towatari M, Kiyoi H et al. Tandem-duplicated Flt3 constitutively activates STAT5 and MAP kinase and introduces autonomous cell growth in IL-3-dependent cell lines. Oncogene 2000;19:624–631.

48. Whitman S, Archer K, Feng L et al. Absence of the wild-type allele predicts poor prognosis in adult de novo acute myeloid leukemia with normal cytogenetics and the internal tandem duplication of FLT3: a Cancer and Leukemia Group B study. Cancer Res 2001;61:7233–7239.

49. Abu-Duhier F, Goodeve A, Wilson G et al. FLT3 internal tandem duplication mutations in adult acute myeloid leukaemia define a high-risk group. Br J Haematol 2000;111:190–195.

50. Kiyoi H, Naoe T, Nakano Y et al. Prognostic implication of FLT3 and N-RAS gene mutations in acute myeloid leukemia. Blood 1999;93:3074–3080.

51. Kottaridis P, Gale R, Frew M et al. The presence of a FLT3 internal tandem duplication in patients with acute myeloid leukemia (AML) adds important prognostic information to cytogenetic risk group and response to the first cycle of chemotherapy: analysis of 854 patients from the United Kingdom Medical Research Council AML 10 and 12 trials. Blood 2001;98:1752–1759.

52. Schnittger S, Schoch C, Dugas M et al. Analysis of FLT3 length mutations in 1003 patients with acute myeloid leukemia: correlation to cytogenetics, FAB subtype, and prognosis in the AMLCG study and usefulness as a marker for the detection of minimal residual disease. Blood 2002;100:59–66.

53. Thiede C, Steudel C, Mohr B et al. Analysis of FLT3-activating mutations in 979 patients with acute myelogenous leukemia: association with FAB subtypes and identification of subroups with poor prognosis. Blood 2002;99:4326–4335.

54. Yokota S, Kiyoi H, Nakao M et al. Internal tandem duplication of the FLT3 gene is preferentially seen in acute myeloid leukemia and myelodysplastic syndrome among various hematologic malignancies: a study on a large series of patients and cell lines. Leukemia 1997;11:1605–1609.

55. Kiyoi H, Towatari M, Yokota S et al. Internal tandem duplication of the FLT3 gene is a novel modality of elongation mutation which causes constitutive activation of the product. Leukemia 1998;12:1333–1337.

56. Mizuki M, Fenski R, Halfter H et al. Flt3 mutations from patients with acute myeloid leukemia induce transformation of 32D cells mediated by the Ras and STAT5 pathways. Blood 2000;96:3907–3914.

57. Kelly L, Liu O, Kutok J et al. FLT3 internal tandem duplication mutations associated with human acute myeloid leukemias induce myeloproliferative disease in a murine bone marrow transplant model. Blood 2002;99:310–318.

58. Abu-Duhier F, Goodeve A, Wilson G et al. Identification of novel FLT-3 Asp835 mutations in adult acute myeloid leukaemia. Br J Haematol 2001;113:983–988.

59. Yamamoto Y, Kiyoi H, Nakano Y et al. Activating mutation of D835 within the activation loop of FLT3 in human hematologic malignancies. Blood 2001;97:2434–2439.

60. Binns K, Taylor P, Sicheri F et al. Phosphorylation of tyrosine residues in the kinase domain and juxtamembrane region regulates the biologic and catalytic activities of Eph receptors. Mol Cell Biol 2000;20:4791–4805.

61. Rombouts W, Lowenberg B, van Putten WL et al. Improved prognostic significance of cytokine-induced proliferation in vitro in patients with de novo acute myeloid leukemia of intermediate risk: impact of internal tandem duplications in the FLT3 gene. Leukemia 2001;15:1046–1053.

62. Kiyoi H, Naoe T, Yokota S et al. Internal tandem duplication of FLT3 associated with leukocytosis in acute promyelocytic leukemia. Leukemia 1997;11:1447–1452.

63. Stirewalt D, Kopecky K, Meshinchi S et al. FLT3, RAS, and TP53 mutations in elderly patients with acute myeloid leukemia. Blood 2001;97:3589–3595.

64. Christiansen D, Pedersen-Bjergaard J. Internal tandem duplications of the FLT3 and MLL genes are mainly observed in atypical cases of therapy-related acute myeloid leukemia with a normal karyotype and are unrelated to type of previous therapy. Leukemia 2001;15:1848–1851.

65. Horiike S, Yokota S, Nakao M et al. Tandem duplications of the FLT3 receptor gene are associated with leukemic transformation of myelodysplasia. Leukemia 1997;11:1442–1446.

66. Xu F, Taki T, Yang H et al. Tandem duplication of the FLT3 gene is found in acute lymphoblastic leukaemia as well as acute myeloid leukaemia but not in myelodysplastic syndrome or juvenile chronic myelogenous leukaemia in children. Br J Haematol 1999;105:155–162.

67. Liang D, Shih L, Hung I et al. Clinical relevance of internal tandem duplication of the FLT3 gene in childhood acute myeloid leukemia. Cancer 2002;94:3292–3298.

68. Meshinchi S, Woods W, Stirewalt D et al. Prevalence and prognostic significance of Flt3 internal tandem duplication in pediatric acute myeloid leukemia. Blood 2001;97:89–94.

69. Kondo M, Horibe K, Takahashi Y et al. Prognostic value of internal tandem duplication of the FLT3 gene in childhood acute myelogenous leukemia. Med Pediatr Oncol 1999;33:525–529.

70. Iwai T, Yokota S, Nakao M et al. Internal tandem duplication of the FLT3 gene and clinical evaluation in childhood acute myeloid leukemia. The Children's Cancer and Leukemia Study Group, Japan. Leukemia 1999;13:38–43.

71. Xu F, Taki T, Eguchi M et al. Tandem duplication of the FLT3 gene is infrequent in infant acute leukemia. Japan Infant Leukemia Study Group. Leukemia 2000;14:945–947.

72. Levis M, Tse K, Smith B et al. A FLT3 tyrosine kinase inhibitor is selectively cytotoxic to acute myeloid leukemia blasts harboring FLT3 internal tandem duplication mutations. Blood 2001;98:885–887.

73. Levis M, Allebach J, Tse K et al. A FLT3-targeted tyrosine kinase inhibitor is cytotoxic to leukemia cells in vitro and in vivo. Blood 2002;99:3885–3891.

74. Diverio D, Rossi V, Avvisati G et al. Early detection of relapse by prospective reverse transcriptase-polymerase chain reaction analysis of the PML/RARalpha fusion gene in patients with acute promyelocytic leukemia enrolled in the GIMEMA-AIEOP multicenter "AIDA" trial. GIMEMA-AIEOP Multicenter "AIDA" trial. Blood 1998;92:784–789.

75. Lo Coco F, Diverio D, Avvisati G et al. Therapy of molecular relapse in acute promyelocytic leukemia. Blood 1999;94:2225–2229.

76. Gameiro P, Vieira S, Carrara P et al. The PML-RAR alpha transcript in long-term follow-up of acute promyelocytic leukemia patients. Haematologica 2001;86:577–585.

77. Degan M, Mazzocco F, Francia RD et al. Normalizing complementary DNA by quantitative reverse transcriptase-polymerase chain reaction of beta2-microglobulin: molecular monitoring of minimal residual disease in acute promyelocytic leukemia. Diagn Mol Pathol 2000;9:98–109.

78. Applegate T, Iland H, Mokany E et al. Diagnosis and molecular monitoring of acute promyelocytic leukemia using DzyNA reverse transcription-PCR to quantify PML/RARα fusion transcripts. Clin Chem 2002;48:1338–1343.

79. Cassinat B, Zassadowski F, Balitrand N et al. Quantitation of minimal residual disease in acute promyelocytic leukemia patients with t(15;17) translocation using real-time PCR. Leukemia 2000;14:324–328.

80. Tobal K, Moore H, Macheta M et al. Monitoring minimal residual disease and predicting relapse in APL by quantitating PML-RARalpha transcripts with a sensitive competitive RT-PCR method. Leukemia 2001;15:1060–1065.

81. Miyamoto T, Nagafuji K, Akashi K et al. Persistence of multipotent progenitors expressing AML1/ETO transcripts in long-term remission patients with t(8;21) acute myelogenous leukemia. Blood 1996;87:4789–4796.

82. Kusec R, Laczika K, Knobl P et al. AML1/ETO fusion mRNA can be detected in remission blood samples of all patients with t(8;21) acute myeloid leukemia after chemotherapy or autologous bone marrow transplantation. Leukemia 1994;8:735–739.

83. Nucifora G, Larson R, Rowley J. Persistence of the 8;21 translocation in patients with acute myeloid leukemia type M2 in long-term remission. Blood 1993;82:712–715.

84. Barragan E, Bolufer P, Moreno I et al. Quantitative detection of AML1-ETO rearrangement by real-time RT-PCR using fluorescently labeled probes. Leuk Lymphoma 2001;42:747–756.

85. Guerrasio A, Pilatrino C, De Micheli D et al. Assessment of minimal residual disease (MRD) in CBFbeta/MYH11-positive acute myeloid leukemias by qualitative and quantitative RT-PCR amplification of fusion transcripts. Leukemia 2002;16:1176–1181.

86. Buonamici S, Ottaviani E, Testoni N et al. Real-time quantitation of minimal residual disease in inv(16)-positive acute myeloid leukemia may indicate risk for clinical relapse and may identify patients in a curable state. Blood 2002;99:443–449.

87. Marcucci G, Caligiuri M, Dohner H et al. Quantification of CBFbeta/MYH11 fusion transcript by real time RT-PCR in patients with INV(16) acute myeloid leukemia. Leukemia 2001;15:1072–1080.

88. Mitterbauer G, Zimmer C, Fonatsch C et al. Monitoring of minimal residual leukemia in patients with MLL-AF9 positive acute myeloid leukemia by RT-PCR. Leukemia 1999;13:1519–1524.

89. Kottaridis P, Gale R, Langabeer S et al. Studies of FLT3 mutations in paired presentation and relapse samples from patients with acute myeloid leukemia: implication for the role of FLT3 mutations in leukemogenesis, minimal residual disease detection, and possible therapy with FLT3 inhibitors. Blood 2002;100:2393–2398.

90. Ramaswamy S, Golub TR. DNA microarrays in clinical oncology. J Clin Oncol 2001; 20:1932–1941.

91. Golub T, Slonim D, Tamayo P et al. Molecular classification of cancer: class discovery and class prediction by gene expression monitoring. Science 1999;286:531–537.

92. Armstrong S, Staunton J, Silverman L et al. MLL translocations specify a distinct gene expression profile that distinguishes a unique leukemia. Nat Genet 2002;30:41–47.

93. Schoch C, Kohlmann A, Schnittger S et al. Acute myeloid leukemias with reciprocal rearrangements can be distinguished by specific gene expression profiles. Proc Natl Acad Sci USA 2002;99:10008–10013.

94. Virtaneva K, Wright F, Tanner S et al. Expression profiling reveals fundamental biological differences in acute myeloid leukemia with isolated trisomy 8 and normal cytogenetics. Proc Natl Acad Sci USA 2002;98:1124–1129.

Chapter 5

Microarray Analysis: An Essential Tool for Treatment Tailoring in Young Patients with Early Breast Cancer

Marc van de Vijver

Laura van't Veer

Conny Vrieling

Harry Bartelink

Breast-conserving therapy (local tumor excision and sentinel node procedure or axillary lymph node dissection followed by radiotherapy) is now a generally accepted treatment option for patients with early-stage breast cancer. A series of trials have shown that locoregional control and survival rates achieved with this therapy are comparable to those obtained with mastectomy.[1-7] However, several studies[5] demonstrated that young patients with early-stage breast cancer have a worse prognosis than older patients that consists of a higher local recurrence rate and a lower survival rate.[8-10]

Many studies have tried to elucidate the relationship between this worse prognosis and young age at diagnosis. It was reported that younger patients present more frequently with factors known to be associated with a poor prognosis, such as large tumors,[1,2] high-grade tumors,[1-3,5-7] vascular invasion,[3,5] lymph node involvement,[1,2,8] negative hormone receptors,[1,2,5,8-11] tumors with high S-phase fractions,[2,7] and overexpression of p53.[2] The question of whether a combination of these factors can explain the poor prognosis remains unsolved. However, these studies were limited because some examined data accumulated over a long period of time and some of the relevant treatment parameters (e.g., volume of excision, frequency of reexcision, margin evaluation, or radiation dose to the tumor bed) were missing.[5,9,11,12] In a prospective, randomized, phase III trial, the efficacy of an extra boost dose to the tumor bed in reducing the local recurrence rate was investigated. In this trial, 5569 patients were entered; all received breast-conserving surgery. After whole-breast irradiation of 50 Gy, patients were randomly assigned to no further treatment or a 16-Gy boost to the tumor bed.[13] The results confirmed again that young patients had a significantly higher local recurrence rate as well as more frequent distant metastasis than older patients (Figs 5.1 and 5.2). The higher radiation dose appeared to reduce the 5-year local recurrence rate from 20% to 10% for patients younger than 41 years of age

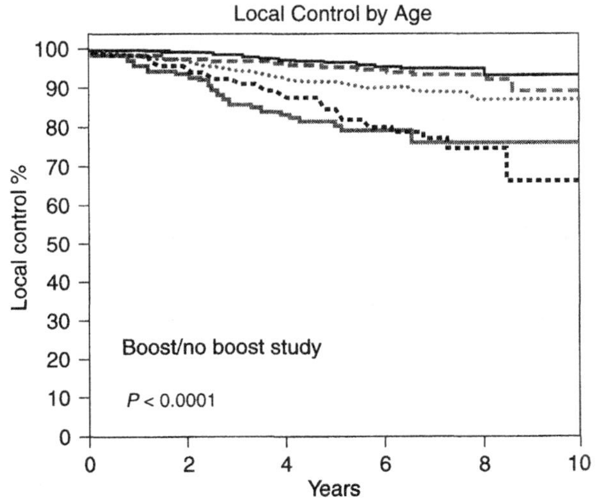

O	N	Number of patients at risk at each time interval						
28	156	137	95	46	9	1	——— ≤ 35	
48	314	285	200	90	17	0	▪▪▪▪▪▪ 36 – 40	
109	1407	1316	912	407	75	0	········· 41 – 50	Age, years
75	1885	1768	1220	525	102	0	▬ ▬ ▬ 51 – 60	
58	1807	1694	1237	518	85	0	——— > 60	

FIGURE 5.1 Survival free of local recurrence according to age. (With permission from Ref. 13)

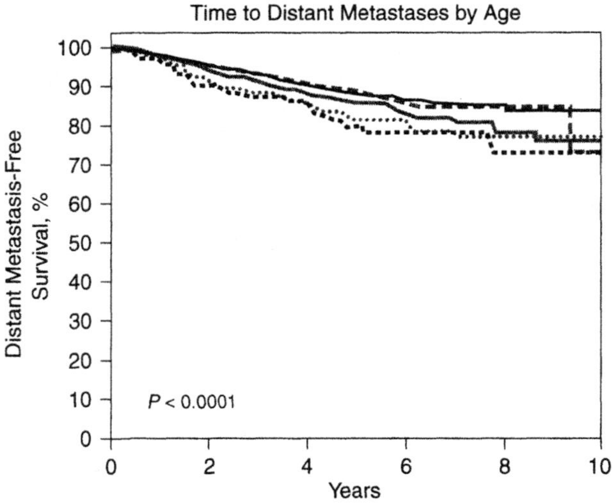

O	N	Number of patients at risk at each time interval						
30	156	135	104	47	10	1	······ ≤ 35	
55	314	287	207	100	21	0	········· 36 – 40	
199	1407	1288	891	405	78	0	—— 41 – 50	Age, years
200	1885	1738	1204	514	98	0	- - - 51 – 60	
198	1807	1661	1200	510	86	0	—— > 60	

FIGURE 5.2 Cumulative incidence of distant metastases according to age. (With permission from Ref. 13)

(Fig. 5.3). The analysis showed that in patients younger than 41 years of age, unfavorable factors were more frequently observed than in older patients. For example, they tended to have larger tumors, the tumors were more often high grade and estrogen receptor (ER) negative. The multivariate analysis of prognostic factors associated with local control demonstrated that only age and use of an additional radiation dose remained significant at a level of 0.001.[14] Similarly, for time to distant metastases, the multivariate analysis demonstrated that young age was an independent unfavorable prognostic factor. An important and unanswered question is why these tumors have such aggressive characteristics when compared with tumors arising in older patients. Furthermore, the known clinical and pathological prognostic factors do not fully explain the unfavorable prognosis for both local control and distant metastases in young patients. As a result of this, all patients younger than 35 years receive a high radiation dose as part of their breast-conserving therapy and they receive adjuvant chemotherapy as part of their treatment.[13,15] However, one may significantly reduce the treatment burden for these young patients if one could better predict which of these young patients do not have such a high local recurrence and/or distant metastasis rate. Such better prediction will very likely be achieved by gene expression profiling

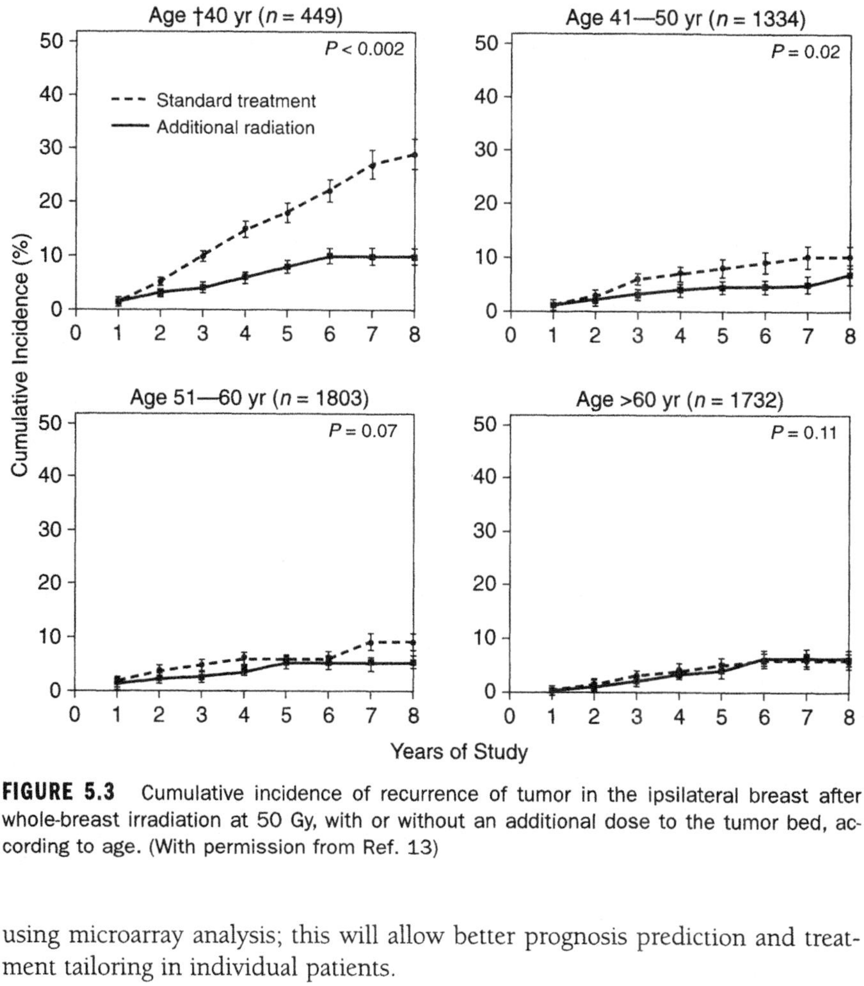

FIGURE 5.3 Cumulative incidence of recurrence of tumor in the ipsilateral breast after whole-breast irradiation at 50 Gy, with or without an additional dose to the tumor bed, according to age. (With permission from Ref. 13)

using microarray analysis; this will allow better prognosis prediction and treatment tailoring in individual patients.

Microarray Analysis

The characteristics of breast carcinomas, including clinical behavior, are largely determined by the expression pattern of genes of several classes. Differences between tumors are the result of differences in expression of regulatory proteins. If it would be possible to look at the association between specific clinical characteristics and the expression of all genes, the effector proteins that are instrumental in these differences could be identified. As a result of the Human Genome Project and the contributions of individual researchers, the nucleotide sequence is available for all 30,000–40,000 genes that are present in the human genome. It is to be expected that the function of the proteins encoded by many of these genes will be elucidated in the coming years. In addition to these developments, the software required to analyze such large and complex data sets is also rapidly evolving.

Microarray analysis allows the study of the level of expression of large numbers of messenger RNAs in a single experiment. A microarray is an orderly arrangement of known or unknown DNA samples attached to a solid support. One array may contain many thousands of spots and can be obtained by many methods. The probes attached to the solid support can be small oligonucleotides, complementary DNAs (cDNAs), or genomic sequences. The array may be formatted by photolithographic synthesis of oligonucleotides in situ, or the DNA samples may be applied directly to the array surface by pins, nibs, or inkjet technology. The target sequence hybridized to probes on the array may be radioactively or fluorescently labeled.

Investigators at Stanford University have developed a microarray analysis that uses cDNAs microspotted on glass slides; this technique has been used to study the level of expression of large numbers of messenger RNAs in cell lines and tumors.[16-19] In brief, messenger RNA from cells to be analyzed is isolated and reverse transcribed in the presence of red-fluorescent nucleotides. Fluorescent cDNA is then mixed with a green fluorescent–labeled standard, and the mixture is hybridized to the microarray. Using a fluorescent scanner, the level of fluorescence is computerized, and for each cDNA on the microarray, the level of gene expression relative to the standard is determined and transferred to a database. By use of software specifically developed for microarray analysis, the level of expression for many thousands of genes can be compared in different tumor samples.

An advantage of microarray analysis is that the expression level of a large set of genes can recognize specific properties of cells; this characteristic has been given the operational definition "expression signatures."[20] A gene expression signature can be defined by the cell type in which its component genes are expressed (e.g., T-cell signature) or by the biologic process in which its component genes are known to function (e.g., proliferation signature). If this approach is taken in the analysis of breast tumor samples, the amount of stromal cells and tumor infiltrating inflammatory cells and the proliferative signature of the tumor cells can be determined. Hedenfalk et al[21] have performed microarray analysis using RNA from samples of primary tumors from seven carriers of the *BRCA1* mutation, seven carriers of the *BRCA2* mutation, and seven patients with sporadic cases of breast cancer. By permutation analysis of multivariate classification functions, the investigators showed that the gene-expression profiles of tumors with *BRCA1* mutations, tumors with *BRCA2* mutations, and sporadic tumors differed significantly from each other. An analysis of variance between the levels of gene expression and the genotype of the samples identified 176 genes that were differentially expressed in tumors with *BRCA1* mutations and in tumors with *BRCA2* mutations. These findings indicate that functional differences exist between breast tumors with *BRCA1* mutations and those with *BRCA2* mutations. Another important implication of these findings is that in tumors with unknown

BRCA1 or *BRCA2* mutational status, gene expression profiling can be used to determine the likelihood that such a mutation is present.

Perou et al obtained microarray portraits of a set of 65 surgical specimens of human breast tumors from 42 individuals.[17] There was considerable variation in the pattern of gene expression among the tumors. This variation could be partly due to changes in the levels of certain cell types within the tumors, such as endothelial cells, stromal cells, adipose-enriched normal breast cells, B and T lymphocytes, and macrophages. Once genes characteristic of these cell types had been excluded, the authors selected a subset of 496 genes, called the "intrinsic" gene set, that still showed considerable variation in expression levels between different tumors. When variations in level of expression within the genes were used to order the tissue samples, a striking division of the tumors into ER-positive and ER-negative categories occurred. Interestingly, the ER-positive group was characterized by the expression of many genes specific to breast luminal cells. The ER-negative tumors could be further divided into several subgroups. A subgroup of six tumors had an expression pattern that was characteristic of breast basal (myoepithelial) cells, whereas another subgroup was partially characterized by high levels of expression of genes associated with overexpression of the *HER2* oncogene.

In collaboration with Rosetta Inpharmatics, (Kirkland, WA), we have studied a large series of breast carcinomas.[15] Rosetta Inpharmatics has developed a highly flexible next-generation DNA microarray platform. The in situ synthesized arrays use a glass support on which oligonucleotides are formed by use of standard phosphoramidite chemistry. In addition, Rosetta has developed a powerful bioinformatics software package (named the "Resolver") to interpret DNA microarray data sets.

In a first set of analysis, we have collected a set of breast carcinomas with distinctive characteristics:

- 18 carcinomas from patients with BRCA1 germline mutations
- two carcinomas from patients with *BRCA2* germline mutations
- from carcinomas < 5 cm of lymph node-negative patients younger than 55 years
- 34 from patients who experienced distant metastases within 5 years
- 44 from patients who had not experienced local or distant metastases at a follow-up of ≥ 5 years

Using unsupervised two-dimensional hierarchical cluster analysis, we found two main tumor clusters. These two clusters differed with respect to ER status, indicating that gene expression pattern differs dramatically in ER-positive tumors and ER-negative tumors. It is known from other studies that carcinomas in patients with *BRCA1* germline mutations are almost all ER negative. As expected, most *BRCA1*-associated tumors clustered in the group of ER-negative tumors.

We also performed supervised cluster analysis, comparing tumors from patients who experienced distant metastases with those who remained disease free. To identify reliably "good" and "poor" prognostic tumors, we employed a powerful supervised classification method. The correlation coefficient of the expression for each significantly regulated gene with disease outcome was calculated. After several steps of optimization, 70 genes were identified (Fig. 5.4). The ex-

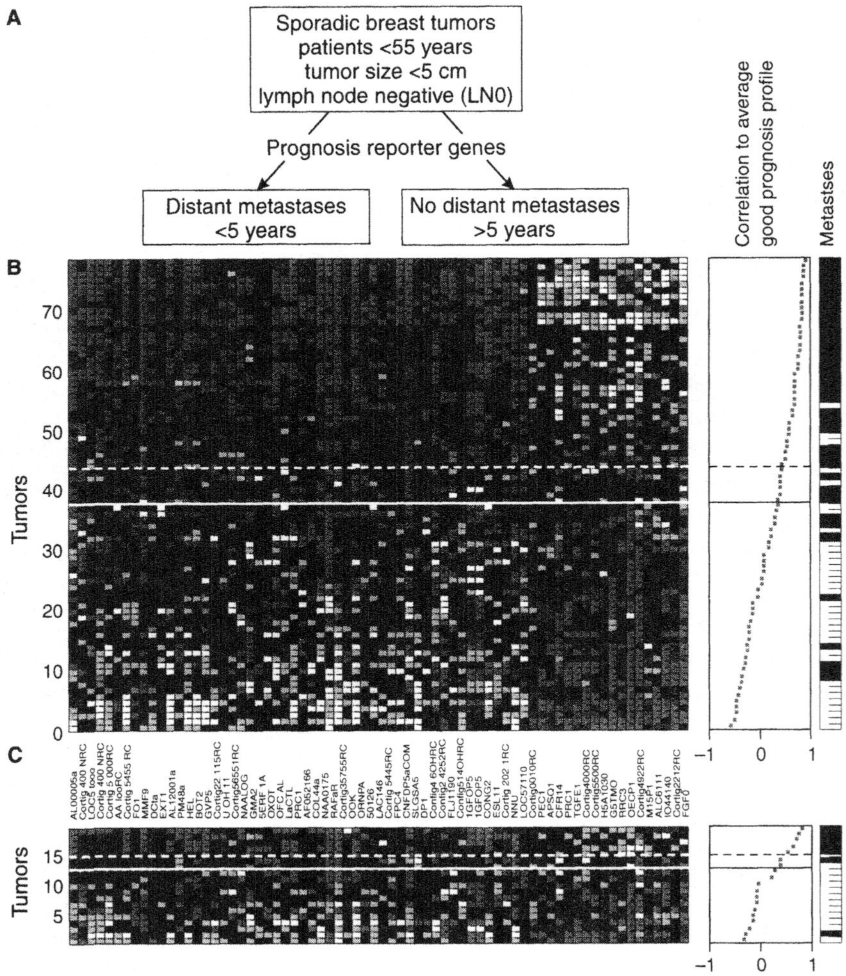

FIGURE 5.4 Supervised classification on prognosis signatures. (With permission from Ref. 15)

pression pattern of this set of 70 genes correctly predicted the actual outcome of disease for 65 of the 78 patients (83%), with five poor-prognosis patients and eight good-prognosis patients were not correctly classified by gene expression signature. Using an optimized sensitivity threshold resulted in 15 misclassifications; three poor-prognosis tumors were classified as "good prognosis," and 12 good-prognosis tumors were classified as "poor prognosis." Genes involved in cell cycle, invasion and metastasis, angiogenesis, and signal transduction are significantly unregulated in the poor-prognosis signature (e.g., *cyclin E2, MCM6,* metalloproteinases *MMP9* and *MP1, RAB6B, PK428, ESM1,* and the *VEGF*-receptor *FLT1*).

The next step was to study the prognostic value of the classifier in a series of 295 patients with breast carcinoma.[22]

One hundred eighty tumors had a poor-prognosis signature and 115 tumors had a good-prognosis signature. Overall, 10-year survivals for the poor- and the good-prognosis signature groups were 54.6% (SE 4.4%) and 94.5% (SE 2.6%), respectively. Distant metastasis-free probabilities for the poor- and the good-prognosis signature groups were 50.6% (SE 4.5%) and 85.2% (SE 4.3%), respectively, at 10 years. The hazard ratio for distant metastases of poor- versus the good-prognosis signature is estimated to be 5.1 (95% confidence interval: 2.9–9.0, $P < 0.001$) and retains its significance in lymph node-negative and lymph node-positive subgroups separately when the 61 tumors from the training series were excluded (Fig. 5.5). Multivariable Cox regression analysis reveals that the prognosis profile is a strong independent predictor of disease outcome.

In this way, we have validated the prognosis profile in lymph node–negative and lymph node–positive breast cancer. This profile proved to be the strongest predictor of prognosis for breast cancer and can be used to optimize adjuvant therapy selection in premenopausal breast cancer patients.

Tumor size is a major parameter used in the NIH consensus criteria for adjuvant therapy selection. However, our data show that the ability to develop distant metastases is only partially dependent on tumor size and suggest that metastatic capacity in many tumors is an early and inherent genetic property. Our findings argue against the widely accepted model that metastatic potential is acquired relatively late during multistep tumorigenesis.[23] The notion that metastatic ability in breast cancer is programmed early in tumorigenesis allows prognostic testing for disease outcome, which is likely to be beneficial. Conversely, early onset of metastatic capability theoretically limits the benefit of early detection and intervention in breast cancer. Furthermore, our findings suggest that the molecular mechanism leading to hematogenic (distant) metastases is distinct from lymphogenic (regional) spread of tumor cells and indicate that our prognosis profile is independent of lymphogenic metastases. This is based on our experimental observation that the prognosis profile is strongly predictive of hematogenic metastases, both in lymph node–negative and in lymph node–positive patients.

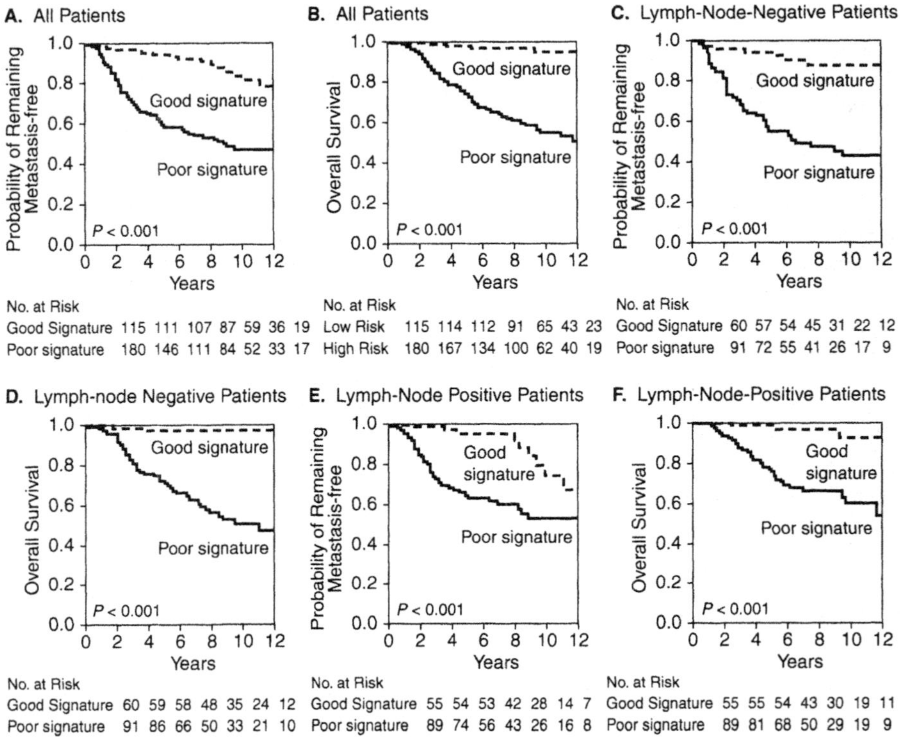

FIGURE 5.5 Kaplan-Meier analysis of the probability that patients would remain free of distant metastases and the probability of overall survival among all patients (panels A, and B, respectively), patients with lymph node-negative disease (panels C and D, respectively), and patients with lymph-node positive disease (panels E and F, respectively) according to whether they had a good-prognosis or a poor-prognosis signature. The *P* values were calculated with use of the log-rank test. (With permission from the Ref. 22.)

FUTURE DEVELOPMENTS

To validate the possibility of microarray use in treatment tailoring, we will perform microarray analysis of all breast carcinomas at the microarray facility of the Netherlands Cancer Institute. We are currently developing a high-throughput facility, and we will implement quality control to perform diagnostic microarray analysis. On each breast cancer sample, we will analyze the expression of the 70 genes of the prognosis gene expression profile we have previously identified. Based on this gene expression pattern, tumors will be assigned to the good-prognosis or the poor-prognosis profile group. In addition, we will correlate the expression pattern of all genes to other clinical endpoints, most importantly local recurrence, response to hormonal treatment, and chemotherapy. Radiotherapy and adjuvant systemic treatment will be validated and later tailored according to gene expression pattern trials. (Fig. 5.6).

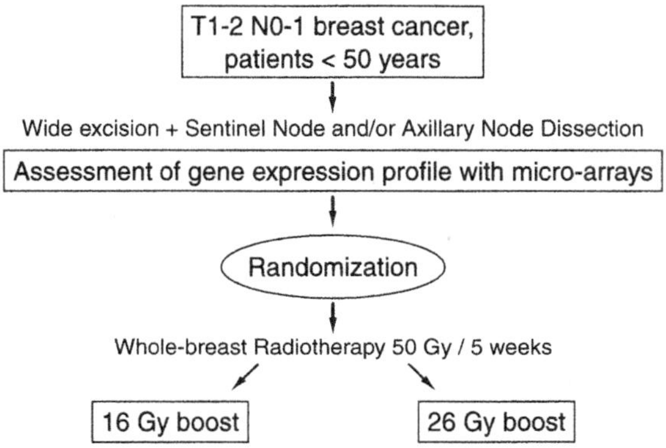

FIGURE 5.6 Design of a randomized phase III trial to prospectively validate the value of microarrays in predicting the need for more aggressive radiotherapy in an individual patient.

REFERENCES

1. Bonnier P, Romain S, Charpin C et al. Age as a prognostic factor in breast cancer: relationship to pathologic and biologic features. Int J Cancer 1995;62:138–144.
2. Albain KS, Allred DC, Clark GM. Breast cancer outcome and predictors of outcome: are there age differentials? J Natl Cancer Inst Monogr 1994;16:35–42.
3. De la Rochefordière A, Asselain B, Campana F et al. Age as prognostic factor in premenopausal breast carcinoma. Lancet 1993;341:1039–1043.
4. Kollias J, Elston CW, Ellis IO et al. Early-onset breast cancer: histopathological and prognostic considerations. Br J Cancer 1997;75:1318–1323.
5. Nixon AJ, Neuberg D, Hayes DF et al. Relationship of patient age to pathologic features of the tumor and prognosis for patients with stage I or II breast cancer. J Clin Oncol 1994;12:888–894.
6. Winchester DP, Osteen RT, Menck HR. The National Cancer Data Base report on breast carcinoma characteristics and outcome in relation to age. Cancer 1996;78:1838–1843.
7. Marcus JN, Watson P, Page DL et al. Pathology and heredity of breast cancer in younger women. J Natl Cancer Inst Monogr 1994;16:23–34.
8. Crowe JP, Gordon NH, Shenk RR et al. Age does not predict breast cancer outcome. Arch Surg 1994;129:483–488.
9. Halverson KJ, Perez CA, Taylor ME et al. Age as a prognostic factor for breast and regional nodal recurrence following breast conserving surgery and irradiation in stage I an II breast cancer. Int J Radiat Oncol Biol Phys 1993; 27:1045–1050.

10. Remvikos Y, Magdelenat H, Dutrillaux B. Genetic evolution of breast cancers III: age-dependent variations in the correlations between biological indicators of prognosis. Breast Cancer Res Treat 1995;34:25–33.
11. Fowble BL, Schultz DJ, Overmoyer B et al. The influence of young age on outcome in early stage breast cancer. Int J Radiat Oncol Biol Phys 1994;30:23–33.
12. Recht A, Connolly JL, Schnitt SJ et al. The effect of young age on tumor recurrence in the treated breast after conservative surgery and radiotherapy. Int J Radiat Oncol Biol Phys 1988;14:3–10.
13. Bartelink H, Horiot JC, Poortmans P et al. Recurrence rates after treatment of breast cancer with standard radiotherapy with or without additional radiation. N Engl J Med 2001;345;1378–1387.
14. Sarrazin D, Lê MG, Arriagada R et al. Ten-year results of a randomized trial comparing a conservative treatment to mastectomy in early breast cancer. Radiother Oncol 1989;14:177–184.
15. van't Veer LJ, Dai H, van de Vijver MJ et al. Gene expression profiling predicts clinical outcome of breast cancer. Nature 2002;415:530–536.
16. Sorlie T, Perou CM, Tibshirani R et al. Gene expression patterns of breast carcinomas distinguish tumor subclasses with clinical implications. Proc Natl Acad Sci USA 2001;98:10869–10874
17. Perou CM, Sorlie T, Eisen MB et al. Molecular portraits of human breast tumors. Nature 2000;406:747–752.
18. Ross DT, Scherf U, Eisen MB et al. Systematic variation in gene expression patterns in human cancer cell lines. Nat Genet 2000;24:227–235.
19. Perou CM, Jeffrey SS, van de Rijn M et al. Distinctive gene expression patterns in human mammary epithelial cells and breast cancers. Proc Natl Acad Sci USA 1999;96:9212–9217.
20. Pollack JR, Perou CM, Alizadeh AA et al. Genome-wide analysis of DNA copy-number changes using cDNA microarrays. Nat Genet 1999;23:41–46.
21. Hedenfalk I, Duggan D, Chen Y et al. Gene-expression profiles in hereditary breast cancer. N Engl J Med 2001;344:539–548.
22. van de Vijver MJ, Yuhong DH, van't Veer LJ et al. A gene expression signature as a predictor of survival in breast cancer. N Engl J Med 2002;347:1999–2009.
23. Bernards R, Weinberg RA. A progression puzzle. Nature 2002; 22:418:823.

Chapter 6

Vascular Targeted Molecular Imaging and Therapy

King C. P. Li

Samira Guccione

Mark D. Bednarski

A critical early step in many inflammatory or immune responses is the promotion of leukocyte adhesion to the vascular endothelium. The realization that unique molecules called cell adhesion molecules are expressed by endothelial cells during various physiologic and disease processes has led to extensive research in characterizing and manipulating these molecules.[1-5] Multiple endothelial ligands and receptors are now known to be up-regulated during various pathologies[6,7] and can potentially serve as molecular targets for diagnostic and/or therapeutic agents. There are many well-known physiologic barriers to the delivery of macromolecules, particles, and monoclonal antibodies to specific tissues in vivo. A blood-borne molecule that enters the circulation of the target tissue reaches the target cells via (1) distribution through vascular space, (2) transport across the microvascular wall, and (3) transport through the interstitial space. During this journey, these materials may bind nonspecifically to proteins or other tissue components, bind specifically to the targets, and/or be metabolized. The experience obtained from years of immunoscintigraphy research suggests that even in the ideal case, only 0.001% to 0.01% of intravenously administered monoclonal antibodies will reach and bind to target tissues in humans.[8] To reach the target sites on the surface of the endothelium, monoclonal antibodies and ligands do not need to be transported across the microvascular wall or through the interstitial space, dramatically decreasing the chances of losing these agents to metabolism and to nonspecific binding to proteins and other tissue components. Because of the significance and accessibility of endothelial receptors, they are superb molecular targets for new diagnostic and therapeutic agents. This chapter summarizes our results in designing a platform technology that allows us to deliver different therapeutic and diagnostic agents to activated endothelium by use of antibodies and ligands as the targeting moieties.

POLYMERIZED NANOPARTICLES AS A DELIVERY VEHICLE FOR ENDOTHELIAL RECEPTORS

The ideal vehicle for targeted delivery to endothelial receptors should have the following properties: (1) biocompatibility; (2) sufficiently long intravascular half-life to allow for repeated passage through, and interactions with, the activated endothelium; (3) ability to have ligands and proteins conjugated on the surface in multivalent configuration to increase the affinity and avidity of interactions with endothelial receptors; (4) ability to have functional groups for high-affinity surface metal chelation; (5) ability to encapsulate drugs; and (6) capability to have both imaging and therapeutic agents loaded on the same vehicle. Liposomes have been extensively studied as drug delivery vehicles and stealth liposome–encapsulated doxorubicin (Doxil) is now commercially available.[9-12] However, a major drawback of conventional liposomal particles is their lack of stability. It is difficult for these particles to withstand the chemical modifications needed to attach antibodies and ligands to their surface. Therefore, despite their attractiveness, we feel that the use of conventional liposomes in receptor-targeted imaging would be problematic. We have chosen to develop polymerized nanoparticles (NPs) rather than conventional liposomes as our targeting vehicle because they are rigid and therefore do not easily fuse with cell membranes, and they possess surface functional groups that can be used to attach other targeting molecules and sufficient numbers of metal ions. Polymerized NPs are composed of amphiphilic lipid molecules with polar head groups and hydrophobic tails that form aggregated bilayer type structures in aqueous solution.[13,14] A functional group (diacetylene) can be incorporated into the tail portion of the lipids, which on irradiation with ultraviolet light, cross-link, polymerizing the lipids into structurally stable particles. These particles then serve as a scaffold for the attachment of antibodies, ligands, contrast ions, and therapeutic agents for imaging and therapy.[15,16] Moreover, the size distribution and rigidity of these particles can be chosen to avoid rapid clearance by the reticuloendothelial system, and the particle surface can be modified with ethylene glycol to further increase intravascular recirculation times.[13,14]

PARAMAGNETIC POLYMERIZED NANOPARTICLES AS TARGETED MRI CONTRAST AGENTS

Magnetic resonance imaging (MRI) provides exquisite morphologic information for diagnosing and monitoring many diseases. However, the lack of specificity of the signal contrast on magnetic resonance images limits its use in many situations. This has stimulated the development of contrast agents for MRI. Contrast agents that can bind to cell surface molecules can, in principle, be used to image the presence of cell surface markers in a manner similar to that of standard histological techniques. MRI, however, operates on living systems and thereby allows analysis of cell surface changes in vivo and in nearly real time. Changes due to pharmacological interventions, physiologic control, and progress of disease as they relate to the expression and changes in cell surfaces at the molecular level can be investigated without having to sacrifice the animal subjects or sample tissues using image-guided biopsies. The advantages of MRI using targeted contrast agents over immunoscintigraphy include higher spatial resolution and no ionizing radiation. The disadvantage is the difficulty in attaching sufficiently high concentrations of metal ions to cell surface receptors so that they are detectable by MRI. With polymerized NPs, a large number of paramagnetic metal ions can be bound to the surface of each NP, increasing the concentration of metal ions that can be attached to each cell surface receptor by five to six orders of magnitude. Therefore, we began to investigate the possibility of using paramagnetic polymerized NPs as potential targeted MRI contrast agents.

Paramagnetic Polymerized Nanoparticles: Synthesis and Characterization

We have designed and constructed a unique paramagnetic particle based on the use of polymerizable lipid molecules. Amphiphilic lipid molecules that contain a polar head group and a hydrophobic tail group often form aggregated bilayer-type structures in aqueous solutions similar to cell membranes. We have incorporated a functional group (diacetylene) into the tail portion of a lipid that forms NPs that will polymerize on irradiation with ultraviolet light (Fig. 6.1). As opposed to conventional liposomes, polymerized NPs are more structurally stable particles.[13,14] These NPs then serve as a scaffold for the attachment of both paramagnetic contrast agents and targeting groups. We have successfully synthesized and characterized paramagnetic polymerized NPs and have studied the use of these NPs as MRI contrast agents.

The NPs are uniquely suited as a scaffold for targeted contrast agents because their size can be readily controlled, targeting groups can be easily attached to their surface, and they are well tolerated in vivo (Fig. 6.2). The control of surface group functionality can be used to avoid phagocytosis by the reticuloendothelial system. In addition, the density of metal atoms that generate the contrast in MRI

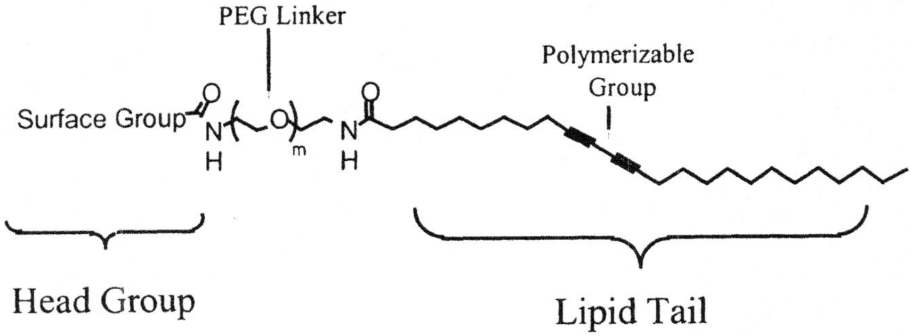

FIGURE 6.1 Schematic diagram demonstrating the basic structures of the lipid structure used in the formation of the polymerized nanoparticles. The lipids contain a functional head group, a polymerizable group (diacetylene), and a lipid tail.

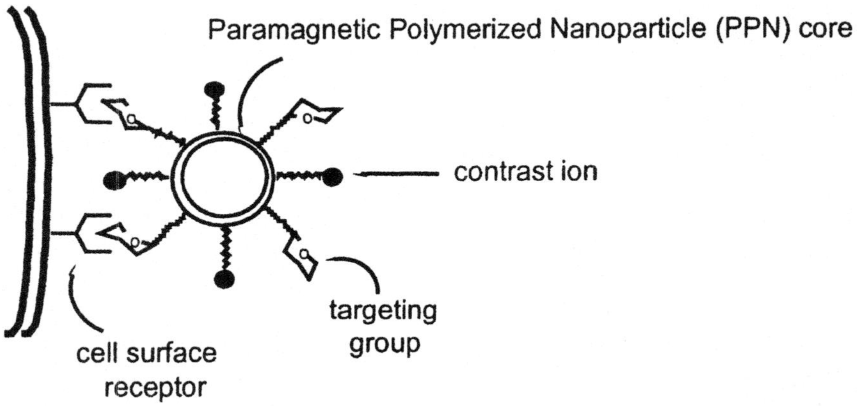

FIGURE 6.2 Diagram illustrating how paramagnetic polymerized nanoparticles with targeting groups on the surface can theoretically interact with cell surface receptors in a multivalent fashion

can be varied by simply changing the lipid composition before the formation and polymerization of the particle.

Lipid Synthesis

The construction of NPs begins with the synthesis of a unique lipid-containing pentacosadiynoic acid (PDA) conjugated to diethylenetriamine pentaacetic acid (DTPA) via a variable-length polyethylene glycol (PEG) linker (Fig. 6.1). These amphipathic molecules have metal chelates as head groups connected to a lipid tail that contains a polymerizable diactylene moiety. The linker length can be controlled by the choice of commercially available polyethylene glycol derivatives. In addition to providing unusual versatility as a spacer, the use of PEG link-

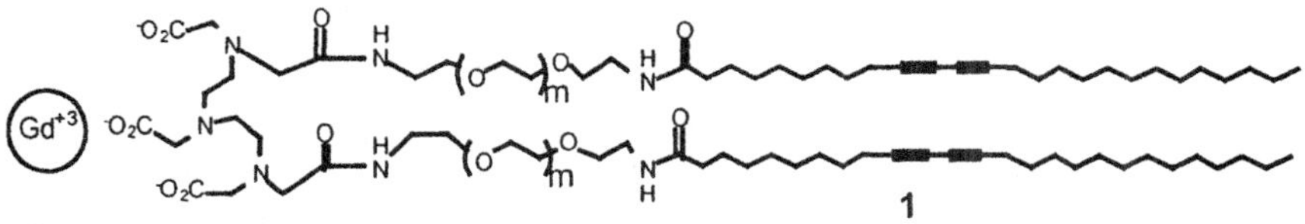

1

FIGURE 6.3 Diagram illustrating the chemical structure of a polymerizable lipid with a gadolinium diethylenetriamine pentaacetic acid (Gd-DTPA) head group.

ers on the surface of NPs has the potential of increasing recirculation of these particles in the blood pool by evasion of the reticuloendothelial system. Specifically, we have synthesized compound 1 by reacting the lipid (PDA) with the linker (PEG_3-$(NH_2)_2$) via the NHS ester, then reacting this conjugate with DTPA dianhydride to form DTPA-bis(PEG_3-PDA)diamide (Fig. 6.3). This is followed by treatment with gadolinium trichloride ($GdCl_3$) to form a neutral amphophilic gadolinium chelate 1 (m = 1).

This compound is then mixed with a "matrix lipid" of diacetylenic phosphatidyl choline (DAPC, 2) in order to control the surface density of the metal on the NP. The matrix lipid (DAPC) is well known to form polymerizable NPs under various conditions and was chosen to closely mimic the topology of native cell membranes. To ensure the miscibility of the two lipids, we conducted Langmuir-Blodgett trough experiments on mixtures of compound 1 and DAPC. In these experiments, the lipid mixture, in organic solvent, is applied to the surface of a trough of water. After the organic solvent evaporates, the surface is compressed via a movable Teflon dam, and the surface pressure is measured as a function of surface area. The resulting pressure-area isotherms exhibit plateaus as the lipids undergo phase transitions, the pressure of which can be interpreted to determine the miscibility of the lipid components. Our experiments show that compound 1 is miscible with DAPC up to 15 mol %, above which the pressure-area isotherm shows evidence of phase separation of the two compounds.

Formation of Paramagnetic Polymerized Nanoparticles

To form the NPs, compound 1 is doped into the DAPC matrix in organic solvent. The organic solvent is removed by evaporation, and the dried lipid film is hydrated to a known lipid density (15 mM of total lipid) with the desired aqueous buffer, generally distilled water. The resulting suspension is sonicated at temperatures above the gel-liquid crystal phase transition for DAPC (T_m = 37°C) with a probe-tip sonicator. This produces a nearly clear, colorless solution of emulsified lipid vesicles, or NPs (Fig. 6.4).

We have determined by transmission electron microscopy that these nanoparticles are 150–200 nm in diameter. Their size can be reduced by extrusion of the suspension through polycarbonate filters with well-defined porosity at

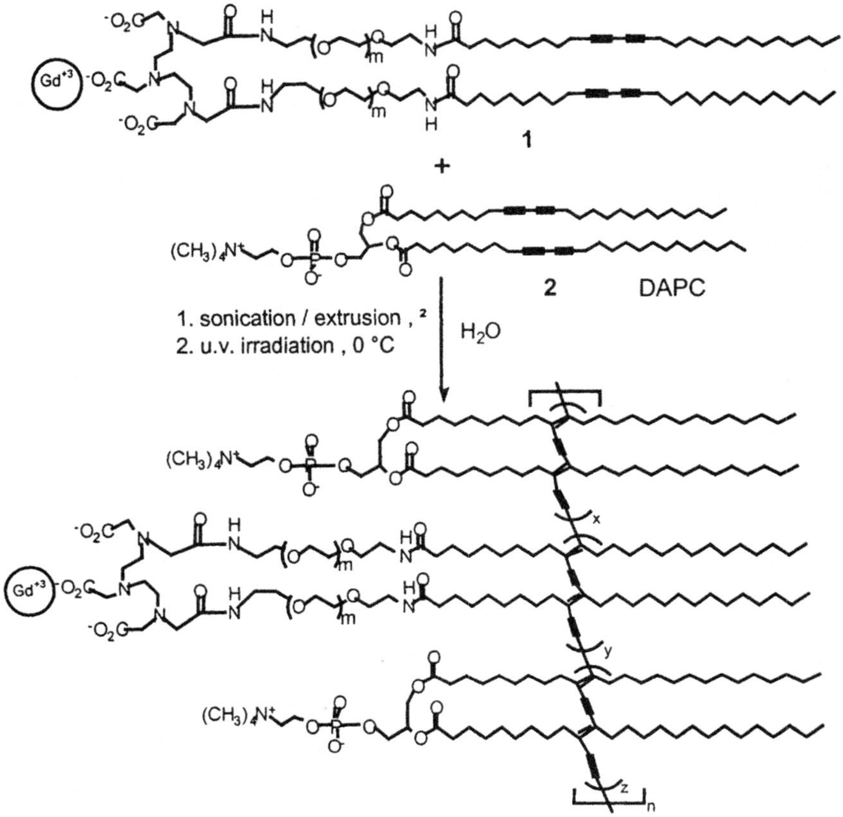

FIGURE 6.4 Diagram illustrating the formation of a paramagnetic polymerized nanoparticle.

temperatures greater that the T_m. After forming NPs of the desired size by extrusion, they are polymerized by cooling the solution to 4°C on a bed of wet ice and irradiating the solution at 254 nm with a hand-held ultraviolet lamp. The resulting NPs are orange, having two visible absorption bands centered at 490 and 510 nm arising from the conjugated ene-yne diacetylene polymer.[13]

Antibody-Conjugated Polymerized Nanoparticle Synthesis and Characterization

To conjugate monoclonal antibodies to NPs, we constructed a particle containing biotinylated lipids. Via biotin molecules on the particle surface, an avidin bridge was utilized to attach biotinylated antibodies (Fig. 6.5).[15,16] NPs containing 0.5% biotinylated lipid (2), 29.5% Gd(+3) chelator lipid (1b), 10% amine-terminated lipid (6), and 60% filler lipid (PDA) (4) were formed as outlined in

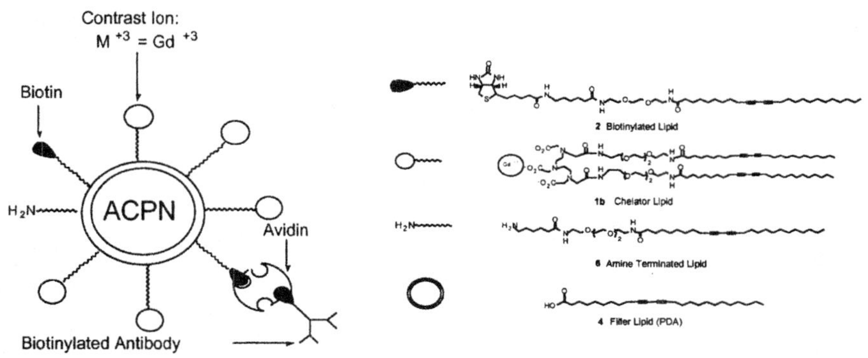

FIGURE 6.5. Schematic representation of an antibody-conjugated polymerized nanoparticle (ACPN).

the previous section. The resulting NPs are dark blue, with absorption bands at 544, 588, and 638 nm (absorption maxima, λ_{max}), but gentle heating turns them red (absorption maxima at 498 and 538 nm). All NPs used in our studies were converted to the red form.

IMAGING OF INTEGRIN UP-REGULATION IN TUMOR NEOVASCULATURE

Tumor-Induced Angiogenesis

Currently, the diagnosis and treatment of solid tumors usually begins at a late stage, when many years of cancer progression have already occurred, and most patients already have occult or overt metastasis. As early as in 1975, Folkman[22] put forward the now-classic postulate that tumors beyond 1-2 mm in size depend on the growth of new vessels, or angiogenesis. There is also increasing evidence that angiogenesis plays an important role in malignant transformation. Because a vascular supply is essential for the growth of malignant tumors and for the development of metastasis, if tumor-induced angiogenesis can be detected in vivo, the diagnosis of solid tumors can be made many years before the capacity of the tumors has been unleashed. Angiogenic factors are hypothesized to directly impact vascular cell adhesion events, which are thought to play a significant role in angiogenesis.[17,18] The adhesion receptor integrin $\alpha_v\beta_3$ has been identified as a marker of angiogenic vascular tissue and may be a useful diagnostic or therapeutic target for diseases characterized by neovascularization, such as cancer. Because angiogenesis is common to all cancers, this marker may be useful for detecting and monitoring cancers. A monoclonal antibody (LM609) directed to $\alpha_v\beta_3$, has been demonstrated to promote tumor regression by inducing apoptosis of angiogenic blood vessels in human melanomas and breast cancers in SCID mouse/human chimeric models.[19,20] LM609 is ideally suited for incorporation into antibody-conjugated polymerized nanoparticles (ACPNs) to be used for in vivo MRI detection of tumor-induced angiogenesis.

Target-Specific MRI for Detection of Integrin Up-Regulation in Tumor Neovasculature

In order to test the hypothesis that LM609-labeled ACPNs can be used to detect $\alpha_v\beta_3$ up-regulation in tumor neovasculature, we inoculated V2 carcinoma cells into the thigh muscle or subcutaneously into the flanks of New Zealand white rabbits. Imaging experiments were carried out when a palpable tumor (approximately 1–3 cm) was established. For in vivo MRI studies, rabbits were injected intravenously with either 5 mL/kg of LM609-labeled ACPNs (1 mg of antibody/kg, 0.005 mmol of Gd^{+3}/kg) or control ACPNs with isotype-matched control antibodies. MRI was performed using an extremity coil in a 1.5 T GE Signa MR imager. The following MRI parameters were: repetition time, TR = 300 milliseconds, echo time, TE = 18 milliseconds, number of excitations = 2, field of view = 16 cm, 256 × 256 matrix, section thickness = 3 mm. Magnetic resonance images were obtained immediately before contrast injection and immediately, 30 minutes, 1 hour, and 24 hours after contrast injection in the coronal plane. The tumor tissues were harvested for immunohistochemical studies immediately after the MRI experiments. Figure 6.6 illustrates the magnetic resonance findings of a V2 carcinoma–carrying rabbit injected with LM609-labeled ACPNs. Immediately, 30 minutes, and 1 hour after contrast injection, no noticeable enhancement of the tumor or tumor margin occurred, compared with the precontrast image (A), whereas at 24 hours after contrast injection (B), enhancement of the

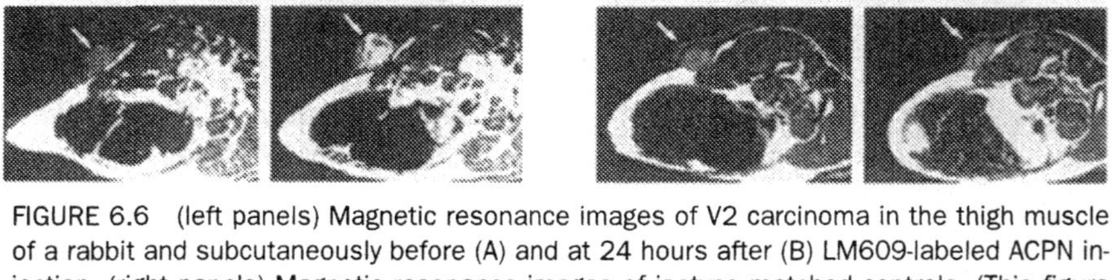

FIGURE 6.6 (left panels) Magnetic resonance images of V2 carcinoma in the thigh muscle of a rabbit and subcutaneously before (A) and at 24 hours after (B) LM609-labeled ACPN injection. (right panels) Magnetic resonance images of isotype matched controls. (This figure is adapted with permission from Sipkins DA, Cheresh DA, Kazemi MR et al. Detection of tumor angiogenesis in vivo by $\alpha_v\beta_3$-targeted magnetic resonance imaging. Nat Med 1998;4:623–626.)

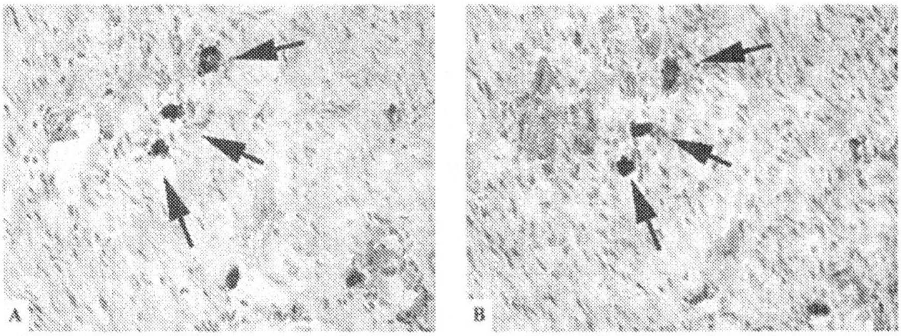

FIGURE 6.7 Immunohistochemical slides taken at the tumor margin of the same rabbit shown in Figure 6.6. **A**, Staining using anti-$\alpha_v\beta_3$ antibodies; **B**, staining using polyclonal anti-mouse antibodies, which should bind to the LM609 antibodies on the antibody-conjugated polymerized liposomes (ACPNs). *Arrows* indicate the most prominently stained areas. (Adapted with permission from Sipkins DA, Cheresh DA, Kazemi MR et al. Detection of tumor angiogenesis in vivo by $\alpha_v\beta_3$-targeted magnetic resonance imaging. Nat Med 1998;4:623–626.)

tumor margin is clearly visible. Low-contrast enhancement 24 hours after contrast injection was observed with the isotype control ACPNs in both tumor models (compare images C with D in Fig. 6).

Figure 6.7 illustrates immunohistochemical slides taken at the tumor margin of the same rabbit shown in Figure 6.6. Figure 6.7A was stained using anti-$\alpha_v\beta_3$ antibodies, and Figure 6.7B was stained using polyclonal anti-mouse antibodies, which should bind to the LM609 antibodies on the ACPNs. The stained regions in Figure 6.7A and Figure 6.7B are identical, showing that the LM609-labeled ACPNs have indeed localized to the sites of $\alpha_v\beta_3$ up-regulation. Therefore, immunohistochemistry results validated that enhancement seen on MRI enhanced with LM609-labeled ACPNs corresponded to sites of activated endothelium with $\alpha_v\beta_3$ up-regulation. In addition, the ACPNs are localized to the vessels and are not distributed throughout the tumor cells.

TARGET-SPECIFIC IMMUNOSCINTIGRAPHY FOR THE DETECTION OF INTEGRIN UP-REGULATION IN TUMOR NEOVASCULATURE

We have also investigated imaging of a solid tumor with LM609 ACPNs labeled with indium 111 (^{111}In). LM609-^{111}In ACPNs were injected intravenously into rabbits with Vx2 carcinoma in their thighs. Scintigraphic imaging was then performed using 100 nm of LM609-^{111}In ACPNs. The tumor volume was approximately 3 cm^3 when the imaging experiments were carried out. Scintigraphic imaging was performed over a 72-hour period and showed accumulation of 22% of the total injected radiation in the tumor at 72 hours, relative to 3% for the ^{111}In NPs, which lack the LM609 antibody. The accumulation of the ACPNs represents approximately 1% of the injected dose per gram of tumor tissue. The target-to-background ratio of the dose to the tumor vasculature is extremely high because of confinement of the ACPNs to the tumor vasculature, which represents a small fraction of the total tumor mass, which in turn is a small fraction of the total body mass. The blood pool half-life was 18 hours for the LM609-^{111}In ACPNs and was similar to the that of the ^{111}In NPs without antibody.

USING POLYMERIZED NANOPARTICLES FOR TARGET-SPECIFIC THERAPY

The concept of angiogenesis in cancer biology was introduced in the 1970s, and since the seminal work by Folkman,[22] tumor vasculature has been a primary target for antiangiogenic strategies. Systemic accessibility of tumor blood vessels is an important advantage over therapeutic approaches that target tumor cells. Antiangiogenic approaches have included: (1) liposomal doxorubicin (Doxil) as a nonspecific antiproliferative agent, which has also been shown to be an active antiangiogenesis agent; (2) combination angiostatin/endostatin treatment as a highly specific antiangiogenic endothelial therapy; (3) thalidomide, an agent that selectively blocks vascular endothelial growth factor and bFGF basic fibroblast growth factor induced endothelial cell activation, proliferation, and migration; or (4) stromelysin (MMP-3) inhibitors, a group of drugs that block the breakdown of basement membrane and extracellular matrix needed for tumor vessel growth. These approaches have had limited success in early phases of clinical trials because of the systemic dosages necessary to achieve efficacy and the difficulty that imaging modalities have accessing the in vivo therapeutic effects of these therapies.[23] A new approach to antiangiogenic therapy is to specifically target the drug to the tumor vasculature through tumor-specific endothelial cell-surface receptors. Before treatment with targeted agents, patients would be screened for these molecular targets by use of clinical molecular imaging approaches. In addition, higher doses can further be delivered to the tumor endothelium if the drug can partition inside the endothelial cells via endocytosis or enzymatic modification (intracellular trapping). Further amplification of the pharmaceutical agent can be accomplished by use of gene delivery, since its transcription and translation inside the cell provides higher amounts of the drug at the target site. Finally, gene transfer and expression can be followed up in vivo by use of new clinical molecular imaging modalities.

We have tried to use all of these strategies to induce apoptosis of the tumor vasculature by developing a targeted NP that can bind tumor vasculature with high specificity, can transport genetic material into the tumor endothelium, and can be monitored by use of molecular imaging techniques. NPs were formulated with small-molecule conjugates for targeting and with cationic materials for binding a plasmid of choice (Fig. 6.8). To target tumor vasculature, we used an integrin antagonist (IA) that binds the integrin $\alpha_v\beta_3$ with high specificity (manuscript in preparation). This integrin plays a key role in endothelial cell survival

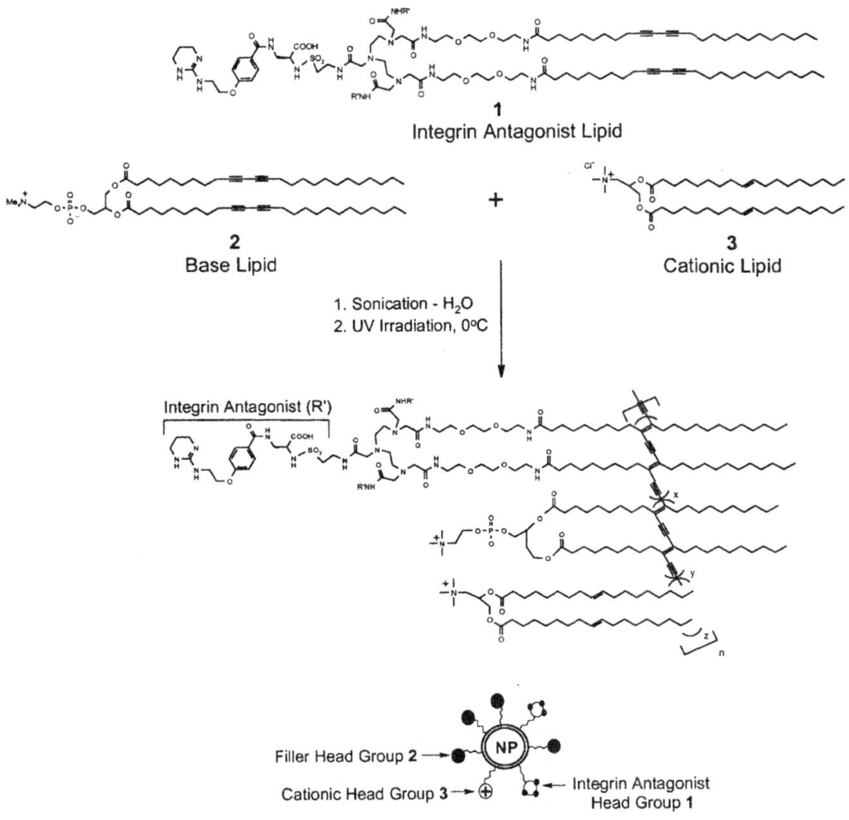

$4\alpha_v\beta_3$-NP

FIGURE 6.8 Formation of targeted nanoparticles (NPs) for gene delivery to the tumor endothelium. (Reprinted with permission from Hood JD, Bednarski MD, Frausto R et al. Tumor regression by targeted gene delivery to the neovasculature. Science 2002;296:2404–2407.)

during angiogenesis in vivo.[24] To induce apoptosis of the tumor endothelium, a plasmid with the mutant form of *Raf-1* was used for gene delivery by use of a targeted NP/plasmid complex. The disruption of the Ras-Raf-MEK-ERK pathway suppresses angiogenesis in vivo, and suppression of *Raf-1* activity has been reported to promote apoptosis.[25,26] This mutant form of *Raf-1* fails to bind adenosine triphosphate (ATP^{μ}-Raf), and has a dominant negative effect.

The screening for successful gene transfer and expression using optical molecular imaging techniques was essential for the design of successful materials before therapeutic agents were developed.[27] In vitro experiments confirmed the selective delivery of luciferase to $\alpha_v\beta_3$-positive cells in tissue culture using NPs

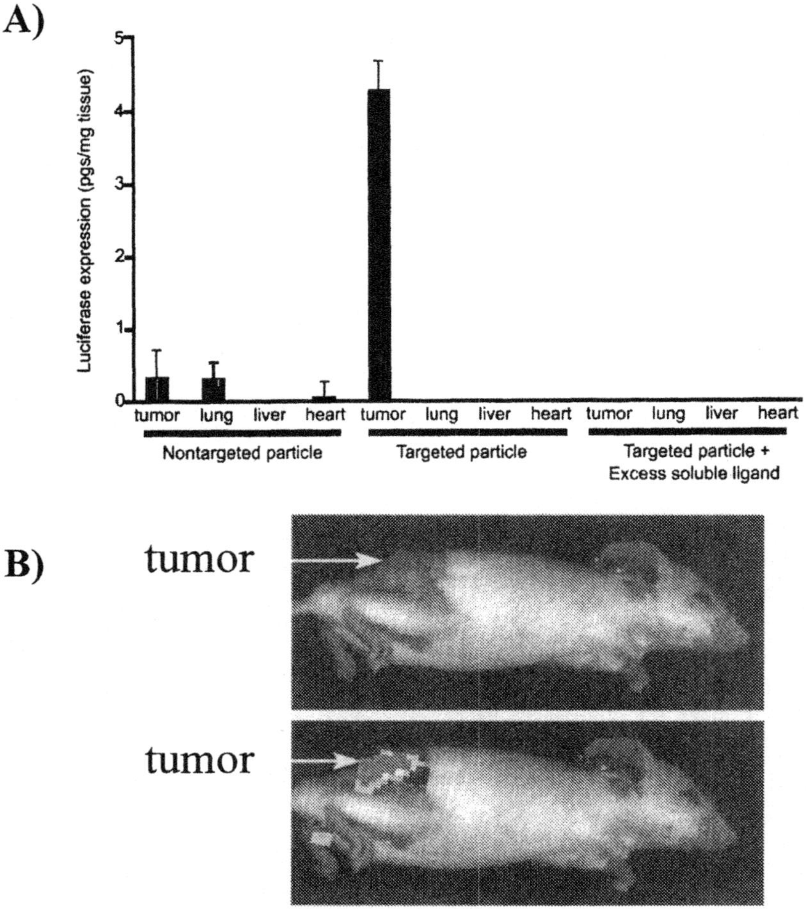

FIGURE 6.9 Evaluation of successful tumor targeting and gene expression using luciferase. **A,** In vitro quantitation of luciferase expression 24 hours after transfection with targeted nanoparticle (NP)/luciferase plasmid. **B,** In vivo imaging of luciferase expressing cells at the tumor site. (Part A of this figure adapted with permission from Hood JD, Bednarski MD, Frausto R et al. Tumor regression by targeted gene delivery to the neovasculature. Science 2002;296:2404–2407.)

with integrin antagonist (IA-NP). In vivo experiments successfully targeted and delivered the systemically introduced NP-gene complex to the angiogenic tumor-associated blood vessels by use of the gene-encoding firefly luciferase. After 24 hours, maximum luciferase expression was detected in the tumor, and minimal expression occurred in the heart and lung of the treated mice (Fig.6.9).

The therapeutic efficacy of this targeted NP/plasmid complex (IA-NP/Raf(-)) was evaluated by systemic injection of the complex in six mice bearing established 400-mm^3 M21-L tumors; these tumors do not express the integrin $\alpha_v\beta_3$. Control groups received systemic injections of the nontargeted complex (nt-

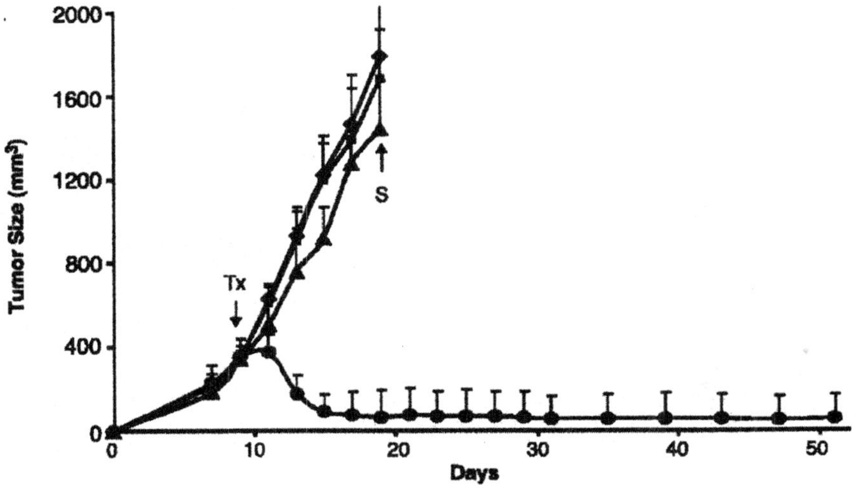

FIGURE 6.10 Tumor size measurements as a function of time. ◆ PBS, phosphate-buffered saline; ● NP-plasmid, nanoparticle-plasmid; ▲ blocking experiment; ■ targeted NP-Raf(-) plasmid. Tx, treatment; S, sacrifice. (Adapted with permission from Hood JD, Bednarski MD, Frausto R et al. Tumor regression by targeted gene delivery to the neovasculature. Science 2002;296:2404–2407.)

NP/Raf(-)), or phosphate-buffered saline (six mice with established 400-mm^3 M21-L tumors per group). Finally, a blocking experiment was performed with the co-injection of IA-NP/Raf(-) and a 20-fold molar excess of the soluble integrin antagonist. Control mice injected with phosphate-buffered saline or nt-NP/Raf(-) formed large tumors (> 1200 mm^3) within 25 days and were euthanized (Figs. 6.10 and 6.11). However, mice injected with a single injection of IA-NP/Raf(-) showed rapid tumor regression (Figs. 6.10 and 6.11), with four of the six mice showing no evidence of tumor 6 days after NP/raf treatment. The two remaining mice showed a > 95% reduction in tumor mass. Because the M21-L tumors lack $\alpha_v\beta_3$, the anti-tumor effect is based on targeting tumor endothelium and does not directly target tumor cells. It is significant that the tumor regressions were sustained for > 250 days, suggesting that the indirect effect of this approach may be widespread. Injection of excess soluble $\alpha_v\beta_3$ ligand completely blocked the anti-tumor effect of IA-NP/Raf(-) (Fig. 6.10).

Therefore, targeted delivery of the mutant *Raf-1* plasmid to the tumor endothelium resulted in a significant regression of tumor volume that was sustained for more than 270 days. These effects were based on the ability of the IA-NP/plasmid complex to promote apoptosis of the angiogenic endothelium.[28] Further evaluation of the therapeutic effect of this NP complex was tested in established syngeneic pulmonary and hepatic metastases of colon carcinoma. Murine CT-26 carcinoma cells were injected either intravenously or intrasplenically into Balb/C mice. This results in pulmonary or hepatic metastases, respectively. These metastases were allowed to establish for 10 days before treatment with the NP/gene

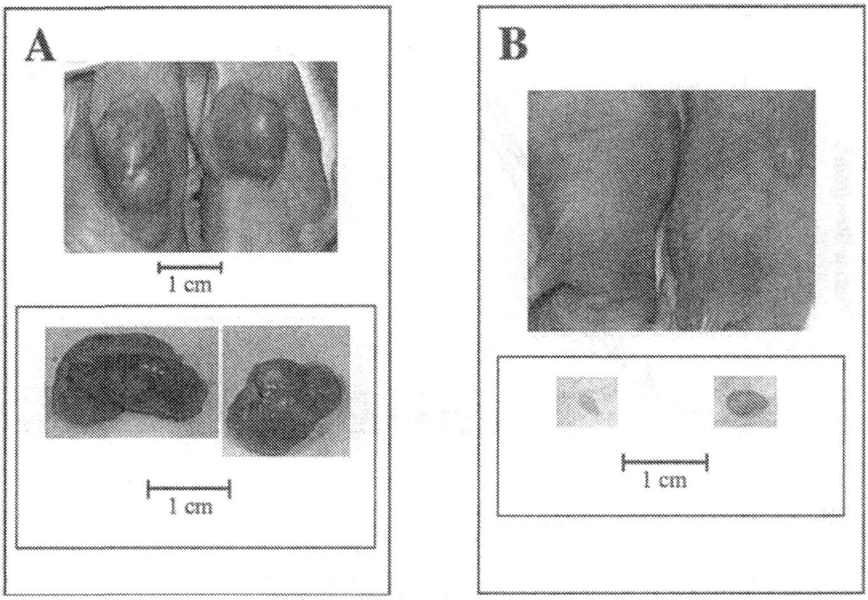

FIGURE 6.11 M21-L murine melanoma tumors control animals (*left*), animals treated with a single injection of integrin antagonist (IA)-NP-Raf(-) complex (*right*). (Adapted with permission from Hood JD, Bednarski MD, Frausto R et al. Tumor regression by targeted gene delivery to the neovasculature. Science 2002;296:2404–2407.)

complexes. Control mice were treated with phosphate-buffered saline, IA-NP complexed to a control vector, or an untargeted nt-NP/Raf(-). These control mice showed extensive tumor burden in their lungs or livers (Figs. 6.12 and 6.13). However, mice treated with IA-NP/Raf(-) had little or no visible tumor metastases, and there was a drastic reduction of the wet lung or liver weight (Figs. 6.12 and 6.13). Blocking experiments in which mice received a coinjection of IA-NP/Raf(-) and a 20-fold molar excess of the soluble targeting ligand showed tumor burden similar to that in control mice (Figs. 6.12 and 6.13).

In summary, significant and sustained tumor regressions can be achieved in mice by systemic delivery of targeted NP/gene complexes that target the tumor endothelium. There are several advantages to the approach we have developed here to facilitate clinical development. First, the NPs have a multivalent targeting capacity that can incorporate a wide array of ligands for targeted therapy. In this study, we used an IA targeting the integrin $\alpha_v\beta_3$ for selective delivery of genes to the tumor angiogenic blood vessels, but other targets can easily be evaluated. Second, we can use in vivo molecular imaging techniques to ensure NP targeting and gene expression in tumors before initiating therapy. As described earlier in this chapter, a similar particle containing gadolinium and the anti-$\alpha_v\beta_3$ targeting antibody LM609 has been successfully used to image angiogenic blood vessels in tumor-bearing rabbits.[15] Third, many plasmids are developed for gene therapy,

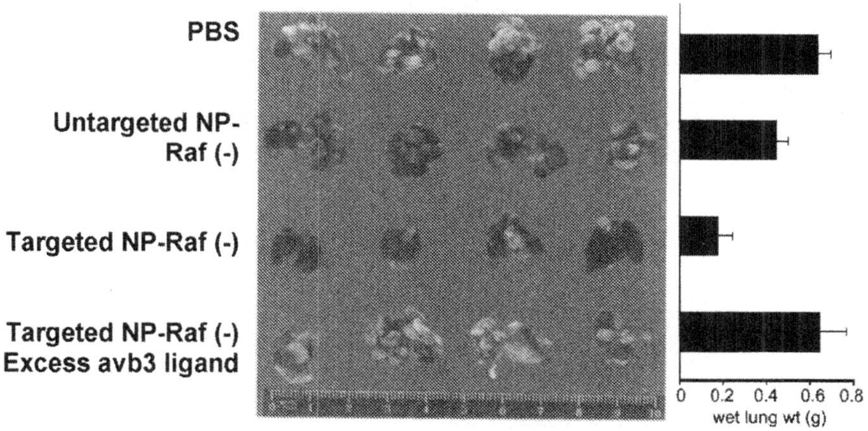

FIGURE 6.12 Representative hepatic metastases of treated and control mice with average wet weight from each experimental group shown on the right. (Adapted with permission from Hood JD, Bednarski MD, Frausto R et al. Tumor regression by targeted gene delivery to the neovasculature. Science 2002;296:2404–2407.)

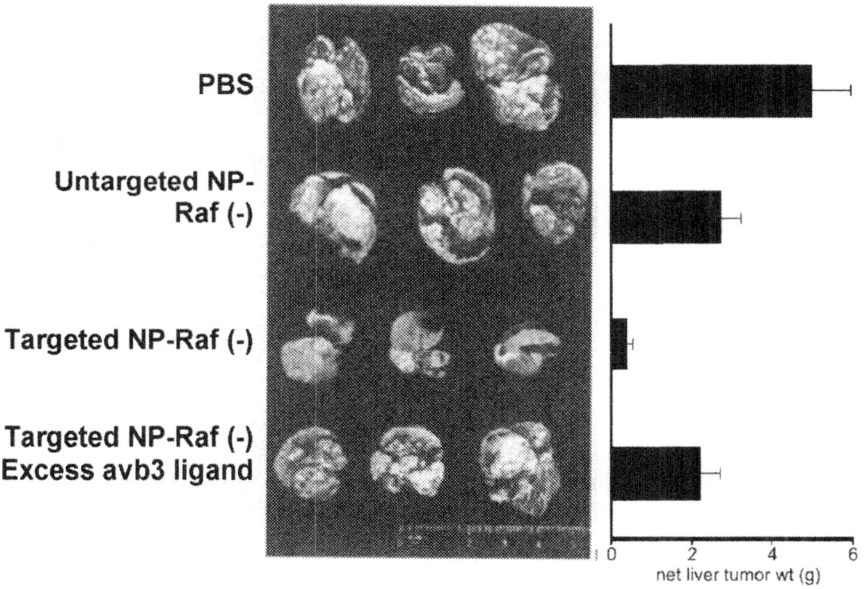

FIGURE 6.13 Representative lung metastases of treated and control mice with average wet weight from each experimental group shown on the right. (Adapted with permission from Hood JD, Bednarski MD, Frausto R et al. Tumor regression by targeted gene delivery to the neovasculature. Science 2002;296:2404–2407.)

and the efficacy of these plasmids can be evaluated by use of this vascular-targeted NP delivery system. Here, a dominant negative gene was used, with the mutant *Raf-1* gene influencing the signaling cascades of two prominent angiogenic growth factors, basic fibroblast growth factor and vascular endothelial growth factor.[29] Studies are in progress to further develop this technology for clinical oncology.

REFERENCES

1. Harlan JM, Liu DY, eds. Adhesion: Its Role in Inflammatory Disease. New York: W.H. Freeman, 1992.
2. Lasky LA. Selectins: interpreters of cell-specific carbohydrate information during inflammation. Science 1992;258:964–969.
3. Osborn L. Leukocyte adhesion to endothelium in inflammation. Cell 1990;62:3–6.
4. Springer TA. Adhesion receptors of the immune system. Nature 1990;346:425–434.
5. Stoolman L. Adhesion molecules controlling lymphocyte migration. Cell 1989;56:907–910.
6. Stoolman LM. LEC-CAMS (Selectins): Lectin-like receptors involved in leukocyte recruitment. In: Fukuda M, ed. Cell Surface Carbohydrates and Cell Development. Boca Baton, FL: CRC Press, 1992:71–98.
7. Simionescu N, Simionescu ME. Endothelial Cell Biology in Health and Disease. New York: Plenum Press, 1988.
8. Gohr-Rosenthal S, Schmitt-Willich H, Ebert W et al. The demonstration of human tumors on nude mice using gadolinium-labelled monoclonal antibodies for magnetic resonance imaging. Invest Radiol 1993;28:789–795.
9. Brandl M. Liposomes as drug carriers: a technological approach. Biotechnol Annu Rev 2001;7:59–85.
10. Lasic DD, Vallner JJ, Working PK. Sterically stabilized liposomes in cancer therapy and gene delivery. Curr Opin Mol Ther 1999;1:177–185.
11. Harrington KJ. Liposomal cancer chemotherapy: current clinical applications and future prospects. Expert Opin Investig Drugs 2001;10:1045–1061.
12. Park JW. Liposome-based drug delivery in breast cancer treatment. Breast Cancer Res 2002;4:95–99.
13. Storrs RW, Tropper FD, Li HY et al. Paramagnetic polymerized liposomes: synthesis, characterization and applications for magnetic resonance imaging. J Am Chem Soc 1995;117:7301–7306.
14. Storrs RW, Tropper FD, Li HY et al. Paramagnetic polymerized liposomes as new recirculating MR contrast agents. J Magn Reson Imaging 1995;5:719–724.
15. Sipkins DA, Cheresh DA, Kazemi MR et al. Detection of tumor angiogenesis in vivo by $\alpha_v\beta_3$-targeted magnetic resonance imaging. Nat Med 1998;4:623–626.
16. Sipkins DA, Gijbels K, Tropper FD et al. ICAM-1 expression in autoimmune encephalitis visualized using magnetic resonance imaging. J Neuroimmunol 2000;104:1–9.
17. Folkman J. The role of angiogenesis in tumor growth. Semin Cancer Biol 1992;3:65–71.
18. Kohn EC, Liotta LA. Molecular insights into cancer invasion: strategies for prevention and intervention. Cancer Res 1995;55:1856–1862.

19. Brooks PC, Clark RAF, Cheresh DA. Requirement of vascular integrin $\alpha_v\beta_3$ for angiogenesis. Science 1994;264:569–571.

20. Brooks PC, Stromblad S, Klemke R et al. Antiintegrin $\alpha_v\beta_3$ blocks human breast cancer growth and angiogenesis in human skin. J Clin Invest 1995;96:1815–1822.

21. Bednarski MD, Lee DW, Yun AJ et al. In vivo imaging of tumor angiogenesis: studies using polymerized vesicles co-labeled with indium and LM609 targeting alpha(v)beta(3) on endothelium [abstract]. Radiology 2000;217(SS):112.

22. Folkman J. Tumor angiogenesis: a possible control point in tumor growth. Ann Intern Med 1975;82:96–100.

23. Ellis LM, Liu W, Ahmad SA et al. Overview of angiogenesis: biologic implications for antiangiogenic therapy. Semin Oncol 2001:28:94–104.

24. Eliceiri BP, Cheresh DA. Adhesion events in angiogenesis. Curr Opin Cell Biol 2001;13:563–568.

25. Wickham TJ, Mathias P, Cheresh DA et al. Integrins alpha v beta 3 and alpha v beta 5 promote adenovirus internalization but not virus attachment. Cell 1993;73:309–319.

26. Felding-Habermann B, Mueller BM, Romerdahl CA et al. Involvement of integrin alpha v gene expression in human melanoma tumorigenicity. J Clin Invest 1992;89:2018–2022.

27. Contag CH, Jenkins D, Contag FR et al. Use of reporter genes for optical measurements of neoplastic disease in vivo. Neoplasia 2000;2:41–52.

28. Hood JD, Bednarski MD, Frausto R et al. Tumor regression by targeted gene delivery to the neovasculature. Science 2002;296:2404–2407.

29. Takeshita S, Tsurumi Y, Couffinahl T et al. Gene transfer of naked DNA encoding for three isoforms of vascular endothelial growth factor stimulates collateral development in vivo. Lab Invest 1996;75:487–501.

Chapter 7

New Approaches to the Prevention of GVHD and the Induction of GVL Activity After Allogeneic Stem Cell Transplantation

Ana Kostic

Stanley R. Riddell

Allogeneic hematopoietic stem cell transplantation (HSCT) is curative for a subset of patients with hematologic malignancies and for patients with inherited diseases of the hematopoietic system.[1] Acute graft-versus-host disease (GVHD), characterized by epithelial damage in the skin, gastrointestinal (GI) tract, and/or liver, is the major complication of HSCT.[2] On the basis of studies in murine models, Billingham[3] identified three factors that were essential for GVHD: (1) the graft must contain a sufficient number of immunologically competent cells, (2) the host must appear foreign to the graft and must be capable of stimulating donor cells, and (3) the host must be incapable of generating an effective immune response against the graft. T cells were identified as the critical "immunologically competent cells" in the graft, and major histocompatibility antigens (human leukocyte antigen [HLA] in humans) or minor histocompatibility antigens (mHAgs), which are presented in association with HLA molecules, were identified as the "foreign" determinants on recipient cells. Donor T cells also mediate graft-versus-leukemia (GVL) activity, as inferred from the fact that the rate of leukemia relapse for patients who received allogeneic HSCT was lower than that of patients who received syngeneic HSCT.[4] Indeed, the GVL effect associated with allogeneic HSCT represents the clearest demonstration that human malignancies can be eradicated by immunologic means. However, GVHD contributes to significant mortality after HSCT, and major improvements in survival, particularly for patients with advanced disease, will require both a reduction in GVHD and an augmentation of the GVL effect. This chapter reviews recent advances in our understanding of the complex cellular interactions involved in the pathogenesis of GVHD that are being translated into novel approaches to prevent GVHD, as well as advances in the identification of antigens expressed by leukemic cells that hold promise for selectively augmenting GVL activity.

GRAFT VERSUS HOST DISEASE

Approaches that are now used for the prevention of GVHD after allogeneic HSCT include the use of immunosuppressive drugs that interfere with T-cell activation and function, and the depletion of donor T cells from the stem cell graft. Currently available immunosuppressive drugs are effective in preventing GVHD in only a subset of patients and interfere with immunologic reconstitution and the GVL effect, resulting in infection and relapse.[5] The elimination of donor T cells from the stem cell graft is the most effective approach for preventing GVHD, but it increases the risk of graft rejection, profoundly delays immune reconstitution, and abrogates the GVL effect.[6] Thus, new approaches for preventing GVHD are needed to improve transplantation outcome.

Pathogenesis of GVHD

Major and Minor Histocompatibility Antigens Are Targets of Donor T Cells

The critical molecules recognized by donor T cells that mediate GVHD are the HLA class I and II molecules, which are encoded by genes on chromosome 6 and are ligands for engagement by $\alpha\beta^+$ T cells. Class I HLA molecules are expressed in association with β_2-microglobulin on all nucleated cells, whereas class II HLA molecules are constitutively expressed only on a subset of hematopoietic cells, including antigen-presenting cells (APCs). The HLA molecules contain a peptide-binding groove and display peptides derived from both self and foreign proteins to T cells. $CD8^+$ T cells recognize peptides derived from the proteosomal degradation of intracellular proteins and presented at the cell surface bound to class I HLA molecules.[7] CD4+ T cells recognize peptides derived by lysosomal degradation of endogenous or phagocytosed exogenous proteins and presented at the cell surface bound to class II HLA molecules.[8] The display of self-peptides contributes to the development of a T-cell repertoire that is tolerant to host cells, whereas the display of foreign peptides derived from pathogens provides for activation of T cells that recognize infected cells.

In the setting of unmodified allogeneic HSCT, the stem cell inoculum contains mature donor CD8+ and CD4+ T cells that may recognize HLA/peptide complexes displayed on recipient cells as "foreign." The most severe forms of GVHD occur after HLA-mismatched HSCT.[9] However, GVHD still occurs in 35%–70% of HLA-identical patients, depending on the age of the patient, the patient's disease status, the conditioning regimen, and whether the donor is related or unrelated.[1] This is due to recognition of recipient mHAgs, which are unique peptides presented by class I and II HLA molecules and derived from recipient proteins that differ in amino acid sequence with the homologous donor proteins as a result of polymorphism in the genome.[10]

Role of APCs in the Induction of T-Cell Responses in GVHD The requisite event in the development of GVHD is the activation and expansion of donor T cells specific for recipient minor or major histocompatibility antigens. The initiation of T-cell responses occurs in secondary lymphoid organs and requires interaction of naive T cells with specialized APCs, such as dendritic cells (DCs), activated B cells, and monocyte/macrophages. DCs are the most potent APC and are strategically located in tissues where, in their immature form, they are proficient at capturing and processing antigen from infected or damaged cells.[11] DC maturation can be induced by pathogens or cytokines and is characterized by expression of CCR-7, which promotes trafficking to secondary lymphoid organs and up-regulation of HLA, costimulatory, and adhesion molecules that provide for efficient presentation of antigen to T cells.[11] In murine models of allogeneic HSCT, both CD4+ and CD8+ T cells contribute to GVHD, although the CD8+ T-cell subset consistently induces the most severe forms of GVHD.[12]

A recent study in a murine model examined whether CD8+ T cells that mediate GVHD were activated in vivo by host APCs that persisted after the conditioning regimen or were "cross-primed" by donor APCs that had taken up recipient antigens.[13] Chimeric mice were generated to have deficient class I major histocompatibility complex (MHC) expression only on hematopoietic cells, including APCs, and were then transplanted with bone marrow containing both T cells and normal APCs from MHC-matched, multiple mHAg–mismatched donors. GVHD failed to develop in these mice, demonstrating an essential role for host APC in the induction of T-cell responses to recipient mHAgs.[13] The contribution of various subsets of host APC remains to be elucidated; however, these findings suggest that the development of strategies to eliminate or inactivate host APCs before transplantation may provide a novel approach for reducing GVHD.

Role of T-Cell Costimulation in GVHD The signal delivered by engagement of the T-cell receptor with MHC/peptide complexes on APC alone is not sufficient for the activation, expansion, and differentiation of antigen-specific T cells.[14] This requires a second signal delivered simultaneously through costimulatory receptor/ligand interactions between the T cell and the APC. The most studied costimulatory pathway involves the CD28 molecule on T cells and its CD80 and CD86 ligands on APC. CD80 and CD86 bind to CD28 and, in conjunction with a T-cell receptor signal, result in tighter formation of the immunological synapse, increased expression of the antiapoptotic protein BcL-X_L, enhanced transcription and stability of interleukin-2 (IL-2) messenger RNA, and increased IL-2 production, which together promote T-cell proliferation and survival.[14-16] However, T-cell receptor engagement in the absence of a CD28 signal induces a state of T-cell unresponsiveness or anergy, suggesting that blockade of this signal could promote tolerance.[14] CD80 and CD86 also bind CTLA-4, which is not constitutively expressed on naive T cells but is up-regulated upon their activation and has a higher affinity for binding its ligands than CD28.[17] CTLA-4 serves as a negative regulator of both CD4 and CD8 T cell responses by inhibiting IL-2 production and cell cycle progression, suggesting that under some circumstances APCs also negatively regulate T-cell responses.[17] Studies in rodent models of allogeneic HSCT have evaluated whether CD28 costimulation is required for the induction of GVHD. Transplantation of allogeneic T cells from CD28 knockout mice, or inhibition of CD80/86 with a soluble CTLA-4-Ig fusion molecule or monoclonal antibodies, reduced the severity of GVHD.[18-20] These results defined an important role for costimulation in GVHD and suggested that blockade of CD28 may be applicable to human transplantation.

Multiple other costimulatory ligands on APCs, including CD40, 4-1BB, OX40, LIGHT, and B7H, have been identified, and their individual and collective role in regulating the function, differentiation, and survival of T cells is only beginning to be revealed.[21-26] Studies in murine models have already shown that interactions between several of these ligands and their receptors on T cells are involved in the pathogenesis of GVHD (Table 7.1). Inhibition of some coreceptors, such as ICOS, may have either a positive or a negative effect on T-cell responses, depending on whether the inhibitor is delivered in the priming or in the effector phase.[25] Additional studies are likely to shed further light on these signaling pathways and their contributions to T-cell activation, expansion, and differentiation and may identify strategies that are suitable for clinical application. Recent studies in mice have already begun to explore whether combined blockade of costimulatory pathways, particularly those that have greater activity for promoting either $CD4^+$ or $CD8^+$ T-cell responses, might have synergistic effects. Blockade of the CD40-CD40L interaction alone by administration of anti CD40L mAb inhibited the proliferation and function of host-reactive $CD4^+$ T cells and provided partial protection from GVHD.[27] Similarly, blockade of LIGHT/HVEM interactions with soluble lymphotoxin β receptor-immunoglobulin (Ig) fusion

TABLE 7.1 Role of Individual Costimulatory Molecules in GVHD

T cell	APC	Result of Inhibition/Blockade	References
CD28	CD80/C8D6	↓	14, 18–20
CD40L	CD40	↓	22, 27
4-1BBL	4-1BB	↓	23
OX40L	OX40	↓	24
HVEM	LIGHT	↓	26
ICOS	B7H	↓in acute GVHD, ↑ in chronic GVHD	21, 25

Abbreviations: APC, antigen-presenting cell; GVHD, graft-versus-host disease.

protein (LTβR-Ig) inhibited anti-host CD8+ T-cell function and provided partial protection from GVHD.[26] Combined treatment with both anti-CD40L mAb and LTβR-Ig provided more effective prevention of GVHD than either agent alone and resulted in persistent anergy in host-reactive CD8+ T cells.[28] These findings suggest that manipulation of costimulatory signaling pathways that regulate priming, differentiation, and effector function of T cells, either ex vivo in the stem cell graft or in the patient, will be a promising approach for reducing GVHD.

Role of Tissue Damage in Initiating APC Activation of T Cells The conditioning regimen administered to the recipient before transplantation, which is essential to suppress host immunity and allow engraftment of donor cells, also contributes to the development of GVHD.[29] The high-dose chemotherapy and/or total body irradiation that is typically used causes extensive epithelial damage and disrupts the normal physiologic barrier to pathogens. Injury to the GI tract is particularly important because it permits translocation of bacterial lipopolysaccharides and other constituents into the circulation and regional lymphatics. Lipopolysaccharides and bacterial peptidoglycans activate monocytes via Toll-like receptors and induce the production of tumor necrosis factor-α, IL-1, and IL-12, which may contribute to direct tissue injury. They are also important for signaling the maturation of DCs, ensuring that they will be highly effective in presenting host antigens to incoming donor T cells.[30] A recent study, which addressed the location of the host lymphoid compartment where donor T cells mediating GVHD are activated, provided additional evidence for the principle role of the GI tract in GVHD pathogenesis. In this experimental model, infiltration of donor T cells into the Peyer's patch lymphoid tissue, which is the major site of luminal antigen and microorganism sampling, was essential for the induction of GVHD.[31] The results suggest that approaches that reduce the toxic effects of conditioning may have important modulating effects on the tempo of activation of donor T cells that cause GVHD.

T-Cell Effector Mechanisms in GVHD The activation of alloreactive T cells in lymphoid tissue by APCs initiates a complex cascade of events that includes the production of cytokines and chemokines, the up-regulation of cytolytic molecules such as perforin, granzyme B, and Fas ligand, and the proliferation, differentiation, and emigration of T cells to tissue sites. An increasing number of cytokines have been shown to be up-regulated in GVHD, either by elevated serum levels or inferred from analysis of tissue RNA levels. The administration of individual cytokines or cytokine inhibitors to modulate these effects in murine models of GVHD has often provided conflicting results, perhaps because these molecules have pleiotropic effects on T cells, APCs, and tissue cells and may activate different pathways, depending on the timing of administration.[32]

One area that may be amenable to clinical manipulation and has been extensively studied in murine models is $CD4^+$ T-cell cytokine production. $CD4^+$ T cells can differentiate into either Th1 cells that produce interferon gamma and IL-2, or Th2 cells that produce IL-4 and IL-10, and it is possible to influence this polarization in vitro and in vivo.[33] Thus, several studies have examined how these distinct subsets of $CD4^+$ T cells may contribute to GVHD. These studies have used a variety of approaches, including anticytokine antibodies, knockout mice lacking either the IL-4 or the interferon gamma genes, and cytokine infusions. The general conclusion is that Th1 cells have a dominant role in GVHD, although Th2 cells are also capable of mediating GVHD.[34-37] A recent study addressed this issue using donor mice that were transgenic for the HSV-TK gene under the transcriptional regulation of either the IL-4 or the IL-2 promoter to permit the selective ablation of Th2 or Th1 cells in the recipient after transplantation using ganciclovir. Cohorts of mHAg-mismatched mice were transplanted with bone marrow and T cells from either IL-4TK or IL-2TK mice, and ganciclovir was administered after transplantation. Ablation of the appropriate $CD4^+$ Th subset was confirmed, and GVHD resolved in both cohorts of mice, suggesting that both Th subsets contributed to GVHD. Taken together, these results suggest that strategies to influence T-cell polarization after human HSCT are likely to have only a modest effect on GVHD.[38]

The role of cytolytic effector mechanisms in GVHD has also been examined in murine models. Perforin/granzyme B and Fas ligand mediate cytolysis of target cells by independent mechanisms, and both have a role in the tissue injury mediated by alloreactive T cells.[39] Initial studies showed that perforin-mediated effects were important in models of class I MHC disparity, where $CD8^+$ T cells mediate GVHD, and FasL-mediated injury predominated in models of class II disparity, where $CD4^+$ T cells mediate GVHD.[40] However, FasL-mediated cytotoxicity is critical in hepatic GVHD, even when it is mediated by $CD8^+$ T cells, implying that if selective inhibition of FasL/Fas interactions could be safely accomplished, it may be possible to reduce GVHD in some organ sites.[41] This approach is conceptually attractive because GVL effects are dependent on perforin/granzyme B in murine models, and disrupting FasL/Fas interactions might preserve GVL activity.[42,43] However, additional studies are needed to determine whether the GVL effect against human leukemias is solely dependent on perforin/granzyme B.

Regulation of T-Cell Responses in GVHD There is now substantial evidence that autoreactive T-cell responses are suppressed by a subset of $CD4^+$ $CD25^+$ regulatory T cells (Trs), which inhibit CD4 and CD8 T-cell activation by various mechanisms.[42-45] These Trs also suppress T-cell responses to malignancy, and there is increasing evidence that they promote tolerance in GVHD.[46,47] In murine models, $CD4^+$ $CD25^+$ T cells are potent inhibitors of allogeneic responses in vitro, and removal of this subset from the stem cell graft or use of T cells from mice that are deficient in CD25 accelerates the development of GVHD.[47-49] Of interest, the CD28 pathway appears to be critical for the generation or activation of Trs, suggesting that co-stimulatory blockade has the potential to interfere with the generation of regulatory subsets of cells that may be important in tolerance.[50]

Novel Biologic Strategies for Prophylaxis of GVHD in Clinical HSCT

Lymphocyte depletion of the graft and pharmacologic prophylaxis with methotrexate and cyclosporin or tacrolimus have been the main modalities employed for GVHD prevention, but both have significant limitations. Newer immunosuppressive drugs, such as mycophenolate mofetil and sirolimus, are now being used clinically, and it is conceivable that new combinations of agents with differing modes of action will improve their efficacy. In addition, a variety of new biologic approaches based on insights derived from studies of GVHD pathogenesis are now being subjected to clinical trials or are poised for clinical development in the near future (Fig. 7.1).

Depletion of Donor T Cells or Host APCs The depletion of T cells from the donor graft can be accomplished by various methods, including antibody purging, $CD34^+$ selection, and physical separation. Although T-cell depletion effectively prevents GVHD without the morbidity associated with immunosuppressive drugs, its use has not resulted in improved survival. The limitations of global T-cell depletion include increased graft rejection, delayed immune reconstruction and infections, and relapse due to loss of the GVL effect.[6] Several T-cell depletion strategies are now being investigated that involve delayed infusion of subsets of donor T cells or preservation of some T cells in the graft to improve immune reconstitution and GVL activity.

T-Cell Depletion with Delayed Infusion of $CD4^+$ T Cells One approach is to administer a T-cell depleted graft and then infuse a limited number of donor $CD4^+$ T cells after the recipient has recovered from the conditioning regimen. This strategy was in part based on animal studies that showed that $CD4^+$ T cells alone were less effective in causing GVHD but could mediate some GVL activ-

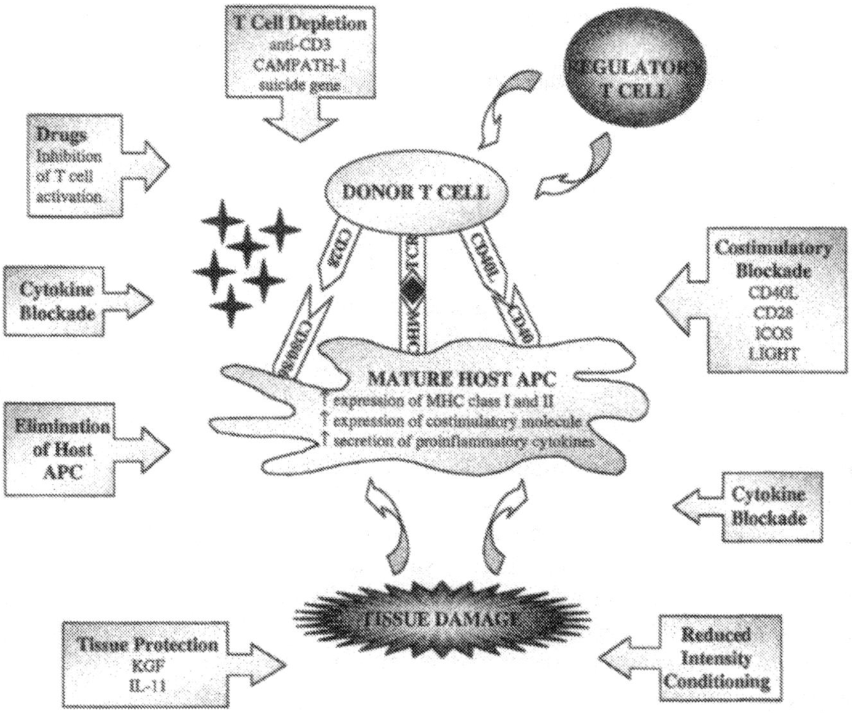

FIGURE 7.1 Potential sites of intervention for prevention of graft-versus-host disease (GVHD). The critical role of the interaction between the donor T cell and host antigen-presenting cells (APC) has identified a number of potential interventions that interfere with the activation, expansion, and differentiation of alloreactive T-cell responses.

ity.[43] A study of this approach in a small number of patients showed a low incidence of GVHD and preservation of GVL activity, particularly in CML, which is exquisitely sensitive to the GVL effect.[51]

Selective Depletion of Alloreactive T Cells Several groups have developed approaches that specifically remove alloreactive donor T cells. This typically involves coculturing donor T cells with irradiated recipient mononuclear cells in vitro, which induces activation markers on alloreactive T cells, such as CD25 and CD69, that can be used as targets for depletion by immunomagnetic isolation or with an immunotoxin.[52,53] The latter approach has recently been used in a clinical trial of HLA-mismatched HSCT in children. Only 2/15 recipients developed grade II GVHD, and there was evidence of T-cell immune reconstitution to viruses.[53] However, three of the five patients with malignancies experienced relapse, suggesting that future trials will need to carefully determine whether the GVL effect is retained with this approach.

Elimination of Alloreactive Donor T Cells Using Suicide Genes A third approach to T-cell depletion is to use retrovirus-mediated gene transfer to introduce a suicide gene into donor T cells in order to permit their ablation in vivo by administration of a nontoxic drug. The most extensively studied suicide gene is the herpes simplex virus thymidine kinase (TK) gene, which renders cells susceptible to ganciclovir. There are two published trials of suicide gene therapy in HSCT. In the first trial, TK-modified T cells were given only after the development of lymphoproliferative disease induced by Epstein-Barr virus or relapse. In the second trial, the TK-modified T cells were infused simultaneously with a T cell–depleted, HLA-identical sibling HSCT.[54,55] In both studies, GVHD developed in a subset of patients, and in most of these patients, ganciclovir administration ablated TK^+ T cells and resolved GVHD.[54,55] These results are encouraging, but several limitations were also apparent. In the second trial, 3/12 patients experienced Epstein-Barr virus lymphoproliferative disease, raising concerns about the repertoire and functional competence of the TK-modified T cells that were administered with the donor stem cells.[55] TK has also been shown to be immunogenic, which can lead to the premature elimination of the gene-modified T cells and an inadequate GVL effect. These issues may be resolved by the use of alternative transduction and culture methods, and by the development of nonimmunogenic suicide genes.[56,57] However, serious safety issues related to retrovirus-mediated gene transfer have recently been raised by the report of T-cell leukemia in a patient treated for X-linked SCID with gene-modified stem cells.[58] Thus, the potential risks and benefits of this approach may need to be reconsidered.

Depleting Host APC The demonstration in murine models that GVHD requires host APCs has suggested that strategies to delete or modulate APCs before transplantation may have a role in prevention. In a murine allogeneic HSCT model, depletion of host DCs can be accomplished by administering an anti-CD11c mAb.[13] Although a similar reagent has not yet been tested in humans, the Campath-1 mAb, which has been used extensively ex vivo and in vivo for T-cell depletion to prevent GVHD, recognizes CD52, a molecule that is expressed on both lymphocytes and some subsets of APC.[59] The administration of Campath-1 before transplantation rapidly depleted circulating DCs without affecting the recovery of donor DCs,[60] suggesting a second mechanism by which this reagent may be effective in preventing GVHD. However, because of its T cell–depleting properties, Campath-1 delays T-cell reconstitution and increases the risk of infection.[61] Thus, the development of more selective agents for ablating host APCs is eagerly awaited.

The critical role of host APCs in GVHD was also suggested by studies in haploidentical HSCT recipients. GVHD is a major concern after haploidentical HSCT, and for these transplants to be successful, donor T cells must be rigorously depleted from the stem cell inoculum. Ruggeri and coworkers[62] observed that haploidentical HSCT recipients that lacked the class I killer immunoglobulin domain receptor (KIR) ligands for donor natural killer (NK) cells developed less GVHD than recipients that expressed KIR ligands for donor NK cells. The possibility that this effect might be due to NK-mediated deletion of host APCs was addressed in a murine model. The infusion of purified NK cells into mice that lacked ligands for inhibitory receptors on the donor NK cells eliminated the need for conditioning and eliminated recipient APCs. Remarkably, the depletion of host APCs also permitted the subsequent infusion of donor T cells without GVHD. In mice whose APCs were KIR ligand compatible with donor NK cells, no reduction in APCs was achieved by NK infusion, and administration of T cells resulted in lethal GVHD.[62] These observations provide further support for the development of strategies to deplete host APCs and suggest that it may be possible to give delayed infusions of donor T cells to reconstitute immunity without severe GVHD in the subset of human haploidentical HSCT recipients that do not express the appropriate HLA molecules to interact with donor KIR.

Induction of Donor T-Cell Tolerance: *Costimulatory Blockade* The critical role of costimulatory molecules in the initiation of T-cell responses that mediate GVHD revealed by studies in murine models has encouraged efforts to apply costimulatory blockade to induce T-cell tolerance after human HSCT. The first efforts at preventing GVHD involved blockade of CD28 signaling in recipients of haploidentical HSCT.[63] In this trial, donor bone marrow was cultured ex vivo with irradiated recipient mononuclear cells in the presence of CTLA-4-Ig, a soluble form of CTLA-4 that binds with high affinity to CD80 and CD86 and inhibits interaction with CD28. This approach reduced the frequency of functional alloreactive T cells in the stem cell inoculum, and engraftment was achieved in all evaluable patients, with only three of 12 patients experiencing GVHD.[63] Larger trials are needed to confirm these preliminary results and to further analyze whether specific and selective tolerance to host antigens can be achieved with this approach. As discussed previously, many other costimulatory molecules are the focus of active research in animal models, and blockade of individual pathways alone or in combination may soon be translated to the clinical setting.

Cytokines or Regulatory T Cells to Induce T-Cell Tolerance The use of cytokines such as IL-10 and transforming growth factor-beta (TBF-β), which induce alterations in biochemical signaling in T cells that are similar to costimulatory blockade, has been investigated as a method to induce specific T-cell tolerance to alloantigens. This approach is effective both in vitro in mixed lymphocyte cultures and in murine transplant models, where ex vivo treatment of the graft prevented the induction of GVHD.[64,65]

Another promising area that is rapidly emerging is the use of immune Tr to induce T-cell tolerance. The infusion of ex vivo expanded donor $CD4^+$ $CD25^+$ Trs has resulted in significant inhibition of GVHD in murine models.[48,49] Human $CD4^+$ $CD25^+$ Trs also inhibit alloreactivity of both naive and memory $CD4^+$ T cells in vitro, and these cells can be expanded in vitro with maintenance of suppressor function.[66] Much remains to be discovered concerning the mechanism or mechanisms by which $CD25^+$ $CD4^+$ T cells function, but current data suggest that further study of the potential to manipulate this immune regulatory cell for GVHD is warranted.

Modulating the Induction Phase of GVHD: Reduced-Intensity Conditioning Studies in murine models illustrated the importance of the cytokine storm that is in part induced by the toxicity of the conditioning regimen.[32] This led to optimism that reducing the intensity of conditioning would be beneficial in reducing GVHD. The development of low-intensity regimens that were sufficiently immunosuppressive to permit engraftment of donor cells has led to a large number of transplantations being performed in older patients. However, preliminary results from these trials suggest that GVHD develops later after transplantation but with a similar incidence to that observed after conventional myeloablative HSCT.[67]

Cytokines That Inhibit Tissue Injury An alternative approach to reduce the cytokine storm is to strengthen the GI mucosal barrier before conditioning to minimize tissue injury and to prevent the entry from the GI lumen of lipopolysaccharides and other mediators that activate APCs. In murine GVHD models, two growth factors, IL-11 and keratinocyte growth factor, were able to prevent GVHD and preserved the GVL effect.[68,69] Both of these agents have progressed to clinical trials, but IL-11 was very toxic and the randomized, placebo-controlled trial examining its efficacy was closed.[70] Disappointing results were also obtained in a trial of an IL-1 receptor antagonist, which was no more effective than placebo in GVHD prevention.[71] Thus, although interruption of the "cytokine storm" is clearly effective in preventing GVHD in murine models, this strategy as currently applied has not been effective in humans.

GRAFT-VERSUS-LEUKEMIA RESPONSES

Experiments in animal models have de-monstrated the potential of immune-based approaches for cancer therapy, and allogeneic HSCT is an example that human malignancies can also be cured by an immunologic modality. The recognition that donor immune cells contained in, or derived from, the stem cell graft contribute to the eradication of malignant cells after HSCT has already led to new approaches in clinical transplantation. Donor lymphocyte infusions (DLIs) are now routinely used to treat patients who experience relapse after transplantation. Most patients who experience recurrence of chronic myelogenous leukemia (CML) after HSCT achieve a complete remission, and a smaller but significant fraction of patients who experience a relapse of multiple myeloma, acute myloid leukemia (AML), myelodysplastic syndrome, and acute lymphoblastic leukemia

(ALL) also respond to DLI.[72-74] Not unexpectedly, GVHD is the major complication of DLI.

A second approach that has evolved from the identification of the GVL effect is the use of low-intensity or nonmyeloablative conditioning, which is not sufficiently cytotoxic to induce tumor regression but suppresses host immunity and facilitates engraftment of donor cells.[75,76] In older patients, nonmyeloablative transplantations can be performed with lower toxicity than that observed with conventional myeloablative HSCT, and antitumor activity is observed in some patients with CML, CLL, multiple myeloma, lymphoma, and renal cell carcinoma.[75-78] However, despite the reduction in tissue damage with the use of less intensive conditioning, GVHD still remains a major complication of this approach. Moreover, for patients with malignancies that are less sensitive to the GVL effect, such as AML, ALL, myelodysplastic syndrome, and high-grade lymphoma, relapse is also a major obstacle to a successful outcome.

Many of the approaches for improved prophylaxis of GVHD discussed earlier are likely to interfere with GVL activity. Thus, a major challenge in allogeneic HSCT is to augment the GVL effect without causing GVHD. There is now evidence that distinct donor effector cells can contribute to GVL activity without causing GVHD, including NK cells, T cells specific for tumor-associated antigens, and T cells specific for a subset of mHAgs. Here, we review recent developments in this area and discuss strategies to selectively augment GVL activity after allogeneic HSCT that are now being introduced into the clinic.

NK Cells

NK cells recognize abnormal or transformed cells as a consequence of the integration of signals delivered through cell surface–activating and cell surface–inhibitory receptors, including KIR, C-type lectins, and natural cytotoxicity receptors.[79] Class I molecules, particularly HLA-C, serve as major ligands for inhibitory NK receptors, and NK cells are important for controlling viruses that down-regulate the expression of class I to evade recognition by $CD8^+$ cytotoxic T cells.[80,81] NK cells are not perceived to have a primary role in GVHD but have now been shown to have a critical role in the GVL effect against myeloid leukemia after allogeneic HSCT from a haploidentical donor.[62,82] In this setting, the depletion of donor T cells to prevent life-threatening GVHD eliminates any contribution of alloreactive T cells to GVL activity. However, if the recipient lacks the appropriate class I HLA-C ligands for the inhibitory KIR on donor cells, NK cells administered with the stem cell graft mediate a potent antileukemic effect against AML and virtually eliminate relapse as a cause of treatment failure.[62] Despite the lack of signaling through inhibitory KIRs, NK cells do not cause GVHD, presumably reflecting a lower sensitivity of normal epithelial cells to NK recognition.[83] Unfortunately, ALL seems resistant to this NK-mediated GVL effect, and this resistance has been attributed to lower expression of adhesion molecules on

ALL.[82] These remarkable results have raised hope that NK cells might also be harnessed after HSCT between HLA-identical individuals. However, in HLA-identical donor/recipient pairs, all donor NK cells express at least one inhibitory receptor that is specific for recipient class I MHC, and a contribution to GVL activity seems unlikely in the context of our present knowledge of NK receptor/ligand interactions.

T Cells Specific for Minor Histocompatibility Antigens

After HLA-identical HSCT, T-cell responses to mHAgs are the primary mediators of GVHD, and they are also critical for the GVL effect. In murine models of HSCT, the administration of allogeneic T cells provided a greater antileukemic effect than syngeneic T cells, suggesting that recognition of mHAgs on leukemic cells contributed to the GVL response.[84] Direct evidence for the antileukemic activity of mHAg-specific T cells was provided by studies in which the adoptive transfer of donor T cells, specific for a single murine mHAg that is abundantly expressed on hematopoietic cells, eradicated leukemic cells without causing GVHD. These data also suggested that differential tissue expression of individual mHAgs might serve as a potential basis for separating GVL effects from those of GVHD.[85,86]

Studies in humans have examined the ability of mHAg-specific T cells isolated from allogeneic HSCT recipients to recognize cells from various tissues. These studies have focused on $CD8^+$ T cells because murine models have suggested that $CD8^+$ T cells are primarily responsible for GVL activity. Some $CD8^+$ T-cell clones that have been isolated from allogeneic HSCT recipients recognize mHAgs that are broadly expressed on both hematopoietic and nonhematopoietic cells, whereas others recognize only hematopoietic cells.[87,88] The mHAg-specific T cells that were specific for hematopoietic lineage–restricted antigens also lysed leukemic cells in vitro and prevented engraftment of human leukemia in immunodeficient mice.[87,89,90] These findings have led to efforts to identify the polymorphic genes that encode such mHAgs to facilitate analysis of their frequency in the population and expression on various tissues in vivo, which should assist in defining appropriate mHAgs to induce a selective GVL effect. Several methods are being used to identify genes that encode human mHAgs. These include elution of antigenic peptides from the cell surface, followed by sequencing with mass spectrometry,[91] complementary DNA (cDNA) expression cloning,[92,93] and genetic linkage analysis.[94] A small number of autosomal and Y chromosome genes that encode mHAgs have now been discovered, and this work has identified potential opportunities to enhance the GVL effect by augmenting T-cell responses to selected mHAgs.

Y-Chromosome Genes That Encode mHAgs (H-Y Antigens) Transplantation of stem cells from a female donor into a male recipient (F→M) is a special situation in which proteins encoded by the Y chromosome that are polymorphic with their X homologues could provide mHAgs involved in GVHD and GVL responses. F→M HSCT is associated with both increased GVHD and a reduced risk of leukemic relapse when compared with HSCT between other donor/recipient gender combinations.[95] However, even after the analysis was controlled for GVHD, the risk of relapse was lower after F→M HSCT, suggesting that mHAgs encoded on the Y chromosome contribute selectively to GVL activity.[96]

Prior studies have identified T-cell responses to the SMCY protein in patients with GVHD.[97] SMCY is encoded by the Y chromosome and is ubiquitously expressed on both hematopoietic and nonhematopoietic cells. Our laboratory has searched for Y-encoded mHAgs that are preferentially expressed on hematopoietic cells and might be responsible for GVL activity in F→M HSCT. $CD8^+$ cytotoxic T lymphocytes (CTLs) were isolated from a male recipient who did not develop GVHD after HSCT from his HLA-identical sister. These recognized a novel H-Y antigen presented by HLA-B8.[93] In vitro, B8/HY-specific CTLs lysed male hematopoietic cells, including AML blasts, but did not lyse nonhematopoietic cells. Investigators using both deletion mapping and cDNA expression cloning mapped the epitope recognized by the B8/HY CTL to the UTY gene on the Y chromosome.[93] This discovery permitted analysis of UTY messenger RNA in various tissues. High levels of UTY transcripts were found in hematopoietic cells, and much lower, but still detectable, levels were observed in nonhematopoietic tissues.[93] Although the expression of UTY is not entirely selective for hematopoietic cells, the absence of GVHD in the recipient suggests that the level of gene expression in nonhematopoietic tissues may be less than the threshold necessary for T-cell recognition.

Several UTY peptides, which bind to HLA-A*0201 and are polymorphic with UTX, were identified by use of computer algorithms that predict peptides likely to bind to common class I MHC molecules and are also recognized by T cells after F→M HSCT.[98] Studies of the ability of CTLs specific for other UTY epitopes to recognize hematopoietic and nonhematopoietic cells are in progress to determine whether targeting UTY may be broadly applicable for promoting a GVL effect after F→M HSCT.

mHAgs Encoded by Autosomal Genes Autosomal genes that are selectively expressed on hematopoietic cells and encode mHAgs recognized by T cells have also been discovered by use of peptide elution and cDNA expression cloning. These include KIAA0023 and MYO1G, which encode the HA-1 and HA-2 mHAgs, respectively, that are presented by HLA-A2.[99,100] Both HA-1 and HA-2 have amino acid substitutions when compared with the homologous donor peptides, and they are selectively expressed in hematopoietic cells, suggesting that they may be appropriate targets to promote a GVL effect.[10,99,100] This was questioned when some studies linked HA-1 incompatibility with GVHD, although a recent large study failed to find a significant association with GVHD.[101] Dolstra et al[92] used cDNA expression cloning to identify an autosomal gene, *HB-1*, which encodes an mHAg presented by HLA-B44 and is expressed only in transformed

B cells, including B-ALL. The expression of HB-1 on B-ALL but not in non-hematopoietic cells suggests that it may provide a target for immunotherapy after allogeneic HSCT for ALL in HLA-B44–positive recipients.

These elegant studies have identified human mHAgs that are attractive targets to induce a selective GVL effect but have so far proved difficult to translate into therapeutic approaches in the clinical setting. The major issue is that to target one of these mHAgs, either by the adoptive transfer of T-cell clones or by vaccination, it is essential (1) that the recipient express both the appropriate HLA molecule and the mHAg and (2) that the donor lack the mHAg. The proportion of individuals that express HA-1, HA-2, and HB-1 are 69%, 95%, and 72%, respectively.[92,99,100] Thus, even though HLA-A2 and HLA-B44 are relatively common alleles, the actual number of allogeneic transplant recipients who both express these HLA alleles and are appropriately discordant for one of these three mHAgs with their donor is relatively small. Similarly, the potential utility of UTY is restricted to F→M HSCT and only to those settings in which the recipient expresses HLA molecules for which UTY peptides have been identified. Thus, identification of additional candidate mHAgs is clearly needed, and it is hoped that the development of databases on gene polymorphisms in humans that emanate from the Human Genome Project combined with new bioinformatics techniques will facilitate this effort.

T Cells Specific for Leukemia-Associated Antigens

An alternative approach to augment immunologically mediated antitumor responses after allogeneic HSCT is to target more conventional nonpolymorphic tumor antigens. Recent studies suggest that novel proteins, expressed in tumor cells as a result of chromosome translocations or mutations, or normal proteins, which are overexpressed as a consequence of aberrant differentiation, are potential targets for T cells. Proteins involved in cellular transformation, such as mutated ras and bcr/abl, represent potential tumor-specific targets.[102] Unfortunately, there is little evidence for the activation of T cells that are specific for these proteins in leukemia patients or in those who have undergone allogeneic HSCT.

Several normal proteins that are overexpressed in leukemic cells and may be associated with the malignant phenotype have been identified as potential tumor associated antigens. These include proteinase-3, Wilms tumor protein (WT-1), and survivin.[103] The analysis of genes that are highly expressed in leukemic cells by array techniques is likely to identify additional candidates in this category.[104] The data for proteinase-3 and WT-1 are briefly discussed here because efforts to employ these proteins as targets for therapy have been initiated in the clinic. Proteinase-3 is a serine protease that is expressed during normal differentiation of myeloid cells but is overexpressed (10–25 fold) in CML and AML progenitors. $CD8^+$ T cells reactive with proteinase-3 were initially isolated by stimulating lymphocytes from normal individuals with a synthetic peptide (PR-1) that was selected on the basis of its ability to bind to HLA-A2.[105] These T cells lysed leukemic cells and inhibited leukemic colony formation in vitro but had no effect on normal hematopoietic progenitors.[106] Increased numbers of T cells specific for the PR-1 epitope were found in the blood of HLA-A2–positive patients with CML who responded to allogeneic HSCT, DLI, or interferon therapy, suggesting that these T cells may mediate an antileukemic effect without interfering with normal hematopoiesis in vivo.[107]

The WT-1 protein is also expressed at high levels in acute leukemia and at low or undetectable levels in normal cells. $CD8^+$ T cells reactive with WT-1 have been isolated by in vitro culture of lymphocytes from normal individuals with synthetic peptides corresponding to WT-1 sequences that were predicted to bind to either HLA-A2 or HLA-A24.[108,109] These $CD8^+$ T cells also lyse leukemic cells in vitro without affecting normal hematopoietic colonies, suggesting that they could mediate a selective GVL effect in vivo.[110]

STRATEGIES FOR AUGMENTING GVL RESPONSES WITHOUT GVHD

Several approaches could be used to augment T-cell responses to leukemia-associated antigens or mHAgs expressed on leukemic cells after allogeneic HSCT. The adoptive transfer of T-cell clones of selected specificity is an attractive approach that may permit the establishment of T-cell responses of sufficient magnitude for efficacy. This approach has been effective in reconstituting deficient T-cell responses to CMV in allogeneic HSCT recipients who are at risk for CMV infection,[111] and recent studies using T-cell clones that are specific for antigens expressed by solid tumors have demonstrated therapeutic efficacy.[112] Techniques for eliciting T cells that are specific for leukemia-associated antigens, such as PR-3 and WT-1, from normal donors have been developed, and such cells could be adoptively transferred after allogeneic HSCT to augment GVL activity. Several issues are relevant to the development of this approach, including the difficulty isolating T cells of high avidity to epitopes from these normal self-proteins, the potential for toxicity to normal tissues that may express low levels of antigen, and the absence of a $CD4^+$ Th response to support the survival and function of transferred CTLs.[103] Despite these potential limitations, several laboratories are now poised to evaluate the safety and efficacy of this approach.

The T-cell response to mHAgs has many attributes that suggest that it also can be manipulated effectively by adoptive transfer of T-cell clones to mediate GVL activity. First, mHAgs are highly immunogenic, and most mHAg-specific T-cell clones that have been isolated after allogeneic hematopoietic cell transplantation are of high avidity, increasing the likelihood that they will recognize tumor cells that may express lower levels of MHC and/or antigen. Second, the T-cell response to mHAgs after hematopoietic cell transplantation involves both $CD8^+$ and $CD4^+$ T-cell subsets, providing the opportunity to transfer effector cells that can mediate antileukemic activity by distinct mechanisms. Finally, the T-cell response to mHAgs can be directed at multiple determinants, and this breadth of recognition may prevent the outgrowth of tumor cells that have lost or reduced levels of antigen expression.

The major obstacle that has impeded clinical application of T-cell therapy that targets mHAgs is the lack of a sufficient number of mHAgs that have been molecularly characterized and have been determined to be suitable candidates for therapy, primarily because of the technical complexity of current approaches employed for antigen discovery. It would seem most appropriate to attempt to augment T-cell responses to mHAgs that are strictly expressed on recipient hematopoietic cells to avoid causing GVHD. However, studies in a murine model have suggested that it may be possible to target mHAgs that are not completely limited in their expression to hematopoietic cells.[85] The absence of GVHD could reflect the differential sensitivity of hematopoietic and nonhematopoietic cells to recognition by T cells that are specific for this mHAg in vivo, or the ability of the transferred T cells to survive only long enough to eradicate leukemia but not mount a sustained attack on epithelial tissues. Another issue is the need for culture techniques that rapidly isolate mHAg-specific T cells that would be available for the treatment of patients who experience relapse or for the prophylaxis of patients who are at high risk for relapse. Current approaches rely on isolating the donor T cells from the recipient after transplantation to allow in vivo priming of the response. However, this approach involves a time delay and may not always be successful. Studies using the HA-1 mHAg as a model have shown that it is feasible to isolate HA-1–specific T cells from donor blood by use of dendritic cells pulsed with the HA-1 peptide or transfected with the HA-1 gene as APCs.[113]

It should soon be possible to generate T cells for adoptive transfer that are specific for antigens expressed on leukemic cells and not on tissues that are targets for GVHD. Although this approach for augmenting GVL activity is likely to be useful in many clinical settings, it is anticipated that it might be best combined with novel biologic approaches to prevent GVHD, which alone might compromise GVL activity.

ACKNOWLEDGMENTS

This work was supported by grants from the National Institutes of Health CA18029 and the Leukemia and Lymphoma Society of America. The authors thank Wendy Hilliker for assistance in the preparation of the manuscript.

REFERENCES

1. Appelbaum FR. The current status of hematopoietic cell transplantation. Annu Rev Med 2003;54:491–512.

2. Gratwohl A, Brand R, Apperley J et al. Graft-versus-host disease and outcome in HLA-identical sibling transplantations for chronic myeloid leukemia. Blood 2002;100:3877–3886.
3. Billingham RE. The biology of graft-versus-host reactions. Harvey Lect 1966;62:21–78.
4. Horowitz MM, Gale RP, Sondel PM et al. Graft-versus-leukemia reactions after bone marrow transplantation. Blood 1990;75:555–562.
5. Carlens S, Aschan J, Remberger M et al. Low-dose cyclosporine of short duration increases the risk of mild and moderate GVHD and reduces the risk of relapse in HLA-identical sibling marrow transplant recipients with leukaemia. Bone Marrow Transplant 1999;24:629–635.
6. Ho VT, Soiffer RJ. The history and future of T-cell depletion as graft-versus-host disease prophylaxis for allogeneic hematopoietic stem cell transplantation. Blood 2001;98:3192–3204.
7. Solheim JC. Class I MHC molecules: assembly and antigen presentation. Immunol Rev 1999;172:110–19.
8. Pieters J. MHC class II-restricted antigen processing and presentation. Adv Immunol 2000;75:159–208.
9. Petersdorf EW, Mickelson EM, Anasetti C et al. Effect of HLA mismatches on the outcome of hematopoietic transplants. Curr Opin Immunol 1999;11:521–526.
10. Goulmy E. Human minor histocompatibility antigens: new concepts for marrow transplantation and adoptive immunotherapy. Immunol Rev 1997;157:125–140.
11. Banchereau J, Briere F, Caux C et al. Immunobiology of dendritic cells. Annu Rev Immunol 2000;18:767–811.
12. Korngold R, Sprent J. Variable capacity of L3T4+ T cells to cause lethal graft-versus-host disease across minor histocompatibility barriers in mice. J Exp Med 1987;165:1552–1564.
13. Shlomchik WD, Couzens MS, Tang CB et al. Prevention of graft versus host disease by inactivation of host antigen-presenting cells. Science 1999;285:412–415.
14. Schwartz RH. T cell anergy. Annu Rev Immunol 2003;21:305–334.
15. Boise LH, Minn AJ, Noel PJ et al. CD28 costimulation can promote T cell survival by enhancing the expression of Bcl-XL. Immunity 1995;3:87–98.
16. Powell JD, Ragheb JA, Kitagawa-Sakakida S et al. Molecular regulation of interleukin-2 expression by CD28 co-stimulation and anergy. Immunol Rev 1998;165:287–300.
17. Chambers CA, Kuhns MS, Egen JG et al. CTLA-4-mediated inhibition in regulation of T cell responses: mechanisms and manipulation in tumor immunotherapy. Annu Rev Immunol 2001;19:565–594.
18. Yu XZ, Martin PJ, Anasetti C. Role of CD28 in acute graft-versus-host disease. Blood 1998;92:2963–2970.
19. Blazar BR, Sharpe AH, Taylor PA et al. Infusion of anti-B7.1 (CD80) and anti-B7.2 (CD86) monoclonal antibodies inhibits murine graft-versus-host disease lethality in part via direct effects on CD4+ and CD8+ T cells. J Immunol 1996;157:3250–3259.
20. Blazar BR, Taylor PA, Linsley PS et al. In vivo blockade of CD28/CTLA4: B7/BB1 interaction with CTLA4-Ig reduces lethal murine graft-versus-host disease across the major histocompatibility complex barrier in mice. Blood 1994;83:3815–3825.
21. Liang L, Sha WC. The right place at the right time: novel B7 family members regulate effector T cell responses. Curr Opin Immunol 2002;14:384–390.
22. Blazar BR, Taylor PA, Noelle RJ et al. CD4(+) T cells tolerized ex vivo to host alloantigen by anti-CD40 ligand (CD40L:CD154) antibody lose their graft-versus-host disease lethality capacity but retain nominal antigen responses. J Clin Invest 1998;102:473–482.

23. Blazar BR, Kwon BS, Panoskaltsis-Mortari A et al. Ligation of 4-1BB (CDw137) regulates graft-versus-host disease, graft-versus-leukemia, and graft rejection in allogeneic bone marrow transplant recipients. J Immunol 2001;166:3174–3183.
24. Blazar BR, Sharpe AH, Chen AI et al. Ligation of OX40 (CD134) regulates graft-versus-host disease (GVHD) and graft rejection in allogenic bone marrow transplant (BMT) recipients. Blood 2003;9:9.
25. Ogawa S, Nagamatsu G, Watanabe M et al. Opposing effects of anti-activation-inducible lymphocyte-immunomodulatory molecule/inducible costimulator antibody on the development of acute versus chronic graft-versus-host disease. J Immunol 2001;167:5741–5748.
26. Tamada K, Shimozaki K, Chapoval AI et al. Modulation of T-cell-mediated immunity in tumor and graft-versus-host disease models through the LIGHT co-stimulatory pathway. Nat Med 2000;6:283–289.
27. Blazar BR, Taylor PA, Panoskaltsis-Mortari A et al. Blockade of CD40 ligand-CD40 interaction impairs CD4+ T cell-mediated alloreactivity by inhibiting mature donor T cell expansion and function after bone marrow transplantation. J Immunol 1997;158:29–39.
28. Tamada K, Tamura H, Flies D et al. Blockade of LIGHT/LTbeta and CD40 signaling induces allospecific T cell anergy, preventing graft-versus-host disease. J Clin Invest 2002;109:549–557.
29. Gonzalez M, Quezada SA, Blazar BR et al. The balance between donor T cell anergy and suppression versus lethal graft-versus-host disease is determined by host conditioning. J Immunol 2002;169:5581–5589.
30. Barton GM, Medzhitov R. Control of adaptive immune responses by Toll-like receptors. Curr Opin Immunol 2002;14:380–383.
31. Murai M, Yoneyama H, Ezaki T et al. Peyer's patch is the essential site in initiating murine acute and lethal graft-versus-host reaction. Nat Immunol 2003;13:13.
32. Teshima T, Ferrara JL. Understanding the alloresponse: new approaches to graft-versus-host disease prevention. Semin Hematol 2002;39:15–22.
33. Dong C, Flavell RA. Th1 and Th2 cells. Curr Opin Hematol 2001;8:47–51.
34. Williamson E, Garside P, Bradley JA et al. Neutralizing IL-12 during induction of murine acute graft-versus-host disease polarizes the cytokine profile toward a Th2-type alloimmune response and confers long-term protection from disease. J Immunol 1997;159:1208–1215.
35. Murphy WJ, Welniak LA, Taub DD et al. Differential effects of the absence of interferon-gamma and IL-4 in acute graft-versus-host disease after allogeneic bone marrow transplantation in mice. J Clin Invest 1998;102:1742–1748.
36. Ellison CA, Fischer JM, HayGlass KT et al. Murine graft-versus-host disease in an F1-hybrid model using IFN-gamma gene knockout donors. J Immunol 1998;161:631–640.
37. Nikolic B, Lee S, Bronson RT et al. Th1 and Th2 mediate acute graft-versus-host disease, each with distinct end-organ targets. J Clin Invest 2000;105:1289–1298.
38. Liu J, Anderson BE, Robert ME et al. Selective T-cell subset ablation demonstrates a role for T1 and T2 cells in ongoing acute graft-versus-host disease: a model system for the reversal of disease. Blood 2001;98:3367–3375.
39. van den Brink MR, Burakoff SJ. Cytolytic pathways in haematopoietic stem-cell transplantation. Nat Rev Immunol 2002;2:273–281.
40. Graubert TA, DiPersio JF, Russell JH et al. Perforin/granzyme-dependent and independent mechanisms are both important for the development of graft-versus-host disease after murine bone marrow transplantation. J Clin Invest 1997;100:904–911.
41. Ueno Y, Ishii M, Yahagi K et al. Fas-mediated cholangiopathy in the murine model of graft versus host disease. Hepatology 2000;31:966–974.

42. Schmaltz C, Alpdogan O, Horndasch KJ et al. Differential use of Fas ligand and perforin cytotoxic pathways by donor T cells in graft-versus-host disease and graft-versus-leukemia effect. Blood 2001;97:2886–2895.

43. Hsieh MH, Patterson AE, Korngold R. T-cell subsets mediate graft-versus-myeloid leukemia responses via different cytotoxic mechanisms. Biol Blood Marrow Transplant 2000;6:231–240.

44. Shevach EM. CD4+ CD25+ suppressor T cells: more questions than answers. Nat Rev Immunol 2002;2:389–400.

45. Kursar M, Bonhagen K, Fensterle J et al. Regulatory CD4(+)CD25(+) T cells restrict memory CD8(+) T cell responses. J Exp Med 2002;196:1585–1592.

46. Liyanage UK, Moore TT, Joo HG et al. Prevalence of regulatory T cells is increased in peripheral blood and tumor microenvironment of patients with pancreas or breast adenocarcinoma. J Immunol 2002;169:2756–2761.

47. Cohen JL, Trenado A, Vasey D et al. CD4(+)CD25(+) immunoregulatory T cells: new therapeutics for graft-versus-host disease. J Exp Med 2002;196:401–406.

48. Hoffmann P, Ermann J, Edinger M et al. Donor-type CD4(+)CD25(+) regulatory T cells suppress lethal acute graft-versus-host disease after allogeneic bone marrow transplantation. J Exp Med 2002;196:389–399.

49. Taylor PA, Lees CJ, Blazar BR. The infusion of ex vivo activated and expanded CD4(+)CD25(+) immune regulatory cells inhibits graft-versus-host disease lethality. Blood 2002;99:3493–3499.

50. Johnson BD, Konkol MC, Truitt RL. CD25+ immunoregulatory T-cells of donor origin suppress alloreactivity after BMT. Biol Blood Marrow Transplant 2002;8:525–535.

51. Soiffer RJ, Alyea EP, Hochberg E et al. Randomized trial of CD8+ T-cell depletion in the prevention of graft-versus-host disease associated with donor lymphocyte infusion. Biol Blood Marrow Transplant 2002;8:625–632.

52. Koh MB, Prentice HG, Corbo M et al. Alloantigen-specific T-cell depletion in a major histocompatibility complex fully mismatched murine model provides effective graft-versus-host disease prophylaxis in the presence of lymphoid engraftment. Br J Haematol 2002;118:108–116.

53. Andre-Schmutz I, Le Deist F, Hacein-Bey-Abina S et al. Immune reconstitution without graft-versus-host disease after haemopoietic stem-cell transplantation: a phase 1/2 study. Lancet 2002;360:130–137.

54. Bonini C, Ferrari G, Verzeletti S et al. HSV-TK gene transfer into donor lymphocytes for control of allogeneic graft-versus-leukemia. Science 1997;276:1719–1724.

55. Tiberghien P, Ferrand C, Lioure B et al. Administration of herpes simplex-thymidine kinase-expressing donor T cells with a T-cell-depleted allogeneic marrow graft. Blood 2001;97:63–72.

56. Berger C, Blau CA, Clackson T et al. CD28 costimulation and immunoaffinity-based selection efficiently generate primary gene-modified T cells for adoptive immunotherapy. Blood 2003;101:476–484.

57. Thomis DC, Marktel S, Bonini C et al. A Fas-based suicide switch in human T cells for the treatment of graft-versus-host disease. Blood 2001;97:1249–1257.

58. Hacein-Bey-Abina S, von Kalle C, Schmidt M et al. A serious adverse event after successful gene therapy for X-linked severe combined immunodeficiency. N Engl J Med 2003;348:255–256.

59. Ratzinger G, Reagan JL, Heller G et al. Differential CD52 expression by distinct myeloid dendritic cell subsets: implications for alemtuzumab (Campath-1H) activity at the level of antigen-presentation in allogeneic graft-host interactions in transplantation. Blood 2002;10:10.

60. Klangsinsirikul P, Carter GI, Byrne JL et al. Campath-1G causes rapid depletion of circulating host dendritic cells (DCs) before allogeneic transplantation but does not delay donor DC reconstitution. Blood 2002;99:2586–2591.

61. Chakrabarti S, Avivi I, Mackinnon S et al. Respiratory virus infections in transplant recipients after reduced-intensity conditioning with Campath-1H: high incidence but low mortality. Br J Haematol 2002;119:1125–1132.

62. Ruggeri L, Capanni M, Urbani E et al. Effectiveness of donor natural killer cell alloreactivity in mismatched hematopoietic transplants. Science 2002;295:2097–2100.

63. Guinan EC, Boussiotis VA, Neuberg D et al. Transplantation of anergic histoincompatible bone marrow allografts. N Engl J Med 1999;340:1704–1714.

64. Zeller JC, Panoskaltsis-Mortari A, Murphy WJ et al. Induction of CD4+ T cell alloantigen-specific hyporesponsiveness by IL-10 and TGF-beta. J Immunol 1999;163:3684–3691.

65. Boussiotis VA, Chen ZM, Zeller JC et al. Altered T-cell receptor + CD28-mediated signaling and blocked cell cycle progression in interleukin 10 and transforming growth factor-beta-treated alloreactive T cells that do not induce graft-versus-host disease. Blood 2001;97:565–571.

66. Jonuleit H, Schmitt E, Stassen M et al. Identification and functional characterization of human CD4(+)CD25(+) T cells with regulatory properties isolated from peripheral blood. J Exp Med 2001;193:1285–1294.

67. Feinstein L, Storb R. Nonmyeloablative hematopoietic cell transplantation. Curr Opin Oncol 2001;13:95–100.

68. Hill GR, Cooke KR, Teshima T et al. Interleukin-11 promotes T cell polarization and prevents acute graft-versus-host disease after allogeneic bone marrow transplantation. J Clin Invest 1998;102:115–123.

69. Panoskaltsis-Mortari A, Lacey DL, Vallera DA et al. Keratinocyte growth factor administered before conditioning ameliorates graft-versus-host disease after allogeneic bone marrow transplantation in mice. Blood 1998;92:3960–3967.

70. Antin JH, Lee SJ, Neuberg D et al. A phase I/II double-blind, placebo-controlled study of recombinant human interleukin-11 for mucositis and acute GVHD prevention in allogeneic stem cell transplantation. Bone Marrow Transplant 2002;29:373–377.

71. Antin JH, Weisdorf D, Neuberg D et al. Interleukin-1 blockade does not prevent acute graft-versus-host disease: results of a randomized, double-blind, placebo-controlled trial of interleukin-1 receptor antagonist in allogeneic bone marrow transplantation. Blood 2002;100:3479–3482.

72. Collins RH Jr, Shpilberg O, Drobyski WR et al. Donor leukocyte infusions in 140 patients with relapsed malignancy after allogeneic bone marrow transplantation. J Clin Oncol 1997;15:433–444.

73. Porter DL, Collins RH Jr, Hardy C et al. Treatment of relapsed leukemia after unrelated donor marrow transplantation with unrelated donor leukocyte infusions. Blood 2000;95:1214–1221.

74. Levine JE, Braun T, Penza SL et al. Prospective trial of chemotherapy and donor leukocyte infusions for relapse of advanced myeloid malignancies after allogeneic stem-cell transplantation. J Clin Oncol 2002;20:405–412.

75. Champlin R, Khouri I, Shimoni A et al. Harnessing graft-versus-malignancy: non-myeloablative preparative regimens for allogeneic haematopoietic transplantation, an evolving strategy for adoptive immunotherapy. Br J Haematol 2000;111:18–29.

76. Niederwieser D, Maris M, Shizuru JA et al. Low-dose total body irradiation (TBI) and fludarabine followed by hematopoietic cell transplantation (HCT) from HLA-matched or mismatched unrelated donors and postgrafting immunosuppression with cyclosporine and mycophenolate mofetil (MMF) can induce durable complete chimerism and sustained remissions in patients with hematological diseases. Blood 2002;3:3.

77. Childs R, Chernoff A, Contentin N et al. Regression of metastatic renal-cell carcinoma after nonmyeloablative allogeneic peripheral-blood stem-cell transplantation. N Engl J Med 2000;343:750–758.

78. Khouri IF, Saliba RM, Giralt SA et al. Nonablative allogeneic hematopoietic transplantation as adoptive immunotherapy for indolent lymphoma: low incidence of toxicity, acute graft-versus-host disease, and treatment-related mortality. Blood 2001;98:3595–3599.

79. Farag SS, Fehniger TA, Ruggeri L et al. Natural killer cell receptors: new biology and insights into the graft-versus-leukemia effect. Blood 2002;100:1935–1947.

80. Storkus WJ, Alexander J, Payne JA et al. Reversal of natural killing susceptibility in target cells expressing transfected class I HLA genes. Proc Natl Acad Sci USA 1989;86:2361–2364.

81. Cerwenka A, Lanier LL. Natural killer cells, viruses and cancer. Nat Rev Immunol 2001;1:41–49.

82. Ruggeri L, Capanni M, Casucci M et al. Role of natural killer cell alloreactivity in HLA-mismatched hematopoietic stem cell transplantation. Blood 1999;94:333–339.

83. Zijlstra M, Auchincloss H Jr, Loring JM et al. Skin graft rejection by beta 2-microglobulin-deficient mice. J Exp Med 1992;175:885–893.

84. Korngold R, Leighton C, Manser T. Graft-versus-myeloid leukemia responses following syngeneic and allogeneic bone marrow transplantation. Transplantation 1994;58:278–287.

85. Fontaine P, Roy-Proulx G, Knafo L et al. Adoptive transfer of minor histocompatibility antigen-specific T lymphocytes eradicates leukemia cells without causing graft-versus-host disease. Nat Med 2001;7:789–794.

86. Meunier MC, Roy-Proulx G, Labrecque N et al. Tissue distribution of target antigen has a decisive influence on the outcome of adoptive cancer immunotherapy. Blood 2003;101:766–770.

87. Warren EH, Greenberg PD, Riddell SR. Cytotoxic T-lymphocyte-defined human minor histocompatibility antigens with a restricted tissue distribution. Blood 1998;91:2197–207.

88. de Bueger M, Bakker A, Van Rood JJ et al. Tissue distribution of human minor histocompatibility antigens. Ubiquitous versus restricted tissue distribution indicates heterogeneity among human cytotoxic T lymphocyte-defined non-MHC antigens. J Immunol 1992;149:1788–1794.

89. Faber LM, van der Hoeven J, Goulmy E et al. Recognition of clonogenic leukemic cells, remission bone marrow and HLA-identical donor bone marrow by CD8+ or CD4+ minor histocompatibility antigen-specific cytotoxic T lymphocytes. J Clin Invest 1995;96:877–883.

90. Bonnet D, Warren EH, Greenberg PD et al. CD8(+) minor histocompatibility antigen-specific cytotoxic T lymphocyte clones eliminate human acute myeloid leukemia stem cells. Proc Natl Acad Sci USA 1999;96:8639–8644.

91. den Haan JM, Sherman NE, Blokland E et al. Identification of a graft versus host disease-associated human minor histocompatibility antigen. Science 1995;268:1476–1480.

92. Dolstra H, Fredrix H, Maas F et al. A human minor histocompatibility antigen specific for B cell acute lymphoblastic leukemia. J Exp Med 1999;189:301–308.

93. Warren EH, Otterud BE, Linterman RW et al. Feasibility of using genetic linkage analysis to identify the genes encoding T cell-defined minor histocompatibility antigens. Tissue Antigens 2002;59:293–303.

94. Warren EH, Gavin MA, Simpson E et al. The human UTY gene encodes a novel HLA-B8-restricted H-Y antigen. J Immunol 2000;164:2807–2814.

95. Gratwohl A, Hermans J, Niederwieser D et al. Female donors influence transplant-related mortality and relapse incidence in male recipients of sibling blood and marrow transplants. Hematol J 2001;2:363–370.

96. Randolph SB, Gooley TA, Warren EH et al. Impact of donor/patient gender on relapse and graft versus host disease in matched related hematopoietic stem cell transplant. Blood 2002;100:546a.

97. Mutis T, Gillespie G, Schrama E et al. Tetrameric HLA class I-minor histocompatibility antigen peptide complexes demonstrate minor histocompatibility antigen-specific cytotoxic T lymphocytes in patients with graft-versus-host disease. Nat Med 1999;5:839–842.

98. Randolph SB, Warren EH, Riddell SR. Identification of novel minor histocompatibility antigen encoded by the Y chromosome gene, UTY. Blood 2002;100.

99. den Haan JM, Meadows LM, Wang W et al. The minor histocompatibility antigen HA-1: a diallelic gene with a single amino acid polymorphism. Science 1998;279:1054–1057.

100. Pierce RA, Field ED, Mutis T et al. The HA-2 minor histocompatibility antigen is derived from a diallelic gene encoding a novel human class I myosin protein. J Immunol 2001;167:3223–3230.

101. Lin MT, Gooley T, Hansen JA et al. Absence of statistically significant correlation between disparity for the minor histocompatibility antigen-HA-1 and outcome after allogeneic hematopoietic cell transplantation. Blood 2001;98:3172–3173.

102. Clark RE, Dodi IA, Hill SC et al. Direct evidence that leukemic cells present HLA-associated immunogenic peptides derived from the BCR-ABL b3a2 fusion protein. Blood 2001;98:2887–2893.

103. Molldrem JJ, Komanduri K, Wieder E. Overexpressed differentiation antigens as targets of graft-versus-leukemia reactions. Curr Opin Hematol 2002;9:503–508.

104. Golub TR. Genomic approaches to the pathogenesis of hematologic malignancy. Curr Opin Hematol 2001;8:252–261.

105. Molldrem J, Dermime S, Parker K et al. Targeted T-cell therapy for human leukemia: cytotoxic T lymphocytes specific for a peptide derived from proteinase 3 preferentially lyse human myeloid leukemia cells. Blood 1996;88:2450–2457.

106. Molldrem JJ, Clave E, Jiang YZ et al. Cytotoxic T lymphocytes specific for a nonpolymorphic proteinase 3 peptide preferentially inhibit chronic myeloid leukemia colony-forming units. Blood 1997;90:2529–2534.

107. Molldrem JJ, Lee PP, Wang C et al. Evidence that specific T lymphocytes may participate in the elimination of chronic myelogenous leukemia. Nat Med 2000;6:1018–1023.

108. Ohminami H, Yasukawa M, Fujita S. HLA class I-restricted lysis of leukemia cells by a CD8(+) cytotoxic T-lymphocyte clone specific for WT1 peptide. Blood 2000;95:286–293.

109. Bellantuono I, Gao L, Parry S et al. Two distinct HLA-A0201-presented epitopes of the Wilms tumor antigen 1 can function as targets for leukemia-reactive CTL. Blood 2002;100:3835–3837.

110. Gao L, Bellantuono I, Elsasser A et al. Selective elimination of leukemic CD34(+) progenitor cells by cytotoxic T lymphocytes specific for WT1. Blood 2000;95:2198–2203.

111. Walter EA, Greenberg PD, Gilbert MJ et al. Reconstitution of cellular immunity against cytomegalovirus in recipients of allogeneic bone marrow by transfer of T-cell clones from the donor. N Engl J Med 1995;333:1038–1044.

112. Yee C, Thompson JA, Byrd D et al. Adoptive T cell therapy using antigen-specific CD8+ T cell clones for the treatment of patients with metastatic melanoma: in vivo persistence, migration, and antitumor effect of transferred T cells. Proc Natl Acad Sci USA 2002;99:16168–16173.

113. YMutis T, Verdijk R, Schrama E et al. Feasibility of immunotherapy of relapsed leukemia with ex vivo-generated cytotoxic T lymphocytes specific for hematopoietic system-restricted minor histocompatibility antigens. Blood 1999;93:2336–2341

Chapter 8

Mammographic Screening: A Key Factor in the Control of Breast Cancer

Làszló Tabár

Robert A. Smith

Bedrich Vitak

Ming-Fang Yen

Tony Hsiu-Hsi Chen

Jane Warwick

Jonathan P. Myles

Stephen W. Duffy

Since the late 1980s, there has been broad agreement, with few dissenters, that mammographic screening significantly and substantially reduced mortality from breast cancer. This was based on the findings of the eight randomized trials of breast screening worldwide.[1-9] Figure 8.1 shows the results of these with respect to breast cancer mortality. The combined result is a significant 24% reduction in breast cancer mortality in women aged 40–74 years in association with invitation to screening. Overviews of age-specific effects of screening show a significant 18% reduction in breast cancer mortality with invitation to screening in women aged 40–49 years and a significant 27% reduction in women aged 50–74 years.[10,11] A sizeable proportion of the evidence comes from the Swedish Two-County Trial of mammographic screening, conducted from 1977 to 1986 in Kopparberg and Östergötland counties in Sweden.

For the most part, this consensus on the benefits of mammographic screening continues to prevail, although it has been questioned by a meta-analysis by that claims to find no benefit of breast cancer screening. Indeed, Gøtzsche and Olsen[12,13] claim that screening causes harm by increasing the rates of radical treatment. In particular, the authors of the meta-analysis asserted that

1. Only two of the randomized trials are of sufficient quality to be considered in reviewing the evidence.
2. Screening leads to more use of radiotherapy, which in turn leads to more cardiovascular deaths. These deaths are not counted when breast cancer mortality is compared between groups invited and those not invited to screening.
3. For this reason and others, the use of breast cancer mortality as an endpoint is biased in favor of screening.
4. Screening increases the rates of mastectomy.

In view of these points, the authors concluded that the case for mammographic screening was not established and that future evaluation should be based on all-cause (rather than breast cancer) mortality, including deaths in women who never get breast cancer.

The judgment of quality of the trials is based on observed or alleged imbalances between study and control groups and alleged inconsistencies in reported results. It has been shown, however, that the imbalances referred to are either trivial, including a 1-month imbalance in age between study and control groups in the Gothenburg trial; or are fully adjusted for in analysis, such as the social class imbalance in the Edinburgh trial; or both, such as the 5-month age imbalance in favor of the control group in the Swedish Two-County Trial.[6,9,14,15]

Inconsistencies have been shown to be either trivial or not inconsistencies at all. For example, alleged inconsistent reporting of deaths was due to the difference between an expert panel's judgment of cause of death and that recorded on the routine death certificate, or to larger numbers of deaths with longer follow-up.[16] The judgment of study quality is therefore dubious at best. Any review of the randomized controlled trials should be evenhanded and include all the available evidence.

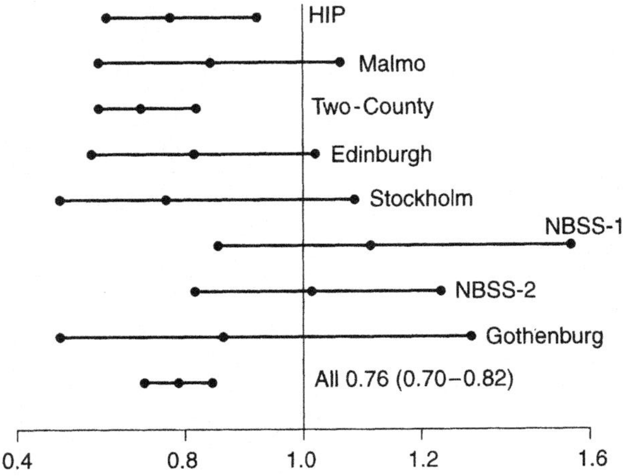

FIGURE 8.1 Relative rates of breast cancer death in the eight randomized trials of breast cancer screening, using primary sources where available, secondary otherwise.

The assertion that screening leads to more radiotherapy seems to be based on what Gøtzsche and Olsen[12,13] thought *should* happen rather than on what *did* happen. In a detailed survey of treatment in the Kopparberg part of the Swedish Two-County Study, treatment with radiotherapy was more common in the control group than in the group invited to screening.[17] Table 8.1 shows treatment by study arm in Kopparberg. Also, the increased risk of cardiovascular disease with radiotherapy pertains to archaic forms of radiotherapy that are no longer practiced.

The other assertions about cause of death seem similarly ill founded. Indeed, if one considers all causes of death in breast cancer patients (because mammography cannot be expected to affect deaths in women who do not get breast cancer), there was a reduced risk of death from any cause in the group invited to screening.[18] Table 8.2 shows the relative mortality from breast cancer, all other causes, and all causes in breast cancer cases in the Two-County Trial. The conclusions of Olsen and Gøtzsche[13] were based on incorrect statistical analysis that failed to take account of lead time.

There is also no convincing evidence that screening increases the rates of radical surgery, in particular, mastectomy. Mastectomy rates were lower in the group invited to screening in the Two-County Trial (Table 8.1) and indeed have been shown to fall by 40% with the introduction of service screening in Florence.[17,19]

It therefore appears that the consensus among the scientific community was correct. The vast body of evidence indicates a substantial reduction in mortality from breast cancer from mammographic screening. Whether this reduction justifies the financial and human costs of a screening program is a judgment that has

TABLE 8.1 Numbers of Cases Receiving Mastectomy and Adjuvant Radiotherapy, with Rates per 1000 Subjects Randomly Assigned, by Trial Arm (Kopparberg County Swedish Two-County Trial)

Group	Number (Rate/1000) of Breast Cancer Cases Receiving:		Total Subjects
	Mastectomy	Radiotherapy	
Study	475 (12)	433 (11)	38,589
Control	258 (14)	227 (12)	18,582

to be made by individual societies and will depend on the prevailing rates of breast cancer, the availability of facilities and expertise, the costs of these, and numerous other considerations. However, the benefit in terms of reduced breast cancer deaths is not in question.

The time for repeatedly revisiting the trials has gone. The challenge for the future is to evaluate the effects of the service screening programs that are springing up around the world and to pinpoint potential improvements where possible. The remainder of this chapter is devoted to assessing the effect of service screening on breast cancer mortality. In terms of the randomized trial results, however, we can conclude that

- The trials show a reduction in breast cancer mortality of 20%–30%, depending on age, in association with invitation to screening.
- This reduction includes women in the study group who were invited to screening, but declined, and women who undergo screening despite their trial status in the control group.
- The mortality reduction in women who *actually receive* screening is considerably greater than has been suggested. Modern screening programs, often with more intensive regimens than in the randomized trials (more frequent screening, more multiple-view mammography, more multiple reading) should be expected to do better than the trials.

TABLE 8.2 Relative Risks of Death among Breast Cancer Cases, Invited versus Noninvited to Screening (Swedish Two-County Study)

Endpoint	RR	95% CI
Breast cancer deaths	0.69	0.50–0.80
Other-cause deaths	1.12	0.96–1.31
All-cause deaths	0.87	0.78–0.99

RR, relative risk; CI, confidence interval.

ASSESSING THE EFFECT OF SERVICE SCREENING PROGRAMS ON BREAST CANCER MORTALITY: METHODOLOGICAL CONSIDERATIONS

As stated at the end of the last section, the randomized trials of screening show a 20%–30% reduction in breast cancer mortality in association with invitation to screening. The trials have lower age limits, varying from 40–50 years; upper age limits from 50–74 years; attendance rates varying from about 60% to about 90%; interscreening intervals from 1 year to almost 3 years; and various screening regimens (numbers of views, numbers of readers, inclusion of physical examination). Subsequent service screening programs have been designed in light of the results of the trials. Typically, although not invariably, service screening programs have had a 2-year interscreening interval, with a shorter interval for women aged less than 50 years or less than 55 years. Two-view mammography is the standard, and two readers are usually recommended, although human resources do not always allow this. Well-organized programs are usually accompanied by intense quality assurance systems for the surveillance of screening, diagnosis, and treatment.

These represent improvements on the randomized trials. One would therefore expect organized service screening programs to achieve mortality reductions that are greater than those observed in the trials. The problems for evaluation are (1) the measurement of the benefit in the absence of a randomized control group and (2) the derivation of a valid estimate of the benefit in women who are actually screened. The effect of introducing the screening program is analogous to the intention-to-treat effect of invitation to screening that is usually quoted as the primary result of a randomized trial. It is also of interest to calculate the (presumably larger) effect of actually receiving screening, to indicate for a woman invited to screening what benefit she may personally expect from a decision to attend, in terms of her risk of dying from breast cancer. This is complicated by the fact that those who comply with preventive measures tend to be more health conscious and therefore have a lower risk of premature mortality a priori than those who do not comply.

In a randomized trial of screening, the calculation of the effect of the invitation to screening on mortality is relatively simple. The relative risk is

$$RR = \frac{r_1}{r_2}$$

where r_1 is the rate of death from breast cancer in the group randomly assigned to invitation to screening, and r_2, the rate in the group randomly assigned to no invitation. That is,

$$r_1 = \frac{d_1}{p_1}$$

where d_1 is the number of deaths in the invited group, and p_1, either the population or person-years at risk. A similar formula applies to r_2. The percentage mortality reduction can be calculated as

$$P_r = 100 \times (1 - RR)$$

In the case of a service screening program, we wish to calculate

$$RR = \frac{r_1}{r_2}$$

where in this case, r_1 is the death rate from breast cancer pertaining to the screening program, and r_2, an estimate of the rate that would be expected if the screening did not take place. Calculation of both r_1 and r_2 is problematic. Consider first the more simple problem, that of estimating r_1.

Suppose that in a certain area, a mammographic screening program was introduced for women aged 40–69 years in 1990 and that we wish to derive an intention-to-treat estimate. In the first instance, we might use as the appropriate death rate pertaining to the screening program

$$r_1 = \frac{d_{90}}{p_{90}}$$

where d_{90} is the number of breast cancer deaths in the age group aged 40–69 years in 1990–1999, and p_{90}, the corresponding person-years. There are various deficiencies in this estimate. First, screening does not simply start instantaneously on New Year's Day 1990 for the entire eligible population. It may take, say, 2 years to invite all eligible women. Thus, in this population in 1990 and 1991, about half will not have been invited to screening. In addition, tumors will have been diagnosed clinically in 1990 and 1991 in women who were not yet invited to screening that subsequently resulted in breast cancer death during the period of observation. More importantly, a large proportion of the deaths from breast cancer in 1990–1999 will have been from tumors diagnosed before 1990, and whose prognosis could not possibly have been affected by screening. Figure 8.2 shows the proportion, by year in the decade spanning 1978 to 1987, of breast cancer deaths in Kopparberg County from tumors that were diagnosed in that decade. In the decade as a whole, more than 50% of the deaths were from tumors diagnosed before 1978. In 1990–1999, as a result of improved survival, the proportion diagnosed before the decade began would be even larger. Deaths would also be counted within the age group 40–69 years that are from tumors diagnosed before the age of 40, and other deaths occurring after age 69 would not be counted in the 40–69 age range that nonetheless resulted from tumors that were diagnosed in the age range 40–69 years.

Therefore, the death rate pertaining to the screening program should ideally be from tumors diagnosed in the epoch of the screening program and in the age

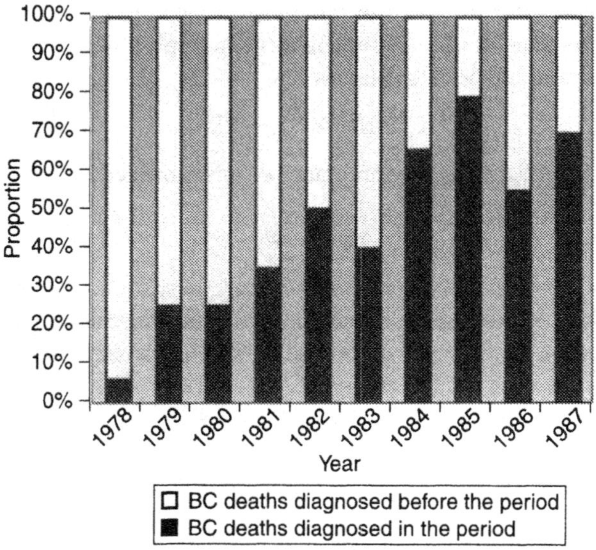

FIGURE 8.2 Proportion of breast cancer deaths from 1978–1987. The data are from Kopparberg County, from tumors diagnosed in the period.

group targeted for screening. With individual invitation data, one approach is to divide the cancers into those diagnosed before invitation and those diagnosed after invitation. Another approach using aggregate data is to pick a common calendar period cut-off that trades off numbers invited before the date and numbers not invited after (one might prefer to base this decision on numbers screened rather than numbers invited). Thus, suppose invitations started in October 1989, with 12% of the eligible population being invited by the end of 1989, 71% by the end of 1990, and 100% by the end of 1991. If we choose the beginning of 1990 as the start date, there is considerable contamination in the first year by persons not yet invited, and if we pick the beginning of 1992, there is no contamination of the invited period, but considerable contamination of the last year of the noninvited period by invitation. It would therefore seem reasonable to select the beginning of 1991 as the cut-off date. The 9-year period of follow-up would only have 12/9 = 1.3% contamination, and a comparable 9-year preinvitation period would have approximately 71/9 = 7.9% contamination.

Both of these strategies are illustrated below, but first one should consider r_2, the expected mortality rate in the absence of screening. In the case of individual entry dates, one can use the deaths from cancers diagnosed in 1990 and 1991 in women who were not yet invited and compare them with deaths from cancers diagnosed contemporaneously or afterward in invited women. The advantages of this strategy are that the comparison is exactly between invited and uninvited women as in the randomized trials, it is only partly confounded by epoch of diagnosis, and there is no self-selection bias from the generally better outcome of compliers compared with noncompliers, because the comparison is between invited and noninvited subjects. The major disadvantage is that usually it only takes 1–3 years to invite the population, so there is only a small amount of preinvitation data. Also, care needs to be taken in allowing equivalent follow-up of the cancers diagnosed in invited and uninvited women, and in calculating the relevant person-years denominators for the rates.

Now consider the strategy of adopting a common cut-off date that involves minimal contamination. The mortality rate associated with the screening program might be

$$r_{91} = \frac{d_{91}}{p_{91}}$$

where d_{91} represents the deaths occurring in 1991–1999 from tumors diagnosed within 1991–1999 and diagnosed at ages 40–69 years, and p_{91} represents the total person-years of observation in 1991–1999 in ages 40–69 years. For the expected death rate in the absence of screening, various possibilities might be considered. If there is a neighboring community with no screening program, the corresponding rates of deaths from tumors diagnosed in the same period and the same age group might be a reasonable estimate. Usually, however, a "control" area in the same country is not available, because different areas in the same country have tended to introduce screening within a few years of each other. If such a geographic control were available, one would need to consider breast cancer mortality rates in the two areas before 1991, in case there are underlying differences in the risk of death from breast cancer between the two areas that are unrelated to screening.

If a contemporaneous control area is unavailable, one might consider a before-and-after comparison. Again, suppose one took the cut-off of 1991 to avoid substantial contamination of postscreening and prescreening periods. There is a 9-year screening period in which the average follow-up of tumors diagnosed in that period would be approximately 4.5 years. One might be tempted to simply have as long a prescreening period as possible, but this would be a mistake. Apart from long-term changes unrelated to screening that might take place before the screening period, the nonconstant annual fatality rate after diagnosis means that a longer prescreening period would confer a different mortality rate in the two periods, even if the screening had no effect at all. One would therefore be well advised to use 1982–1990 as the comparison period, because it is as long as and occurs immediately before the screening period. In making such a before-after comparison, it is necessary to consider:

- There are changes in breast cancer survival over time for reasons other than the screening, such as improvements in awareness, therapy, and management.
- If there is substantial screening contamination in the nominally prescreening period, some deaths will apparently be avoided in the later period, not be-

cause the case did not prove fatal but because it was diagnosed before 1991 as a result of the screening.

- The length of the screening period is likely to affect the observed mortality reduction; because it takes several years for the effect of screening to be reflected in mortality rates, shorter periods are likely to lead to underestimation of the benefit.

The first of these considerations may be estimated from changes in mortality strictly within the prescreening period.[20] Another possibility is to compare the mortality reduction in the age group targeted for screening with that observed in an age group in which screening did not take place in either epoch.[21] For the second method, an adjustment to the person-years may be used to correct for the bias, with such an adjustment based on the numbers screened and the estimates of the average lead time from the literature.[20] The third involves another consideration besides symmetry of duration of the periods compared—that the period of screening observation, and therefore the prescreening period, should be as long as possible.

Other considerations that may arise are the necessity to adjust for self-selection bias if one is restricting comparison to those actually screened, and the possibility that mortality changes over time as a consequence not of changes in case survival but of changes in incidence. These are dealt with by example in a later section in this chapter.

EVALUATION OF SERVICE SCREENING: TWO EXAMPLES

Using examples from Italy and Sweden, we can illustrate the two approaches to selection of nominal screening periods. The first example, the Florence breast screening program, uses individual invitation data so that a comparison is made between deaths from tumors diagnosed partly contemporaneously in invited and not-yet-invited women in the same area.[22] The second, from seven counties in Sweden, involves the use and selection of a common cut-off point within each county and demonstrates a simple before-and-after comparison.

Use of Individual Invitation Data in the Florence Program

Figure 8.3 illustrates the design and evaluation of the Florence program. The population size in the eligible age range of 50–69 years was 59,947. The program aimed to deliver two-view mammography every 2 years, although the interval slipped to 2.3 years in practice. Invitation started in late 1990 and was completed in early 1993. During this period, 372 tumors were diagnosed in women who were not yet invited, with 164,742 person-years of observation. From 1990 to 1996, 750 tumors were diagnosed in women who had received an invitation to screening, with 254,890 person-years of observation. Both sets of tumors were followed up *for the same period of time,* to a maximum of 8 years and an average of approximately 5 years, but the person-years pertain to the period of diagnosis.

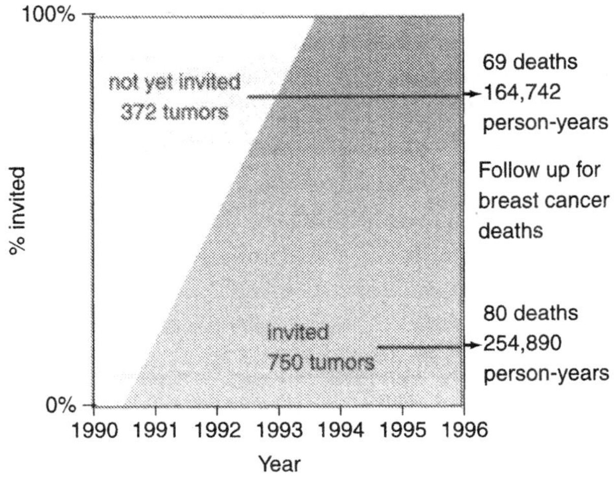

FIGURE 8.3 Evaluation of the Florence program on the basis of individual invitation dates.

The relative risk of breast cancer mortality pertaining to invitation to screening was

$$RR = \frac{80/254{,}890}{69/164{,}742} = 0.75$$

with a 95% confidence interval of 0.54–1.04. Thus, invitation to screening was associated with a 25% reduction in mortality from breast cancer, a finding that was of borderline significance. If one compares screened with unscreened women, a significant 37% mortality reduction is observed; however, this is affected by selection bias. The true reduction associated with actually receiving screening lies somewhere between the 25% and the 37%. An illustration of correcting for selection bias is shown in the section The Effect of Actually Receiving Screening (below).

Service Screening in Seven Counties in Sweden: Cut-Off Dates and Before-After Comparisons

In this study, seven Swedish counties with screening programs targeting about 300,000 women aged 40–69 years were included for evaluation. Two-view mammography was mainly used. The screening interval was an average of 2 years and did not vary a great deal from county to county. Dates of introduction of screening varied between counties, and as one would expect, invitation of the entire population took different lengths of time to complete in the different screening programs. Cut-off dates were chosen on the basis of coverage by actual screening rather than by invitation. Table 8.3 shows the cut-off dates chosen and the consequent contamination rates in the by county and period. Note that the

TABLE 8.3 Nominal Starting Dates of Screening and Contamination Rates in the Seven Swedish Counties

County	Nominal Starting Date	Contamination Before (% Screened)	Contamination After (% Not Screened)
Dalarna	1978	0.5	25
Gävleborg	1984	0[a]	16
Södermanland	1990	0.7	23
Uppsala	1989	3	18
Värmland	1994	3	27
Västmanland	1989	14	8
Örebro	1989	4	36

[a]Some sporadic screening with very long intervals took place in this county before 1984.

contamination rates in the screening period are higher than in the prescreening. This is inevitable. In the nominal prescreening period, contamination is due mainly to the choice of a cut-off date, which trades off the inclusion of some of the earliest screens in the program in the prescreening period with inclusion of not-yet-screened women in the screened period. Few women have received screening in the prescreening period. In the screening period, however, there is a sizeable minority who choose not to attend screening. These are categorized as contamination regardless of the choice of cut-off date.

Table 8.4 illustrates the periods of observation for each county. The durations of the screening (and therefore the prescreening) periods range from 5 to 20 years.

Our r_1 figures for each county consist of the numbers of breast cancer deaths within the screening period from tumors diagnosed within the screening period in women aged 40–69 years, divided by the person-years for the screening period in the age group 40–69 years. The r_2 figures are calculated in the same way but from the prescreening period.

Note that for one county, Västmanland, there was substantial prescreening contamination. We therefore need to adjust for the fact that in the screening period, some breast cancer deaths may not be counted, not because the deaths were prevented, but because the diagnosis time was advanced to the prescreening period as a result of the screening contamination therein. We correct for this by an adjustment to the person-years. Table 8.5 shows the average populations in Västmanland, breast cancer deaths, and person-years in the two periods. The uncorrected relative risk is

$$RR_u = \frac{85/470{,}961}{112/448{,}442} = 0.72$$

In the last year of the nominal prescreening period, 20,037 women were actually screened. The average lead time (i.e., number of years by which detection and

TABLE 8.4 **Periods of Study (Shaded Areas Represent Periods Not Studied)**

1958	1978	1998
(shaded)	Värmland prescreening, 1989–1993	Värmland screening, 1994–1998
(shaded)	Södermanland prescreening, 1981–1989	Södermanland screening, 1990–1998
(shaded)	Uppsala prescreening, 1979–1988	Uppsala screening, 1989–1998
(shaded)	Västmanland pre-screening, 1979–1988	Västmanland screening, 1989–1998
(shaded)	Örebro prescreening, 1979–1988	Örebro screening, 1989–1998
(shaded)	Gävleborg prescreening and screening, 1984–1998	
Dalarna prescreening, 1958–1977	Dalarna screening, 1978–1997	(shaded)

[a] Shaded areas represent periods not studied.

treatment move forward) in this age group is 3.4 years.[3] We might then expect that 3.4 × 20,037 = 68,126 person-years worth of tumors would be omitted from the screening period as a result of the screening in the prescreening period. We therefore subtract 68,126 from the person-years in the screening period, giving 402,835 as our person-years. The corrected relative risk is thus

$$RR_c = \frac{85/402{,}835}{112/448{,}442} = 0.84$$

TABLE 8.5 **Data for Västmanland County and Results With and Without Lead Time Correction**

Period	Average Population	Breast Cancer Deaths	Person-Years	Uncorrected RR (95% CI)	Corrected RR (95% CI)
Prescreening	44,844	112	448,442	1.00	1.00
Screening	47,096	85	470,961	0.72 (0.54–0.96)	0.84 (0.64–1.12)

RR, relative risk; CI, confidence interval.

TABLE 8.6 **Results of Evaluation of Screening in Seven Counties in Sweden by Before-After Comparison**

Counties	Period	Breast Cancer Deaths	Person-Years	Corrected RR (95% CI)
Those with ≤ 10 years of screening	Prescreening	489	1,870,007	1.00
	Screening	421	2,017,511	0.82 (0.72–0.94)
Those with > 10 years of screening	Prescreening	680	1,823,057	1.00
	Screening	454	1,797,819	0.68 (0.60–0.77)
All 7 counties	Prescreening	1169	3,693,064	1.00
	Screening	875	3,815,330	0.75 (0.68–0.82)

Table 8.6 shows the results for the seven counties stratified by duration of the screening period, and for all seven counties combined. The relative risks are corrected for the lead time in Västmanland as described earlier. They also take into account other complexities in the data that are not described here for considerations of simplicity of presentation. For details, see Duffy et al.[20] The results show a significant 32% reduction in breast cancer mortality in the screening period compared with the prescreening period in those counties with a history of more than 10 years of screening (RR = 0.68, 95% CI 0.60–0.77, $P < 0.001$) and a significant 18% reduction in those counties with 10 years or less of screening (RR = 0.82, 95% CI 0.72–0.94, $P = 0.004$). This illustrates the fact that it takes some years for a screening program to exhibit its full effect on mortality from the disease. For all seven counties combined, there was a significant 25% reduction in mortality (RR = 0.75, 95% CI 0.68–0.82, $P < 0.001$).

Examination of changes in mortality in the prescreening periods showed an average reduction in breast cancer mortality of 1% per year. This in turn suggests an 11% reduction in breast cancer mortality between the prescreening and screening periods that is caused by reasons other than screening. Thus, most of the observed reduction in mortality is due to early detection.

These are the mortality reductions associated with the policy of offering screening. Because the contamination rates, which mainly result from nonattendance in the screening period, average more than 20% and indeed are as high as 36% in one county, the benefit of actually receiving screening must be considerably higher. This is illustrated in Figure 8.4, which shows cumulative mortality during the 10-year study period from one of the counties, Dalarna. The mortality is from incident tumors within the periods as before. The figure shows the cumulative mortality for the 10 years immediately preceding screening (1968–1977) and the 10 years during which the entire population aged 40–59 years was invited to screening (1988–1997), omitting the period during which the Two-County Trial was ongoing (1978–1987). The figure illustrates how the mortality reduction builds up over

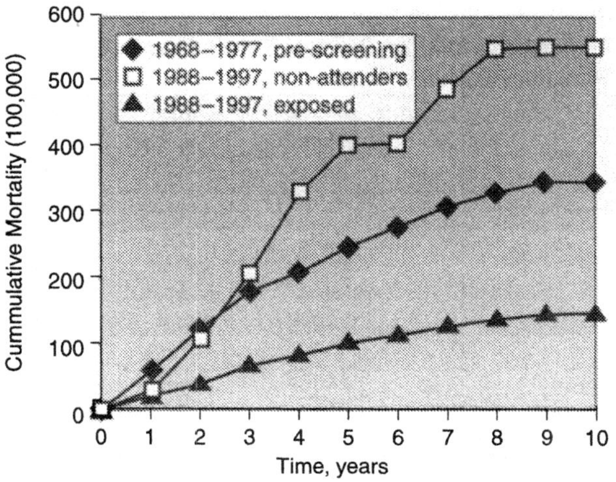

FIGURE 8.4 Cumulative mortality from breast cancer by period for women aged 40–69 years in Dalarna (formerly Kopparberg) County.

time and shows the greater benefit in women who actually received screening—a significant 60% reduction in breast cancer mortality *in screened women* in the screening period compared with those in the prescreening period. It also illustrates the problem of self-selection bias, in that the nonattenders in the screening period have a 49% greater mortality than the uninvited women in the prescreening period. Clearly, this does not mean that breast cancer survival has actually deteriorated over time in unscreened populations. On the contrary, it demonstrates the phenomenon previously described that those who comply with a preventive measure tend to be healthier a priori than those who do not, and that noncompliers tend to be at particularly high risk of premature mortality, for a variety of attitudinal, lifestyle, and socioeconomic reasons. Thus, both the observed increase in mortality in the unscreened women and the reduced mortality in the screened women are likely to be overestimates. Also, the comparison does not take into account an underlying increase in mortality due to increased incidence of breast cancer. The next section obtains age-specific estimates of the effect of organized service screening on breast cancer mortality, adjusting for potential biases from self-selection and changes in incidence.

THE EFFECT OF ACTUALLY RECEIVING SCREENING, ADJUSTED FOR SELF-SELECTION BIAS AND INCIDENCE TRENDS

To demonstrate the long-term effect of mammographic screening on breast cancer mortality, with corrections for self-selection bias and incidence trends, we obtained incidence and mortality data in the 40 years spanning 1958–1997 from the two counties that made up the Swedish Two-County Trial: Dalarna (formerly called Kopparberg) and Östergötland counties. During the period 1958–1977,

TABLE 8.7 Unadjusted Breast Cancer Incidence and Mortality from Incident Tumors, with Relative Risks of Breast Cancer Death by Period and Screening Exposure Status

Period Screening Exposure	Person Years (1000's)	Breast Cancer Cases (Rate/10^5)	Breast Cancer Deaths (Rate/10^5)	RR	95% CI
1958–1977, unscreened	2416	3151 (130.5)	1129 (46.7)	1.00	-
1978–1997, screened	1647	3594 (218.3)	401 (24.4)	0.52	0.46–0.59
1978–1997, unscreened	752	1308 (173.9)	457 (60.8)	1.30	1.16–1.45
1978–1997, all	2399	4902 (204.4)	858 (35.8)	.77	0.70–0.85

there was no screening apart from a small percentage of the population in late 1977. From late 1977 to 1984, in the Swedish Two-county Trial, 58% of the population (aged 40–69 years and indeed aged 70–74 years) were randomly assigned to invitation to screening. The screening interval was 2 years for those aged 40–49 years and 2.75 years for those aged 50 or more. From approximately 1985–1987, the control group members were invited to screening, and the trial closed thereafter. From 1988–1997, the entire population aged 40–69 years in the two counties was invited to screening, with a 1.5-year interval for women aged 40–54 years and a 2-year interval for women aged 55 years or more.

As before, our focus of attention is the breast cancer mortality rate in the screening period (1978–1997) from tumors diagnosed within that period and at ages 40–69 years, compared with the corresponding mortality rate in the prescreening period (1958–1977). Table 8.7 shows the breast cancer incidence and mortality as both rates and absolute numbers within the prescreening and screening periods. The incidence figures show a substantial increase with time, in common with the rest of the world. In the screening period, the figures are further stratified by whether or not the subjects were exposed to screening. There was a significant 48% reduction in breast cancer mortality in the screened women in the screening period compared with those in the prescreening. In the unscreened women, there was a significant 30% increase in breast cancer mortality. In the screening period as a whole (both screened and unscreened women combined), there was a significant 23% reduction in mortality. Figure 8.5 shows the corresponding cumulative mortality rates.

Adjustment for Changes in Incidence

To adjust for changes in incidence, we can divide the mortality rates in the two periods by the corresponding incidence rates. It could be argued, however, that

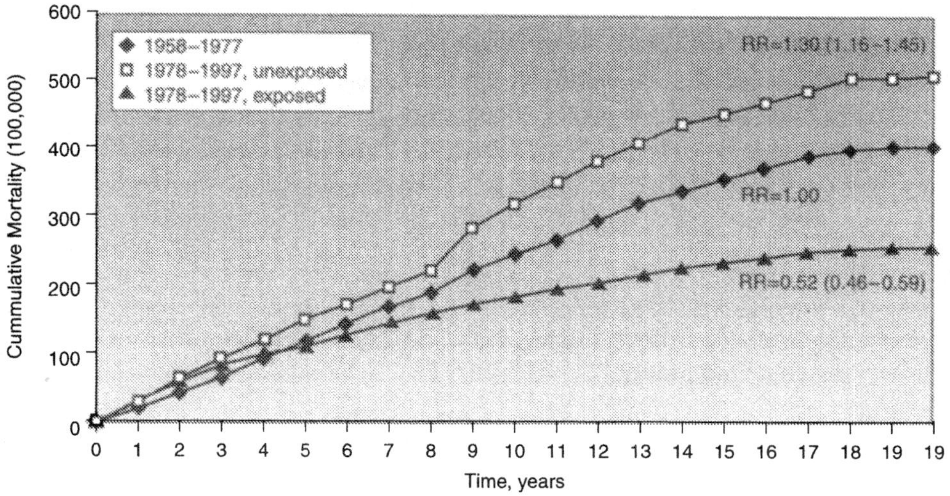

FIGURE 8.5 Cumulative mortality from incident tumors diagnosed in women aged 40–69 years by 20-year period and screening exposure in Dalarna (formerly Kopparberg) and Östergötland counties.

some of the increased incidence observed in the screening period is artificial and results from anticipated cases as a result of the screening, because screening detects many tumors that may have been detected up to 4 years in the future. We therefore divide the mortality rates in the screening period not by the overall incidence rates, but by the rates in the unscreened women (which cannot have been artificially inflated by screening) in the screening period.

Thus, for example, the relative risk for the screened women in the screening period compared with those in the prescreening period is

$$RR = \frac{24.4/173.9}{46.7/130.5} = 0.39$$

This indicates a significant 61% reduction in breast cancer mortality in the screened women (RR = 0.39, 95% CI 0.34–0.45), after adjustment for changes in breast cancer incidence. The relative risk for the unscreened women in the screening period compared with those in the prescreening period is

$$RR = \frac{60.8/173.9}{46.7/130.5} = 0.98$$

This indicates a nonsignificant 2% reduction in breast cancer mortality in the unscreened women compared with those in the prescreening period (RR = 0.98, 95% CI 0.86–1.12), with the value being adjusted for changes in breast cancer incidence. For the entire population in the postscreening period (screened and unscreened combined), the relative risk is

$$RR = \frac{35.8/173.9}{46.7/130.5} = 0.58$$

Thus, there was a significant 42% reduction in mortality in the screening period, regardless of screening status, relative to the prescreening period (RR = 0.58, 95% CI 0.34–0.45), after the value was adjusted for changes in incidence.

Figure 8.6 shows the corresponding survival by period and screening exposure. Standard errors of the relative risk estimates presented earlier can be calculated as shown by Tabár et al.[23] Figure 8.7 shows the three incidence-adjusted relative risks with 95% confidence intervals. The incidence adjustment cannot be artificially inflated by screening, because it is calculated from the unscreened women in both periods.

Adjustment for Self-Selection Bias

The relative risks quoted in the previous section are adjusted for trends in incidence over the 20-year period, but when mortality from breast cancer is stratified by screening status, a further correction for self-selection bias is necessary to take into account the fact that noncompliers tend to have higher premature death rates, and compliers lower premature death rates, than the general population, independently of screening. We first consider adjusting the relative risk for the screening-exposed women for self-selection bias. Suppose RR is the relative risk for the screened women in the screening period compared with those in the prescreening period, corrected for incidence but not for self-selection bias; p is the proportion of women who comply with the invitation to screening; and D is the relative risk among noncompliers compared with an *uninvited* population. Duffy et al[24] show how D can be estimated as 1.36 from the randomized trials of breast screening. There are two possible measures of relative risk that are corrected for self-selection bias. The first is the intention to treat estimate associated with invitation to screening, RR_I, where

$$RR_I = pRR + (1 - p)\,D$$

The derivation and standard error of RR_I are given by Tabár et al.[21]

The second measure is the estimate of the relative risk associated with actually being screened in those who *would* comply if invited. This is an adaptation of the service screening evaluation of the noncompliance adjustment for randomized trials of screening, which was developed by Cuzick et al.[25] It estimates the risk of mortality in patients who comply compared with the risk in an uninvited population who would have complied if they had been invited. If RR, p, and D are defined as they were earlier, the selection bias–corrected relative risk associated with actually being screened is RR_S, where

$$RR_S = \frac{pRR}{(1 - (1 - p)D)}$$

This is a re-expression of the estimate derived by Duffy et al.[24]

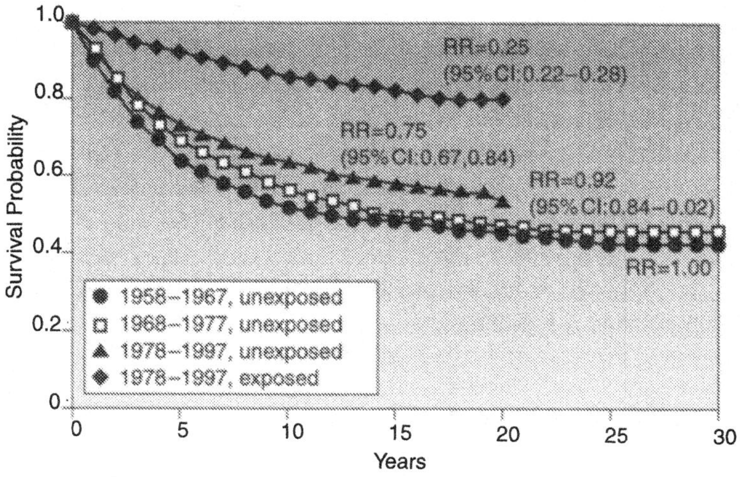

FIGURE 8.6 Survival of breast cancer patients aged 40–69 years at diagnosis, by period and screening exposure.

Adjustment for self-selection bias in the unscreened women is simpler. During 1978–1997, 43% of the unscreened person-years are the result of noncompliance and 57% are the result of being randomly assigned to no invitation in the Two-County Trial during 1977–1984. If RR_{NS} is the relative risk for the unscreened women in the screening period compared with those in the prescreening period,

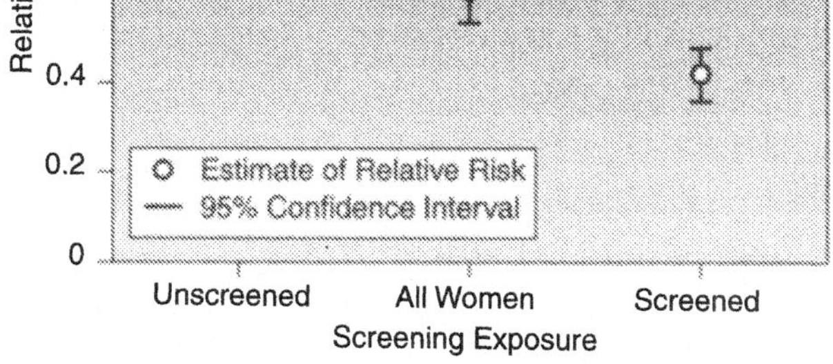

FIGURE 8.7 Incidence-adjusted relative risks for breast cancer mortality in the screening period compared with prescreening values, stratified by screening exposure.

corrected for incidence but not for self-selection bias, then RR_{NC}, which is the relative risk corrected for both incidence and self-selection bias,[21] is

$$RR_{NC} = \frac{RR_{NS}}{0.57 \times 1 + 0.43 \times D}$$

This is the estimated reduction in mortality that would have happened in the general population if screening had not taken place.

Figure 8.8 shows the relative risks corrected for both changes in incidence and self-selection bias. There was a significant 58% reduction in breast cancer mortality associated with actually being screened (*RR* = 0.42, 95% CI 0.36–0.49) and a significant 46% reduction associated with invitation to screening (*RR* = 0.54, 95% CI 0.48–0.61), a finding that is consistent with the significant 42% reduction observed in the population as a whole (*RR* = 0.58, 95% CI 0.51–0.65). In the unscreened women in the screening period, there was a nonsignificant 15% reduction (*RR* = 0.85, 95% CI 0.69–1.05), suggesting a decrease of 1% per year in breast cancer mortality rates, independently of screening. This is consistent with previous results[20] and suggests that about 64% of the mortality reduction observed in the population as a whole is due to screening and about 74% of the reduction in the screened women is due to screening.

Because of the particular interest in the age group 40–49 years,[26] we also calculated the incidence and selection bias–corrected relative risks for this age group. These are shown in Figure 8.9. The results are very similar to those for aged 40–69 years as a whole, with a significant 60% reduction in breast cancer mortality that was associated with actually being screened (*RR* = 0.40, 95% CI 0.26–0.61) and a significant 48% reduction that was associated with invitation (*RR* = 0.52, 95% CI 0.40–0.67). The unscreened women in the screening period showed a nonsignificant 19% reduction (*RR* = 0.81, 95% CI 0.60–1.09), again consistent with a 1% reduction in breast cancer mortality per year, independently of screening. This suggests that 58% of the mortality reduction in the population and 68% of the reduction in the screened women is due to screening. These results indicate that the shorter interscreening interval in women aged less than 55 years is yielding benefits in the younger women that are comparable with those in the older women.

DISCUSSION

A range of observed or predicted mortality reductions from service screening have been reported by other researchers. Most pertain to invitation to screening rather than actually receiving screening. Other researchers in Sweden have estimated various mortality reductions, but a 30% reduction with invitation to

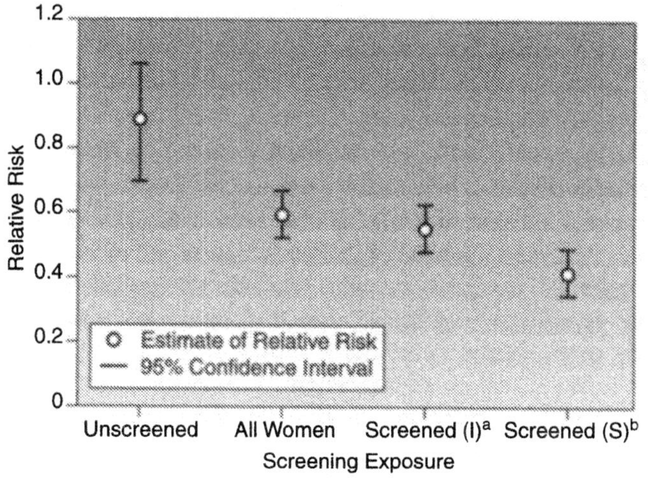

FIGURE 8.8 Relative mortality from incident breast cancers in the screening period compared with prescreening values, adjusted for incidence and self-selection bias, in women aged 40–69 years at diagnosis.

screening is typical.[27-29] In the United Kingdom, Blanks et al[30] reported only a 6% reduction, but this is qualified by the fact that it includes large numbers of deaths in nominally screened cohorts, from tumors diagnosed before screening was available, issues that heavily dilute the true reduction. Another study in the United Kingdom that strictly separates tumors into invited and not-yet-invited

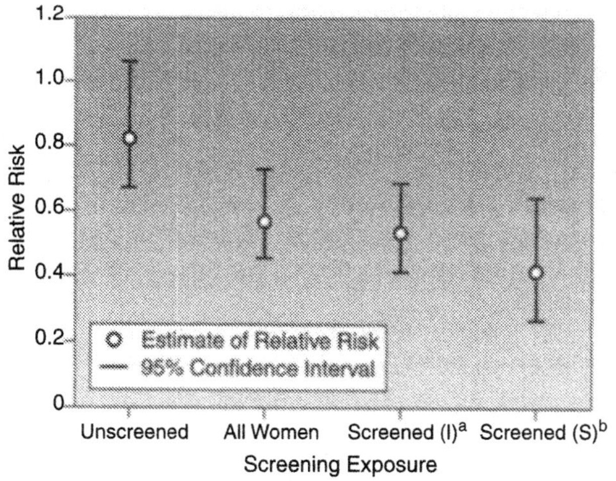

FIGURE 8.9 Relative mortality from breast cancers in the screening period compared with prescreening values, adjusted for incidence and self-selection bias, in women aged 40–49 years at diagnosis.

subjects predicted a 19% reduction with invitation to screening, based on the tumor size, node status, and grade of breast cancers.[31] As already described, the Florence program reported a 25% reduction with invitation to screening and a 37% reduction with actual screening.[22]

Our estimates tend to be higher than those of others partly because of a high level of organization, interdisciplinary cooperation, good compliance, and relatively short interscreening intervals. Another reason may be our ability to define breast cancer deaths on the basis of time of diagnosis and to determine who was actually exposed to screening and who was not. The misclassification of cases that were never invited to screening before diagnosis as being exposed to screening (because death occurred after the screening program was initiated) leads to spectacular underestimation of the benefit. It is interesting to observe that in evaluating any other intervention, it is generally appreciated that linking the outcome to be prevented to the intervention received is crucial. For some reason, this rather obvious fact does not seem to be understood in the evaluation of breast cancer screening.

CONCLUSIONS

In the methodology of evaluation of service screening, the following conclusions can be drawn:

- Before-after comparisons, with suitable safeguards against bias, provide a powerful tool for evaluating the impact of service screening on breast cancer mortality.
- In estimating the mortality reduction associated with screening, it is important to link the outcome, which is death from breast cancer, directly to the invitation to, or the actual exposure to, screening.
- It is therefore vital to obtain data on date of diagnosis as well as on date of death.
- To estimate the effect of actually receiving screening, we need information on who has been screened and who has not, in both the population at risk and the breast cancer death cases.
- Methods are available to correct such evaluation for potential biases, including self-selection for screening and changes in incidence, treatment, awareness, or management.
- Longer periods of evaluation are preferable because 1) they provide more data and hence more precise estimates and 2) a longer period gives screening more chance to manifest its full effect on mortality.

In terms of our knowledge of the effect of mammographic screening on breast cancer mortality, we conclude that

- The randomized, controlled trials show a significant benefit of invitation to screening, reflected in the 20%–30% reduction in breast cancer mortality.
- This benefit is attained and often exceeded in modern, organized service screening.
- The benefit of actually receiving screening in such organized service screening programs is much larger: 40%–60% reduction in breast cancer mortality.
- This benefit can be achieved in women in their forties if a short (18 months or less) interscreening interval is used.

REFERENCES

1. Shapiro S, Strax P, Venet L. Periodic breast cancer screening in reducing mortality from breast cancer. J Am Med Assoc 1971;215:1777–1785.
2. Shapiro S. Periodic screening for breast cancer: the HIP randomized controlled trial. Monogr Natl Cancer Inst 1997;22:27–30.
3. Tabár L, Vitak B, Chen HH et al. The Swedish Two-County Trial twenty years later: updated mortality results and new insights from long-term follow-up. Radiol Clin North Am 2001;38:625–651.
4. Andersson I, Nystörm L. Mammography screening. J Natl Cancer Inst 1995;87: 1263–1264.
5. Frisell J, Lidbrink E, Hellstrom L et al. Follow-up after 11 years: update of mortality results in the Stockholm mammographic screening trial. Breast Cancer Res Treat 1997;45:263–270.
6. Bjurstam N, Björneld L, Duffy SW et al. The Gothenburg Breast Screening Trial: first results on mortality, incidence and mode of detection for women ages 39-49 years at randomisation. Cancer 1997;80:2091–2099.
7. Miller AB, To T, Baines CJ, Wall C. The Canadian National Breast Screening Study: update on breast cancer mortality. Monogr Natl Cancer Inst 1997;22:37–41.
8. Miller AB, To T, Baines CJ et al. Canadian National Breast Screening Study-2: 13-year results of a randomized trial in women aged 50-59 years. J Natl Cancer Inst 2000;92:1490–1499.
9. Alexander FE, Anderson TJ, Brown HK et al. 14 years of follow-up from the Edinburgh randomized trial of breast-cancer screening. Lancet 1999;353:1903–1908.
10. Kerlikowske K. Efficacy of screening mammography among women aged 40 to 49 years and 50 to 69 years: comparison of relative and absolute benefit. Monogr Natl Cancer Inst 1997;22:79–86.
11. Hendrick RE, Smith RA, Rutledge JH et al. Benefit of screening mammography in women aged 40-49: a new meta-analysis of randomized controlled trials. Monogr Natl Cancer Inst 1997;22:87–92.
12. Gøtzsche PC, Olsen O. Is screening for breast cancer with mammography justifiable? Lancet 2000;355:129–134.
13. Olsen O, Gøtzsche PC. Cochrane review on screening for breast cancer with mammography. Lancet 2001;358:1340–1342.
14. Nixon RM, Prevost TC, Duffy SW et al. Some random effects models for the analysis of cluster randomized trials: application to the Swedish two-county trial of breast cancer screening. J Epidemiol Biostat 2000;5:349–358.

15. Tabár L, Fagerberg G, Duffy SW et al. The Swedish two-county trial of mammographic screening for breast cancer: recent results and calculation of benefit. J Epidemiol Community Health 1989;43:107–114.

16. Duffy SW, Tabár L, Smith RA. The mammographic screening trials: commentary on the recent work by Olsen and Gøtzsche. CA Cancer J Clin 2002;52:68–71.

17. Tabár L, Chen HH, Duffy SW et al. Primary and adjuvant therapy, prognostic factors and survival in 1053 breast cancers diagnosed in a trial of mammography screening. Jpn J Clin Oncol 1989;29:608–616.

18. Tabár L, Duffy SW, Yen MF et al. All-cause mortality among breast cancer patients in a screening trial: support for breast cancer mortality as an endpoint. J Med Screening; in press.

19. Paci E, Duffy SW, Giorgi D et al. Are breast cancer screening programmes increasing rates of mastectomy? Observational study. Br Med J 2002;325:418.

20. Duffy SW, Tabár L, Chen HH et al. The impact of organized mammography service screening on breast carcinoma mortality in seven Swedish counties: a collaborative evaluation. Cancer 2002;95:458–469.

21. Tabár L, Vitak B, Chen HH et al. Beyond randomized controlled trials: organized mammography screening substantially reduces breast carcinoma mortality. Cancer 2001;91:1724–1731.

22. Paci E, Duffy SW, Giorgi D et al. Quantification of the effect of mammographic screening on fatal breast cancers: the Florence programme 1990-96. Br J Cancer 2002;87:65–69.

23. Tabár L, Yen MF, Vitak B et al. Mammography service screening and mortality among breast cancer cases: results of 20-year follow-up before-after introduction of screening. Lancet; submitted.

24. Duffy SW, Cuzick J, Tabár L et al. Correcting for non-compliance bias in case-control studies to evaluate screening programmes. Appl Stat 2002;51:235–243.

25. Cuzick J, Edwards R, Segnan N. Adjusting for non-compliance and contamination in randomised screening trials. Stat Med 1997;16:1017–1029.

26. Ringash J. Preventive health care, 2001 update: screening mammography among women aged 40-49 years at average risk of breast cancer. Can Med Assoc J 2001;164:469–476.

27. Törnberg S, Carstensen J, Hakulinen T et al. Evaluation of the effect on breast cancer mortality of population-based mammography screening programmes. J Med Screening 1994;1:184–187.

28. Lenner P, Jonsson H. Excess mortality from breast cancer in relation to mammography screening in northern Sweden. J Med Screening 1997;4:6–9.

29. Jonsson H, Nyström L, Törnberg S et al. Service screening with mammography of women aged 50-69 years in Sweden: effects on mortality from breast cancer. J Med Screening 2001;8:152–160.

30. Blanks RG, Moss SM, McGahan CE et al. Effect of NHS breast screening programme on mortality from breast cancer in England and Wales, 1990-8: comparison of observed with predicted mortality. Br Med J 2000;321:665–669.

31. McCann J, Duffy SW, Day NE. Predicted long-term mortality reduction associated with the second round of breast screening in East Anglia. Br J Cancer 2001;84:423–428.

Chapter 9

Radiolabeled Octreotide for Treatment of Endocrine and Other Tumors

Irvin M. Modlin

Kevin D. Lye

Mark Kidd

Since the advent of nuclear medicine in the 1930s, the field has seen steady progress in the discovery, invention, and utilization of radiobiologic compounds. John Lawrence, recognized as the father of nuclear medicine, initiated radiopharmacology in 1937 by treating a leukemia patient with an isotope of phosphate. Dynamic imaging of the gastrointestinal system followed shortly thereafter, with Joseph Hamilton's use of radioactive sodium to demonstrate how consumed foods enter and traverse the human body. This process was predicated by the development of the cyclotron by John's brother Ernest Lawrence and was followed by Hal Anger's invention of the scintillation camera, the predecessor of today's positron emission tomography (PET) and single-photon emission computed tomography (SPECT) imaging systems (Fig. 9.1). After the identification later of the somatostatin receptor and the development of long-acting somatostatin analogues, the integration of nuclear medicine, oncologic therapy, and the

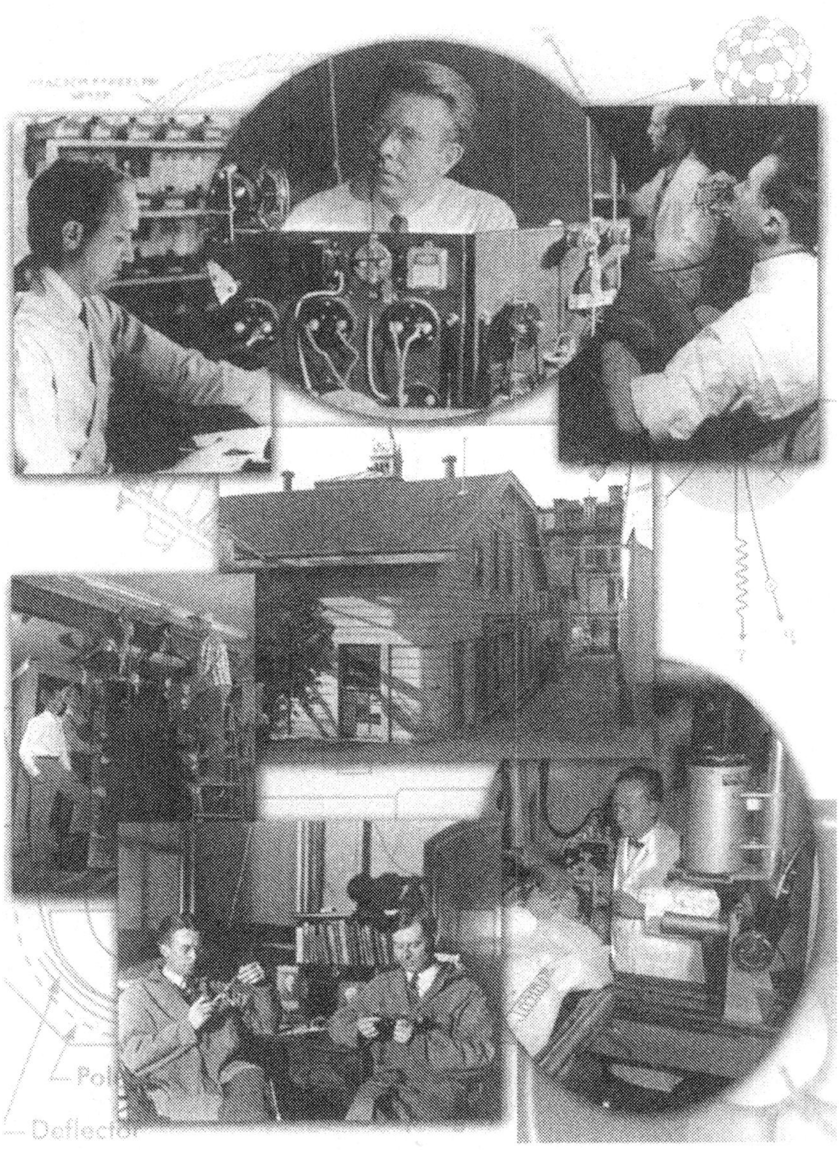

FIGURE 9.1 The nascence of radiopharmaceuticals. John Lawrence (*top left*), considered the father of modern radiotherapy, became interested in the biologic effects of neutrons during a 1935 visit to the University of California at Berkeley and was persuaded in 1936 to join the Radiation Laboratory (*center*) by his brother Ernest Orlando Lawrence (*top center*), who invented the cyclotron after arriving there in 1928. Soon after John Lawrence began his search for useful radioisotopes, he was able to generate ^{24}Na efficiently by bombarding rock salt with deuterons. Joseph Hamilton (*top right*), shown here drinking radiosodium in 1939, capitalized on the behavior of this substance and its convenient half-life of 15 hours to make it useful in medical diagnosis and therapy: "My medical friends tell me that the properties of radiosodium are almost ideal for many medical applications, such as the treatment of cancer." John Lawrence predicted that use of ^{24}Na would supersede that of radium. Hamilton

"Continued"

gastrointestinal system is now practiced with receptor-based radiotherapy (RBRT) targeting neuroendocrine and other diseases.

The need for additional methods and types of cancer therapy is evidenced by the overwhelmingly poor rate of long-term tumor control in metastatic and inoperable primary disease for most tumor types that are treated with conventional radiotherapy and chemotherapeutic regimens. The clinical application of recent discoveries in cellular biology promises improved safety and efficacy in a novel method of highly selective, easily administered, tumor-targeted radiotherapy; the nonisotopic delivery compounds themselves offer therapeutic and symptomatic benefit. This chapter reviews the basis of somatostatin analogue–related RBRT, examines the various analogues now in use and under investigation, and discusses the principal radioisotopes used for tumoricidal energy delivery. New developments in site- and disease-specific therapy are presented, as is a summary of recently identified potential side effects of RBRT, concluding with some reflections on the future of this technology.

OVERVIEW

Somatostatin is an endogenous tetradecapeptide hormone found in neuroendocrine cells of the pancreas, gastrointestinal tract, and nervous system. Initially known as somatotropin-release–inhibiting factor, somatostatin inhibits cell proliferation, down-regulates angiogenesis, and plays a role in immunomodulation and neurotransmission. The effects of somatostatin are mediated through the somatostatin receptor subset of the G protein family.[1,2] Five principal somatostatin

---

would down a solution of the isotope, after which Lawrence would track its course through his body. The drama of this burgeoning technology was enhanced at presentations in which Lawrence received fresh supplies of ^{24}Na by air mail, delivered to a lecture hall equipped with an awaiting scintigraph apparatus. Although radiosodium did not fulfill Lawrence's hopes, other isotopes found important applications in medicine: ^{32}P was employed for treatment of leukemia, polycythemia vera, and Hodgkin's disease, ^{131}I is still used in the treatment of thyroid disease, and ^{60}Co plays a role in cancer therapy. The development by Hal Anger (*lower right*) of the Anger (or scintillation) camera was a quantum leap for medical imaging, enabling the detection of gamma rays emitted by radioactive isotopes. This device is a direct forebear of today's PET and SPECT imaging systems. The three-ton steel door (*middle left*) for a human body radiation counting room was hoisted into place at Berkeley in 1960. The idea for a "heavy ion" machine was originated by Dr. Glen T. Seaborg and Albert Ghiorso, who conferred with Drs. Ernest Lawrence and Luis W. Alvarez. This group discussed building a machine to accelerate a beam composed of the nuclei of atoms up to ^{40}Ar; Ernest Lawrence (*at left, in lower left*) and Jesse W. Beams discuss the project in an unnamed laboratory at Yale University. The heavy ion machine, designed jointly by the University of California Radiation Lab (now Lawrence Berkeley National Laboratory) and Yale, became the precursor to modern linear accelerators. (Images courtesy of the Ernest Orlando Lawrence Berkeley National Laboratory.) PET, positron emission tomography; SPECT, single-photon emission computed tomography.

TABLE 9.1 Somatostatin Receptor–Expressing Tumors

APUDoma	Meningioma
Astrocytoma	Neuroblastoma
Breast carcinoma	Non-Hodgkin's lymphoma
Carcinoid	Non–small cell lung cancer
Central nervous system	Paraganglioma
Exocrine pancreas	Pheochromocytoma
Gastrinoma	Pituitary tumor
Glucagonoma	Prostate
Graves' disease of the thyroid	Pulmonary tumors
Graves' ophthalmopathy	Renal cell carcinoma
Hodgkin's disease	Sarcoidosis
Insulinoma	Sarcoma
Low-grade glioma	Small cell lung cancer
Lymphoma	Tuberculosis
Medullary thyroid carcinoma	Wegener's granulomatosis
Melanoma	

receptor subtypes have been identified and characterized. Of these receptors, somatostatin receptor type 2 ($hSST_R2$) appears to be overexpressed most commonly in human tumors. These receptors are expressed in neuroendocrine tumors, such as carcinoids, gastrinomas, pituitary tumors, endocrine pancreatic tumors, and paragangliomas; sarcoidosis and primary tissues involved with autoimmune diseases may also express sufficiently high numbers of somatostatin receptors to facilitate receptor-based imaging (Table 9.1).

Although several radioligands have been implemented on the basis of peptide receptor recognition throughout the past decade, and although multiple preclinical and clinical studies confirm the potential for their use in diagnosis as well as treatment of cancer patients, an optimal radiopeptide formulation has yet to be developed for RBRT. Receptor-based scintigraphy and its evolutionary counterpart, receptor-based radioisotope therapy, have undergone a tremendous surge in research and development over the past few years. New techniques employing isotopes of varying radioemittive energies and therapeutic radii enhance tumoricidal activity with acceptable toxicity profiles.

The logical successor to peptide-receptor scintigraphy, the labeling of molecules avid for somatostatin receptors with radionuclides emitting tumoricidal particles, is under intense scrutiny. Radiotherapy with labeled peptides that release alpha or beta particles as well as Auger or conversion electrons has been described in several studies. This mode of therapy is gaining acceptance and should be considered for eradication of metastatic disease, either as adjuvant therapy after surgical excision of somatostatin receptor–positive tumors for metastatic disease or as primary therapy for patients unable or unwilling to undergo surgery.

SOMATOSTATIN AND ITS ANALOGUES

Somatostatin

Initially identified in the rat,[3,4] a peptide inhibiting the release of growth hormone was serendipitously detected by Krulich and associates in 1968 during studies of the distribution of growth hormone–releasing factor in the mutrine hypothalamus. Table 9.2 includes a chronology of seminal events in the history of neuroendocrine disease and somatostatin analogue therapy preceding and succeeding this discovery.[6-18]

The biosynthesis of somatostatin has been studied extensively. Located on chromosome 3q in humans, somatostatin I is a highly conserved gene found within most vertebrates[19] that encodes preprosomatostatin, a protein of 116 amino acids.[20] Preprosomatostatin is cleaved into prosomatostatin (ProS), a 92-residue prohormone.[21] Depending on the cells in which ProS is expressed, its C-terminus is differentially processed into one of two bioactive peptides: somatostatin-14 (S-14) and somatostatin-28 (S-28). The former of these is the C-terminal 14 amino acids of the latter (Fig. 9.2A and B). In intestinal endocrine cells, S-28 peptide sequences are generated in numbers equal to those of $ProS_{1\text{-}64}$, suggesting a primary posttranslational proteolysis. S-14 is found in gastric and islet D cells (among others) and may arise either with concomitant formation of $ProS_{1\text{-}78}$ or indirectly from cleavage of S-28.

Native somatostatin is a cyclic peptide interconnected with disulfide bonds between its two cysteine residues. It has been demonstrated, however, that an equivalent linear sequence of the amino acids found in S-14 confers equivalent biologic activity, suggesting that the cyclic formation is not essential for receptor recognition.[22]

Continued work has expanded the initially simple concept of somatostatin as a peptide with the regulation of growth hormone secretion as its main function. It is known that somatostatin acts as a neurotransmitter in the brain. In addition to reducing the secretion of growth hormone, somatostatin inhibits the release of dopamine, norepinephrine, thyrotropin-releasing hormone, thyroid-stimulating hormone, corticotropin-releasing hormone, and somatostatin itself.[19] Although adrenocorticotropic hormone release is not suppressed in normal subjects, adrenocorticotropic hormone is inhibited by somatostatin in patients with Addison's disease or adrenocorticotropic hormone–secreting tumors. Within the gastrointestinal tract, somatostatin inhibits gut exocrine secretion, including that of gastric acid, pepsin, bile, and colonic fluid. Gut motor activity, including gastric emptying, gallbladder contraction, and small intestine segmentation (the to-and-fro mixing of chyme) are also inhibited by somatostatin. Secretion of gastrin, gut glucagon, secretin, and cholecystokinin are inhibited by somatostatin as well.[23] Additional effects of somatostatin[24,25] are described in Table 9.3; it is not difficult to appreciate why the term "somatostatin" is now considered rather archaic.

TABLE 9.2 Carcinoid Disease and the Development of Somatostatin Analogues

Year	Event
1867	Langhans[6] first describes a gut tumor with carcinoid characteristics.
1888	Lubarsch[7] records specific details of an intestinal tumor resembling a carcinoid.
1890	Ransom[8] provides the first comprehensive descriptions of the classical symptoms of what is later regarded as the carcinoid syndrome.
1907	Oberndorfer[9] first uses the word *karzinoide* to distinguish neoplasms that he believed were benign from malignant adenocarcinoma.
1914	Gosset and Masson[10] recognize carcinoids as endocrine-related tumors.
1953	Lembeck[13] demonstrates the presence of serotonin in carcinoid tissue.
1954	Thorson et al[14] analyze and propose the carcinoid syndrome.
1968	Krulich et al[5] describe an unexpected inhibitor of rat growth hormone release, concluding that "it is still too early to be certain of the physiological significance of this factor."
1969	Hellman and Lernmark[11] identify a factor in extracts of pigeon pancreatic islets which inhibits insulin release.
1973	Brazeau et al[12] isolate and sequence a cyclic tetradecapeptide inhibitory of human growth hormone, dubbing it "somatotropin-release inhibiting factor."
1977	Roger Guillemin and Andrew Schally are awarded the Physiology or Medicine Nobel Prize for discoveries concerning peptide hormone production within the brain, work that had led to their earlier isolation of somatostatin.
1977	Itakura et al[17] fuse a synthesized somatostatin gene to an *Escherichia coli* plasmid, harvesting the first functional human gene product produced through genetic engineering.
1978	Thulin et al[15] and Frölich et al[16] describe the use of somatostatin to control symptoms associated with carcinoid syndrome.
1982	Bauer et al[26] describe synthesis of the octapeptide SMS 201-995 (later named octreotide), noting its selectivity and potency above that of native somatostatin.
1985	Radiolabeled octreotide facilitates autoradiography of somatostatin receptors.[18]
1988	FDA approves octreotide acetate for diarrhea associated with intestinal cancer.
1992	Radiolabeled octreotide therapy trials begin.
1994	FDA approves [^{111}In]pentetreotide for scintigraphic localization of primary and metastatic neuroendocrine tumors bearing somatostatin receptors.
1998	FDA approves long-acting repeatable octreotide.

Abbreviation: FDA, Food and Drug Administration.

TABLE 9.3 Actions of Somatostatin

Processes inhibited by somatostatin
Absorption of carbohydrates
ADH-regulated water absorption
Enterologic motor activity, including gastric emptying, gallbladder contraction, small intestinal segmentation
Proliferation of lymphocytes, T cells, inflammatory, intestinal mucosal, cartilage, and bone-precursor cells
Angiogenesis
Angiotensin II–stimulated aldosterone secretion
ACTH secretion in Addison's disease patients or those with ACTH-producing tumors
Acetylcholine-stimulated catecholamine secretion from the renal medulla
Gastric acid secretion
Gastrin release
Histamine release by enterochromaffin-like cells
Inflammatory cascade
Parietal cell secretion of hydrochloric acid
Prolactin secretion in acromegaly
Release of calcitonin from thyroid parafollicular cells
Release of cytokines IL-6, IFN-γ
Release of dopamine from midbrain
Release of growth factors IGF-1, EGF, PDGF, VEGF
Release of norepinephrine, TRH, CRH, and endogenous somatostatin from the hypothalamus
Release of renin stimulated by hypovolemia
Secretion of gastric acid, pepsin, bile, colonic fluid
Secretion of glucagon
Secretion of growth hormone
Secretion of insulin
TSH-stimulated release of T_3 and T_4
Processes stimulated by somatostatin
Intestinal migrating motor complex activity
Vasoconstriction of the splanchnic circulation

Abbrevations: ADH, antidiuretic hormone; EGF, epidermal growth factor; IGF, insulin-like growth factor; PDGF, platelet-derived growth factor; IFN, interferon; TSH, thyroid stimulating hormone; ACTH, adrenocorticotropic hormone; CRH, corticotropin-releasing hormone; IL, interleukin; VEGF, vascular endothelial growth factor TRH, thynotropin releasing hormone; T_3, triiodothyronine; T_4, thyroxine.

Data from references 4, 19, 24, and 25.

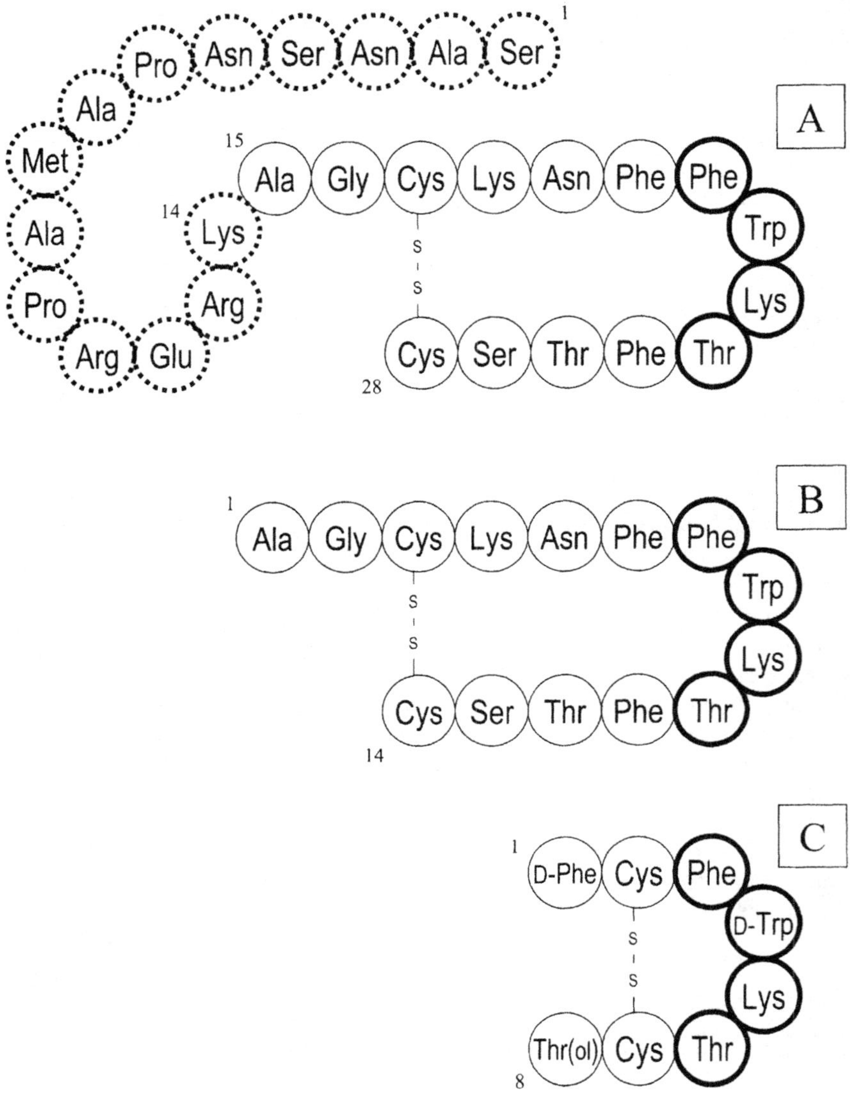

FIGURE 9.2 Amino acid sequences of the native human somatostatins and octreotide. Somatostatin-28 (A) is cleaved from the 92-residue prosomatostatin (ProS) by a trypsin-like peptidase; somatostatin-14 (B) may be simultaneously cleaved from ProS in a similar fashion, or it may be processed from somatostatin-28 at a later time. Octreotide (C), the archetypal somatostatin analogue, echoes the cysteine–cysteine disulfide bonds found in the native molecule and maintains the principal residues thought to be critical to somatostatin-receptor binding (Phe–Trp–Lys–Thr).

TABLE 9.4 Somatostatin Analogue Peptide Sequence

Name[a]	Peptide 1	2	3	4	5	6	7	8
Octreotide (OC)	D-Phe	Cys	Phe	D-Trp	Lys	Thr	Cys	Thr
Tyr^3-octreotide (TOC)	D-Phe	Cys	Tyr	D-Trp	Lys	Thr	Cys	Thr
Tyr^3-octreotate (TATE)	D-Phe	Cys	Tyr	D-Trp	Lys	Thr	Cys	Thr-OH
Lanreotide (LAN)	D-β-Nal	Cys	Tyr	D-Trp	Lys	Val	Cys	$Thr-NH_2$
Vapreotide (VAP)	D-Phe	Cys	Tyr	D-Trp	Lys	Val	Cys	$Trp-NH_2$
Seglitide	(N-Me)	Ala	Tyr	D-Trp	Lys	Val	Phe	
Depreotide		(N-Me)Phe	Tyr	D-Trp	Lys	Val	Hcy	

Abbreviations: Thr-OH, threoninol; N-Me, methylamino; β-Nal, D-3(2-napthyl)alanine

[a]Except for seglitide and depreotide, each analogue is cyclized with double-sulfide bonds between cysteine residues at positions 2 and 7.

Octreotide and Octreotate

Octreotide is a synthetic cyclic octapeptide; six of its eight amino acids are connected through a disulfide bond to form a ring structure similar to (but smaller than) that of the native somatostatins (Table 9.4). The sequence Phe-Trp-Lys-Thr is found within the ring portion of both molecules, although the specific *dextro* isomer of tryptophan is substituted into octreotide in this subsequence (Fig. 9.2C). In somatostatin and its analogues, these four residues are essential for receptor-specific binding.

Analogues of somatostatin have been under investigation for at least two decades. Many such agents are derivatives of octreotide, which was first synthesized[26] in 1982 (Table 9.2). The clinical usefulness of octreotide is facilitated by stereoisomer substitution at its first and fourth amino acids, which confers a half-life 80 times that of the 1 to 3 minutes of native somatostatin. The further substitution of tyrosine for phenylalanine in the three-position[27] and conversion of the *C*-terminus from an alcohol to a carboxylic acid[28] changes octreotide to Tyr^3-octreotate and improves the targeting of certain somatostatin-rich tissues. Conformational changes modifying the receptor-binding properties of these compounds may be effected by the addition of various conjugates and radioisotopes.[29]

Lanreotide and Long-Acting Repeatable Octreotide

Like long-acting repeatable octreotide, lanreotide is a depot formulation of a somatostatin analogue for intramuscular injection. Lanreotide requires more frequent administration than long-acting repeatable octreotide and has been used as a somatostatin receptor ligand in scintigraphic neuroendocrine tumor imaging. The structure of lanreotide is closely related to that of octreotide, having the same number of amino acids; D-Phe^1 is replaced by D-3(2-napthyl)alanine, Phe^3 by Tyr, and Thr^6 by Val. There is some evidence of improved diagnostic capacity with lanreotide-based imaging compared to that with octreotide-based compounds for certain tumor types.[30]

SOMATOSTATIN RECEPTORS

Somatostatin Receptor Subtypes

Although five human somatostatin receptor ($hSST_R$) genes have been identified, there are six somatostatin receptor subtypes; the messenger RNA transcribed from the SST_R2 gene can be spliced to produce receptors SST_R2A and SST_R2B, distinct (though similar) products with unique carboxyl-terminal sequences.[31] Each of the six somatostatin receptor subtypes consists of seven transmembrane domains with an overall amino acid sequence homology of approximately 50%. Most of the intersubtype differences are found within the intra- and extracellular domains, giving rise to the distinct properties and effects elicited with individual receptor subtype activation.

All somatostatin receptors bind the native somatostatin peptides S-28 and S-14, as well as the newly identified cortistatins.[32] The general affinity of these receptors for peptide analogues and nonpeptide ligands and the recent development of highly receptor-specific analogues[33] make it possible to differentiate the receptor subtypes and determine their individual functions. Much work is underway in the development of such singly specific somatostatin analogues. The first iodinatable SST_R1-selective analogue, CH-288, is the dodecapeptide *des*-$AA^{1,5}$-(Tyr^2, D-Trp^8, $IAmp^9$)somatostatin.[34] (The nomenclature *des* indicates the deletion of residues 1 and 5 from the native S-14 peptide after the parenthesized amino acid substitutions are made; IAmp represents 4-(*N*-isopropyl)-aminomethylphenylalanine.)

Tumor Expression of Somatostatin Receptors

Homogenate binding studies and in vitro somatostatin receptor autoradiography demonstrate that somatostatin receptors are expressed by various endocrine and nonendocrine human tumors (Table 9.1). A strong correlation has been demonstrated between in vitro analyses of somatostatin receptors with in vivo imaging by radiolabeled octreotide, and clinical studies have shown that radiolabeled octreotide may identify at least 80% of known gastroenteropancreatic endocrine tumor sites and up to 90% of carcinoid tumors.[1]

Although neuroendocrine tumors demonstrate high-density expression of somatostatin receptors, other tumors, including breast and renal cell carcinomas, lymphomas, and gliomas, frequently express significant levels of somatostatin receptors as well. Because the level of expression of somatostatin receptors is the key to tumor localization, the specificity of somatostatin analogues for the localization of tumors expressing $hSST_R2$ has prompted studies using higher doses of radioactivity with therapeutic intent. Early results from Krenning and associates[35]

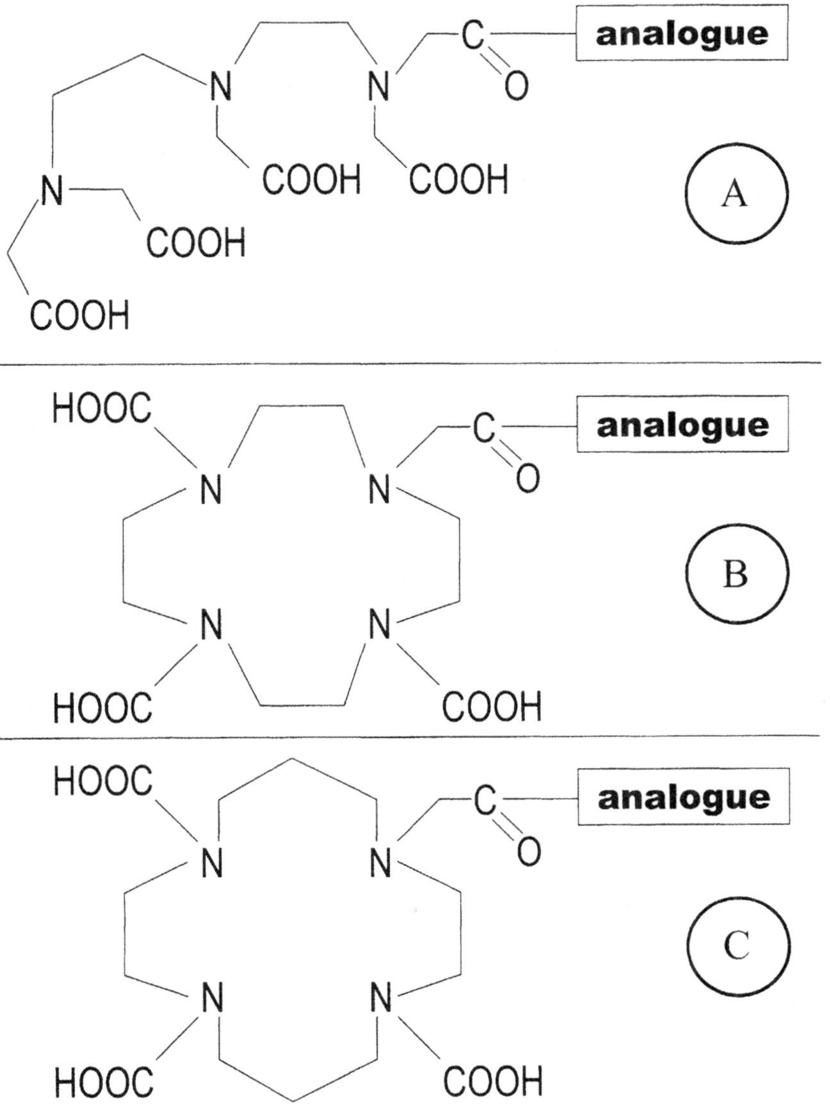

FIGURE 9.3 Principal chelator molecules used in receptor-based radiotherapy. A, DTPA. B, DOTA. C, TETA.

TABLE 9.5 Chelator Molecules

Abbrevation	Definition
DTPA	diethylene-triamine-pentaacetic acid
DOTA	1,4,7,10-tetra-azacyclo-dodecane–1,4,7,10-tetraacetic acid
TETA	1,4,8,11-tetra-azacyclo-tetradecane–N,N′,N″,N‴-tetraacetic acid
DO4Pr	1,4,7,10-tetra(carboxyethyl)-1,4,7,10-tetraazacyclododecane
DO3A1Pr	1,4,7-*tris*(carboxymethyl)-10-(carboxyethyl)-1,4,7,10-tetraazacyclododecane

suggested the feasibility of such treatment, and their initial experiences revealed no significant clinical side effects other than transient declines in counts of lymphocytes and platelets.

CHELATOR MOLECULES

Although somatostatin analogues are able to selectively target somatostatin receptor (SST_R)-expressing tissues, none alone is currently able to deliver to tissues the isotopes typically employed for the delivery of therapeutic radiation. Complex chelating molecules, which themselves are typically bound to one of the terminal peptides of the somatostatin analogue, are able to sequester and deliver the energy-emitting isotopes (Fig. 9.3).

The most commonly employed chelator molecules currently in use are diethylene-triamine-pentaacetic acid (DTPA) and 1,4,7,10-tetra-azacyclo-dodecane–1,4,7,10-tetraacetic acid (DOTA). Additional chelators, including 1,4,8,11-tetra-azacyclo-tetradecane–N,N′,N″,N‴-tetraacetic acid (TETA), are listed in Table 9.5.

By combining the various somatostatin analogues with these isotope chelators, numerous radioligands have been developed for in vivo diagnostic and radiotherapeutic use (Table 9.6). Reubi and colleagues[36] have used cell lines engineered for individual somatostatin receptor subtype expression to analyze the

TABLE 9.6 Chelator–Peptide Conjugates

Abbrevation	Definition
DTPAOC	DTPA-octreotide (pentetreotide)
DOTAOC	DOTA-octreotide
TETAOC	TETA-octreotide
DOTATOC	DOTA-Tyr^3-octreotide
DTPATATE	DTPA-Tyr^3-octreotate
DOTATATE	DOTA-Tyr^3-octreotate
DOTALAN	DOTA-lanreotide (MAURITIUS)
DOTAVAP	DOTA-vapreotide

TABLE 9.7 Affinity Profiles of Selected Somatostatin Analogues for Human Somatostatin Receptors

Peptide	$hSST_R1$	$hSST_R2$	$hSST_R3$	$hSST_R4$	$hSST_R5$
Somatostatin-28	5.2 ± 0.3	2.7 ± 0.3	7.7 ± 0.9	5.6 ± 0.4	4.0 ± 0.3
CH-288	23 ± 2	> 10,000	> 1000	> 10,000	> 1000
Octreotide	> 10,000	2.0 ± 0.7	187 ± 55	> 1000	22 ± 6
DTPAOC	> 10,000	12 ± 2	376 ± 84	> 1000	299 ± 50
In-DTPAOC	> 10,000	22 ± 3.6	182 ± 13	> 1000	237 ± 52
DOTAOC	> 10,000	14 ± 3	27 ± 9	> 1000	103 ± 39
Y-DOTAOC	> 10,000	20 ± 2	27 ± 8	> 10,000	57 ± 22
Ga-DOTAOC	> 10,000	7.3 ± 1.9	120 ± 45	> 1000	60 ± 14
DOTATOC	> 10,000	14 ± 2.6	880 ± 324	> 1000	393 ± 84
Y-DOTATOC	> 10,000	11 ± 1.7	389 ± 135	> 10,000	114 ± 29
Ga-DOTATOC	> 10,000	2.5 ± 0.5	613 ± 140	> 1000	73 ± 21
DTPATATE	> 10,000	3.9 ± 1	> 10,000	> 1000	> 1000
In-DTPATATE	> 10,000	1.3 ± 0.2	> 10,000	433 ± 16	> 1000
DOTATATE	> 10,000	1.5 ± 0.4	> 1000	453 ± 176	547 ± 160
Y-DOTATATE	> 10,000	1.6 ± 0.4	> 1000	523 ± 239	187 ± 50
Ga-DOTATATE	> 10,000	0.2 ± 0.04	> 1000	300 ± 140	377 ± 18
DOTALAN	> 10,000	26 ± 3.4	771 ± 229	> 10,000	73 ± 12
Y-DOTALAN	> 10,000	23 ± 5	290 ± 105	> 10,000	16 ± 3.4
DOTAVAP	> 10,000	29 ± 7	419 ± 104	743 ± 190	80 ± 19
Y-DOTAVAP	> 10,000	12 ± 2	102 ± 25	778 ± 225	20 ± 2.3

Abbreviations: $hSST_R$, human somatostatin receptor; IC_{50}, inhibitory concentration of 50%; SEM, standard error of the mean.

All values are IC_{50} ± SEM in nM. IC_{50} is the concentration of ligand that causes half-maximal inhibition of somatostatin-14 binding to engineered cells that express individual somatostatin receptors; lower values indicate stronger complex–receptor affinities. Nonisotopic metal chelates were used.

Adapted from reference 34.

in vitro binding characteristics of unlabeled and radiolabeled DOTA-octreotide, DOTA-Tyr³-octreotate, DOTA-lanreotide, DOTA-vapreotide, and DTPA-Tyr³-octreotate; Table 9.7 presents the receptor affinity profiles of these and other compounds.

Recent work has demonstrated novel modifications to the chelators now in use that yield isotope loading rates up to 2000-fold over that of DOTA, although actual yields have proved to be much less than the theoretical maxima.[37] Such agents, including 1,4,7,10-tetra(carboxyethyl)–1,4,7,10-tetra-azacyclo-dodecane (DO4Pr) and 1,4,7-*tris*(carboxymethyl)–10-(carboxyethyl)–1,4,7,10-tetra-azacyclo-dodecane (DO3A1Pr), may be used in the future for improved energy delivery.

Preliminary investigations have used isotopic halogens for the delivery of radiation in receptor-based radiotherapy. Carbohydration may allow direct radiolabeling of somatostatin analogues, allowing them to serve as the isotope chelators themselves. This process may even improve the pharmacokinetics of peptide delivery.[38] Early murine experiments comparing iodinated maltotriose-Tyr^3-octreotate with its unglycated congener have demonstrated diminished renal uptake and improved tumor uptake.

CURRENT AND FUTURE RADIOISOTOPES

There are approximately 275 isotopes of the 82 stable elements. If an atom with an artificial combination of neutrons and protons is generated, the unstable atom is called a *radioactive isotope* or *radioisotope*. The most common means for radioisotope generation is through neutron activation in a nuclear reactor, which involves the capture of a neutron by the nucleus of an atom, thus resulting in a neutron-rich isotope. Alternatively, protons may be introduced to the nucleus of an atom within a cyclotron, thereby creating a net deficiency of neutrons (and hence a proton-rich isotope).

In this state, stability of the radioisotope nucleus is usually achieved through emission of an alpha or beta particle. These particles may be accompanied by the emission of electromagnetic radiation or gamma rays; such is the process of radioactive decay.

Beta Electrons

The particle penetrance of beta decay is between that of alpha and gamma decay. Beta electrons (from isotopes such as ^{131}I and ^{90}Y) can penetrate about 1 cm of tissue before being brought to a halt by electrostatic forces.

Auger Electrons

The term *Auger effect,* attributed to the work in 1931 by the French physicist Pierre V. Auger (1899–1993), describes the process in which an ionized atom emits a second electron rather than a photon. Such ejected Auger electrons are typically of only a few thousand electron-volts in energy because this process occurs principally in elements of low atomic number. The effective radius of travel of these electrons is typically less than 100 nm. As such, Augur emitters (e.g., ^{111}In) are effective only if they are internalized within a cell.[39]

Gamma Electrons

A very highly charged gamma ray is produced when a parent isotope falls into a lower energy state. Gamma radiation is the most penetrating of all types; such photons can pass through the body and can cause damage by ionizing all molecules in their paths. ^{131}Iodine and ^{111}In also exhibit gamma decay.

Primary Radioisotopes

Although ^{111}In has thus far been the most frequently used therapeutic isotope for somatostatin-labeled radiotherapy trials, ^{90}Y, with its distinct radioemission profile, has also been tested in several series.

^{111}Indium At present, this isotope is the basis of the radiolabeled octreotide therapy regimen. With a half-life of 2.83 days and gamma decay by electron capture, ^{111}In has been bound to numerous somatostatin analogues, including octreotide and its substituted cousin octreotate. It is likely that ^{111}In will maintain its place in the therapeutic arsenal while newer agents and radioisotopes are evaluated.

Preclinical trials with ^{111}In-labeled octreotide have demonstrated high levels of neuroendocrine tumor uptake with promising dose-dependent responses in tumor size. De Jong and associates[40] reported on a series of patients treated with [^{111}In]DTPA^{0}-octreotide resulting in therapeutic effects in 21 of 40 evaluable patients, including remission and stabilization of disease. Modlin et al[1] used [^{111}In]pentetreotide as well as to treat 30 patients with SST_R-expressing gastroenteropancreatic (GEP) malignancies, with symptomatic stability or improvement in 80%. Anthony and colleagues[39] described similar benefits from [^{111}In]DTPA^{0}-octreotide therapy for 16 of 26 evaluable patients with otherwise untreatable GEP tumors; only mild and temporary myelodysplastic side effects had been identified through follow-up of over 48 months.

^{90}Yttrium With a half-life of 2.67 days, beta-emitting ^{90}Y has been explored as a therapeutic agent for somatostatin receptor–positive tumors. The recent development of the somatostatin ligand DOTA-D-Phe^{1}-Tyr^{3}-octreotide (DOTATOC) has been lauded for its stability and easy labeling with ^{90}Y, and animal models demonstrate the therapeutic promise of this agent. De Jong et al[41] report complete control of pancreatic tumors implanted into the flanks of rats when they were treated with 370 MBq of [^{90}Y]DOTA^{0}-Tyr^{3}-octreotide, although no animals with tumors greater than 14 cm^{2} demonstrated complete response with full tumor eradication.

In a series of 30 patients with histologically proven cancer, Paganelli and colleagues[42] have demonstrated complete or partial tumor mass reduction in 23% of cases, with an additional 64% showing stable disease. High becquerel activities of [^{90}Y]DOTATOC (up to 7.8 GBq) were administered with low evidence of myelotoxicity; cumulative radiation dose to the kidneys was a limiting factor.

Waldherr and associates[43] recently presented a phase II human trial evaluating the palliative effect of [^{90}Y]DOTATOC on the carcinoid syndrome in 41 patients with neuroendocrine GEP and bronchial tumors. Eighty-one percent of these patients had progressive disease that was resistant to conventional therapy. Administration of 6 GBq/m^{2} in four divided doses over the course of several months resulted in an overall response rate of 24%, which increased to 36% for patients with endocrine pancreatic tumors alone. One patient (2%) demonstrated complete remission, while partial remission, minor response, and stability of disease occurred in 22%, 12%, and 49%, respectively. Eighty-three percent of patients with carcinoid syndrome symptoms noted a significant reduction in their symptoms. All patients with morphine-dependent tumor-related pain reported a reduction in pain score. Emesis (23%) and pancytopenia (5%) were the most significant side effects. The impending publication of further human clinical trials will provide additional evaluation of ^{90}Y as a valuable therapeutic radioisotope.

Alternative Isotopes

Several isotopes have been examined for their potential as effective radiotherapy delivery vehicles. Lutetium and rhenium may soon evolve to the forefront of the therapeutic arsenal, and isotopes of technetium, iodine, copper, and gallium are on various portions of their respective therapeutic utility curves.

^{177}Lutetium Attempts to increase the therapeutic index for radiopharmaceuticals have led to a search for optimal radioisotopes and somatostatin-receptor ligands. Radiation doses from high-energy particles are limited by the risk of myelosuppression from circulating and accumulated agents.[44] The progression from iodine-, technetium-, and indium-tagged somatostatin analogues has recently shed light on lutetium.[45]

As an emitter of beta and gamma particles, ^{177}Lu effects significant tumor regression when it is bound to DOTA^0-Tyr^3-octreotate in rat models.[46] When compared with [^{111}In]octreotide, uptake is three to four times higher in most somatostatin receptor–positive tumors. The spleen and kidneys received the highest absorbed doses of radiation from ^{177}Lu; intravenous administration of amino acids reduced kidney exposure by a mean of 47%. Higher absorbed doses with relatively equivalent dosages to critical organs may lead lutetium to the forefront as the therapeutic agent of choice.

The half-life of reactor-produced lutetium is 6.64 days,[47] making it useful for *in situ* receptor-mediated brachytherapy. Tissue penetration range is lower in ^{177}Lu than in ^{90}Y; this may be beneficial for the treatment of small neuroendocrine tumors because the therapeutic-dose exposure of cells distant from the bound and internalized somatostatin receptors can be minimized. Cure rates in rat models are strongly correlative to initial tumor size;[48] single- or dual-dose treatments have resulted in cure rates of 75%–100% for pancreatic tumors $\leq$ 1 cm in diameter, whereas cure rates of only 40%–50% occurred in rats with larger tumors.

^{188}Rhenium Rhenium-labeled compounds can be produced through a double-ligand transfer reaction from perrhenate;[49] isotopic ^{188}Re itself is eluted from a ^{185}tungsten generator. Although it has a relatively short half-life of 16.8 hours,[50] this rhenium isotope has been used to label somatostatin analogues for tumor imaging and localization.[51] The beta- and gamma-emission profile of ^{188}Re makes it potentially attractive for therapeutic applications as well.[52] The rhenium moiety itself may enhance the binding selectivity of peptide ligands for somatostatin receptors.[53]

Studies in the mid-1990s examined the safety and therapeutic potential of ^{188}Re coupled to the somatostatin analogue RC-160 (vapreotide). More recently, vapreotide has been posited as an inhibitor of inflammation,[54] oral cancer,[55] and murine-grafted human epithelial ovarian carcinoma.[56,57] Zamora et al[58] tested intralesional and intracavity injection of the labeled analogue and uncoupled ^{188}Re in three mouse lines with prostate, mammary gland, and small cell lung carcinomas. Free ^{188}Re did not accumulate in normal tissues and was excreted rapidly through the urinary bladder; tumors that did not bind the labeled analogue showed no therapeutic benefit.

Hosono and colleagues[59] have examined the localization of small cell lung carcinoma xenografts in athymic mice by use of ^{188}Re- and ^{111}In-labeled octreotide. Although tumor uptake of the rhenium and indium compounds was found to be equivalent, the tumor-to-blood ratio for the ^{111}In compound was nearly 10 times that of the ^{188}Re compound, suggesting that indium may ultimately be a safer and more efficacious agent for tumor localization.

^{99m}Technetium Technetium-labeled compounds have been used for many years for nuclear medicine studies such as the bone scan and scintimammography. As the most widely used radioisotope in medicine, ^{99m}Tc plays a role in more than half of all nuclear medicine procedures. ^{99m}Tc has a short half-life of 6 hours,[50] which allows localization and imaging studies to be performed without allowing significant radiation accumulation within the patient. There is no high-energy beta emission from this technetium isotope, and the low-energy gamma rays that are emitted are detectable by gamma cameras for planar and three-dimensional imagery. Its role in the treatment of endocrine disease is often that of an imaging or localization precursor before definitive therapy, whether radiopharmacologic or surgical.

The relative ease of use and common availability of ^{99m}Tc in the nuclear medicine department of most hospitals makes it an attractive candidate for somatostatin analogue labeling. The technetium isotope is washed in solution from a lead-encased tube of ^{99}molybdenum, which itself has half-life of 66 hours. The molybdenum generator is returned to a nuclear reactor for recharging or exchange approximately every 2 weeks.

Research in Kyoto has demonstrated the relative stability of certain somatostatin analogues under the extreme conditions that may be needed for ^{99m}Tc-labeled compound creation.[60] However, octreotide cannot be labeled with ^{99m}Tc, because the ring structure of the former is susceptible to the cleavage reaction necessary for labeling with the latter.[61] Depreotide, another small, synthetic peptide, contains the same Tyr–D-Trp–Lys–Val amino acid sequence found in lanreotide and vapreotide in a cyclated structure that is free of disulfide bonds, making it amenable to ^{99m}Tc labeling. Vapreotide has been labeled with ^{99m}Tc by Amartey and associates[62] and has been evaluated using a process measuring its affinity for receptors expressed on HTB-121 breast cancer cell lines. Further studies with additional analogues will be needed to compare the efficacy of technetium with that of its indium counterparts.

Iodine Isotopes Iodine isotopes have a long history in the field of radiopharmaceuticals. Iodine is used most often for scintigraphy and treatment of iodine-avid thyroid tissue, and recent studies have demonstrated an analogous application of ^{123}I and ^{131}I to the detection and treatment of neuroendocrine tumors. Kaltsas et al[63] note that although scintigraphy with [^{111}In]pentetreotide is usually more sensitive for such lesions, scintigraphy with [^{123}I]meta-iodobenzylguanidine may occasionally demonstrate lesions that are not evident with [^{111}In]pentetreotide. [^{131}I]meta-iodobenzylguanidine (MIBG) therapy, based on a positive [^{123}I]MIBG scan, can produce significant improvement in symptoms and serum hormone levels and can moderate tumor regression or stabilization in patients with metastatic neuroendocrine tumors. As such, tumor detection and treatment with iodine isotopes may be an alternative or additional therapeutic option. A combination of both indium and iodine radionuclides is one possible regimen worth investigating for refractory cases.

^{64}Copper Isotopic copper (half-life, 12.7 hours[64]) has been under examination as a useful ligand label for somatostatin analogues for several years.[65] Recent research has explored the use of copper as an alternative imaging agent; compounds such as [^{64}Cu]TETA-octreotide have been shown (in small sample populations) to have superior tumor sensitivity to that of [^{111}In]DTPA-octreotide.[66]

More recently, Lewis and associates[67] compared DOTA-Tyr^3-octreotide and DOTA-Tyr^3-octreotate, each labeled with either ^{90}Y or ^{64}Cu, for absorbed doses in human organs and rat tumors. Although this study demonstrated comparable tumor to normal tissue dose ratios for the yttrium– and copper–octreotide compounds, the octreotate derivatives with either isotope delivered higher absorbed doses to tumors than the doses of their octreotide analogues. Complete tumor regression and improved survival times after treatment with [^{64}Cu]TETA-Tyr^3-octreotate in rats with pancreatic tumors have been shown in other experiments by the same group.[68]

In a separate rat model, [^{64}Cu]TETA-D-Phe^1-octreotide has been shown by Anderson and colleagues[65] to bind to the somatostatin receptor with five times the affinity of [^{111}In]octreotide and to have a desirable clearance profile (renal clearance with rapid excretion). However, the role of isotopic copper in the treatment of somatostatin-expressing tumors remains elusive and bears additional investigation.

^{68}Gallium Early studies involving gallium-labeled somatostatin analogues were presented in 1994.[69,70] More recent studies have addressed the applicability of

^{68}Ga-bound somatostatin analogues for imaging neuroendocrine tumors. Hofmann et al[71] used a high-yield preparation protocol with [^{68}Ga]DOTA-Tyr^3-octreotide to demonstrate 100% detection of 40 known lesions in eight patients, compared with 85% detection by [^{111}In]octreotide. Interestingly, the gallium compound gave a 100:1 tumor to nontumor activity ratio for central nervous system lesions, whereas the indium compound ratio was only 10:1.

Although indium-labeled octreotide has shown success in SPECT imaging of somatostatin receptor–positive neurinomas and neurofibromas, this method has limited sensitivity for detecting small meningiomas. Labeling octreotide compounds with a photon emitter affords the increased spatial resolution and biodistribution analyses associated with PET scanning. As such, Henze and associates[72] labeled (1,4,7,10-tetraazacyclododecane-N,N′,N″,N‴)-tetraacetate-D-Phe1-Tyr3-octreotide (DOTATOC) with the positron-emitting nuclide ^{68}Ga (half-life, 1.13 hours) to facilitate the analysis of three patients with a total of eight meningiomata ranging in diameter from 7 to 25 mm. After injection, all tumors were clearly identified with a high tumor-to-background ratio and good correlation with previously obtained conventional tomography. This experience suggests that ^{68}Ga-labeled octreotide may be another valuable tool for the identification of somatostatin receptor–positive tumors, including small meningiomata.

RADIOPHARMACEUTICALS: ANALOGUE-CHELATOR-ISOTOPE COMPLEXES

Radiolabeled octreotide has been used for more than a decade as an imaging agent and, more recently, has been used as a therapeutic agent for otherwise untreatable tumors that express somatostatin receptors. Distinct chemical production processes are used for the conjugation of chelator molecules to specific somatostatin analogues; the radioisotope is typically mixed with this lyophilized compound immediately before administration.

Receptor Affinity

Most human tumors express at least one of the known human somatostatin receptor subtypes.[51] Neuroendocrine tumors frequently overexpress $hSST_R2A$,[73] whereas intestinal adenocarcinomas tend to overexpress one or both of $hSST_R3$ or $hSST_R4$. The $hSST_R$ binding characteristics of somatostatin ligand analogues can thus be used to selectively target specific tumor tissues if the expressed receptor profile can be determined. As shown in Table 9.7, although DTPA-octreotide (DTPAOC) binds with high affinity to $hSST_R2$ and with moderate affinity to $hSST_R3$ and $hSST_R5$, it does not significantly bind to $hSST_R1$ or $hSST_R4$. DOTA-lanreotide (DOTALAN) binds to $hSST_R2$ and $hSST_R5$ with high affinity and to $hSST_R3$ with moderate affinity, and it does not significantly bind to $hSST_R1$ or $hSST_R4$.[36] Other somatostatin analogues with particular affinities to various

TABLE 9.8 Human Somatostatin Receptor Binding Affinities

Ligand	hSSTR1	hSSTR2	hSSTR3	hSSTR4	hSSTR5
Somatostatin-14	0.4	0.1	0.3	0.8	0.6
Octreotide	200	0.6	10	> 1,000	7
[^{111}In]DTPAOC	> 1,0000	1.5	30	> 1,000	1
[^{111}In]DTPATOC	> 1,000	1.5	250	> 1,000	1
[^{67}Ga]DOTATOC	> 10,000	2.5	600	> 1,000	70
DOTATATE	> 10,000	1.5	> 1,000	453	547
[^{90}Y]DOTATATE	> 10,000	1.6	> 1,000	523	187
[^{67}Ga]DOTATATE	> 10,000	0.2	> 1,000	300	377
DOTALAN	154	0.3	15	2.5	0.4
[^{90Y}]DOTALAN	215	4.3	5.1	3.8	10
[^{99m}Tc]depreotide	> 1,000	1	1.5	> 1,000	2

Abbreviations: Abbreviations: $hSST_R$, human somatostatin receptor; IC_{50}, inhibitory concentration of 50%; SEM, standard error of the mean.

All values are IC_{50} ± SEM in nM. IC_{50} is the concentration of ligand that causes half-maximal inhibition of somatostatin-14 binding to engineered cells that express individual somatostatin receptors. Lower values indicate stronger complex–receptor affinities. Isotopic metal chelates were used. The absolute values here cannot be compared with those in Table 9.7.

Adapted from reference 78.

$hSST_R$ subtypes are also finding increased clinical utility: [^{99m}Tc]depreotide (Table 9.8) and [^{99m}Tc]-6-hydrazinopyridine-3-carboxylic acid (HYNIC) octreotide and are now used for imaging of neuroendocrine tumors and nonsmall cell lung cancer.[51,74,75]

Affinity for $hSST_R2$ has been found to be markedly improved for gallium-labeled DOTA-Tyr^3-octreotide when compared with the same yttrium-labeled compound.[76] Although strong affinity for $hSST_R2$ occurs for [^{111}In]DTPA-Tyr^3-octreotate and [^{90}Y]DOTA-Tyr^3-octreotate, [^{68}Ga]DOTA-Tyr^3-octreotate binds to $hSST_R2$ with a considerably higher affinity. Improvement in $hSST_R3$ affinity of up to 30-fold occurs for unlabeled or ^{90}Y-labeled DOTA-octreotide when compared with its tyrosine^3-substituted analogues. With their similar $hSST_R$ binding profiles, [^{111}In]DOTA-lanreotide is a sensitive radioligand for tumor diagnosis, whereas the higher-energy [^{90}Y]DOTA-lanreotide is suitable for receptor-mediated radionuclide therapy. However, an über-radiopeptide formulation does not yet exist.

The highest affinity for $hSST_R5$ among all compounds tested by Virgolini and colleagues[77,78] was found in [^{90}Y]DOTA-lanreotide, although this compound had lesser affinities for $hSST_R3$ and $hSST_R4$. In their studies, substitution of DTPA by

DOTA yielded significant increases in $hSST_R3$ and $hSST_R5$ binding affinities in yttrium-labeled octreotide, lanreotide, and vapreotide compounds.

It is likely that these observed alterations in receptor subtype affinity are secondary to subtle steric changes as well as to the regional charges and hydrophilic alterations imparted to the somatostatin analogues by these chelator compounds. The various radii of the radioisotopes themselves may play a role in the coordinate geometry of the complexes as a whole, as demonstrated by the improved receptor affinities with [^{68}Ga]DOTA, when compared with [^{90}Y]DOTA in both Tyr^3-octreotide and Tyr^3-octreotate. These and similar observations must be used in the development of future peptide radioligands.

Internalization of Receptor-Bound Somatostatin Analogues

The technique of in vivo somatostatin receptor scintigraphy for $hSST_R$-positive tumors provides visualization within 24–48 hours after intravenous injection of the radiolabeled [^{111}In]DTPA^0-D-Phe^1-octreotide. The effectiveness of radiolabeled scintigraphy and receptor-mediated radiotherapy relies on the finding that somatostatin receptors, once bound with the appropriate ligand, are internalized and become associated with cytoplasmic organelles, such as the Golgi apparatus, lysosomes, and secretory granules.[79] This provides an extended residence time of radioactivity on or within such neuroendocrine tumors. Hofland et al[80] noted that [^{125}I]DOTA^0-Tyr^3-octreotide is internalized to a degree five times that of [^{125}I]DTPA^0-Tyr^3-octreotide in human insulinoma cells. Furthermore, the latter compound provided a tumor : background radioactivity ratio ranging from 274:1 up to 623:1, depending on the tumor tissue type; this suggests that such internalization provides suitable targeting for receptor-guided radiotherapy or radioguided surgery.

Diagnostic Radiopharmaceuticals

The observation that certain organs and tissues selectively absorb particular chemicals or elements has been noted by physicians, chemists, and physicists for decades. Radiopharmacy has used this information by attaching isotopes to biologically active substances with the goal of incorporating the traceable marker into a known biochemical process. Diagnostic and therapeutic radiopharmaceutical agents have undergone significant development and refinements over the past decade; various isotope ligands and somatostatin analogues have been investigated in the search for optimal imaging and therapeutic profiles. Pentetreotide can easily be labeled with ^{111}In and is currently commercially available for the scintigraphic localization of tumors expressing somatotstatin receptors. The [^{90}Y]DTPA linkage is less stable than that of [^{111}In]DTPA; however, ^{90}Y does form a highly stable complex with DOTA, rendering it a more suitable delivery vehicle for therapeutic radiation doses.[81]

Therapeutic Radiopharmaceuticals

Auger and conversion electrons, which have a very short particle range (3–100 nm) and limited tissue penetration, are emitted by ^{111}In. Studies have demonstrated that isotope-coupled somatostatin analogues are internalized in somatostatin receptor–positive tumor cells.[82] There is evidence that lysosomal compartments may be one area in which the internalized receptors are sequestered, but the ^{111}In itself is translocated to the perinuclear area and into the nucleus.[83] The potential therapeutic efficacy of radiation from isotopes bound to octreotide or other somatostatin analogues may be limited (on a micro-, rather than a pico-, scale) to the region of the binding site. Such physical specifications may improve the efficacy of this targeted therapy by minimizing the tissue distribution of irradiation.

Diagnostic Imaging

Intraoperative identification of somatostatin receptor–positive tumor burden using a radioisometric probe is of demonstrable benefit for gastrinomas and small tumors with high concentrations of appropriate receptors.[84] Patients are injected with [^{111}In]DTPA^{0}-octreotide immediately before surgery; audible cues from a gamma probe provide assistance in identifying relative scintillation counts of diseased tissue both in vivo and after resection.

Recurrence of tumor burdens expressing somatostatin receptors is evaluable with [^{111}In]DTPA0-octreotide; this radiopharmaceutical has demonstrated high overall sensitivity for the localization of neuroendocrine tumors.[30] Inclusion of somatostatin-receptor imaging in localization or staging for several neuroendocrine tumor types has been shown to provide significant advantages in cost effectiveness, patient management, and quality of life and may lead to a change in treatment plan in up to 40% of patients.[84] Evaluation of somatostatin-receptor imaging in patients with breast cancer, malignant lymphomas, granulomatous diseases, and other tumors is underway.

Multimodality Capture and Display

Gamma particle scintigraphy has long been used in the field of radioisotope-labeled somatostatin analogues; PET, with the incorporation of appropriate isotopes, is experiencing an increase in modern clinical use. Information garnered from either of these modalities is maximized when it is taken in context with data from conventional computed tomography (CT) or magnetic resonance imaging. One group has touted the potential for improved monitoring of thoracoabdominal disease progression or regression by the coaxial superposition and display of data from planar SPECT and conventional CT slices.[85] More recently, new transmission and emission tomography hardware, which is capable of simultaneously acquiring SPECT and CT images,[86] has been used to plan (and occasionally alter) surgical intervention for patients with neuroendocrine tumors and thyroid carcinomas. Advantages of transmission and emission tomography may include improved anatomic localization of otherwise obscure somatostatin receptor–positive tumors, demonstration of unsuspected bone involvement, and differentiation of physiologic uptake from tumor uptake.

Bioactive Molecules

For decades, various isotopes have been used in nuclear medicine to image tumors of multiple types. The mechanisms of tracer uptake may be through specific mechanisms or binding properties. Useful isotopic compounds such as [^{123}I]- or [^{121}I]meta-iodobenzylguanidine and [^{111}In]pentetreotide emit gamma particles for scintigraphic imaging by external cameras. Additional techniques, such as radiolabeled monoclonal antibodies and [^{18}F]fluorodeoxyglucose PET, may be supplanted by positron-emitting tracers such as ^{11}C bound to the serotonin precursor 5-hydroxytryptophan for the detection of carcinoid tumors.[87] Similarly, [^{11}C]-L-3,4-dihydroxyphenylalanine (L-DOPA) may prove to be superior for visualizing small endocrine pancreatic tumors, although its usefulness for differentiating small cell and nonsmall cell lung carcinomas has been questioned.[88] It seems likely that any of these bioactive molecules may eventually be labeled with higher-energy radioemitters for site-selective delivery of therapeutic radiation.

THERAPEUTIC OPTIONS

In 1990, Harris[89] commented on the prospects of radiolabeled octreotide in the treatment of GEP and other tumors. In the years after the finding that receptors for vasoactive intestinal peptide and somatostatin are overexpressed in certain tumor cell lines, ^{123}I and ^{99m}Tc were the initial agents of choice for the scintigraphic diagnosis of neuroendocrine tumors, small primary adenocarcinomas, and liver metastases.[90]

Departments of nuclear medicine play prominent roles in the research, development, and administration of radiopharmaceuticals such as ^{111}In- and ^{90}Y-labeled somatostatin analogues.[91] This noninvasive, targeted tumor therapy has developed in tandem with sentinel lymph node detection and handheld gamma probes[92] and provides a less invasive means of disease staging. Analysis and control of chemotherapy necessitate careful monitoring of the effects of chemotherapeutic drugs on normal organ function. However, nuclear medicine studies should always be interpreted along with the information obtained from other imaging tests to ensure maximal amplification of patient care.

Both somatostatin receptor imaging in patients with endocrine pancreatic cancer and [^{18}F]fluorodeoxyglucose PET imaging in patients with nonendocrine pancreatic cancer play an important role in the detection or confirmation of the presence of pancreatic masses.[93] Each modality has a role in tumor staging and provides information regarding the suitability of an individual for surgery. Such imaging can assist clinicians in the selection of available systemic therapeutic options.

Chemotherapy and Biotherapy For Neuroendocrine Tumors

Medical treatment for neuroendocrine tumors is guided by the properties of the tumor in question; options for therapy have historically included chemotherapy, somatostatin analogues, and interferon-α. Endocrine pancreatic tumors, lung carcinoids, and highly proliferative neuroendocrine tumors are typically responsive to chemotherapy. Partial remissions in 40%–60% of patients with advanced disease treated with regimens of streptozotocin combined with 5-fluorouracil and doxorubicin have generated median survivals of about 2 years. Anaplastic endocrine pancreatic tumors and lung carcinoids have been countered with cisplatinum–etoposide regimens.[94]

Slowly proliferating tumors, such as midgut carcinoids, demonstrate much poorer response rates with the same combinations of cytotoxic agents; short-lasting responses are common in less than 10% of patients. In such patients, treatment with biologic agents such as interferon-α has shown promise.[94] Subcutaneous doses of 3 to 9 million units of interferon-α three to seven times per week have resulted in improvement of serum biochemical markers in 50% of patients and long-term reduction of tumor size (lasting up to 3 years) in 15% of patients.

The treatment of neuroendocrine tumors of the gut and pancreas has been supplemented by somatostatin analogues for quite some time. Most currently available somatostatin analogues target somatostatin receptor subtypes 2 and 5 and demonstrate low affinity for subtype 3. Octreotide is now approved in the United States for the reduction of growth hormone and insulin-like growth factor-1 in acromegaly, the suppression of severe diarrhea and flushing associated with malignant carcinoid syndrome, and the treatment of profuse watery diarrhea associated with vasoactive intestinal peptide-secreting tumors. Standard doses of 100–300 (μg/day provide relief of symptoms in approximately 60% of patients; improvement in serum biochemical markers is noted in up to 70% of patients. However, fewer than 5% of patients demonstrate significant and long-lasting improvement in tumor burden with this therapy alone.[94] Long-acting formulations of somatostatin analogues do significantly improve the quality of life in such patients.

Peptide Receptor Radionuclide Therapy: Preclinical Experiences

A variety of tumors expressing somatostatin receptors are identifiable with peptide receptor scintigraphy using the radiolabeled somatostatin analogue

[^{111}In]DTPA^0-octreotide. This sensitive and specific technique is used to localize primary tumors and metastases of neuroendocrine and other cancers. Peptide receptor radionuclide therapy, through the administration of high doses of ^{111}In- or ^{90}Y-labeled octreotide analogues, has shown to be of benefit in treatment of appropriate tumors. Investigations by De Jong and colleagues[95] of the radiotherapeutic effect of ^{90}Y- and ^{111}In-labeled DOTA^0-Tyr^3-octreotide as well as [^{111}In]DTPA^0-octreotide have been undertaken in Lewis rats with somatostatin receptor–positive pancreatic tumors in either the flank or the liver. Thirty rats with end-stage disease were treated up to a maximal cumulative radiation dose of about 74 GBq. Rats with flank tumors required at least two 111-MBq injections of [^{111}In]DOTA^0-Tyr^3-octreotide to achieve a tumor response; 40% of the animals demonstrated complete tumor remission after a 10-month follow-up period. One or two injections of [^{90}Y]DOTA^0-Tyr^3-octreotide yielded stability of disease. Rats with liver tumors receiving doses of 370 MBq of [^{111}In]DTPA^0-octreotide or 93 MBq of [^{90}Y]DOTA^0-Tyr^3-octreotide showed inhibition of growth of somatostatin receptor–positive metastases. Follow-up of these animals for up to 2 years demonstrated no major clinical side effects; transient declines in platelet counts and lymphocytes were noted. Therapeutic efficacy was documented as well: of 21 animals with progressive disease receiving a cumulative dose of more than 20 GBq of [^{111}In]DTPA^0-octreotide, eight showed stabilization of disease, and six additional subjects showed a reduction in tumor size. Better results were noted in animals with tumors that demonstrated higher accumulations of the radioligand.

Radionuclide Therapy

The benefits of radionuclide therapy are conferred when there is a significantly higher and constant radiation dose delivered to the target tissue relative to normal and surrounding tissue. Pretherapy dosimetry studies are used to determine the relative absorption of radiation in tissues and organs and to evaluate maximum tolerable doses. Cremonesi et al[96] demonstrated the safety profile of the ^{90}Y-labeled somatostatin analogue DOTATOC. Biologic clearance of the ^{90}Y-labeled agent was evaluated with serial blood samples and complete urine collections obtained up to 48 hours after injection. Biodistribution was examined with several whole-body scintigrams. Prompt radioisotope clearance from the blood, principally by renal excretion, was noted by the finding of low total-body, or background, irradiation. This study and several others demonstrate that high levels of [^{90}Y]DOTATOC can be administered with acceptable radiation doses to unaffected organs.

Palliative benefit has been obtained from [^{131}I]MIBG therapy, especially in patients with demonstrably elevated concentrations of tumor radioactivity on initial scintigraphy. Several trials have shown how receptor-mediated in situ radiotherapy has brought clinical benefit and radiologic evidence of tumor regression to patients with neuroendocrine disease who have failed to respond to conventional therapeutic modalities.[97] A measured progression from cell-line testing through animal models to human safety trials can be seen throughout the literature of the past decade, with the demonstration of this sequence for almost every novel radioisotope or ligand that has come under investigation.[95,98] Concern exists in some circles about the existence of a reliable, steady supply of therapeutic radionuclides in quantities sufficient for both research and routine clinical use.[99]

Several studies have examined somatostatin analogues with multireceptor affinities. The novel radiopharmaceuticals [^{111}In]- and [^{90}Y]DOTA-lanreotide as well as [^{111}In] DOTATOC and [^{90}Y]DOTATOC have shown encouraging results in the localization and treatment of $hSST_R$-positive tumors. Initial results with the yttrium-labeled versions of these compounds has suggested benefit with radionuclide receptor–based radiotherapy, which may ultimately be cost-effective when compared with conventional radiotherapy or chemotherapy.[100]

Because of its $hSST_R$ binding profile, [^{90}Y]DOTA-lanreotide has been used for receptor-mediated radionuclide therapy. Having previously demonstrated that [^{111}In]DOTA-lanreotide is an acceptable imaging agent for neuroendocrine tumors, Virgolini and colleagues[78] reported clinical evidence of the therapeutic potential of [^{90}Y]DOTA-lanreotide, itself dubbed MAURITIUS (Multicenter Analysis of a Universal Receptor Imaging and Treatment Initiative, a eUropean Study). An early study using MAURITIUS included 25 patients with advanced cancer (refractory to conventional antineoplastic treatments) in whom pretreatment dosimetry and imaging with [^{111}In]DOTA-lanreotide were performed. With this agent, occult tumor sites that were not otherwise identified with conventional imaging (CT, magnetic resonance imaging, or bone scan) were identified in six patients with carcinoid tumors, one patient with prostate cancer, and one patient with lymphoma.[78] All patients with gastrointestinal cancers demonstrated liver metastases. No severe hematological toxicity or change in renal or liver function reulting from [^{111}In]DOTA-lanreotide therapy was reported.

Later, in a series of more than 60 patients treated with 10 GBq of [^{90}Y]DOTA-lanreotide, radiologic evidence of disease stability was documented in 35% of patients, and regression of disease was noted in 15%.[51] No acute or chronic severe hematologic toxicity or change in renal or liver function parameters due to [^{90}Y]DOTA-lanreotide was reported. More recent updates regarding this trial have suggested that tumor stability occurred in up to 41% of 154 treated patients and tumor regression occurred in 14%.[77]

The Rotterdam group[101] (Krenning et al) have accumulated the largest series of patients treated with various radiolabeled somatostatin analogues; this group has carefully examined the issue of radiation dose tolerability. In a series of 50 patients with malignant, progressive, or symptomatic somatostatin receptor–positive tumors, divided doses totaling 4.7 to 160 GBq of [^{111}In]DTPA^0-octreotide were administered over the course of 4 to 6 months. Forty patients receiving cumulative doses greater than 20 GBq were evaluable. CT evaluation of tumor sizes before and after therapy suggested a treatment benefit in 19 patients, manifested by mild tumor regression or stability of lesion volume. Categorization by tumor grade showed a positive therapeutic effect of ^{111}In therapy in nine of 10 patients with grade 4 tumors and lesser effects (44% and 33%) for patients with tumor grades 3 and 2, respectively.

Analysis of serum biochemical markers in this study by Krenning et al[19] revealed a correlation between chromogranin A and CT response: increasing chromogranin A corresponded with increasing lesion volume on CT imaging, whereas stable or decreasing chromogranin A was accompanied with stable or decreasing tumor volume on CT. Side effects for the above radioisotope therapy were mild and transient, in general, but were statistically significant as well. Mean platelet counts dropped from baseline levels of $311 \pm 30 \times 10^9$/L to just greater than 100×10^9/L after 70 to 90 GBq of [^{111}In]DTPA^0-octreotide. Transient decreases in mean white blood cell counts and hemoglobin were similarly identified. More severe toxicities were rarely encountered: three patients receiving more than 100 GBq of [^{111}In]DTPA^0-octreotide experienced myelodysplastic syndrome, acute myeloid leukemia, or both; this radioactivity count was suggested as the maximal tolerable dose of this agent in light of such bone marrow toxicity. Severe renal toxicity, including markedly elevated serum creatinine and significantly diminished creatinine clearance, was not noted.

The results of this phase I clinical trial examining the role of [^{111}In]DTPA^0-octreotide in patients with advanced neuroendocrine tumors are comparable to those of earlier studies.[97,102,103] Additional findings suggest that this agent is, overall, poorly effective for end-stage patients and those with large tumors. However, further work by Krenning and colleagues[40] has employed [^{90}Y]DOTA-Tyr^3-octreotide and [^{177}Lu]DOTA-Tyr^3-octreotate in similar phase I trials. Of 92 patients treated with the former, 20% demonstrated a partial response, and an additional 60% maintained stability of their disease burden. Complete remission of symptoms was noted in several patients with either malignant insulinoma or gastrinoma. Early reporting on 18 of 63 patients treated with divided doses of [^{177}Lu]DOTA-Tyr^3-octreotate suggests that this analogue may have the highest tumor uptake of any of the widely employed radiolabeled somatostatin analogues. Excellent tumor-to-kidney accumulation ratios, with tumor shrinkage occurring in 6% of patients, tumor stability in 44%, and partial remission of disease in 39%, suggest that this compound is yet another promising vehicle for the therapy of otherwise untreatable SST_R2-positive tumors.

Radioguided Surgery

Hand-held gamma-detecting probes have been used in the localization of in situ $hSST_R$-expressing tumor during open surgical procedures.[82,92] In some cases, this is the only means by which the tumor in question can be identified, even after ultrasound, CT, superselective angiography, and endoscopic ultrasound have been performed.[104] Radioguided surgery after isotope-labeled octreotide administration allows localization of small insulinomas, identification of occult neoplasms, and verification of the completeness of surgical excision in the field and in the excised tissue. Unfortunately, the background emission from both kidney and liver, combined with the lack of ideal handheld collimators, has limited intraoperative localization.

DISEASE- AND SITE-SPECIFIC ADVANCES

Somatostatin receptor imaging has been examined in patients with a wide variety of diseases, including gastrinomas, endocrine pancreatic tumors, pituitary tumors, paragangliomas, and carcinoids.[84] Other diseases in which somatostatin receptors may also be expressed, such as sarcoidosis and autoimmune diseases, have been explored as well. More studies examining breast cancer, malignant lymphomas, and other granulomatous diseases are underway. The use of radiolabeled somatostatin analogues as a therapeutic modality does not yet have a well-established base, although animal models and human protocols are beginning to provide additional information about the safety and efficacy of such agents for this purpose.

Novel murine models of xenografted human non–small cell lung tumors have been used to address the possibility of somatostatin receptor induction to enhance binding of ^{90}Y-labeled somatostatin analogues.[105] Early in vivo results suggest significantly longer median tumor quadrupling times in animals with vector-induced receptor overexpression.

Antiangiogenesis

The affinity of radiolabeled somatostatin analogues to receptors expressed in angiogenic tumor vessels has raised the question of correlation between Auger electron emission and antitumor activity. Neuroblastoma tumor fragments expressing $hSST_R2$, when treated with an ^{111}In-labeled somatostatin analogue, demonstrate inhibited growth and angiogenesis.[106] A portion of the antiangiogenic response to isotopically labeled somatostatin analogues is likely derived from the analogue itself; octreotide has been shown to inhibit the expression of vascular endothelial growth factor and matrix metalloproteinase-2 in murine models;[107] the latter of these is involved in angiogenesis in the breakdown of basement membranes, facilitation of neovascularization, and tubule formation. These effects of octreotide on angiogenesis[108] may evolve into an effective in situ radiotherapy modality.

In fact, Gulec and colleagues[109] reported an in vitro model of human placental vein tissue treated with a radiolabeled somatostatin analogue. Proliferating endothelial cells express $hSST_R2$, and the SST_R2-avid [^{111}In]pentetreotide was used to treat disks of human placental vein that were placed in culture. Although

[^{111}In]pentetreotide did not completely block the initiation of angiogenic sprouting, neovascular growth was significantly decreased in comparison to control groups, including those treated with unlabeled pentetreotide. It is postulated that both Auger electron and gamma radiation effects contributed to the observed angiotoxicity. An increased receptor-profile selectivity or an altered radiation profile will no doubt improve on these results in the future.

GEP tumors

Carcinoid tumors express high levels of $hSST_R2$, making such tumors principal targets for receptor-based radiotherapy. In a recent trial, Modlin et al[1] treated 39 patients who had otherwise recalcitrant neuroendocrine tumors with SST_R2-avid [^{111}In]pentetreoetide to examine the tolerability and safety of accumulated doses up to 1200 mCi. Patients with unresectable advanced malignancy, at least one tumor-bearing site documented by [^{111}In]pentetreotide uptake, and no further conventional therapeutic options were included in the study. Of treated patients with GEP tumors, 80% demonstrated stability or improvement in symptomatology, and 77% demonstrated stability or modest improvement over serial radiographic examinations. Fifty-six percent of patients with evaluable hormone markers demonstrated stable levels or a significant decrease in one or more measured markers. The major observed toxicities were myelosuppresion, including leukopenia, thrombocytopenia, and anemia. Alterations in renal function (acute renal tubular necrosis) occurred in only one patient (2.5%).

Anthony et al[39] reported on a series of patients with carcinoid or pancreatic islet cell tumors treated with at least two monthly intravenous injections of 180 mCi of [^{111}In]pentetreotide; these investigators have shown a clinical benefit in 16 (62%) of 26 patients. Significant tumor necrosis was noted in 27%; 81% of patients demonstrated decreased hormonal markers. Side effects included transient leukocytopenia, thrombocytopenia, and anemia. These trials and others highlight the potential of receptor-mediated radiotherapy to avoid the dramatic adverse consequences of long-term cytotoxic therapy or external-beam irradiation for inoperable neuroendocrine disease.

Other studies have examined the role of yttrium-based chelate–analogue complexes in the treatment of carcinoid disease. Divided doses totaling 7.4 GBq of [^{90}Y]DOTATOC have been administered to patients with progressive neuroendocrine tumors by Waldherr and colleagues,[110] yielding low rates of either complete remission or progression of disease (5% and 8%, respectively) but a notable incidence of partial remission and stability of disease (18% and 69%, respectively). Of patients with carcinoid syndrome, significant reductions in symptoms such as diarrhea, cutaneous flushing, and wheezing were noted (83%, 46%, and 63%, respectively). As in the Modlin et al[1] trial, the principal side effects included transient leukopenia, anemia, and renal insufficiency.

Gastrinomas, often located in the head of the pancreas and often metastatic at time of detection, can be difficult to localize. Although octreotide-mediated scintigraphy has been shown to confirm or provide additional details in gastrinoma identification,[111,112] experience with receptor-mediated radiotherapy for these tumors has been scant, and efficacy trials are underway.[113] One case report[114] has described tumor regression in a patient with metastatic gastrinoma from four divided 1-GBq doses of [^{90}Y]DOTA-lanreotide administered over a 6-month period.

Pancreas

Octreotide-based scintigraphy can be useful for the identification of somatostatin receptor–expressing tumors of the pancreas, which may be amenable to long-term symptom control by nonradiolabeled somatostatin analogue therapy.[115] Additionally, investigation into the suitability of ^{90}Y-labeled DOTA-lanreotide for patients with neuroendocrine tumors of the pancreas has suggested its potential for use as therapy for otherwise untreatable disease.[114,116]

Lung

Small cell lung cancer and bronchial carcinoid tumors express somatostatin receptors. Recent work suggests that therapy with radiolabeled somatostatin analogues may improve outcomes in patients with solid tumors such as these when compared with treatment with traditional chemotherapy alone.[117] Both somatostatin receptor–positive and somatostatin receptor–negative lung tumors have shown inhibition from somatostatin analogues.

Thymus

High uptake of indium-labeled octreotide has occurred in tumors of the thymus. In contrast to carcinoid and other neuroendocrine tumors, high levels of $hSST_R3$ have been identified in thymic tumors by immunohistochemical means.[118] This may play a role in the future development of receptor-specific ligands for this tumor type.

Breast

Neuroendocrine tumors of the breast that express $hSST_R$ have been targeted with [^{90}Y]DOTA-D-Phe^1-Tyr^3-octreotide; phase I trials have established safety and tolerability for a fixed-dose regimen of three cycles each of 120 mCi and have demonstrated significant tumor shrinkage.[119] Other ligands, such as DOTA-lanreotide, may have superior binding profiles to breast tumors and may prove efficacious in such therapy.[116]

Thyroid

Early experience with receptor-mediated radionuclide therapy using [^{90}Y]DOTA-TOC against nonmedullary thyroid cancer has been disappointing. Görges et al[120] reported failure of tumor control in three such patients, with total treatment doses approaching 37 GBq. It appears that traditional surgical or iodine-based radioablative procedures have yet to be supplanted.

Ovary

Human ovarian cancers have recently been shown to express $hSST_R1$ with high frequency (65%), as well as $hSST_R2$, $hSST_R3$, and, to a lesser extent, $hSST_R5$ (65%, 41%, and 24%, respectively).[121] The presence of these subtypes may be exploited in the future by subtype-specific radiolabeled ligands complexed with somatostatin analogues.

Pituitary

The observation of in vivo uptake of [^{64}Cu]TETA-Tyr^3-octreotate in somatostatin-rich pituitary tissue in rat[28] and primate[27] models suggests that improved radioligand specificity may lead to the development of an effective therapeutic agent for primary or metastatic pituitary disease.

Malignant Melanoma

Lum and colleagues[122] analyzed $hSST_R$ subtypes within 23 melanomas of 17 patients and found expression of $hSST_R1$ in 96% of tumors, $hSST_R2$ in 83%, $hSST_R3$ in 61%, $hSST_R4$ in 57%, and $hSST_R5$ in 9%. Although octreotide scintigraphy identified only 63% of all tumors, those that are imaged may be susceptible to somatostatin analogues radiolabeled with high-energy isotopes, potentially making available a new means of therapy. In fact, ^{90}Y-labeled lanreotide compounds have demonstrated high binding affinities for melanoma call lines[116]; further trials are needed.

Merkel Cell Tumors

Also known as trabecular cancer or neuroendocrine cancer of the skin, Merkel cell cancer is a rare entity that typically appears in hair follicles or as firm, painless skin lumps on or just beneath the skin. The precise cause of Merkel cell cancer is not known; most cases occur in white patients between the seventh and ninth decades of life.

Surgery and external-beam radiotherapy are the principal treatments for Merkel cell carcinoma; the cancer grows rapidly and often metastasizes to other parts of the body, with spread to the regional lymph nodes and commonly to the liver, bone, lungs, and brain. Treatment of micrometastatic Merkel cell tumors may be performed as adjuvant therapy or for recurrent disease. ^{111}In-labeled octreotide has recently been described for the scintigraphic visualization of primary and noncutaneous metastatic disease[123]; therapeutic trials may be forthcoming if more specific receptor-binding ligands can be devised.

Sarcoidosis

Receptors for somatostatin have been identified in the inflammatory lesions of patients with sarcoidosis and other granulomatous diseases. The recent elucidation of $hSST_R2$ as the predominantly expressed receptor subtype in patients with sarcoidosis, Wegener's granulomatosis, and giant-cell arteritis,[124] and the subsequent successful treatment of one such patient with a somatostatin analogue, are early evidence that $hSST_R2$-specific radiolabeled analogues may some day be of therapeutic use for such disease processes.

Oncogenic Osteomalacia

Mesenchymal tumors are the most common cause of oncogenic osteomalacia[125]; this hypophosphatemic syndrome is identified by defects in bone mineralization, reduced serum calcitriol concentrations, and hypophosphatemia due to excessive phosphaturia. Mesenchymal tumors, which often are small, slow growing, and situated in unusual locations, have been shown to express somatostatin receptors.[126] Scintigraphic imaging with [^{111}In]pentetreotide has been used to facilitate surgical treatment of the condition; for widespread, diffuse, or otherwise unresectable disease, high-energy isotopes bound to somatostatin analogues may provide equally effective therapy.

Endocrine Ophthalmopathy

A subset of patients with active endocrine ophthalmopathy and orbital somatostatin receptor expression, as identified by [^{111}In]pentetreotide scintigraphy, have been treated with biweekly intramuscular lanreotide.[127] Promising results occurred in patients treated at an early stage. It is possible that radiolabeled pentetreotide or another analogue complex may improve or extend results in such patients. The fact that the orbit and its contents are a common site for metastatic carcinoid disease[128] suggests the possibility that radiopharmaceutical therapy with ^{111}In- or ^{90}Y-labeled somatostatin analogues will be undertaken in the future.

Central Nervous System

Treatment of central nervous system tumors with intrathecal injections of ^{90}Y-labeled DTPA was discussed in 1976.[129] However, these early trials (before the development of somatostatin analogues) failed to demonstrate effective remission in most patients. Even after octreotide and metal-chelating complexes such as DTPA became available, enthusiasm for receptor-mediated radiotherapy for central nervous system lesions has been tempered by the intact blood–brain barrier,[130] which prevents these compounds from reaching the target $hSST_R2$. However, these receptors are expressed in tumors such as medulloblastoma, central primitive neuroectodermal tumors, neurocytoma, gangliocytoma, olfactory neuroblastoma, and paraganglioma.[131] Medulloblastoma cell proliferation inhibition by octreotide has been demonstrated, and ^{68}Ga-labeled DOTATOC preparations demonstrate excellent tumor-to-nontumor contrast for central nervous system imaging. Therefore, highly selective, high-energy compounds for such lesions are plausible. Cavalla et al[131] and Koper et al[132] pointed out that any trial with somatostatin analogues in patients with meningiomata (located outside the blood-brain barrier) should be undertaken with great caution; such compounds have been shown to increase thymidine incorporation into cultured meningioma cells by 21%–49%, suggesting an increase in DNA synthesis.

SIDE EFFECTS OF RADIOISOTOPE THERAPY

Adverse effects from isotopic somatostatin analogue therapy may arise from the analogue itself or from the energy emitted by the associated radiolabel. Somatostatin analogues themselves may induce reduced glucose tolerance, nausea, abdominal cramps, diarrhea, fat malabsorption, and flatulence.[134] Although the onset of such symptoms is typically a few hours after the initial analogue injection, they usually subside within 10 to 14 days, even with continued analogue treatment. An increased incidence of cholesterol gallstones occurring with long-term somatostatin analogue therapy[134] has been described in the literature.

Phase I and II trials for the agents in question have addressed the safety of patients exposed to varying activities of these radiolabeled pharmaceuticals. In most cases, transient prompt or delayed myelosuppression has been identified as the principal morbidity; thrombocytopenia and decrements in renal function have also been noted. Caplin and associates[135] noted side effects such as short-lived decrements in circulating lymphocytes and platelets as well as a slight reduction in glomerular filtration rate in a small number of patients with known disseminated neuroendocrine tumors who were treated with multiple doses of between 1.3 and 4.6 GBq of [^{111}In]octreotide administered over a 12-month period.

However, concern about radiation accumulation and exposure and its effects on renal function has its merit in the concentration and excretion of most radiolabeled somatostatin analogues by the renal system. Moll and colleagues[136] described five of 29 patients (17%) treated with [^{90}Y]DOTA-D-Phe^1-Tyr^3-octreotide (mean cumulative dose, 165.4 ± 36.4 mCi/m^2) who experienced biopsy-proven thrombotic microangiopathy within 3 months of the final ^{90}Y administration. All five patients experienced increasing serum creatinine values; three patients had end-stage renal failure within 6 months, and the other two experienced chronic renal insufficiency. Renal biopsies confirmed the presence of thrombotic microangiopathy identical in appearance to lesions seen after external-beam radiotherapy. Ultimately, this nephrotoxicity must be weighed against the benefits of such therapy in these otherwise untreatable patients.[137]

Additional consideration must be given to the potential radiation exposure to health care workers and family members of patients undergoing high-energy radioisotope therapy. The Nuclear Regulatory Commission provides extensive guidelines for the handling and disposal of isotope-containing materials, fluids, and tissues.

FUTURE CONSIDERATIONS

The future of receptor-based scintigraphy and isotopic therapy will be enhanced with forthcoming imaging hardware, which will provide improved gamma particle sensitivity and dramatically higher resolution, thus ensuring earlier detection of smaller lesions. Continued advances in computer processing power will allow manipulation of more data, including multimodality overlays for improved anatomic correlations with surrounding tissues and structures.

Isotopes of optimal tissue penetration and emitted energies will be identified, multiple isotopes may be bound to larger chelating molecules, and treatment with several receptor-specific moieties will be used. Amplification of somatostatin receptor expression on tumor cells will be effected with adenoviral or other vectors, thereby increasing the isotopic energy delivery to such lesions. Current management guidelines for GEP and neuroendocrine tumors (Fig. 9.4) will continue to evolve.

The coupling of new or additional functional moieties onto current or novel ligands will broaden the therapeutic arsenal at the command of the treating physician. The creation of less toxic, deliverable analogues of free-radical radiosensitizers, such as misonidazole, attached to somatostatin-avid ligands, will enhance the tumoricidal properties of today's regimen of agents. Improved knowledge of the inconstant somatostatin receptor profile during and after the course of radiochemotherapy administration will allow the development of more precise isotopic regimens. With the introduction of highly tissue-specific compounds, renewed interest in ^{10}boron neutron capture therapy will allow the evolution of binary cancer treatments that combine intravenously delivered agents and external neutron beam activation. To supplement the solid-tumor–destroying beta-emitting radioisotope conjugates that are already in use, short-lived alpha-emitting radioisotopes (such as ^{149}terbium, ^{211}astatine, ^{213}bismuth, and ^{225}actinium) bound to appropriate receptor ligands will target, sequester, and destroy individual tumor cells intravascularly during the process of metastasis itself.

Although improved resolution of scintigraphy scanners will afford higher-resolution imaging, continued developments in simultaneous transmission and emission tomography will hone the correlation of anatomic data and receptor-expressing tissues beyond that which can be easily ascertained from each modality

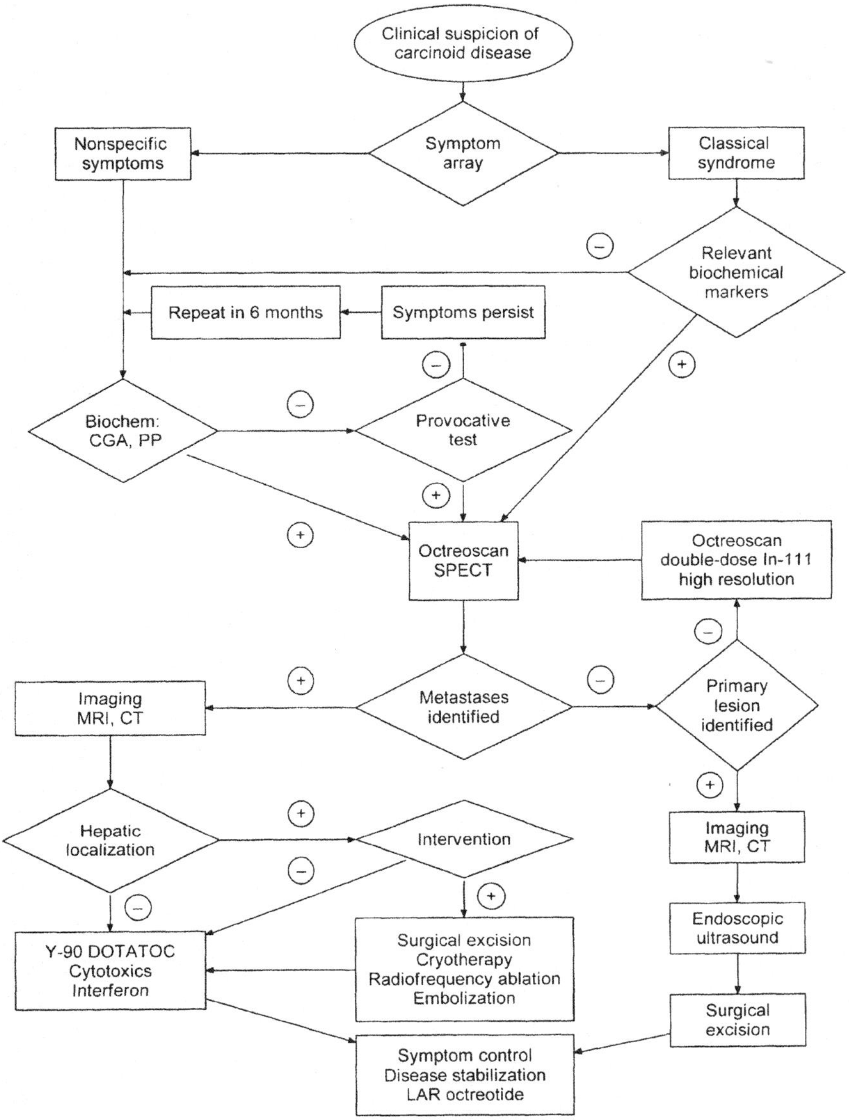

FIGURE 9.4 A diagnostic and therapeutic algorithm for the management of suspected carcinoid disease. The tenets of this process are applicable to neuroendocrine disease in general. The identification of elevated biochemical markers (chromogranin A [CGA]; pancreatic polypeptide [PP]) warrant scintigraphic imaging, likely with [^{111}In]DTPA-octreotide. The identification of a primary lesion should be pursued if it is not readily evident on the initial scan. Diffuse and otherwise inoperable metastases may be addressed with intravenous receptor-based isotopic therapy, traditional cytotoxic regimens, or biologic modifiers, such as interferon and long-acting repeatable (LAR) octreotide.

in isolation. Dual- or multiple-isotopic SPECT imaging will expand beyond the realm of prostatic disease and improve the treatment of patients with endocrine carcinomata, highlighting multiclonal tumor nests with disparate somatostatin receptor profiles.

Sadly, the nirvana of approaching receptor-mediated radiotherapy with per-tumor absolute site specificity (and sensitivity) remains elusive. The stream of useful radioisotopes and ligands that have come into clinical use over the past decade will continue to flow as a result of diligent work by dedicated nuclear chemists, medical physicists, core laboratory personnel, and clinicians. With continued trials and research, it is not unreasonable to assume that metastatic disease, and perhaps primary tumors, will someday be identified with genome-predictive scintigraphic screening while in the kilocellular range and be promptly obliterated with the intravenous administration of a personally tailored radioisotope cocktail!

REFERENCES

1. Modlin I, Murren J, Cornelius E et al. The utility of octreotide and isotopes in the diagnosis and treatment of neuroendocrine tumors (NETs). J Gastroenterol Hepatol 2002;17[suppl]:A80.
2. Afargan M, Janson ET, Gelerman G et al. Novel long-acting somatostatin analog with endocrine selectivity: potent suppression of growth hormone but not of insulin. Endocrinology 2001;142:477–486.
3. Krulich L, Dhariwal APS, McCann SM. Stimulatory and inhibitory effects of purified hypothalamic extracts on growth hormone release from rat pituitary in vitro. Endocrinology 1968;83:783–790.
4. Lamberts SW, van der Lely AJ, de Herder WW et al. Octreotide. N Engl J Med 1996;334:246–254.
5. Krulich L, Dhariwal AP, McCann SM. Stimulatory and inhibitory effects of purified hypothalamic extracts on growth hormone release from rat pituitary in vitro. Endocrinology 1968;83:783–790.
6. Langhans T. Ueber einen drusenpolyp im ileum. Virchows Arch 1867;38:559–560.
7. Lubarsch O. Ueber den primaren Krebs des Ileum, nebst Bemerkungen uber das gleichzeitige Vorkommen von Krebs und Tuberkolose. Virchows Arch 1888;111:280–317.
8. Ransom WB. A case of primary carcinoma of the ileum. Lancet 1890;2:1020–1023.
9. Oberndorfer S. Karzenoide tumoren des dünndarms. Frankf Zschr Pathol 1907;1:426–430.
10. Gosset A, Masson P. Tumeurs endocrines de l'appendice. Presse Med 1914;25:237–239.
11. Hellman B, Lernmark Å. Inhibition of the in vitro secretion of insulin by an extract of pancreatic alpha-1 cells. Endocrinology 1969;84:1484–1488.
12. Brazeau P, Vale W, Burgus R et al. Hypothalamic polypeptide that inhibits the secretion of immunoreactive pituitary growth hormone. Science 1973;179:77–79.
13. Lembeck F. 5-Hydroxytryptamine in a carcinoid tumor. Nature 1953;172:910–911.
14. Thorson Å, Biörck G, Björkman G et al. Malignant carcinoid of the small intestine with metastases to the liver, valvular disease of the heart (pulmonary stenosis and tricuspid regurgitation without septal defects) peripheral vasomotor symptoms, bronchoconstriction, and an unusual type of cyanosis: a clinical and pathologic syndrome. Am Heart J 1954;47:795–817.

15. Thulin L, Samnegard H, Tyden G et al. Efficacy of somatostatin in a patient with carcinoid syndrome. Lancet 1978;2:43.
16. Frölich JC, Bloomgarden ZT, Oates JA et al. The carcinoid flush: provocation by pentagastrin and inhibition by somatostatin. N Engl J Med 1978;299:1055–1057.
17. Itakura K, Hirose T, Crea R et al. Expression in Escherichia coli of a chemically synthesized gene for the hormone somatostatin. Science 1977;198:1056–1063.
18. Maurer R, Reubi JC. Brain somatostatin receptor subpopulation visualized by autoradiography. Brain Research 1985;333:178–181.
19. Patel YC. Somatostatin and its receptor family. Front Neuroendocrinol 1999;20:157–198.
20. Shen LP, Pictet RL, Rutter WJ. Human somatostatin I: sequence of the cDNA. Proc Natl Acad Sci USA1982;79:4575–4579.
21. Ensinck JW, Baskin DG, Vahl TP et al. Thrittene, homologous with somatostatin-28(1-13), is a novel peptide in mammalian gut and circulation. Endocrinology 2002;143:2599–2609.
22. Harris AG. Somatostatin and somatostatin analogues: pharmacokinetics and pharmacodynamic effects. Gut 1994;35[3 suppl]:S1–S4.
23. Reichlin S. Somatostatin. N Engl J Med 1983;309:1495–1501.
24. Reichlin S. Neuroendocrine-immune interactions. N Engl J Med 1993;329:1246–1253.
25. Buscail L, Vernejoul F, Faure P et al. Regulation of cell proliferation by somatostatin. Ann Endocrinol 2002;63[2 pt 3]:2S13–2S8.
26. Bauer W, Briner U, Doepfner W et al. SMS 201–995: a very potent and selective octapeptide analogue of somatostatin with prolonged action. Life Sci 1982;31:1133–1140.
27. Lewis JS, Srinivasan A, Schmidt MA et al. In vitro and in vivo evaluation of ^{64}Cu-TETA-Tyr3-octreotate: a new somatostatin analog with improved target tissue uptake. Nucl Med Biol 1999;26:267–273.
28. Lewis JS, Lewis MR, Srinivasan A et al. Comparison of four ^{64}Cu-labeled somatostatin analogues in vitro and in a tumor-bearing rat model: evaluation of new derivatives for positron emission tomography imaging and targeted radiotherapy. J Med Chem 1999;42:1341–1347.
29. Reichert DE, Norrby PO, Welch MJ. Molecular modeling of bifunctional chelate peptide conjugates: 1. Copper and indium parameters for the AMBER force field. Inorg Chem 2001;40:5223–5230.
30. Virgolini I, Patri P, Novotny C et al. Comparative somatostatin receptor scintigraphy using ^{111}In-DOTA-lanreotide and ^{111}In-DOTA-Tyr3-octreotide versus ^{18}FDG-PET for evaluation of somatostatin receptor-mediated radionuclide therapy. Ann Oncol 2001;12[suppl 2]:S41–S45.
31. Schonbrunn A. Somatostatin receptors: present knowledge and future directions. Ann Oncol 1999;10[suppl 2]:S17–21.
32. Spier AD, de Lecea L. Cortistatin: a member of the somatostatin neuropeptide family with distinct physiological functions. Brain Res Brain Res Rev 2000;33:228–241.
33. Rohrer SP, Birzin ET, Mosley RT et al. Rapid identification of subtype-selective agonists of the somatostatin receptor through combinatorial chemistry. Science 1998;282:737–740.
34. Reubi JC, Schaer JC, Waser B et al. A selective analog for the somatostatin sst1-receptor subtype expressed by human tumors. Eur J Pharmacol 1998;345:103–110.
35. Krenning EP, de Jong M, Kooij PP et al. Radiolabelled somatostatin analogue(s) for peptide receptor scintigraphy and radionuclide therapy. Ann Oncol 1996;10[suppl 2]:S23–S29.
36. Reubi JC, Schar JC, Waser B et al. Affinity profiles for human somatostatin receptor subtypes SST1-SST5 of somatostatin radiotracers selected for scintigraphic and radiotherapeutic use. Eur J Nucl Med 2000;27:273–282.
37. Keire DA, Jang YH, Li L et al. Chelators for radioimmunotherapy: I. NMR and ab initio calculation studies on 1,4,7,10-tetra(carboxyethyl)-1,4,7,10-tetraazacyclododecane (DO4Pr)

and 1,4,7-*tris*(carboxymethyl)-10-(carboxyethyl)-1,4,7,10-tetraazacyclododecane (DO3A1Pr). Inorg Chem 2001;40:4310–4318.

38. Wester HJ, Schottelius M, Scheidhauer K et al. Comparison of radioiodinated TOC, TOCA and Mtr-TOCA: the effect of carbohydration on the pharmacokinetics. Eur J Nucl Med Mol Imaging 2002;29:28–38.

39. Anthony LB, Woltering EA, Espenan GD et al. Indium-111–pentetreotide prolongs survival in gastroenteropancreatic malignancies. Semin Nucl Med 2002;32e:123–132.

40. De Jong M, Valkema R, Jamar F et al. Somatostatin receptor-targeted radionuclide therapy of tumors: preclinical and clinical findings. Semin Nucl Med 2002;32:133–140.

41. de Jong M, Breeman WA, Bernard BF et al. Tumor response after [^{90}Y-DOTA^{0},Tyr^{3}]octreotide radionuclide therapy in a transplantable rat tumor model is dependent on tumor size. J Nucl Med 2001;42:1841–1846.

42. Paganelli G, Zoboli S, Cremonesi M et al. Receptor-mediated radiotherapy with ^{90}Y-DOTA-D-Phe^{1}-Tyr^{3}-octreotide. Eur J Nucl Med 2001;28:426–434.

43. Waldherr C, Pless M, Maecke HR et al. The clinical value of [90Y-DOTA]-D-Phe1-Tyr3-octreotide (90Y-DOTATOC) in the treatment of neuroendocrine tumours: a clinical phase II study. Ann Oncol 2001;12:941–945.

44. Buchsbaum DJ, Rogers BE, Khazaeli MB et al. Targeting strategies for cancer radiotherapy. Clin Cancer Res 1999;5[suppl 10]:3048S–3055S.

45. Breeman WA, de Jong M, Kwekkeboom DJ et al. Somatostatin receptor-mediated imaging and therapy: basic science, current knowledge, limitations and future perspectives. Eur J Nucl Med 2001;28:1421–1429.

46. Kwekkeboom DJ, Bakker WH, Kooij PP et al. [^{177}Lu-DOTA0-Tyr^{3}]octreotate: comparison with [111In-DTPA]octreotide in patients. Eur J Nucl Med 2001;28:1319–1325.

47. Lewis JS, Wang M, Laforest R et al. Toxicity and dosimetry of (177)Lu-DOTA-Y3-octreotate in a rat model. Int J Cancer 2001;94:873–877.

48. de Jong M, Breeman WA, Bernard BF et al. [^{177}Lu-DOTA(0),Tyr^{3}] octreotate for somatostatin receptor-targeted radionuclide therapy. Int J Cancer 2001;92:628–633.

49. Spradau TW, Katzenellenbogen JA. Protein and peptide labeling with (cyclopentadienyl)tricarbonyl rhenium and technetium. Bioconjug Chem 1998;9:765–772.

50. Le Bideau F, Salmain M, Top S et al. New and efficient routes to biomolecules substituted with cyclopentadienyltricarbonylrhenium and -technetium derivatives. Chem Eur J 2001;7:2289–2294.

51. Virgolini I, Traub T, Novotny C et al. New trends in peptide receptor radioligands. Q J Nucl Med 2001;45:153–159.

52. Bender H, Zamora PO, Rhodes BA et al. Clinical aspects of local and regional tumor therapy with ^{188}Re-RC-160. Anticancer Res 1997;17:1705–1712.

53. Pearson DA, Lister-James J, McBride WJ et al. Somatostatin receptor-binding peptides labeled with technetium-99*m*: chemistry and initial biological studies. J Med Chem 1996;39:1361–1371.

54. Kurnatowska I, Pawlikowski M. Anti-inflammatory effects of somatostatin analogs on zymosan-induced earlobe inflammation in mice: comparison with dexamethasone and ketoprofen. Neuroimmunomodulation 2001;9:119–124.

55. Dasgupta P, Singh AT, Mukherjee R. Lipophilization of somatostatin analog RC-160 with long chain fatty acid improves its anti-proliferative activity on human oral carcinoma cells in vitro. Life Sci 2000;66:1557–1570.

56. Chatzistamou I, Schally AV, Varga JL et al. Antagonists of growth hormone-releasing hormone and somatostatin analog RC-160 inhibit the growth of the OV-1063 human epithelial ovarian cancer cell line xenografted into nude mice. J Clin Endocrinol Metab 2001;86:2144–2152.

57. Yano T, Radulovic S, Osuga Y et al. Inhibition of human epithelial ovarian cancer cell growth in vitro by somatostatin analog RC-160. Oncology 2000;59[suppl 1]:45–49.

58. Zamora PO, Bender H, Gulhke S et al. Pre-clinical experience with Re-188–RC-160, a radio-labeled somatostatin analog for use in peptide-targeted radiotherapy. Anticancer Res 1997;17:1803–1808.

59. Hosono M, Hosono MN, Haberberger T et al. Localization of small-cell lung cancer xenografts with iodine-125–, indium-111–, and rhenium-188–somatostatin analogs. Jpn J Cancer Res 1996;87:995–1000.

60. Uehara T, Arano Y, Ono M et al. The integrity of the disulfide bond in a cyclic somatostatin analog during ^{99m}Tc complexation reactions. Nucl Med Biol 1999;26:883–890.

61. Menda Y, Kahn D. Somatostatin receptor imaging of non-small cell lung cancer with 99mTc depreotide. Semin Nucl Med 2002;32:92–96.

62. Amartey JK, Parhar RS, Al-Jammaz I. Synthesis and preliminary evaluation of Tc-99*m*-labeled somatostatin analog (RC-160) using "3+1" mixed ligand approach. Nucl Med Biol 2001;28:225–233.

63. Kaltsas GA, Mukherjee JJ, Grossman AB. The value of radiolabelled MIBG and octreotide in the diagnosis and management of neuroendocrine tumours. Ann Oncol 2001;12[suppl 2]:S47–S50.

64. Bass LA, Wang M, Welch MJ et al. In vivo transchelation of copper-64 from TETA-octreotide to superoxide dismutase in rat liver. Bioconjug Chem 2000;11:527–532.

65. Anderson CJ, Pajeau TS, Edwards WB et al. In vitro and in vivo evaluation of copper-64–octreotide conjugates. J Nucl Med 1995;36:2315–2325.

66. Anderson CJ, Dehdashti F, Cutler PD et al. 64Cu-TETA-octreotide as a PET imaging agent for patients with neuroendocrine tumors. J Nucl Med 2001;42:213–221.

67. Lewis JS, Laforest R, Lewis MR et al. Comparative dosimetry of copper-64 and yttrium-90–labeled somatostatin analogs in a tumor-bearing rat model. Cancer Biother Radiopharm 2000;15:593–604.

68. Lewis JS, Lewis MR, Cutler PD et al. Radiotherapy and dosimetry of 64Cu-TETA-Tyr3-octreotate in a somatostatin receptor-positive, tumor-bearing rat model. Clin Cancer Res 1999;5:3608–3616.

69. Smith-Jones PM, Stolz B, Bruns C et al. Gallium-67/gallium-68–[DFO]-octreotide—a potential radiopharmaceutical for PET imaging of somatostatin receptor-positive tumors: synthesis and radiolabeling in vitro and preliminary in vivo studies. J Nucl Med 1994;35:317–325.

70. Stolz B, Smith-Jones PM, Albert R et al. Biological characterisation of [^{67}Ga] or [^{68}Ga]–labelled DFO-octreotide (SDZ 216-927) for PET studies of somatostatin receptor positive tumors. Horm Metab Res 1994;26:453–459.

71. Hofmann M, Maecke H, Borner R et al. Biokinetics and imaging with the somatostatin receptor PET radioligand (68)Ga-DOTATOC: preliminary data. Eur J Nucl Med 2001;28:1751–1757.

72. Henze M, Schuhmacher J, Hipp P, Kowalski J, Becker DW, Doll J, Macke HR, Hofmann M, Debus J, Haberkorn U. PET imaging of somatostatin receptors using. Journal of Nuclear Medicine 2001; 42(7):1053-1056.

73. Pilichowska M, Kimura N, Schindler M et al. Somatostatin type 2A receptor immunoreactivity in human pancreatic adenocarcinomas. Endocr Pathol 2001;12:147–155.

74. Menda Y, Kahn D. Somatostatin receptor imaging of non-small cell lung cancer with ^{99m}Tc depreotide. Semin Nucl Med 2002;32:92–96.

75. Bangard M, Béhé M, Guhlke S et al. Detection of somatostatin receptor-positive tumours using the new ^{99m}Tc-tricine-HYNIC-D-Phe^{1}-Tyr^{3}-octreotide: first results in patients and comparison with 111In-DTPA-D-Phe1-octreotide. Eur J Nucl Med 2000;27:628–637.

76. Froidevaux S, Eberle AN, Christe M et al. Neuroendocrine tumor targeting: study of novel gallium-labeled somatostatin radiopeptides in a rat pancreatic tumor model. Int J Cancer 2002;98:930–937.

77. Virgolini I, Britton K, Buscombe J et al. ^{111}In- and ^{90}Y-DOTA-lanreotide: results and implications of the MAURITIUS trial. Semin Nucl Med 2002;32:148–155.

78. Virgolini I, Kurtaran A, Angelberger P et al. "MAURITIUS": tumour dose in patients with advanced carcinoma. Digest Liver Dis 1999;31[suppl 2]:S227–S230.

79. Hofland LJ, van Koetsveld PM, Waaijers M et al. Internalisation of isotope-coupled somatostatin analogues. Digestion 1996;57[suppl 1]:2–6.

80. Hofland LJ, Breeman WA, Krenning EP et al. Internalization of [DOTA^0,^{125}I,-Tyr^3]octreotide by somatostatin receptor-positive cells in vitro and in vivo: implications for somatostatin receptor-targeted radio-guided surgery. Proc Assoc Am Phys 1999;111:63–69.

81. Chinol M, Bodei L, Cremonesi M et al. Receptor-mediated radiotherapy with 90Y-DOTA-D-Phe^1-Tyr^3-octreotide: the experience of the European Institute of Oncology Group. Semin Nucl Med 2002;32:141–147.

82. Hofland LJ, Breeman WA, Krenning EP et al. Internalization of [DOTA0,125I-Tyr3]octreotide by somatostatin receptor-positive cells in vitro and in vivo: implications for somatostatin receptor-targeted radio-guided surgery. Proc Assoc Am Phys 1999;111:63–69.

83. Janson ET, Westlin JE, Ohrvall U et al. Nuclear localization of 111In after intravenous injection of [^{111}In-DTPA-D-Phe^1]-octreotide in patients with neuroendocrine tumors. J Nucl Med 2000;41:1514–1518.

84. Kwekkeboom D, Krenning EP, de Jong M. Peptide receptor imaging and therapy. J Nucl Med 2000;41:1704–1713.

85. Perault C, Schvartz C, Wampach H et al. Thoracic and abdominal SPECT–CT image fusion without external markers in endocrine carcinomas. J Nucl Med 1997;38:1234–1242.

86. Even-Sapir E, Keidar Z, Sachs J et al. The new technology of combined transmission and emission tomography in evaluation of endocrine neoplasms. J Nucl Med 2001;42:998–1004.

87. Bombardieri E, Maccauro M, De Deckere E et al. Nuclear medicine imaging of neuroendocrine tumours. Ann Oncol 2001;12[suppl 2]: S51–S61.

88. Xing T, Wu F, Brodin O et al. In vitro PET evaluations in lung cancer cell lines. Anticancer Res 2000;20:1375–1380.

89. Harris AG. Future medical prospects for Sandostatin. Metab Clin Exp 1990;39[suppl 2]:180–185.

90. Virgolini I. Mack Forster Award Lecture. Receptor nuclear medicine: vasointestinal peptide and somatostatin receptor scintigraphy for diagnosis and treatment of tumour patients. Eur J Clin Invest 1997;27:793–800.

91. Murray AD, Brooks ME. Nuclear medicine in oncology. J R Coll Surg Edinb 2000;45:110–119.

92. Rodriguez JA, Meyers MO, Jacome TH et al. Intraoperative detection of a bronchial carcinoid with a radiolabeled somatostatin analog. Chest 2002;121:985–988.

93. van Heertum RL, Fawwaz RA. The role of nuclear medicine in the evaluation of pancreatic disease. Surg Clin North Am 2001;81:345–358.

94. Öberg K. Chemotherapy and biotherapy in the treatment of neuroendocrine tumours. Ann Oncol 2001;12[suppl 2]:S111–S114.

95. De Jong M, Breeman WA, Bernard HF et al. Therapy of neuroendocrine tumors with radiolabeled somatostatin-analogues. Q J Nucl Med 1999;43:356–366.

96. Cremonesi M, Ferrari M, Chinol M et al. Dosimetry in radionuclide therapies with ^{90}Y-conjugates: the IEO experience. Q J Nucl Med 2000;44:325–332.

97. McCarthy KE, Woltering EA, Espenan GD et al. In situ radiotherapy with ^{111}In-pentetreotide: initial observations and future directions. Cancer J Sci Am 1998;4:94–102.

98. de Jong M, Bakker WH, Breeman WA et al. Pre-clinical comparison of [DTPA^{0}] octreotide, [DTPA^{0},Tyr^{3}] octreotide and [DOTA^{0},Tyr^{3}] octreotide as carriers for somatostatin receptor-targeted scintigraphy and radionuclide therapy. Int J Cancer 1998;75:406–411.

99. Srivastava S, Dadachova E. Recent advances in radionuclide therapy. Semin Nucl Med 2001;31:330–341.

100. Virgolini I, Traub T, Leimer M et al. New radiopharmaceuticals for receptor scintigraphy and radionuclide therapy. Q J Nucl Med 2000;44:50–58.

101. Valkema R, de Jong M, Bakker WH et al. Phase I study of peptide receptor radionuclide therapy with [In-DTPA]octreotide: the Rotterdam experience. Semin Nucl Med 2002;32:110–122.

102. Tiensuu Janson E, Eriksson B, Öberg K et al. Treatment with high dose [^{111}In-DTPA-D-Phe^{1}]-octreotide in patients with neuroendocrine tumors: evaluation of therapeutic and toxic effects. Acta Oncol 1999;38:373–377.

103. McCarthy KE, Woltering EA, Anthony LB. In situ radiotherapy with ^{111}In-pentetreotide: state of the art and perspectives. Q J Nucl Med 2000;44:88–95.

104. Ressetta G, Geatti O, Pozzetto B et al. An occult pancreatic insulinoma: radio-guided surgery with ^{111}In-octreotide: a case report and review of the literature on pre- and intraoperative diagnosis. Ann Ital Chirurg 2000;71:107–112.

105. Rogers BE, Zinn KR, Lin CY et al. Targeted radiotherapy with [^{90}Y]-SMT 487 in mice bearing human nonsmall cell lung tumor xenografts induced to express human somatostatin receptor subtype 2 with an adenoviral vector. Cancer 2002;94[4 suppl]:1298–1305.

106. Gulec SA, Drouant GJ, Fuselier J et al. Antitumor and antiangiogenic effects of somatostatin receptor-targeted in situ radiation with ^{111}In-DTPA-JIC 2DL. J Surg Res 2001;97:131–137.

107. Wang C, Tang C. Inhibition of human gastric cancer metastasis by ocreotide in vitro and in vivo. Chin Med J 2002;82:19–22.

108. Jenkins SA, Kynaston HG, Davies ND et al. Somatostatin analogs in oncology: a look to the future. Chemotherapy 2001;47[suppl 2]:162–196.

109. Gulec SA, Gaffga CM, Anthony CT et al. Antiangiogenic therapy with somatostatin receptor-mediated in situ radiation. Am Surg 2001;67:1068–1071.

110. Waldherr C, Pless M, Maecke HR et al. Tumor response and clinical benefit in neuroendocrine tumors after 7.4 GBq (90)Y-DOTATOC. J Nucl Med 2002;43:610–616.

111. Bello Arques P, Hervas Benito I, Mateo Navarro A. Scintigraphy with ^{111}In-octreotide in a case of primary hepatic gastrinoma. Rev Esp Med Nucl 2001;20:381–385.

112. Krausz Y, Bar-Ziv J, de Jong RB et al. Somatostatin-receptor scintigraphy in the management of gastroenteropancreatic tumors. Am J Gastroenterol 1998;93:66–70.

113. Caplin ME, Mielcarek W, Buscombe JR et al. Toxicity of high-activity ^{111}In-octreotide therapy in patients with disseminated neuroendocrine tumours. Nucl Med Commun 2000;21:97–102.

114. Leimer M, Kurtaran A, Smith-Jones P et al. Response to treatment with yttrium 90-DOTA-lanreotide of a patient with metastatic gastrinoma. J Nucl Med 1998;39:2090–2094.

115. Turhal NS, Bruckner HW. Pancreatic duct cell carcinoma with positive ^{111}In octreotide uptake. J Exp Clin Cancer Res 2000;19:241–244.

116. Smith-Jones PM, Bischof C, Leimer M et al. DOTA-lanreotide: a novel somatostatin analog for tumor diagnosis and therapy. Endocrinology 1999;140:5136–5148.

117. O'Byrne KJ, Schally AV, Thomas A et al. Somatostatin, its receptors and analogs, in lung cancer. Chemotherapy 2001;47[suppl 2]:78–108.

118. Ferone D, van Hagen MP, Kwekkeboom DJ et al. Somatostatin receptor subtypes in human thymoma and inhibition of cell proliferation by octreotide in vitro. J Clin Endocrinol Metab 2000;85:1719–1726.

119. Smith MC, Liu J, Chen T et al. OctreoTher: ongoing early clinical development of a somatostatin-receptor-targeted radionuclide antineoplastic therapy. Digestion 2000;62[suppl 1]:69–72.

120. Görges R, Kahaly G, Müller-Brand J et al. Radionuclide-labeled somatostatin analogues for diagnostic and therapeutic purposes in nonmedullary thyroid cancer. Thyroid 2001;11:647–659.

121. Halmos G, Sun B, Schally AV et al. Human ovarian cancers express somatostatin receptors. J Clin Endocrinol Metab 2000;85:3509–3512.

122. Lum SS, Fletcher WS, O'Dorisio MS et al. Distribution and functional significance of somatostatin receptors in malignant melanoma. World J Surg 2001;25:407–412.

123. Guitera-Rovel P, Lumbroso J, Gautier-Gougis MS et al. Indium-111 octreotide scintigraphy of Merkel cell carcinomas and their metastases. Ann Oncol 2001;12:807–811.

124. ten Bokum AM, Hofland LJ, de Jong G et al. Immunohistochemical localization of somatostatin receptor sst2A in sarcoid granulomas. Eur J Clin Invest 1999;29:630–636.

125. Rhee Y, Lee JD, Shin KH et al. Oncogenic osteomalacia associated with mesenchymal tumour detected by indium-111 octreotide scintigraphy. Clin Endocrinol 2001;54:551–554.

126. Jan de Beur SM, Streeten EA, Civelek AC et al. Localisation of mesenchymal tumours by somatostatin receptor imaging. Lancet 2002;359:761–763.

127. Pichler R, Maschek W, Holzinger C. Therapy with somatostatin analogs in patient with orbitopathy and positive Octreoscan. Acta Med Austriaca 2001;28:99–101.

128. Isidori AM, Kaltsas G, Frajese V et al. Ocular metastases secondary to carcinoid tumors: the utility of imaging with [^{123}I]meta-iodobenzylguanidine and [^{111}In]DTPA pentetreotide. J Clin Endocrinol Metab 2002;87:1627–1633.

129. Smith S, Thomas RM, Steere HA et al. Therapeutic irradiation of the central nervous system using intrathecal ^{90}Y–DTPA. Br J Radiol 1976;49:141–147.

130. Haldemann AR, Rosler H, Barth A et al. Somatostatin receptor scintigraphy in central nervous system tumors: role of blood-brain barrier permeability. J Nucl Med 1995;36:403–410.

131. Cavalla P, Schiffer D. Neuroendocrine tumors in the brain. Ann Oncol 2001;12[suppl 2]:S131–S134.

132. Koper JW, Markstein R, Kohler C et al. Somatostatin inhibits the activity of adenylate cyclase in cultured human meningioma cells and stimulates their growth. J Clin Endocrinol Metab 1992;74:543–547.

133. Harris AG. Octreotide in the treatment of disorders of the gastrointestinal tract. Drug Invest 1992;4:1–54.

134. Moschetta A, Stolk MF, Rehfeld JF et al. Severe impairment of postprandial cholecystokinin release and gall-bladder emptying and high risk of gallstone formation in acromegalic patients during Sandostatin LAR. Aliment Pharmacol Ther 2001;15:181–185.

135. Caplin ME, Mielcarek W, Buscombe JR et al. Toxicity of high-activity ^{111}In-octreotide therapy in patients with disseminated neuroendocrine tumours. Nucl Med Commun 2000;21:97–102.

136. Moll S, Nickeleit V, Mueller-Brand J et al. A new cause of renal thrombotic microangiopathy: ^{90}yttrium-DOTATOC internal radiotherapy. Am J Kidney Dis 2001;37:847–851

137. Otte A, Weiner SM, Cybulla M. Is radiation nephropathy caused by yttrium-90? Lancet 2002;359:979.

Chapter 10

Current Status of Selective Estrogen Receptor Modulators (SERMs)

Suzanne D. Conzen

Selective estrogen receptor modulators (SERMs) are a class of several structurally diverse molecules, including steroid hormones, that differentially bind to and modulate the estrogen receptor (ER) in a tissue-specific manner. Because of a SERM's ability to act as an estrogen antagonist in breast tissue, these molecules can be potent anticancer agents and have been studied extensively in both the prevention and the treatment of breast cancer. However, the concomitant action of SERMs as potential estrogen agonists in nonbreast tissue, such as bone and endometrium, results in variable effects by individual SERMs on the development of osteoporosis and uterine cancer. On a molecular level, we are only beginning to understand why an individual SERM can act as an ER agonist in one tissue and as an antagonist in another,[1] but it is likely that the change in ER conformation that follows binding by the SERM results in variable interactions with cofactors required for ER-mediated gene regulation.[2] This discovery has led to a resurgence of interest in developing an "ideal" SERM that might have potent antiestrogenic effects in the breast and endometrium and pro-estrogenic effects in the bone and central nervous system. At the same time, the development of

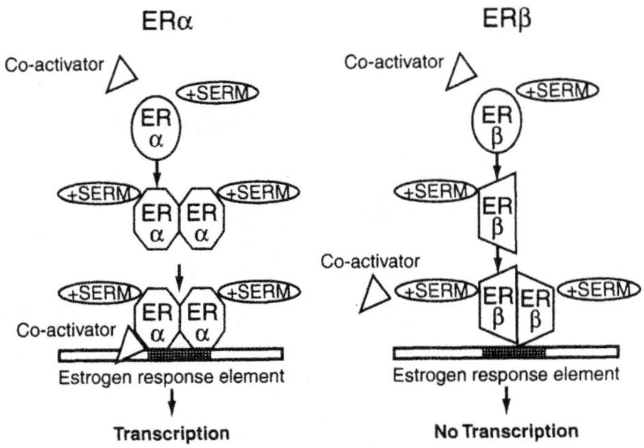

FIGURE 10.1 Model of the molecular basis of the potential differential effects of selective estrogen receptor modulators (SERMs) on estrogen receptor-α (ER-α) versus ER-β. In this conceptual model, binding of a SERM to ER-α creates a conformational change in the ER that favors coactivator binding and results in gene transcription. However, the same SERM can bind to ER-β and result in an alternative conformational change that does not favor ER-β interaction with the coactivator; therefore, no gene transcription results. Differential effects of individual SERMs on ER binding can also result in varied affinities of the ER for corepressors. In addition, the ratio of corepressor to coactivator expression can vary in different target cell types, resulting in cell type–specific gene expression profiles.

aromatase inhibitors (AIs) is challenging the traditional role of SERMs as the gold standard endocrine treatment for early and advanced breast cancer in postmenopausal women.

MOLECULAR MECHANISMS OF SERM ACTION

In the 1970s, tamoxifen was the first SERM to be studied thoroughly in the laboratory and the first to be used in the treatment of breast cancer. As is true with all SERMs, tamoxifen has mixed antagonistic and agonistic effects on the ER. The consequence of tamoxifen binding to an individual ER depends on the ER (α or β isoform) and on the cell type. In fact, within a certain cell type, tamoxifen can act as an estrogen agonist on some genes and an estrogen antagonist on others. This complexity reflects the nature of the interaction of SERMs with ER-α or ER-β; the resulting change in the conformation of the ER on binding to the SERM appears to vary, depending on what cellular environment and specific gene target is being considered (Fig. 10.1).

Our molecular understanding of SERM mechanisms of action has recently increased dramatically because of the knowledge gained from the solution of the ER's three-dimensional structure and because of our better understanding of the mechanisms of ER-mediated gene regulation. In 1998, the structures of the hormone-binding domain of ER-α complexed to estradiol, diethylstilbestrol (DES), tamoxifen, and raloxifene were solved and revealed that the nature of

TABLE 10.1 Overall Efficacy of SERMs in Tamoxifen-Resistant and Hormone-Sensitive Advanced Breast Cancer

Drug	Tamoxifen-Resistant Phase II	Hormone-Sensitive or First-Line Therapy Phase II or III
	ORR (%)	ORR (%)
Tamoxifen	NA	25.3[a]
Toremifene	0–14	24.0[a]
Droloxifene	15	30–51
Idoxifene	9	20
Arzoxifene	3–10	30–36
Raloxifene	0	19
EM-800	14	NA
Fulvestrant	37	17.5–20.7

ORR, overall response rate (complete response + partial response); NA, not available.
[a]Meta-analysis averages (Ref. 16).

these ligands determines the overall change in structure of the receptor after binding.[3,4] The resulting shape of the receptor-SERM complex, in turn, determines the precise interaction of the ER with coactivators and corepressors that are important for individual gene expression. The structure of the ER that is bound to tamoxifen revealed that coactivator binding can be blocked by tamoxifen due to helix 12 of the ER hormone-binding domain moving over and blocking access of the coactivator to the ER. Similarly, the comparative structures of the ER bound to estradiol versus raloxifene revealed that these two compounds bind to the same site within the core of the LBD but demonstrate different binding effects on helix 12. More recently, it was demonstrated that the conformational shape imposed by a specific SERM differs in outcome for a particular gene target depending upon whether the SERM binds to ER-α or ER-β (Fig. 10.1). This implies that a different interaction with the same coactivator or corepressor can result depending on the specific ER isoform that is targeted by an individual SERM.[2] Thus, the emerging picture is that of SERMs binding to ER-α and/or ER-β and producing alternative shapes in the ER binding interfaces with coactivators and corepressors depending on the specific cell type milieu.

The differential gene induction of various SERMs has resulted in a group of drugs that when bound to a receptor have variable effects on a complement of ER-regulated genes. Furthermore, the ability of the ER to interact with a large array of transcriptional regulatory proteins is important because it implies that SERMs can induce differential effects on genes in different cellular contexts based on variable interactions with corepressors and coactivators. It seems likely that the net balance of corepressors and coactivators in a cell as well as the relative proportions of ER-α and ER-β will determine the overall activity of a SERM in any individual cell type (Table 10.1). Therefore, designing SERMs that act as antagonists in breast tissue and in the endometrium and as agonists in brain and bone is the goal of several active pharmaceutical and academic drug discovery programs. Such a compound may have an advantage over the "pure estrogen antagonist" SERMs and the AIs because they could have the beneficial effects of estrogen (e.g., increasing bone density) on some tissues and antagonistic effects in the breast and the uterus.

Because SERMs can act as estrogen antagonists in certain tissues and estrogen agonists in others, a great deal of effort is being placed on understanding and predicting how these molecules achieve their specific effects on different tissues. A SERM that has antiestrogenic effects on the breast but proestrogenic effects on the brain and bone would be ideal. Despite their imperfections, the current SERMS are very effective in their use in ER-positive breast cancer because they act as antagonists to the generally pro-proliferative effects of the ER in mammary epithelial cells. Tamoxifen, the first SERM to gain widespread clinical use and by far the best-studied SERM in clinical conditions, remains the gold standard SERM against which all others are compared.

PHARMACOLOGY OF SERMS

High-Dose Estrogens

DES and other high-dose estrogens were first studied in the late 1970s. The mechanism whereby achieving very high serum concentrations of estrogens inhibits breast cancer growth is not understood, but it may be related to effects that high-dose estrogens have on nuclear receptors other than ER-α and ER-β.[5] The largest study compared DES with tamoxifen in 143 patients being treated for metastatic breast cancer.[6] The 20-year updated results of this trial were recently published and showed that DES ($N = 74$) and tamoxifen ($N = 69$) responses were approximately equal. The overall objective response was 42% for DES and 34% for tamoxifen ($P = .31$), and the median duration of response was 11.8 months for DES and 9.9 months for tamoxifen ($P = .38$). The median survival was 3.0 years for DES, versus 2.4 years for tamoxifen. Thus, duration of response and progression-free survival were not found to be significantly different between DES and tamoxifen. Despite equivalent responses and a favorable duration of response for DES, treatment with DES is more commonly associated with toxicities such as nausea, edema, vaginal bleeding, and cardiac problems. Therefore, tamoxifen currently remains the preferred SERM for the treatment of metastatic breast cancer.

TRIPHENYLETHYLENE SERMS

Tamoxifen

Tamoxifen is a triphenylethylene that was developed more than 30 years ago as a breast cancer treatment.[7] In addition to its anti-estrogenic effects in the breast, tamoxifen lowers cholesterol and increases bone mineral density in postmenopausal women.[8] The National Surgical Adjuvant Breast and Bowel Project (NSABP) P-1 trial showed that tamoxifen was an effective preventive of breast cancer but that there are increased risks of endometrial cancer and thrombosis.[9] Tamoxifen alters the shape of the ER on binding; depending on the cellular context, this change leads to the activation or the repression of ER target genes. Tamoxifen's main mechanism of action in breast tissue is thought to be antagonism of several growth-promoting genes and the induction of a delay in the G_1 phase of the cell cycle in breast epithelial cells.[10]

Tamoxifen acts as an estrogen antagonist in cells of the central nervous system and in the vaginal mucosa, resulting in potentially unpleasant side effects, including hot flashes and vaginal dryness and/or discharge. In addition, tamoxifen is associated with life-threatening complications, such as an increased incidence of blood clots and subsequent pulmonary emboli, presumably due to the pro-estrogenic effects of tamoxifen on the vascular endothelium. For example, the results of the NSABP P-1 trial found that relatively healthy postmenopausal patients receiving tamoxifen (N = 6681) versus placebo (N = 6707) experienced a significantly greater incidence of deep vein thromboses (N = 35 versus 22), pulmonary embolism (N = 18 versus 6), and stroke (N = 38 versus 24). An increased incidence of endometrial cancers and cataracts was also noted in the tamoxifen-treated patients.

Perhaps the most frequently debilitating symptom exacerbated by tamoxifen's anti-estrogenic effects is frequent hot flashes that interrupt a patient's normal activities and sleep cycles. A recent phase III study using the antidepressant medication fluoxetine for the treatment of hot flashes in postmenopausal patients has shown an objective reduction in hot flashes.[11] This trial used a double-blind, randomized, two-period (4 weeks per period), cross-over methodology to study the efficacy of fluoxetine (20 mg/day) for treating hot flashes in women with a history of breast cancer or a concern regarding the use of estrogen (because of breast cancer risk). Another randomized study of a popular treatment for hot flashes, soy, did not result in a significant difference in hot flashes,[12] even though statistically significant levels of genistein, the compound thought to be the active agent in soy milk, was found in the experimental group. Similar results had been noted in an earlier randomized trial of soy tablets versus placebo for the treatment of hot flashes in breast cancer survivors.[13] A randomized trial of black cohosh versus placebo also failed to find a significant effect in alleviating hot flashes.[14] An ongoing Cancer and Leukemia Group B (CALGB) clinical trial is currently evaluating the role of isoflavones and soy in the prevention of hot flashes in women with a history of breast cancer who are receiving concurrent tamoxifen treatment.

Toremifene

Toremifene is similar to tamoxifen in that the only structural difference is a single chlorine atom at position 4 (Fig. 10.2). The inability of toremifene to form DNA adducts in the rat liver may explain why it is not a hepatocarcinogen.[15] As

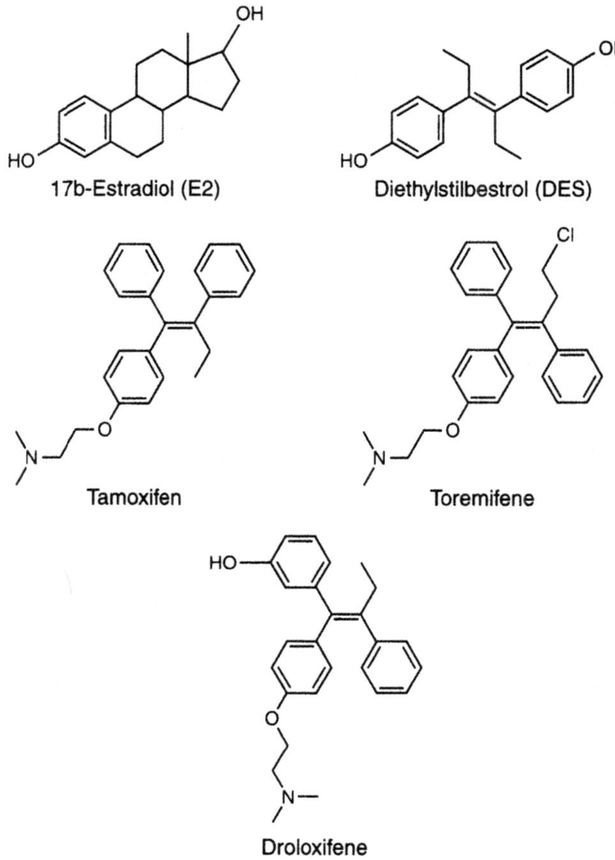

FIGURE 10.2 Chemical structures of estradiol, diethylstilbestrol (DES), and tamoxifen-like selective estrogen receptor modulators (SERMs).

a first-line endocrine therapy for metastatic breast cancer, toremifene has been shown to have response rates that are very similar to those of tamoxifen, ranging from 21% to 38%, in five phase III trials comparing tamoxifen (20–40 mg) with toremifene (40–60 mg).[16] In all studies, toremifene has shown efficacy equivalent to that of tamoxifen for effective response rate, stable disease, time to progression, and overall survival. A recent meta-analysis of 1421 patients from these trials confirmed the lack of difference between tamoxifen and toremifene response rates. Although these studies did not address the question of carcinogenicity from toremifene versus tamoxifen, a Finnish study (N = 899 patients evaluable for safety) assessing the efficacy and safety of toremifene versus tamoxifen in the adjuvant setting for 3 years has found no significant differences in the number of secondary cancers at a short follow-up of 3.4 years.[17] Slightly more vascular complications (deep vein thromboses, cerebrovascular events, and pulmonary embolisms) occurred in tamoxifen-treated patients (5.9%) than in toremifene-treated patients (3.5%) ($P = .11$), whereas bone fractures and vaginal leukorrhea were slightly more common in the toremifene group. The International Breast Cancer Study Group is currently conducting two randomized adjuvant trials evaluating 5 years of toremifene therapy (60 mg/day) versus 5 years of tamoxifen therapy (20 mg/day). Toremifene is approved for the treatment of metastatic breast cancer in the United States and in Europe.

Droloxifene

Droloxifene is 3-hydroxytamoxifen; it has a higher relative binding affinity than tamoxifen for the ER.[18] However, an increased affinity of a SERM for either ER-α or ER-β does not necessarily determine its clinical efficacy. Data on droloxifene and other novel SERMs suggest that a SERM's efficacy is more likely to be determined by its specific effect on ER interactions and that specific cofactors regulate gene transcription. For droloxifene, initial phase I/II studies suggested a 15% response rate in patients who had previously failed to respond to tamoxifen, suggesting that droloxifene exhibits significant non–cross-resistance with tamoxifen, In addition, an early phase II study of droloxifene as a first-line agent showed a response rate of 51% and a median time to progression of 8 months.[19] However, because two randomized phase III studies comparing droloxifene to tamoxifen showed less activity than tamoxifen in hormone-sensitive breast cancer, development of droloxifene has been dropped.[20]

Idoxifene

Idoxifene, like raloxifene, is structurally similar to tamoxifen and has an increased binding affinity for ER-α due to a pyrrolidine side chain with an iodine atom at the 4 position (Fig. 10.2). Pre-clinical experiments were encouraging because idoxifene inhibited the MCF 7 cancer cell line xenograft growth in nude mice more than tamoxifen[21] while showing reduced uterine stimulation.[22] Unfortunately, clinical trials have revealed an increased incidence of uterine prolapse and polyps in idoxifene-treated women, and no major difference in clinical efficacy has been found for idoxifene compared to tamoxifen.[23] Further development of this drug as a breast cancer treatment has therefore been dropped.[24]

SUMMARY OF TAMOXIFEN DERIVATIVES

Although there has been intense interest in developing a tamoxifen-like derivative with less uterine side effects and better efficacy in breast cancer, the ultimate outcome of these attempts has thus far been disappointing. For example, it does not appear that an individual SERM's relatively high affinity for the ER improves its efficacy as an anticancer drug; similarly, a reduced agonist profile in preclinical studies (e.g., less uterine proliferation in a rat uterotrophic model) does not necessarily predict a better safety profile in clinical studies. Conversely, the knowledge that we have gained in the past few years about the structure of ER-α and -β when they are bound to a SERM may allow the rational development of drugs that minimize the pro-proliferative action of the SERMs in the uterus and may maximize the pro-estrogenic effects in the brain and bone.

FIXED-RING SERMS

Raloxifene

Raloxifene is a "fixed-ring" SERM that has a binding affinity for the ER similar to that of tamoxifen (Fig. 10.3). Preclinical studies with raloxifene showed an anti-estrogen effect on rat mammary tumor growth that is equal to that of tamoxifen, but significantly less action as an estrogen in the uterus. However, clinical trials subsequently showed no activity in tamoxifen-resistant patients,[25] and a recent phase II clinical study of raloxifene in metastatic breast cancer showed only a 33% clinical benefit, compared with the 44% occurring with tamoxifen.[26] Thus, raloxifene is not being considered as a treatment for existing breast carcinoma. Instead, it is being developed and marketed as a drug for osteoporosis, which, unlike estrogen, has less pro-estrogenic effects on the breast and uterus. In addition, raloxifene is currently being examined in a breast cancer chemopreventive trial called the Study of Tamoxifen and Raloxifene (STAR) trial.

Arzoxifene (LY-353381)

Arzoxifene is a benzothiophene analogue of raloxifene that has a more favorable therapeutic and safety profile than raloxifene in preclinical studies. Specifically, arzoxifene has exhibited more potent and beneficial effects on bone metabolism than raloxifene and has inhibited the growth of ER-positive breast cancer cells in vitro more potently that raloxifene.[27] Phase II data have revealed relatively low arzoxifene response rates for tamoxifen-resistant patients (10%), although there is a 30% response rate in hormone-sensitive patients and a 17% stable disease rate.[28,29] Based on these data, the use of arzoxifene, 20 mg/day, versus tamoxifen, 20 mg/day, is currently being studied in a large multicenter European phase III clinical trial as a first-line therapy in metastatic breast cancer.

EM-800

EM-800 is a prodrug of the active benzopyrene derivative EM-652 (SCH 57068). EM-652 has an ER binding affinity that is significantly greater than that of tamoxifen or raloxifene. Preclinical studies showed strong antiproliferative effects of EM-800 compared with tamoxifen, and when it was administered to ovariectomized animals, EM-800 prevented bone loss and lowered serum cholesterol and triglyceride levels.[30] A phase II study of 43 women who had not responded to tamoxifen was encouraging and showed a 14% response rate and a 23% rate

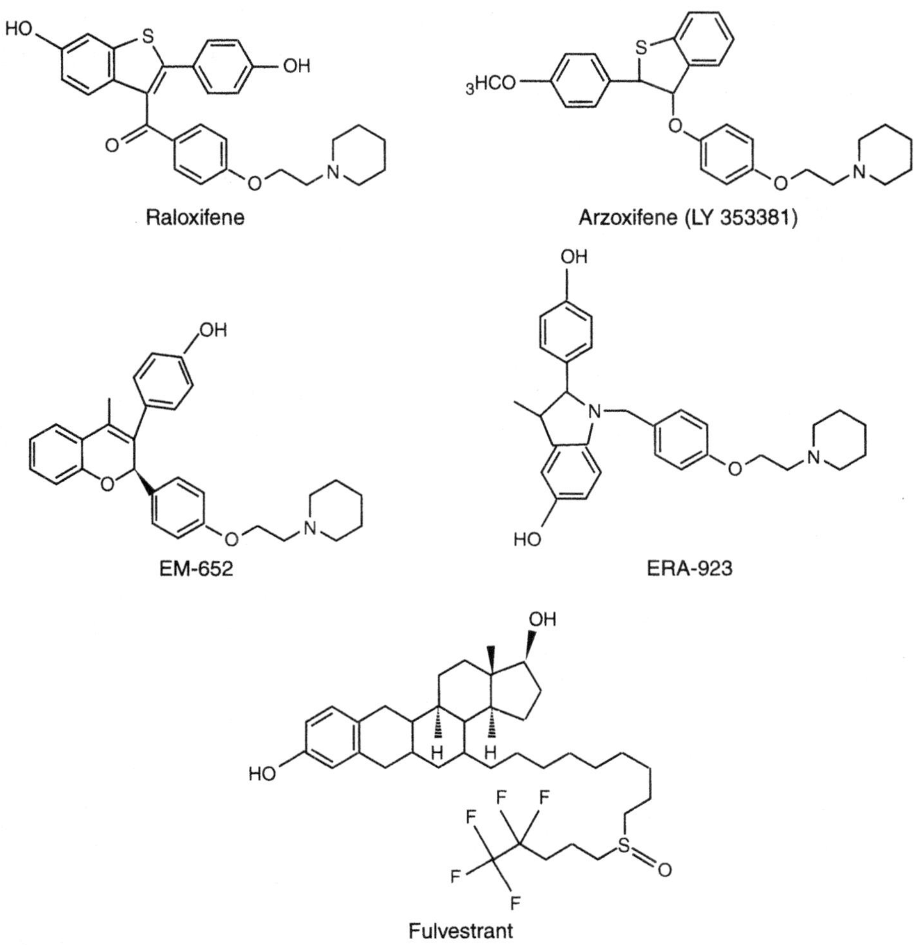

FIGURE 10.3 Chemical structures of second- and third-generation selective estrogen receptor modulators (SERMs).

of stable disease.[31] However, a randomized phase III study in patients with tamoxifen-resistant breast cancer compared EM-800 with the third-generation AI anastrozole; this study has been halted because response rates with EM-800 were lower than those of anastrozole.[24]

ERA-923

ERA-923 is a novel fixed-ring SERM that also has a favorable preclinical profile in comparison with tamoxifen and raloxifene.[32] Unlike tamoxifen, droloxifene, or raloxifene, ERA-923 is not uterotropic in immature rats or ovariectomized mice. A recent pharmacokinetic trial that evaluated the safety and tolerability of once-daily oral ERA-923 (10–200 mg) versus placebo found that subjects taking ERA-

923 had no uterine or ovarian changes, as indicated by transvaginal ultrasound after 28 days of therapy.[33] ERA-923 is currently being evaluated in phase II trials in tamoxifen-resistant breast cancer and as a first-line treatment in ER-positive patients with metastatic breast cancer.[34]

STEROIDAL SERMS ("PURE ANTAGONIST")

Fulvestrant (Faslodex, formerly ICI 182, 780)

Fulvestrant is a derivative of estradiol with a long hydrophobic side chain (Fig. 10.3) and is completely able to block transactivation by the ER. Because of the long bulky side chain at the 7α positions, receptor dimerization appears to be sterically hindered. This drug also appears to induce the degradation of the ER, depleting it from cellular extracts. Furthermore, fulvestrant decreases the number of ER molecules in the nucleus and thus is oftern referred to as an ER "downregulator." The overall result is that the fulvestrant can block tamoxifen and estrogen induction of several common genes. A benefit to fulvestrant is that it is anti-estrogenic in both the breast and the uterus, presumably because instead of causing a conformational change in the ER, fulvestrant initiates the degradation of the ER. The mechanism by which fulvestrant causes the increased degradation is not well understood, but it may be related to the known susceptibility of the ER to ubiquitin-mediated degradation by the proteasome. Degradation may be accelerated on fulvestrant binding because fulvestrant may effect the folding of the ER; misfolded proteins are often targeted for degradation. The end result appears to be a complete suppression of all ER-activated genes.

Fulvestrant is not available as an oral formulation but instead as a long-acting monthly intramuscular injection. Early phase I and II trials suggested that unlike other SERMs, fulvestrant is active in tamoxifen-resistant disease. For example, a small trial of 19 patients with hormone-refractory disease showed that 13 patients had a clinical benefit with a median duration of 25 months, and two demonstrated a partial response and six achieved stable disease.[35] Furthermore, comparison with an historical control group of patients receiving megestrol acetate (Megace) suggested a longer duration of response with fulvestrant (26 versus 14 months, $P = .04$).[36] Two multicenter phase III studies have suggested that fulvestrant is at least as effective as the AI anastrozole in time to disease progression in women with metastatic disease progression who were receiving or had received endocrine therapy.[37,38] Fulvestrant was approved in the United States for metastatic breast cancer in 2002.

SERMS IN BREAST CANCER PREVENTION AND TREATMENT

Prevention Studies

Tamoxifen The first three major chemoprevention trials examining tamoxifen were performed in Britain (Marsden Hospital Trial), Italy (Italian Tamoxifen Prevention Study), and the United States (NSABP Breast Cancer Prevention Trial). Although the Marsden Hospital[39] and the Italian trials[40] do not show a difference between breast cancer prevention in the placebo and tamoxifen arms, the United States trial does. However, several important differences between the trials may help explain their different outcomes.

The British trial was originally designed as a feasibility study to determine the tolerability of tamoxifen in healthy women with a family history of breast cancer. Thus, the trial was relatively small, involving 2494 women of a median age of 47 who received tamoxifen or placebo for up to 8 years. Only 34% of the women were postmenopausal, and these women were allowed the use of estrogen replacement therapy. Estrogen replacement therapy was used during 13% of the tamoxifen medication period. Mean follow-up time in the study was 70 months, and the overall frequency of breast cancers was equivalent.

The Italian trial included healthy hysterectomized women aged 35–70 years and enrolled a total of 5408 women (2708 placebo and 2700 tamoxifen treated). The preliminary study suggests that there was no difference in the incidence of breast cancer between the placebo (22 cases) and the tamoxifen (19 cases) arm.[41] In the 390 women (14%) receiving placebo and receiving hormone-replacement therapy (HRT), eight cases of breast cancer occurred, suggesting that the use of HRT increased the risk of breast cancer. A recent follow-up showed that HRT users who were randomly assigned to tamoxifen therapy had a rate of breast cancer that was close to that of those who had never received tamoxifen, suggesting a benefit for tamoxifen in HRT users but not in hysterectomized women.[41]

The largest trial to date, performed in the United States by the NSABP, showed that tamoxifen reduces the incidence of ipsilateral and contralateral breast cancer by approximately 50%. A total of 13,388 women participated in this trial. Eligibility requirements included women >35 years of age at high risk for developing breast cancer, women > 60 years of age without additional risk factors other than age, and women with a history of lobular carcinoma in situ. No estrogen replacement therapy was permitted. An interim analysis was published in 1998 after a median follow-up of 54.6 months and showed that the tamoxifen-treated group had 86 fewer breast cancers than the placebo group. The data monitoring committee considered that the highly significant reduction in early incidence of breast cancer at the time of this analysis justified the termination of the trial. The greatest levels of benefit were seen in women with lobular carcinoma in situ (relative risk = 0.44) and atypical ductal hyperplasia (relative risk = 0.14), most of whom were premenopausal. The rate of endometrial cancer was increased in the tamoxifen group (risk ratio = 2.53; 95% confidence interval = 1.35–4.97); this increased risk occurred predominantly in women aged 50 years or older. All uterine cancers in the tamoxifen group were stage I (localized disease), and no endometrial cancer deaths had occurred in this group at the time of analysis in 1998. The rates of stroke, pulmonary embolism, and deep-vein thrombosis were also elevated in the tamoxifen treatment group; these events also occurred more frequently in women aged 50 years or older. A recent risk-benefit analysis of this trial concluded that given the side effect profile and characteristics of the subgroup that benefited most in terms of risk reduction, tamoxifen is most beneficial for younger women who have an elevated risk of breast cancer.[42]

In a more recent study, the International Breast Cancer Intervention Study randomized over 7144 women to receive tamoxifen or placebo.[43] Women enrolled had to have an overall increase in risk of two- to threefold based on family history and other risk factors. After a median follow-up of 50 months, 69 breast cancers had been diagnosed in 3578 women in the tamoxifen group and 101 in 3566 in the placebo group (a risk reduction of 32% [95% confidence interval 8–50]; $P = .013$). In this trial, age, degree of risk, and use of hormone-replacement therapy did not affect the reduction. Endometrial cancer was not significantly increased, but thromboembolic events were significantly increased, compared with tamoxifen (particularly after surgery).

In summary, the overall evidence generated by recent prevention trials appears to support a reduction in the incidence of breast cancer in women who are at increased risk, but whether this benefit outweighs the risks and side effects associated with tamoxifen use remains uncertain. Continued follow-up analysis of the ongoing placebo-controlled studies (Marsden, Italian, International Breast Cancer Intervention Study) will allow further analysis of the long-term risks and benefits of tamoxifen in the prevention setting.

Raloxifene Raloxifene is a SERM that was originally developed as a treatment to prevent osteoporosis, but analysis of treatment has suggested a preventive role in breast cancer treatment. In a large North American trial examining the effect of raloxifene on postmenopausal women with osteoporosis as a major endpoint,[44] postmenopausal women with osteoporosis ($N = 7705$) were enrolled in the Multiple Outcomes of Raloxifene Evaluation (MORE) trial and were randomly assigned to receive placebo, raloxifene at 60 mg/day, or raloxifene at 120 mg/day for 4 years. Breast cancer risk was analyzed by the following baseline characteristics indicative of estrogen exposure: previous hormone replacement therapy, prevalent vertebral fractures, estradiol level, bone mineral density, body mass index, and age at menopause. The trial was originally designed with a primary endpoint to measure bone fractures, and the conclusions on the secondary endpoint of examining breast cancer incidence are less powered. At the relatively early follow-up of 3 years, the MORE study results are consistent with the NSABP P-1 trial, showing a significant decrease in the incidence of ductal carcinoma in situ and invasive breast cancer in patients taking tamoxifen. In addition, both studies show a reduction in fracture incidence, an increase in thromboembolic events, and a slight increase in stroke. Neither the NSABP P-1 study nor the raloxifene study showed an impact on cardiovascular mortality in this group of women.

A recent update of the analysis of the MORE trial shows that raloxifene significantly reduces breast cancer risk in both the low-estrogen and the high-estrogen subgroups for all risk factors examined. For example, women with the highest body mass index and those with a family history of breast cancer experienced a significantly greater therapy benefit with raloxifene, compared with the two thirds of patients with a lower body mass index or those without a family history, respectively.[45] These findings imply that increased risk imposed by excessive body fat (presumably due to greater fat-generated estrogen levels) or family history result in a greater benefit from SERM treatment.

In the ongoing STAR trial, raloxifene is being directly compared with tamoxifen. In this study, high-risk postmenopausal women are randomly assigned to either tamoxifen (20 mg/day) or raloxifene (60 mg/day) for 5 years. Results should be available in 2005. The STAR trial should provide a definitive answer about the benefits and side effect profile of these two agents. Ongoing molecular biology projects designed to derive the crystal structure of tamoxifen and raloxifene bound to the ER with peptide structures of cofactors will also shed light on how these drugs can act as mixed agonists and antagonists in various tissues.

In summary, one of the major preventive effects of both tamoxifen and raloxifene is that both of them reduce the incidence of in situ and invasive carcinomas in women who are at relatively high risk for breast cancer. The effects of SERMs appear to be only on ER-positive cells, consistent with the initial findings of a reduction in ER-positive breast cancers and not ER-negative cancers. Further efforts are needed to develop agents that may act as chemoprevention for ER-negative breast cancers.

Adjuvant Treatment of Early Breast Cancer (Ductal Carcinoma In Situ and Invasive Cancers)

The NSABP B-24 involved 1804 women and tested the hypothesis that in ductal carcinoma in situ patients with or without positive tumor specimen margins, lumpectomy, radiation therapy, and tamoxifen would be more effective than lumpectomy, radiation therapy, and placebo in preventing invasive and noninvasive ipsilateral breast tumor recurrences, contralateral breast tumors, and tumors at metastatic sites. This study demonstrated that the administration of tamoxifen after lumpectomy and radiation therapy results in a significant decrease in the rate of all breast cancer events, particularly in invasive cancer.[46] The Early Breast Cancer Trialists Collaborative examined information on 37,000 women in 55 trials comprising about 87% of the worldwide evidence.[41] For trials of tamoxifen treatment for 1, 2, and 5 years of adjuvant tamoxifen, the proportional recurrence reductions produced among these 30,000 women during 10 years of follow-up were 21%, 29%, and 47% respectively, with a highly significant trend toward greater effect with longer treatment. The corresponding proportional mortality reductions were 12%, 17%, and 26%, respectively, and again the test for trend was significant. The benefits appear to be largely irrespective of age, menopausal status, and tamoxifen dose (generally 20 mg/day) and to be unrelated to whether chemotherapy is given. The incidence of endometrial cancer approximately doubled in trials of 1 or 2 years of tamoxifen therapy and approximately quadrupled in trials of 5 years of tamoxifen therapy. Tamoxifen had no apparent effect on the incidence of colorectal cancer or, after exclusion of deaths from breast or endometrial cancer, on any of the other main categories of cause of death. Thus, the overall conclusions of this updated overview are that some years of tamoxifen treatment substantially improve the 10-year survival of both pre- and postmenopausal women with ER-positive tumors.

Recently, a large randomized trial compared the use of the third-generation AI anastrozole (Arimidex) to tamoxifen in the adjuvant setting.[47] The ATAC (Arimidex, Tamoxifen Alone or in Combination) trial was activated in 1996 and closed in 1999 with 9366 postmenopausal breast cancer patients. Postmenopausal patients with invasive operable breast cancer who had completed primary therapy and were eligible to receive adjuvant hormone therapy were randomly assigned to receive anastrozole, tamoxifen, or combination therapy. Median follow-up was 33.3 months, and 7839 (84%) patients were known to be hormone receptor–positive. Disease-free survival at 3 years was 89.4% in patients taking anastrozole and 87.4% in those taking tamoxifen, whereas results with the combination were not significantly different from those with tamoxifen alone. The improvement in disease-free survival with anastrozole occurred in the subgroup of hormone receptor–positive patients, but not the receptor-negative patients. The incidence of contralateral breast cancer was significantly lower with anastrozole than with tamoxifen (odds ratio, 0.42 [0.22–0.79], $P = .007$). Anastrozole caused significantly less endometrial cancer, vaginal bleeding and discharge, cerebrovascular events, venous thromboembolic events, and hot flashes than tamoxifen. However, tamoxifen caused significantly fewer musculoskeletal disorders and fractures than anastrozole. Because the follow-up time is relatively short, the American Society of Clinical Oncologists has recommended that no change be made in the current recommendations for the use of adjuvant tamoxifen unless tamoxifen use is contraindicated (e.g., in a patient with a history of thromboembolic events).[48] The American Society of Clinical Oncologists panel states that they were influenced by the "compelling, extensive, and long-term data available on tamoxifen." Overall, the panel considered the results of the ATAC trial and the extensive supporting data to be very promising but insufficient to change the standard practice from adjuvant treatment with tamoxifen to adjuvant anastrozole. However, in September 2002, the United States Food and Drug Administration approved a supplemental new drug application for anastrozole for the adjuvant treatment of hormone receptor–positive early breast cancer in postmenopausal women.

Metastatic Disease

Three SERMs are approved for the treatment of metastatic breast cancer in the United States: tamoxifen, toremifene, and fulvestrant. Overall, approximately 30% of women treated with these drugs respond to therapy. Interestingly, this benefit applies to both postmenopausal women and premenopausal women with

ER-positive breast cancers. The additional treatment of premenopausal women with ovarian suppression (ovariectomy or luteinizing hormone–releasing hormone agonists) and tamoxifen conferred an advantage over treatment with tamoxifen alone in a meta-analysis of four randomized trials.[49] With a median follow-up of 6.8 years, there was a significant survival benefit and progression-free survival benefit in favor of the combined treatment. The overall response rate was also significantly higher on combined endocrine treatment (stratified Mantel-Haenszel test, $P = 0.03$; odds ratio, 0.67).

Tamoxifen The largest trial to evaluate tamoxifen in advanced breast cancer was conducted by the Australian New Zealand Breast Cancer Trials Group and was begun in 1978. This trial randomly assigned 339 patients to tamoxifen alone, chemotherapy with doxorubicin (50 mg/m^2 intravenously) and cyclophosphamide (750 mg/m^2 intravenously) × six 21-day cycles, or tamoxifen plus chemotherapy.[50] The response rate (complete and partial) for tamoxifen was 22.1%, for chemotherapy alone was 45.1%, and for tamoxifen plus chemotherapy was 51.3%. Despite the differences in response rates, median survival rates were not significantly different ($P = 0.49$).

More recently, the development of AIs has led to comparison of tamoxifen with these agents for treatment of metastatic breast cancer in postmenopausal women. Three clinical trials have already compared tamoxifen with second-generation triazole AIs in large randomized trials. A fourth trial is ongoing, comparing tamoxifen with the steroidal third-generation AI exemestane, a compound that is able to inactivate aromatase completely.

In the first trial, the International Letrozole Study Group trial compared tamoxifen with letrozole in 907 postmenopausal women with advanced breast cancer.[51] The patients had to have ER-positive, PR-positive or ER/PR-unknown tumors to be eligible. Patients may have undergone a single prior endocrine therapy for advanced disease. The overall response rate was (30% versus 20% $P = 0.0006$) in favor of letrozole. Letrozole also had a superior median time to progression (41 weeks versus 26 weeks, $P = 0.0001$). No survival data have been reported.

Two additional large randomized trials have compared tamoxifen, 20 mg daily, with anastrozole, 1 mg daily, for the treatment of metastatic breast cancer. One trial was conducted in Europe, Australia, New Zealand, South America, and South Africa (Tamoxifen or Arimidex Randomized Group Efficacy and Tolerability [TARGET] trial) and the other in the United States and Canada (the North American trial). The international TARGET study randomly assigned 688 postmenopausal women with metastatic breast cancer who were hormone receptor–positive or whose receptor status was unknown.[52] Patients who had undergone previous adjuvant tamoxifen therapy were permitted to enter the trial if the therapy had been stopped at least 12 months earlier; however, no previous hormone therapy for metastatic disease was allowed. Objective response rates were similar: 32.9% for anastrozole and 32.6% for tamoxifen. Clinical benefit rates (complete response + partial response stabilization rates of greater than 24 weeks) were equivalent. Median times to progression were also similar: 8.3 months for tamoxifen and 8.2 months for anastrozole.

The second large randomized trial (the North American Trial) comparing the two drugs also showed equivalent results, except that anastrozole had a greater clinical benefit (59% versus 46%).[37] Anastrozole also had a longer median time to progression (11.1 vs 5.6 months, $P = .005$). Overall, both treatments were well tolerated; however, thromboembolic events (4.1% vs 8.2%) and vaginal bleeding (1.2% vs 3.8%) were reported in fewer patients in the anastrozole group than in the tamoxifen group. Of the 119 patients on this trial whose disease progressed after initial anastrozole therapy and received subsequent tamoxifen, 38 achieved disease stabilization for 24 weeks or more. These data suggest that tamoxifen may be successful after AI treatment, although additional studies need to be performed to address the question of optimal sequencing of hormone therapy in advanced disease.

Neoadjuvant Treatment

Neoadjuvant hormone therapy has recently gathered much support because of the publication of a well-designed, multi-institutional trial comparing tamoxifen with the AI letrozole.[53] The Letrozole 024 Neoadjuvant Trial involved 337 postmenopausal women in 55 centers who had ER- or PR-positive locally advanced breast cancer. Patients were randomly assigned to receive letrozole, 2.5 mg/day, or tamoxifen, 30 mg/day, in a double-blinded study. Letrozole responses occurred in 55% of patients, compared with only 36% of patients taking tamoxifen ($P < .001$). In addition, more patients underwent breast-conserving surgery after treatment with letrozole (45%) compared with tamoxifen (35%). Tumor specimens were banked prospectively in this trial and were used to determine whether ErbB1 (epidermal growth factor receptor) and ErbB2 (HER2/Neu) expression affected the efficacy of tamoxifen treatment.[54] The frequency of tumors expressing ErbB1 or ErbB2 as well as ER was 15.2%, and letrozole was indeed much more effective than tamoxifen in this subset of tumors (88% vs 21%), $P = 0.0004$).[55] These data suggest that increased epidermal growth factor receptor expression may be one mechanism whereby ER-positive breast cancers become resistant to SERM activity.[56]

FUTURE DIRECTIONS IN SERM THERAPY

Although several novel SERMs have gone through preclinical and clinical testing in the past decade, most of these compounds have been found to be non–cross-resistant with tamoxifen and therefore have not been added to the treatment choices for ER-positive breast cancer. The predicted three-dimensional structure of the ligand-binding domain of the ER suggests that the non–cross-resistance of some SERMs (e.g., fulvestrant and possibly arzoxifene) is probably due to functional differences in the ER conformation that results following SERM binding. These three-dimensional effects alter the ER's interaction with corepressors and coactivators, resulting in changes in gene expression that vary significantly between individual SERMs. The AIs also appear to have significant non–cross-resistance with tamoxifen and may be superior to tamoxifen for the first-line treatment of advanced disease in postmenopausal women. As the results of the ATAC trial mature, the AIs may also become the treatment of choice for adjuvant therapy for postmenopausal women.

In premenopausal women, the question of whether ovarian suppression with AI treatment or ovarian suppression with or without tamoxifen is the better treatment for metastatic breast cancer is still under study. In the near future, an international trial will address the question of adjuvant therapy with ovarian suppression with or without AI or tamoxifen in premenopausal women (G. Fleming, personal communication, 2002). The International Breast Cancer Study Group's Suppression of Ovarian Function Trial will randomly assign 3000 patients to treatment with tamoxifen alone for 5 years, tamoxifen with ovarian suppression (gonadotropin-releasing hormone analogue, radiotherapeutic ablation, or surgical oophorectomy), or exemestane with ovarian suppression. The answers to these important adjuvant therapy questions are likely to lead to improved endocrine therapy for premenopausal women in the neoadjuvant and metastatic settings as well. In the prevention setting, the benefits of current SERMs to particular subgroups of women who are at increased risk for breast cancer will continue to be studied carefully so that the appropriate high-risk patients can be identified for prevention strategies. In addition, the benefits of novel SERMs that have fewer detrimental side effects (e.g., less agonist activity in the endometrium) will continue to be evaluated in prevention trials, such as the STAR and MORE studies. Finally, the combined use of SERMs with other prevention strategies, such as cyclooxygenase inhibitors and retinoids, is likely to be implemented as new information that is relevant to the control of breast cancer is translated from the laboratory to the clinic.[57]

REFERENCES

1. Osborne CK, Zhao H, Fuqua SA. Selective estrogen receptor modulators: structure, function, and clinical use. J Clin Oncol 2000;18:3172–3186.
2. Shiau A, Barstad D, Radek J et al. Structural characterization of a subtype-selective ligand reveals a novel mode of estrogen receptor antagonism. Nat Struct Biol 2002;9:359–364.
3. Shiau A, Barstad D, Loria P et al. The structural basis of estrogen receptor/coactivator recognition and the antagonism of this interaction by tamoxifen. Cell 1998;95:927–937.
4. Brzozowski AM, Pike AC, Dauter Z et al. Molecular basis of agonism and antagonism in the oestrogen receptor. Nature 1997;389:753–758.
5. Tremblay GB, Kunath T, Bergeron D et al. Diethylstilbestrol regulates trophoblast stem cell differentiation as a ligand of orphan nuclear receptor ERR beta. Genes Dev 2001;15:833–838.

6. Peethambaram P, Ingle J, Suman V et al. Randomized trial of diethylstilbestrol vs. tamoxifen in postmenopausal women with metastatic breast cancer: an updated analysis. Breast Cancer Res Treat 1999;54:117–122.
7. Harper M, Walpole A. A new derivative of triphenylethylene: effect on implantation and mode of action in rats. J Reprod Fertil 1967;13:101–119.
8. Love RR, Mazess RB, Barden HS. Effects of tamoxifen on bone mineral density in postmenopausal women with breast cancer. N Engl J Med 1992;326:852–856.
9. Fisher B, Costantino JP, Wickerham DL et al. Tamoxifen for prevention of breast cancer: Report of the National Surgical Adjuvant Breast and Bowel Project P-1 study. J Natl Cancer Inst 1998;90:1371–1388.
10. Dhingra K. Selective estrogen receptor modulation: the search for an ideal hormonal therapy for breast cancer. Cancer Invest 2001;19:649–659.
11. Loprinzi C, Sloan J, Perez E et al. Phase III evaluation of fluoxetine for treatment of hot flashes. J Clin Oncol 2002;20:1578–1583.
12. Van Patten CL, Olivotto IA, Chambers GK et al. Effect of soy phytoestrogens on hot flashes in postmenopausal women with breast cancer: a randomized, controlled clinical trial. J Clin Oncol 2002;20:1449–1455.
13. Quella S, Loprinzi C, Barton D et al. Evaluation of soy phytoestrogens for the treatment of hot flashes in breast cancer survivors: a North Central Cancer Treatment Group trial. J Clin Oncol 2000;18:1068–1074.
14. Jacobson JS, Troxel AB, Evans J et al. Randomized trial of black cohosh for the treatment of hot flashes among women with a history of breast cancer. J Clin Oncol 2001;19:2739–2745.
15. Hard G, Latropoulos M, Jordan K et al. Major difference in the hepatocarcinogenicity and DNA adduct forming ability between toremifene and tamoxifen in female Crl:CD(BR) rats. Cancer Res 1993;53:4534–4541.
16. Pyrhonen S, Ellmen J, Vuorinen J et al. Meta-analysis of trials comparing toremifene with tamoxifen and factors predicting outcome of anti-estrogen therapy in postmenopausal women with breast cancer. Breast Cancer Res Treat 1999;56:133–143.
17. Holli K, Valavaara R, Blanco G et al. Safety and efficacy results of a randomized trial comparing adjuvant toremifene and tamoxifen in postmenopausal patients with node-positive breast cancer. J Clin Oncol 2000;18:3487–3494.
18. Roos W, Oeze L, Loser R et al. Antiestrogenic action of 3-hydroxytamoxifen in the human breast cancer cell line MCF-7. J Natl Cancer Inst 1983;71:55–59.
19. Haarstad H, Lonning PE, Gundersen S et al. Influence of droloxifene on metastatic breast cancer as first-line endocrine treatment. Acta Oncol 1998;37:365–368.
20. Dhingra K. Antiestrogens: tamoxifen, SERMs and beyond. Invest New Drugs 1999;17:285–311.
21. Johnston SR, Riddler S, Haynes B et al. The novel anti-oestrogen idoxifene inhibits the growth of human MCF-7 breast cancer xenografts and reduces the frequency of acquired anti-oestrogen resistance. Br J Cancer 1997;75:804–809.
22. Nuttall M, Bradbeer J, Stroup G et al. Idoxifene: a novel selective estrogen receptor modulator prevents bone loss and lowers cholesterol levels in ovariectomized rats and decreases uterine weight in intact rats. Endocrinology 1998;139:5224–5534.
23. Johnston S, Gorbunova V, Lichinister M et al. A multicentre double-blind randomized phase II trial of idoxifene versus tamoxifen as first-line endocrine therapy for metastatic breast cancer. Proc Am Soc Clin Oncol 2001;20:A113.
24. Johnston SRD, Howell A. Endocrine treatment of breast cancer: SERMs. In: Miller WR, Ingle James N, eds. Endocrine Therapy in Breast Cancer. New York: Marcel Dekker, 2002:47–77.

25. Buzdar A, Marcus C, Holmes F et al. Phase II evaluation of LY156758 in metastatic breast cancer. Oncology 1988;45:344–345.

26. Gradishar W, Glusman J, Lu Y et al. Effects of high dose raloxifene in selected patients with advanced breast carcinoma. Cancer 2000;88:2047–2053.

27. Sato M, Turner C, Wang T et al. A novel raloxifene analogue with improved SERM potency and efficacy in vivo. J Pharmacol Exp Ther 1998;287:1–7.

28. Baselga J, Llombart-Cussac A, Bellet M. Double-blind randomized phase II study of a selective estrogen receptor modulator in patients with locally advanced or metastatic breast cancer. Breast Cancer Res Treat 1999;57:A25.

29. Llombart-Cussac A, Bellet M, Guillem-Porta V et al. Efficacy and safety of two doses of the selective estrogen receptor modulator (SERM) LY353381 in locally advanced or metastatic breast cancer (LAMBC): a randomized double blind phase 2 study. Proc Am Soc Clin Oncol 2000;19:157a.

30. Labrie F, Labrie C, Belanger A et al. EM-652 (SCH57068), a pure SERM having complete antiestrogenic activity in the mammary gland and endometrium. J Steroid Biochem Mol Biol 2001;79:213–225.

31 Labrie F, Champagne P, Labrie C et al. Response to the orally active specific antiestrogen EM-800 (SCH-57070) in tamoxifen resistant breast cancer. Breast Cancer Res Treat 1997;42:A211.

32. Greenberger LM, Annable T, Collins KI et al. A new antiestrogen, 2-(4-hydroxy-phenyl)-3-methyl-1-[4-(2-piperidin-1-yl-ethoxy)-benzyl]-1-indol-5-ol hydrochloride (ERA-923), inhibits the growth of tamoxifen-sensitive and -resistant tumors and is devoid of uterotropic effects in mice and rats. Clin Cancer Res 2001;7:3166–3177.

33. Cotreau MM, Stonis L, Dykstra KH et al. Multiple-dose, safety, pharmacokinetics, and pharmacodynamics of a new selective estrogen receptor modulator, ERA-923, in healthy postmenopausal women. J Clin Pharmacol 2002;42:157–165.

34. Johnston SR. Endocrine manipulation in advanced breast cancer: recent advances with SERM therapies. Clin Cancer Res 2001;7:4376s–4387s; discussion 4411s–4412s.

35. Robertson JF. Estrogen receptor downregulators: new antihormonal therapy for advanced breast cancer. Clin Ther 2002;24[suppl A]:A17–30.

36. Robertson J, Howell A, De Friend D et al. Duration of remission to ICI 182,780 compared to megestrol acetate in tamoxifen-resistant breast cancer. Breast 1997;6:186–189.

37. Nabholtz J, Buzdar A, Pollak M et al. Anastrozole is superior to tamoxifen as first-line therapy for advanced breast cancer in postmenopausal women: results of a North American multicenter randomized trial. J Clin Oncol 2000;18:3758–3776.

38. Howell A, Robertson J, Quaresma Albano J et al. Fulvestrant, formerly ICI 182,780, is as effective as anastrozole in postmenopausal women with advanced breast cancer progressing after prior endocrine treatment. J Clin Oncol 2002;20:2296–2403.

39. Powles TJ, Tillyer CR, Jones AL et al. Prevention of breast cancer with tamoxifen: an update on the Royal Marsden Hospital Pilot Programme. Eur J Cancer 1990;26:680–684.

40. Veronesi U, Maisonneuve P, Sacchini V et al. Tamoxifen for breast cancer among hysterectomised women. Lancet 2002;359:1122–1124.

41. Veronesi U, Maisonneuve P, Costa A et al. Prevention of breast cancer with tamoxifen: preliminary findings from the Italian randomised trial among hysterectomised women. Italian tamoxifen prevention study. Lancet 1998;352:93–97.

42. Gail MH, Costantino JP, Bryant J et al. Weighing the risks and benefits of tamoxifen treatment for preventing breast cancer. J Natl Cancer Inst 1999;91:1829–1846.

43. Cuzick J. First results from the International Breast Cancer Intervention Study (IBIS-I): a randomised prevention trial. Lancet 2002;360:817.

44. Cummings SR, Eckert S, Krueger KA et al. The effect of raloxifene on risk of breast cancer in postmenopausal women: results from the more randomized trial. Multiple Outcomes of Raloxifene Evaluation. JAMA 1999;281:2189–2197.

45. Lippman ME, Krueger KA, Eckert S et al. Indicators of lifetime estrogen exposure: effect on breast cancer incidence and interaction with raloxifene therapy in the multiple outcomes of raloxifene evaluation study participants. J Clin Oncol 2001;19:3111–3116.

46. Fisher B, Land S, Mamounas E et al. Prevention of invasive breast cancer in women with ductal carcinoma in situ: an update of the National Surgical Adjuvant Breast Project experience. Semin Oncol 2001;28:400–418.

47. ATAC Trialists Group. Anastrozole alone or in combination with tamoxifen versus tamoxifen alone for adjuvant treatment of postmenopausal women with early breast cancer: first results of the ATAC randomised trial. Lancet 2002;359:2131–2139.

48. Winer E, Hudis C, Burstein HJ et al. American Society of Clinical Oncology technology assessment on the use of aromatase inhibitors as adjuvant therapy for women with hormone receptor-positive breast cancer: status report 2002. J Clin Oncol 2002;20:3317–3327.

49. Klijn JG, Blamey RW, Boccardo F et al. Combined tamoxifen and luteinizing hormone-releasing hormone (LHRH) agonist versus LHRH agonist alone in premenopausal advanced breast cancer: a meta-analysis of four randomized trials. J Clin Oncol 2001;19:343–353.

50. Coates AS, Simpson JF, Forbes JF. A randomized trial in postmenopausal patients with advanced breast cancer comparing endocrine and cytotoxic therapy given sequentially or in combination: the Australian and New Zealand Breast Cancer Trials Group, Clinical Oncological Society of Australia. J Clin Oncol 1986;4:186–193.

51. Mouridsen H, Gershanovish M, Sun Y. Superior efficacy of letrozole versus tamoxifen as first-line therapy for postmenopausal women with advanced breast cancer: results of a phase III study of the International Letrozole Breast Cancer Group. J Clin Oncol 2001;19:2596–2606.

52. Bonneterre J, Buzdar A, Nabholtz J et al. Anastrozole is superior to tamoxifen as first-line therapy in hormone receptor positive advanced breast carcinoma. Cancer 2001; 92:2247–2258.

53. Eiermann W, Paepke S, Appfelstaedt J et al. Preoperative treatment of postmenopausal breast cancer patients with letrozole: a randomized double-blind multicenter study. Ann Oncol 2001;12:1527–1532.

54. Yamauchi H, Stearns V, Hayes DF. The role of c-ERB-2 as a predictive factor in breast cancer. Breast Cancer 2001;8:171–183.

55. Ellis MJ, Coop A, Singh B et al. Letrozole is more effective neoadjuvant endocrine therapy than tamoxifen for erbB1- and/or erbB2-positive, estrogen receptor-positive primary breast cancer: evidence from a phase III randomized trial. J Clin Oncol 2001;19:3808–3816.

56. Newby J, Johnston S, Smith I et al. Expression of epidermal growth factor receptor and c-erbB2 during the development of tamoxifen resistance in human breast cancer. Clin Cancer Res 1997;3:1643–1651.

57. Sporn MB. Hobson's choice and the need for combinations of new agents for the prevention and treatment of breast cancer. J Natl Cancer Inst 2002;94:242–243.

Chapter 11

Correlation of PET and CT in Clinical Cancer Management

Dominique Delbeke, MD, PhD

James A. Patton, PhD

The rapid advances in imaging technologies are a challenge for both radiologists and clinicians who must integrate these technologies for optimal patient care and outcomes at minimal cost. Multiple indications for functional imaging using ^{18}F-fluorodeoxyglucose (FDG) are now well accepted in oncology, including differentiating benign from malignant lesions, staging malignant lesions, detecting malignant recurrence, and monitoring therapy. The utility of FDG imaging was first demonstrated with the use of dedicated PET with multiple full rings of bismuth germinate detectors. The spectrum of equipment available for FDG imaging now includes dual-head gamma camera systems that are capable of imaging conventional single-photon emitters as well as positron emitters, such as FDG.

The fusion of anatomic and molecular images (FDG computed tomography [CT]) obtained with integrated positron emission tomography (PET) CT systems, taken sequentially in time but without moving the patient from the imaging table, allows optimal coregistration of anatomic and molecular images. This leads to accurate attenuation correction and precise anatomic localization of lesions with increased metabolism. This powerful technology provides a valuable new tool for diagnostic and therapeutic applications. The diagnostic accuracy is improved in approximately 50% of patients because of improved lesion detection on both CT and FDG PET images, better differentiation between physiologic and pathological foci of FDG uptake, and better localization of malignant foci of FDG uptake. This new technology affects the management of 10%–20% of patients by guiding further therapy (biopsy, surgery, and promising clinical applications, including guiding biopsy to the metabolically active sites of the tumors, guiding surgery, and planning intensity-modulated radiation therapy).

INTRODUCTION

The goals of oncologic imaging are lesion detection, lesion characterization, evaluation of extent of the neoplasm, staging for malignant lesions, and assessment of therapeutic response. Staging includes localization of lesion, evaluation of proximity to vessels, and detection of nodal and distant metastases. The rapid advances in imaging technologies are a challenge for both the imaging expert and the clinician who must integrate these technologies for optimal patient care and outcomes at minimal cost. Multiple imaging modalities are available to achieve these goals, including morphologic imaging with ultrasound, CT, magnetic resonance imaging (MRI), and molecular imaging using radiopharmaceuticals.

Since the early 1990s, numerous technologic improvements have occurred in the field of radiologic imaging. These include color Doppler ultrasound, spiral computed tomography (CT) that allows multiphase enhancement techniques, fast MRI, new MRI contrast agents, MRI cholangiopancreatography, and positron emission tomography (PET) using (FDG) as a radiopharmaceutical that provides the capability for imaging glucose metabolism.

Molecular imaging using positron imaging is unique in that positron emitters allow labeling of radiopharmaceuticals that closely mimic endogenous molecules and there is continuous development of new biologic tracers. Because of its ability to demonstrate glucose metabolism and its longer, more practical half-life (110 minutes) compared with those of other positron emitters, FDG is the most frequently used tracer in oncology. Although FDG shares some of the limitations of single-photon emitters, the relatively high ratio of tumor-to-background contrast seen with most malignant lesions accounts for the high reported sensitivity and specificity of FDG imaging compared with CT.

Improvements in the distribution of FDG by commercial companies have now made FDG available to many medical centers. Multiple indications for molecular imaging using FDG are now well accepted in the fields of neurology, cardiology, and oncology.[1] It has been well established that various malignant tumors avidly accumulate FDG. This is due, in part, to increased numbers of glucose transporter proteins and increased intracellular enzyme levels of hexokinase and phosphofructokinase, among others, which promote glycolysis.[2-5] FDG PET imaging can be used to exploit the metabolic differences between benign and malignant cells for imaging purposes.[6,7] Although variations in uptake are known to exist among tumor types, elevated uptake of FDG has been demonstrated in numerous primary malignant tumors.[8,9] Therefore, various indications for FDG imaging have been investigated: differentiation of benign from malignant lesions, staging of malignant lesions, detection of malignant recurrence, and monitoring of therapy. Nowadays, the major indication for FDG PET imaging is staging and restaging of malignant tumors, leading to detection of unsuspected metastases in 25%–30% of patients and major changes in therapy. In two thirds of these cases, unnecessary surgery is avoided, thereby decreasing the number of invasive procedures and increasing the cost-effectiveness of health care.[10-12]

The clinical utility of FDG imaging was first established by use of dedicated PET tomographs equipped with multiple rings of bismuth germinate oxide detectors, but a spectrum of equipment is now available for positron imaging, including gamma camera–based PET that is capable of imaging conventional single-photon emitters as well as positron emitters, such as FDG.[8,9] This new technology was developed to make FDG imaging more widely accessible, first using single-photon emission computed tomography (SPECT) with high-energy collimators, and then using dual-head coincidence detection with multihead gamma cameras, which improved spatial resolution. Most hybrid gamma cameras are now equipped with thallium-activated sodium iodide crystals of increased thickness (up to 1 inch in thickness), which improve sensitivity dramatically. For both gamma camera–based PET and dedicated high-resolution PET, technical developments are still evolving, with better iterative reconstruction algorithms being developed to improve the quality of the images and better systems being developed to correct for attenuation.

Although numerous studies have shown that the sensitivity and specificity of FDG imaging is superior to that of CT in many clinical settings, the inability of FDG imaging to provide anatomic localization remains a significant impairment in maximizing its clinical utility. In addition, FDG is an analogue of glucose, and it is a tracer of glucose metabolism. Therefore, the distribution of FDG is not limited to malignant tissue. It has been well documented in the PET literature that the interpreter must be familiar with the normal pattern and physiologic variations of FDG distribution to avoid misinterpretations.[13,14] To avoid misinterpretation of FDG images, the interpreter must be familiar with clinical data relevant to the patient and to standardize the environment of the patient during the uptake period so as to limit physiologic variations of FDG uptake (e.g., in activated muscular tissue).

High-resolution FDG PET emission scans provide high-resolution images of the distribution of FDG in the body that reflect tissue metabolism at the time of the study. However, interpretation of these emission scans is often complicated by the absence of detailed anatomy in the emission data. The problem of anatomic localization of the foci of abnormal uptake and differentiation of physiologic from pathological foci of uptake is compounded by lower resolution and increased noise in the images of some of some of the systems at the low end of the spectrum. Close correlation of FDG studies with conventional CT scans helps minimize these difficulties. In practice, interpretation is accomplished by visually comparing the emission scans to high-quality anatomic maps, such as those provided by clinical CT scanners. The interpreting physician visually integrates the two image sets to precisely locate a region of increased uptake on the CT scan that was identified on the PET scan. To aid in image interpretation, several techniques have been developed to coregister the FDG PET emission scans with the high-resolution anatomic maps provided by CT.[15]

It has been demonstrated that attenuation effects are much more significant in coincidence imaging than in SPECT because both photons from an annihilation process must pass through the region without interaction. Attenuation effects in coincidence imaging produce regional nonuniformities, distortions of intense structures, and edge effects. The topic of attenuation correction has recently been discussed in an editorial by R.L. Wahl.[16] Attenuation correction has significant advantages for the clinical evaluation of FDG images from oncologic patients, the most important of which is improved anatomic delineation (e.g., mediastinum from lungs, lungs from liver). Therefore, localization of lesion is easier on images with attenuation correction. The second advantage of attenuation correction is the possibility of semiquantitative measurement using the standard uptake value, which may be helpful in some clinical settings. One example is differentiating benign from malignant pulmonary lesions that have diameters greater than twice the resolution of the tomograph; another is monitoring therapy for malignant lesions. In addition, correction for these attenuation artifacts improves the quality of the images and increases image contrast. Quantitative measurements of various physiologic parameters (e.g., perfusion rate and glucose metabolism) by use of kinetic modeling also requires optimal attenuation correction to measure true counts in the region of interest in the body. Correction for attenuation effects can be performed with calculated geometric attenuation for uniform structures that are predictable in shape and content, such as the brain. For the body, various methods have been developed with measured attenuation using radioactive transmission sources. The quality of the image corrected for attenuation effects largely depends on coregistration of the attenuation maps (transmission scan) and emission scan.

Optimal coregistration between anatomic and functional studies is necessary both for optimal attenuation correction and anatomic mapping. Coregistration can be obtained using methods such as fitting techniques and image alignment that relies on coregistration software. These methods offer acceptable fusion images for the brain, which is surrounded by a rigid structure, the skull. For the body, coregistration of two images, often obtained at different points in time, is much more difficult. Identical positioning of the patient on the imaging table is critical, and internal organ peristalsis and motion add to the problem. The recent technical development of integrated PET-CT systems provide CT and FDG PET images obtained in a single imaging setting, allowing optimal coregistration of images. The fusion images provided by these systems allow the most accurate interpretation of both CT and FDG PET studies that can be integrated for optimal patient care. Fusion FDG PET-CT imaging is also a promising tool for optimizing radiation therapy. Because of the high-photon flux of x-rays, CT attenuation maps from these integrated PET-CT systems also allow for optimal attenuation correction of the PET images.

IMAGE FUSION USING CO-REGISTRATION SOFTWARE

One technique requires the generation of three-dimensional surface maps of the two distributions and the use of iterative algorithms to find parameters that optimize the alignment of the two distributions. These parameters are then used to transform one of the two acquired data sets so that it is registered with the second set. This technique provides the best registration for a small rigid body in which the surface is well defined by both modalities, such as the brain.[17]

A second method involves the use of automated algorithms that assume that corresponding pixels in the two images are directly related by a common factor, and iterative optimization algorithms are used to determine this factor by minimizing the variance of the ratio of the adjusted-to-reference images. The application of this technique must be limited to the actual tissue distributions by the use of tissue masks that can be determined by edge-detection algorithms, and it is best suited for registering images from a common modality.[18]

The third technique is an iterative interaction procedure in which a knowledgeable observer uses an interactive mathematical registration algorithm that permits the identification of an initial set of trial transformation parameters, an algorithm that performs the transformation, and techniques for image correlation that permit control and evaluation of the accuracy of the transformation. This technique is the most versatile of the three algorithms and has a wide variety of applications, assuming that sufficient anatomic markers are present in both image sets. However, it is subjective and depends on the skills of the observer.[19] After registration has been accomplished using one of these techniques, images of corresponding anatomic slices can then be overlaid (fused) to provide a precise anatomic location of detected abnormalities. However, these methods often suffer from registration errors as a result of difficulties in patient repositioning and movement of internal organs between scanning sessions.

PET-CT INTEGRATED SYSTEMS

The first prototype of integrated PET-CT system was developed by the group of investigators at the University of Pittsburgh. These investigators have mounted a commercial CT scanner and a commercial dedicated PET scanner on a single support system with a common imaging table (Fig. 11.1).[20] The PET scanner used in this configuration was a Siemens-CTI ART scanner (Fig. 11.1A), a partial-ring system that was previously described in this text. The CT

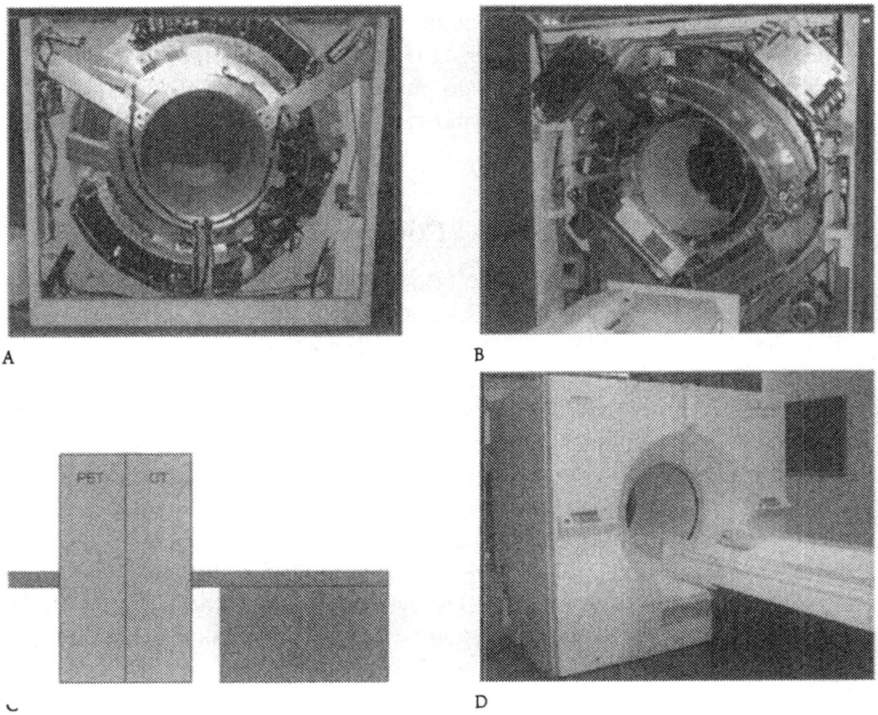

FIGURE 11.1 Partial-ring PET scanner (panel A; Siemens-CTI ART) and a diagnostic CT scanner (panel B; Siemens single-slice, helical scanner) have been coupled to a single rotational gantry and a common imaging table (panel C) to produce an integrated PET-CT scanner (panel D). CT, computed tomography; PET, positron emission tomography. (Courtesy of David Townsend, PhD, University of Pittsburgh, Pittsburgh, PA).

scanner used was a Siemens third-generation, single-slice, helical scanner (Fig. 11.1B). The CT scanner was mounted on the front of a rotational support gantry, and the PET scanner was mounted on the back of the same gantry (Figs. 11.1C and D). The combined gantry has a rotational speed of 30 revolutions per minute. The centers of the two imaging systems are offset axially by 60 cm. A common imaging table is positioned at the front of the gantry and permits an axial travel range of 180 cm. Because of the offsets between the two imaging systems, the system is limited to a maximum axial distance of 100 cm that can be imaged by both systems without moving the patient. The state-of-the-art integrated PET-CT system from Siemens Medical Systems is the Biograph combining the $ECAT_R$ Exact HR+ PET tomography and the Soma tom Emotion multislice CT scanner (CTI PET systems, Knoxville, TN and Siemens Medical Systems, Hoffman Estates, IL).

A similar integrated PET-CT system (Discovery LS) is now being manufactured by General Electric (General Electric Medical Systems, Milwaukee, WI);

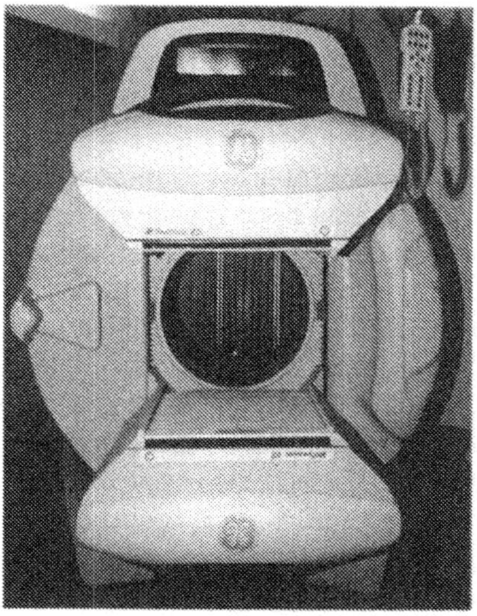

FIGURE 11.2 General Electric Hawkeye, an integrated computed tomographic dual-head scintillation camera with coincidence imaging capability.

this system combines the GE Advance Nxi PET scanner with a light-speed multislice CT unit. In addition, a new PET-CT system (PosiTRACE) is being produced by SMV/General Electric (General Electric Medical Systems, Milwaukee, WI). This system consists of six camera heads with 3/4-inch-thick thallium-activated sodium iodide crystals arranged in a hexagonal array and integrated with a diagnostic CT scanner. This system acquires coincidence data in three-dimensional mode with complete sampling being obtained by rotating the detector system around the patient. More recently, ADAC-Philips Medical Systems has put on the market the PET-CT Gemini (ADAC Laboratories, A Philips Medical Systems Company, Milpitas, CA), which combines the Philips-ADAC Allegro GSO PET system and the Philips MX8000 D multislice CT scanner.

With these integrated systems, a diagnostic CT scan and a PET scan can be acquired sequentially with the patient lying on the imaging table and simply being translated between the two systems. Accurate calibration of the position of the imaging table and the use of common parameters in data acquisition and image reconstruction permit the fusion of images of anatomy and metabolism from the same region of the body that are registered in space and only slightly offset in time. Because the CT scan is actually a high-resolution transmission map, these data can be used to perform a high-quality attenuation correction during image reconstruction of the emission data. Similar advancements have been made in hybrid camera technology. As seen in Fig. 11.2, General Electric has installed an x-ray tube and a linear detector array on a dual-head scintillation camera with coincidence imaging capability (VG Millenium, General Electric

Medical Systems, Milwaukee, WI) to provide attenuation maps and anatomic localization.[21] The x-ray tube and linear detector array are mounted on the slip-ring gantry of the camera and continuously rotate together with the detector heads around the patient in a fixed geometry for data acquisition. The x-ray tube is a low-output tube, and the detector array consists of 384 solid-state detectors (each 1.8 × 28 mm). Because the fan beam is wide enough to cover the full width of the patient, and because the x-ray tube and detector array are in a fixed geometry and rotate together, this system has the characteristics of a low-end, third-generation CT scanner. One CT slice is acquired in 13.6 seconds. As with the integrated PET-CT system, anatomic and metabolic images are acquired sequentially, and the high-photon flux CT images are used for high-quality attenuation correction of the emission data. The CT images and the emission images can also be fused to provide functional images to accurately locate regions of increased metabolic activity. Because this camera can also be used for single-photon imaging, the CT scans can be used for attenuation correction of SPECT images and fusion of anatomic and SPECT images.

ATTENUATION CORRECTION

On images with attenuation correction, lesions are not distorted, and lesions located deeply should have intensity similar to that of superficial lesions. In addition to elimination of attenuation artifacts, improvement occurs in image contrast on images corrected for attenuation artifacts. For images of the brain, models with calculated attenuation correction can be used very accurately and are patient independent. This is not the case for body images because of the variability of the body habitus in different patients and the asymmetry of internal organs. Measured attenuation correction is commonly performed by direct measurement of 511-keV photon attenuation through the body. The transmission scan adds to the length of the study and often requires repositioning of the patient in the gantry of the tomograph, which contributes to coregistration problems and noise in the images. Patient motion during long scanning times is also a problem. If the transmission scan is acquired after FDG administration, quantification errors can occur if no correction is performed. Attenuation correction based on segmentation can produce artifacts if segmentation is inaccurate.

The use of an x-ray tube–based transmission scan provides attenuation-corrected emission images of high quality as a result of the high-photon flux inherent with this technique. Optimal coregistration between attenuation maps and emission images is possible with the use of integrated PET-CT systems when the CT attenuation maps and FDG PET emission images are obtained sequentially in time without moving the patient from the imaging table. Because the FDG emission images have to be acquired during normal breathing, there is still a debate as to whether optimal attenuation maps are provided by attenuation maps obtained with the breath-hold technique or during normal breathing.

CLINICAL IMPACT OF FUSION IMAGES

From the diagnostic point of view, fusion of anatomic and molecular images results in (1) improvement of lesion detection on both CT and FDG PET images; (2) improvement of localization of foci of FDG uptake, resulting in better differentiation of physiologic from pathological uptake and precise localization of the malignant foci. PET-CT fusion images affect the clinical management by guiding further procedures, by excluding the need of further procedures, and by changing both inter- and intramodality therapy. For example, precise localization of metastatic lymph nodes could result in a less invasive and more efficient surgical procedure. PET-CT fusion images have the potential to provide important information to guide the biopsy of a mass to active regions of the tumor and to provide better maps than those obtained with CT alone to modulate the field and the dose of radiation therapy.

Results with the use of fused images of coregistered anatomic and functional data obtained with separate imaging systems support the importance of correlative imaging.[22] Investigators at Rambam Medical Center reported their experience with CT FDG images obtained with a gamma camera–based CT-hybrid PET system.[23] The fusion images changed the interpretation of PET or CT in 45% (75/167) of patients by allowing correct localization of the foci of uptake in 60 patients and by determining that the uptake was physiologic in 15 patients. The management of 17% (29/167) of patients was changed: surgery was cancelled in six patients, surgery was planned in seven patients, and additional chemotherapy or radiation therapy was administered to 15 patients. In another study on 35 patients, image fusion obtained with the same CT-hybrid PET-integrated system allowed precise localization of lesions in the skeleton, in the liver versus the adjacent bowel, and in specific structures of the neck in 31% of patients.[24]

After performing 100 oncology studies using an integrated PET-CT system, the investigators at Pittsburgh University concluded that combined PET-CT image offers significant advantages, including more accurate localization of foci of uptake, distinction of pathological from physiologic uptake, and improvement in guiding and evaluating therapy.[25] More recent studies of 100 patients[26] and 134 patients[27] using integrated PET-CT systems concluded that the diagnostic accuracy of PET is improved in approximately 50% of patients. In the first study, 50% of the equivocal PET findings could be reclassified into the normal or definitely abnormal categories, especially in the region of the neck and the abdomen and pelvis. In the second study, PET-CT fusion images led to better discrimination between benign and malignant foci of uptake and retrospective detection of lesion on CT, leading to a change in therapy in 12% of patients.

Fusion PET-CT images from integrated systems have the potential to change significantly the field of radiation therapy. In a group of 30 patients with various body malignancies who were scheduled to be treated with radiation therapy, the target volumes measured on CT images only were compared with the those measured on fusion PET-CT images.[28] The planned treatment was changed in 63% (19/30) of patients on the basis of PET-CT fusion images, by detection of unsuspected metastases that led to cancellation of radiation therapy (*N* = 5), by changing the therapy from curative to palliative (*N* = 6), by changing the dose (*N* = 9), and by changing the target volume (*N* = 12).

It is also important to be aware of the potentially useful additional information provided by the independent interpretation of a radiologist who is experienced in body imaging of the noncontrasted CT portion of the study obtained with integrated PET-CT systems. An analysis of 250 patients demonstrated that these findings are uncommon (3% of patients) but could be serious enough to warrant alterations in clinical management.[29]

Head and Neck Cancer

A head phantom study for multimodality image registration quality assurance for conformal three-dimensional radiation therapy treatment planning was performed using a fiducial marking system for PET, CT, and MRI. The authors concluded that the registration of CT-CT, CT-MRI, and PET-CT images allowed correlation of anatomic landmarks to within 2 mm.[30]

A study on 21 patients demonstrated the usefulness of FDG PET and CT or MRI fusion images for radiation therapy planning.[31] The images were coregistered using an automatic multimodality image registration algorithm, with the brain being used as an internal reference. The gross tumor volume was determined on the basis of clinical examination and FDG uptake on the fusion images. The clinical target volume was determined following the usual pattern of lymph node spread. The authors concluded that the gross tumor volume was changed in 11% (2/21) of the patients by fusion images. More importantly, parotid gland sparing became possible in 15/21 (71%) patients because fusion images demonstrated absence of abnormal FDG uptake. After a follow-up of 18 months, only 1/21 (4.8%) patients had recurrence.

In a preliminary study of five patients, the investigators at the University of Pittsburgh showed that PET-CT images obtained from an integrated PET-CT system were helpful in distinguishing malignant lesions from normal physiologic FDG uptake in the striated muscles of the head and neck as well as in excretory and bowel activity in the abdomen and pelvis. They also concluded that the technology positively affected patient management through localization for surgical and radiation therapy planning as well as assessment of tumor response to therapy.[32] After performing PET-CT on more than 250 patients, the same group reported a change in management in 20% (14/70) of patients with head and neck cancer.[33]

Chest Tumors: Lung and Esophageal Cancer

In a study of 43 patients with bronchogenic carcinoma, precise localization of lesions was not possible in 18% of patients on PET images alone, but these lesions could be localized to precise anatomic structures on PET-CT fusion images obtained with an integrated PET-CT system.[34]

In a study investigating the usefulness of CT-FDG-PET fusion images for the evaluation of regional lymph node metastases in patients with non–small cell lung cancer, the accuracy of CT alone was 87%, that of FDG PET alone was 91%, and that of visual correlation and fusion was 93%. In the identification of the nodal stage, CT was correct in 50% of patients, PET in 66%, visual correlation in 71%, and fusion in 73%. The authors concluded that the exact localization of metastatic thoracic lymph nodes was improved by visual correlation of CT and PET, but that the fusion images added only marginal benefit over visual correlation.[35]

The value of PET-CT using an integrated system was analyzed in 26 patients referred for suspected recurrent lung cancer. In this study, integrated PET-CT images improved the interpretation of the images in 54% of patients and led to a significant change in management in 27% of them.[36]

The group of investigators at Duke University investigated the utility of FDG PET during CT-based treatment planning for patients with lung cancer. FDG PET data influenced 34% (12/35) of the treatment plans examined and resulted in enlarging portions of the beam aperture up to 15 mm.[37] A more recent study reported on the potential benefit of incorporating PET data into the conventional radiation therapy treatment planning of 11 patients with non–small cell lung cancer.[38] Patients were immobilized in the treatment position for acquisition of both CT and FDG PET images. For all patients, the planned target volume outline was changed on the basis of comparisons of CT images with PET-CT fused images. In 7/11 (64%) patients, the planned target volume was increased by an average of 19% to incorporate distant nodal disease. In the other four patients, the target planned volume was decreased by an average of 18%, excluding atelectasis and trimming the target volume to avoid delivering higher radiation doses to the nearby spinal cord or heart.

Abdominal and Pelvic Tumors

In four patients with recurrent colorectal carcinoma, Fukugana et al[39] correlated FDG PET images coregistered with CT or MRI with pathological examination of the resected specimen. They concluded that in all cases, the preoperative evaluation of tumor recurrence with fusion images provided more useful clinical information for the management of these patients than the anatomic images alone. Illustrative examples are shown in Figures 11.3 and 11.4.

PET-CT fusion images may be particularly important in the abdomen and pelvis. PET images alone may be difficult to interpret, owing to both the absence

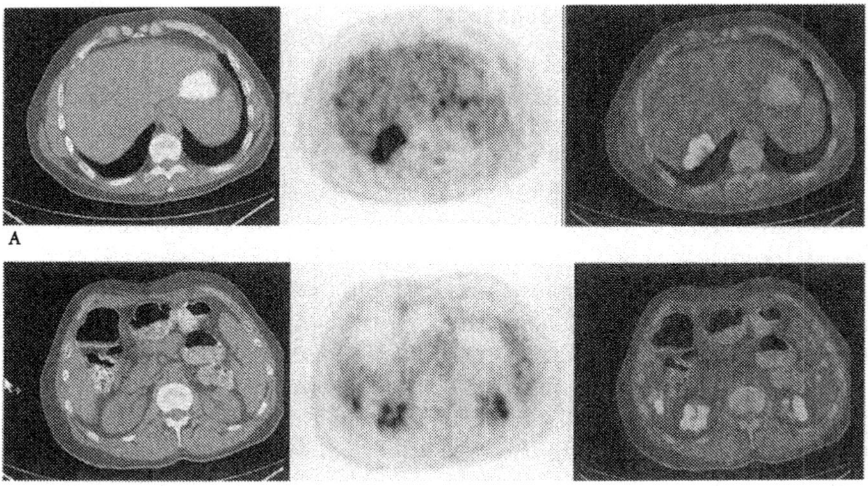

A

B

FIGURE 11.3 This case illustrates the power of fusion images from an integrated PET-CT system for the detection of lesions on FDG PET images, the localization of these lesions on the integrated noncontrasted CT images, and the further identification of these lesions on the diagnostic CT images with intravenous contrast. A 50-year-old man with a history of colorectal cancer presented with rising CEA levels and was referred for a combined CT-FDG PET scan on an integrated system (General Electric Medical Systems, Milwaukee, WI). A and B, Images from the integrated system demonstrated two foci of FDG uptake projecting in the posterior aspect of the right lobe of the liver. *(Continued)*

of anatomic landmarks (other than the kidneys) and the presence of nonspecific uptake in the stomach, bowel, and colon. The usefulness of PET-CT fusion images to differentiated physiologic from pathological FDG uptake in the abdomen had been reported in a study of 28 patients with abdominal tumors[40] and in another study of 10 patients with ovarian malignancies.[41] In both studies, the fusion images were obtained with an integrated PET-CT system.

A more recent study of 46 patients with colorectal cancer referred for FDG PET imaging on an integrated PET-CT system concluded that more definite normal and definitely abnormal lesions (and fewer equivocal lesions) were diagnosed with PET-CT images than with either modality alone. In addition, more lesions could be definitively localized.[42]

LIMITATIONS OF ANATOMICAL-MOLECULAR FUSION IMAGES

Whole-body CT images usually obtained in conjunction with FDG PET images are not equivalent to diagnostic CT scans that involve administration of oral and intravenous contrast agents and precise timing of the acquisition of the images in relationship to the administration of contrast. However, localization of the foci of

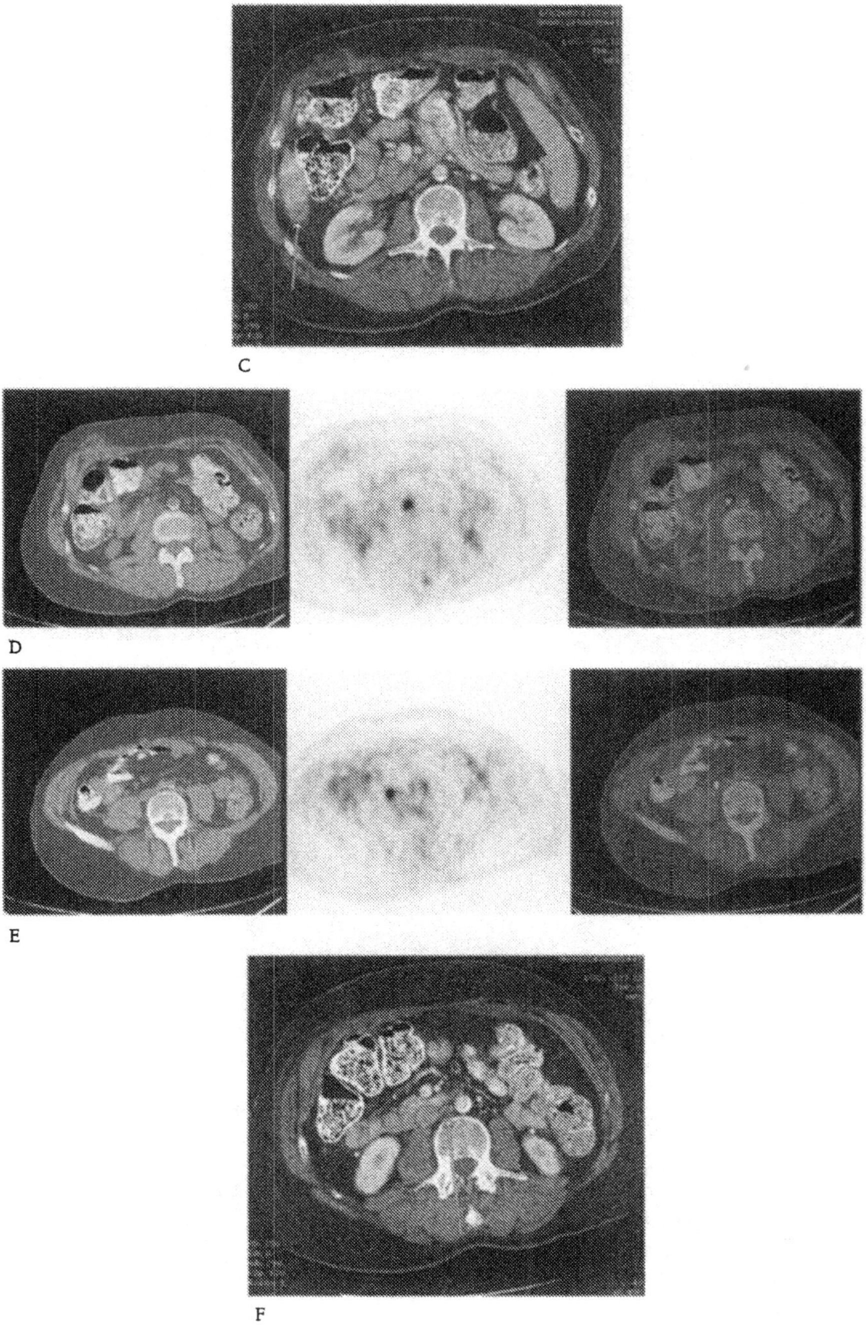

FIGURE 11.3 The larger lesion can be identified on the non-contrasted CT image from the integrated system (A) but the smaller lesion inferiorly (B) can be seen only on a diagnostic CT scan obtained in the portovenous phase of intravenous contrast enhancement (C). D and E, Two foci of FDG uptake are seen in the retroperitoneum, projecting over small soft tissue densities on the noncontrasted CT images. These two lesions can be better identified as lymph nodes (nonenhancing) on the diagnostic CT scan obtained in the portovenous phase of intravenous contrast enhancement (F and G).

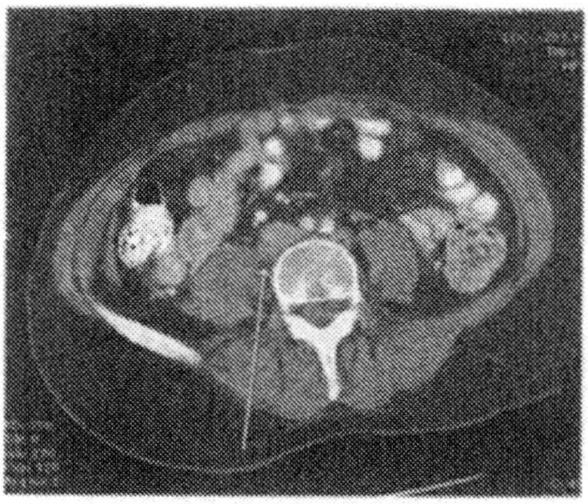

G

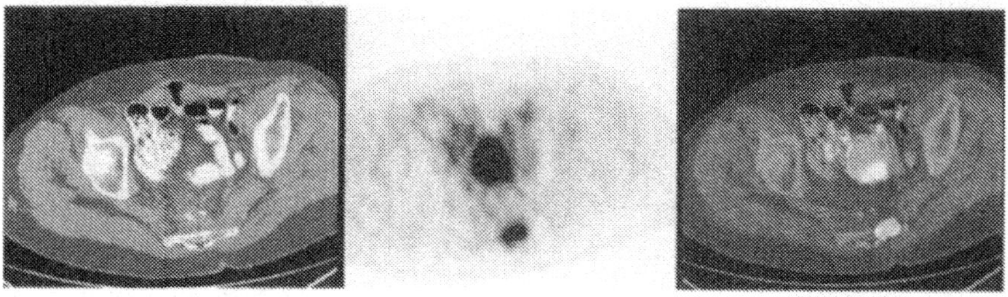

H

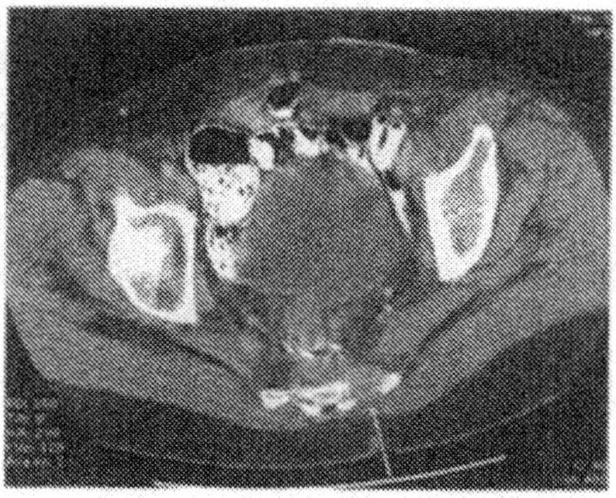

I

FIGURE 11.3 *(Continued)* H, A focus of FDG uptake was also identified, projecting in the presacral region and the sacrum itself, again better identified on the diagnostic CT, indicating local recurrence with sacral involvement. CEA, carcinoembryonic antigen; CT, computed tomography; FDG, ^{18}F-fluorodeoxyglucose; PET, positron emission tomography. (Courtesy of Tennessee Oncology, Nashville, TN)

uptake on the nondiagnostic (integrated) CT images allows precise identification of the CT slice with the abnormality on the diagnostic CT images.

Diagnostic CT images are obtained during breath-holding, whereas PET images and integrated CT images from some systems require several minutes for acquiring the images while the patient breathes normally. This results in some mismatches in location and organ size between the two sets of images, which af-

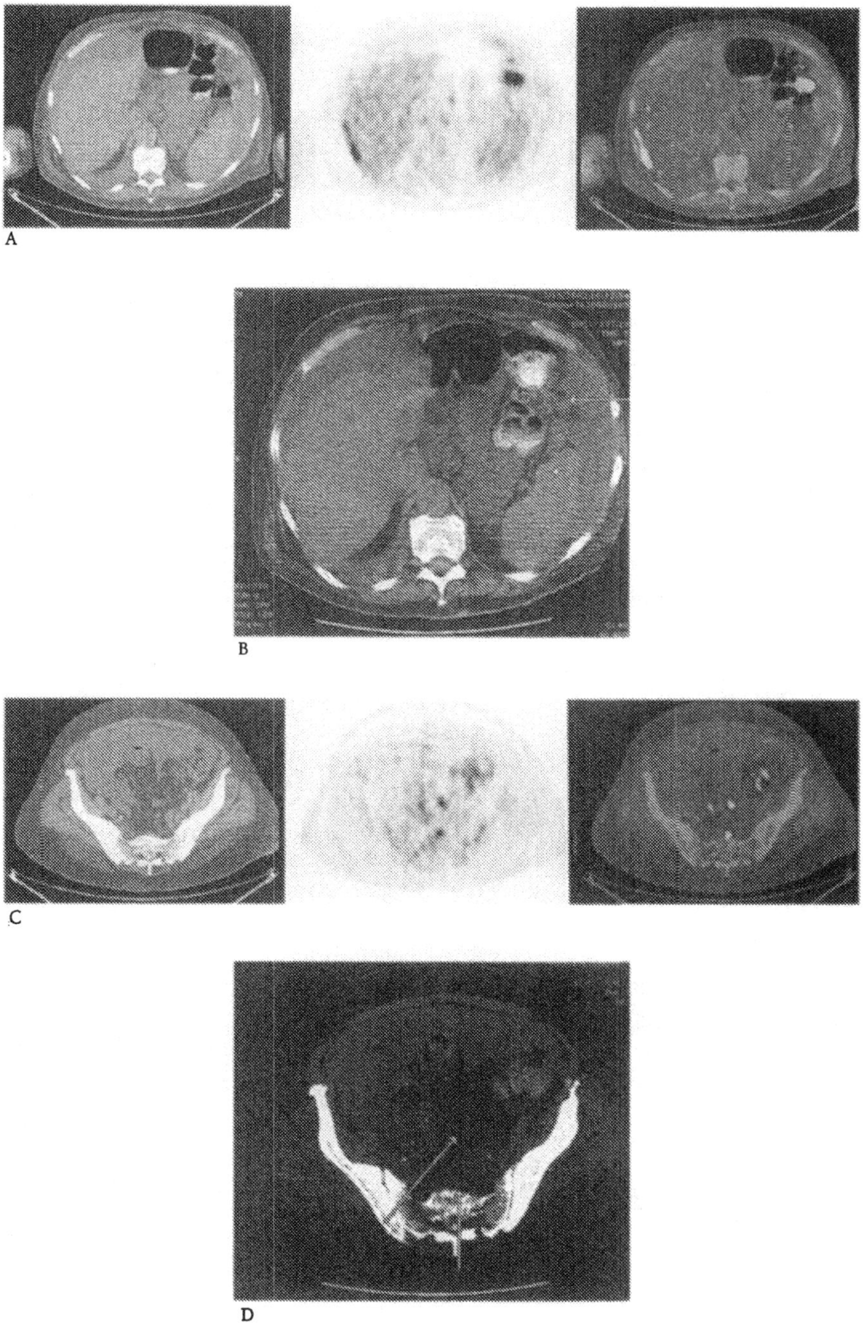

FIGURE 11.4 A 60-year-old female with a history of ovarian cancer presented with rising Ca-125 levels. A and B, FDG PET images from the integrated PET-CT system demonstrated foci of FDG uptake that are most consistent with peritoneal implants. C and D, The integrated CT scan allowed to precisely identify the slice with the lesions that can be identified retrospectively on the diagnostic CT scan. (Courtesy of Tennessee Oncology, Nashville, TN)

fects the quality of the registration.[43] Preliminary studies suggest that respiratory gating may minimize these inaccuracies for localization of lung lesions.[44]

Respiratory motion also has an impact on images with attenuation correction, whether attenuation maps were acquired using a breath-holding technique or not. A study compared localization of lesions on images with attenuation correction using either attenuation maps obtained with ^{68}germanium sources (patient breathing normally) or CT attenuation maps during breath holding. The study describes mislocalization of lesions in 6/275 patients at the base of the lungs or the dome of the liver when the breath-hold technique was used for the attenuation maps.[45]

Unfortunately, integrated PET or SPECT-MRI systems are not available, and for indications that require close comparison of MRI and molecular images, coregistration software is the only alternative.

CONCLUSION

The diagnostic implications of integrated PET-CT imaging include improved detection of lesions on both the CT and the FDG PET images, better differentiation of physiologic from pathological foci of metabolism, and better localization of the pathological foci. This new powerful technology provides more accurate interpretation of both CT and FDG PET images and therefore optimal patient care. PET-CT fusion images affect clinical management by guiding further procedures (biopsy, surgery, radiation therapy), excluding the need for further procedures and changing both inter- and intramodality therapy.

However, this technology does not challenge the need for a diagnostic CT scan with oral and intravenous contrast administration, which are necessary to evaluate the extent of the lesions and their relationship to vascular structures. In patients in whom there is insufficient information to localize a lesion, the data may be used to precisely select the appropriate slice for review from a diagnostic-quality CT scan that matches up with the area of increased metabolism. The combined approach of x-ray attenuation correction and image fusion with FDG imaging is a new and powerful diagnostic tool for nuclear medicine imaging, radiation therapy, and surgical planning.

ACKNOWLEDGMENTS

The authors want to thank Dr. Colin Meyerowitz for providing images for Figures 11.3 and 11.4. These images were obtained on the integrated PET-CT system (Discovery LS, General Electric Medical Systems, Milwaukee, WI) located at Tennessee Oncology in Nashville, Tennessee.

REFERENCES

1. Delbeke D, Martin WH, Patton JA et al, eds. Practical FDG Imaging: A Teaching File. New York: Springer Verlag, 2002.

2. Warburg O. Versuche und uberledbeudem carcinomgewebe (methoden). Biochem Z 1923;142:317–333.

3. Flier JS, Mueckler MM, Usher P et al. Elevated levels of glucose transport and transporter messenger RNA are induced by rats or src oncogenes. Science 1987;235:1492–1495.

4. Monakhov NK, Neistadt EI, Shaylovskii MM et al. Physiochemical properties and isoenzyme composition of hexokinase from normal and malignant human tissues. J Natl Cancer Inst 1978;61:27–34.

5. Knox WE, Jamdar SC, Davis PA. Hexokinase, differentiation, and growth rates of transplanted tumors. Cancer Res 1970;30:2240–2244.

6. Som P, Atkins HL, Bandoypadhayay D et al. A fluorinated glucose analog, 2-fluoro-2-deoxy-2-D-glucose [18F]: nontoxic tracer for rapid tumor detection. J Nucl Med 1980;21:670–675.

7. Gallagher BM, Fowler JS, Gutterson NI et al. Metabolic trapping as a principle of radiopharmaceutical design: some factors responsible for the biodistribution of [18F]2-deoxy-2-fluoro-D-glucose. J Nucl Med 1978;19:1154–1161.

8. Delbeke D. Oncological applications of FDG-PET imaging: brain tumors, colorectal cancer, lymphoma, and melanoma. J Nucl Med 1999;40:591–603.

9. Delbeke D. Oncological applications of FDG-PET imaging. J Nucl Med. 1999;40:1706–1715.

10. Conti PS, Keppler GS, Halls JM. Positron emission tomography: a financial and operational analysis. AJR Am J Roentgenol 1994;162:1279–1286.

11. Valk PE, Pounds TR, Tesar RD et al. Cost-effectiveness of PET imaging in clinical oncology. Nucl Med Biol 1996;23:737–747.

12. Gambhir SS, Hoh CK, Phelps ME et al. Decision tree sensitivity analysis for cost-effectiveness of FDG-PET in the staging and management of non-small-cell lung carcinoma. J Nucl Med 1996;37:1428–1436.

13. Cook GJR, Fogelman I, Maisey MN. Normal physiological and benign pathological variants of 18-fluoro-2-deoxyglucose positron emission tomography scanning: potential for error in interpretation. Semin Nucl Med 1996;26:308–314.

14. Engel H, Steinert H, Buck A et al. Whole body PET: Physiological and artifactual fluorodeoxyglucose accumulations. J Nucl Med 1996;37:441–446.

15. Berger C, Berthold T. Image fusion In: von Schulthess GK, ed. Clinical Positron Emission Tomography (PET). Philadelphia: Lippincott Williams & Wilkins, 2000:41–48.

16. Wahl RL. To AC or not to AC: that is the question. J Nucl Med 1999;40:2025–2027.

17. Pelizzari CA, Chen GT, Spelbring DR et al. Accurate three-dimensional registration of CT, PET, and/or MR images of the brain. J Comput Assist Tomogr 1989;13:20–26.

18. Woods RP, Cherry SR, Mazziotta JC. Rapid automated algorithm for aligning and reslicing PET images. J Comput Tomogr 1992;16:620–633.

19. Pietrzyk U, Herholz K, Fink G et al. An interactive technique for three-dimensional image registration: validation for PET, SPECT, MRI, and CT brain studies. J Nucl Med 1994;35:2011–2018.

20. Beyer T, Townsend DW, Brun T et al. A combined PET/CT scanner for clinical oncology. J Nucl Med 2000;41:1369–1379.

21. Patton JA, Delbeke D, Sandler MP. Image fusion using an integrated dual-head coincidence camera with x-ray tube based attenuation maps. J Nucl Med 2000;41:1364–1368.

22. Alyafei S, Inoue T, Zhang H et al. Image fusion using PACS for MRI, CT, and PET images. Clin Positron Imaging 1999;2:137–143.

23. Israel O, Mor M, Guralnik L et al. The new technology of combined transmission and emission F-18 FDG tomography (FDG-TET) in the diagnosis and management of cancer patients. Clin Positron Imaging 2000;3:143.

24. Delbeke D, Martin WH, Patton JA et al. Value of iterative reconstruction, attenuation correction, and image fusion in the interpretation of FDG PET images with an integrated dual-head coincidence camera and x-ray-based attenuation maps. Radiology 2001;218:163–171.

25. Martinelli M, Townsend D, Meltzer C et al. Survey of results of whole body imaging using the PET/CT at the University of Pittsburgh Medical Center PET facility. Clin Positron Imaging 2000;3:161.

26. Yeung HW, Schoder H, Larson SM. Utility of PET/CT for assessing equivocal PET lesions in oncology: initial experience. J Nucl Med 2002;43:32P.

27. Bar-Shalom R, Keidar Z, Guralnik L et al. Added value of fused PET/CT imaging with FDG in diagnostic imaging and management of cancer patients. J Nucl Med 2002;43:33P.

28. Dizendorf E, Ciernik IF, Baumert B et al. Impact of integrated PETCT scanning on external beam radiation treatment planning. J Nucl Med 2002;43:33P.

29. Osman MM, Cohade C, Fishman E et al. Clinically significant incidental findings on non-contrast CT portion of PET-CT studies: frequency in 250 patients. J Nucl Med 2002;43:307P.

30. Mutic S, Dempsey JF, Bosch WR et al. Multimodality image registration quality assurance for conformal three-dimensional treatment planning. Int J Radiat Oncol Biol Phys 2001;51:255–260.

31. Nishioka T, Shiga T, Shirato H et al. Image fusion between 18FDG-PET and MRI/CT for radiotherapy planning of oropharyngeal and nasopharyngeal carcinomas. Int J Radiat Oncol Biol Phys 2002;53:1051–1057.

32. Kluetz PG, Meltzer CC, Villemagne VL et al. Combined PET/CT imaging in oncology: impact on patient management. Clin Positive Imaging 2000;3:223–230.

33. Meltzer CC, Snyderman CH, Fukui MB et al. Combined FDG PET/CT in head and neck cancer: impact on patient management. J Nucl Med 2001;42:36P.

34. Kamel EM, Goerres G, Dizendorf E et al. Image fusion of whole-body FDG-PET and spiral CT in staging of broncogenic carcinoma. J Nucl Med 2001;42:35P.

35. Vansteenkiste JF, Stroobants SG, Dupont PJ et al. FDG-PET scan in potentially operable non-small cell lung cancer: do anatometabolic PET-CT fusion images improve the localization of regional lymph node metastases? Eur J Nucl Med 1998;25:1495–1501.

36. Keidar Z, Bar-Shalom R, Guralnik L et al. Hybrid imaging using PET/CT with 18F-FDG in suspected recurrence of lung cancer: diagnostic value and impact on patient management. J Nucl Med 2002;43:32P.

37. Munley MT, Marks LB, Scarfone C et al. Multimodality nuclear medicine imaging in three-dimentional radiation treatment planning for lung cancer: challenges and prospects. Lung Cancer 1999;23:105–114.

38. Erdi YE, Rosenzweig K, Erdi AK et al. Radiotherapy treatment planning for patients with non-small cell lung cancer using positron emission tomography (PET). Radiother Oncol 2002;62:51–60.

39. Fukugana H, Sekimoto M, Tasumi M et al. Clinical relevance of fusion images using (18)F-2-fluoro-2-deoxy-D-glucose positron emission tomography in local recurrence of rectal cancer. Int J Oncol 2002;20:691–695.

40. Meltzer CC, Martinelli MA, Beyer T et al. Whole-body FDG PET imaging in the abdomen: value of combined PET-CT. J Nucl Med 2001;42:35P.

41. Meltzer CC, Makhija S, Howden N et al. PET/CT in recurrent ovarian and fallopian tube carcinoma. J Nucl Med 2001;42:284P.

42. Cohade C, Osman M, Leal J et al. Direct comparison of FDG PET and PET-CT imaging in colorectal cancer. J Nucl Med 2002;43:22P.

43. Nakamoto Y, Cohade C, Osman M et al. Comparison of size and location of normal upper abdominal organs on PET and CT using PET/CT. J Nucl Med 2002;43:14P.

44. Cohade C, Osman M, Wahl RL. Accuracy of PET and CT spatial registration of lung lesions with PET-CT. J Nucl Med 2002;43:14P.

45. Osman MM, Cohade C, Nakamoto Y, Wahl RH. Clinically significant inaccurate localization of lesions with PET-CT: frequency in 275 patients. J Nucl Med 2002;43:32P.

Chapter 12

Combined Modality Treatment for Pancreatic Cancer

Douglas B. Evans

Robert A. Wolff

Christopher H. Crane

Peter W.T. Pisters

In 2003, adenocarcinoma of the exocrine pancreas will account for approximately 30,000 deaths in the United States, being the fourth leading cause of cancer-related death for both men and women (following lung, colon, and breast cancers).[1] Exocrine pancreatic cancer is characterized by infiltration of surrounding blood vessels and perineural tissues, spread to regional lymph nodes, and early vascular dissemination. Subclinical metastases are present in most patients at the time of diagnosis, even when findings from imaging studies are normal. Therefore, disease recurrence occurs in 80% to 90% of patients following potentially curative surgery.[2] The understanding that pancreatic cancer is a systemic disease at diagnosis in the overwhelming majority of patients underscores the need for a multimodality approach to patient care. Current clinical trials are studying both new combinations of systemic therapies and the optimal treatment sequencing of chemotherapy, radiation therapy, and surgery. The frequent association of pancreatic cancer with biliary and gastric outlet obstruction, pain, anorexia, and cachexia make quality of life and clinical benefit necessary study endpoints. In this review we focus on recently published and ongoing clinical research in the management of patients with adenocarcinoma of the pancreas. The expanding literature on novel molecular-based strategies for early diagnosis and treatment will be the subject of a subsequent review.

PRETREATMENT STAGING

We currently recommend a computed tomography (CT)-based staging system that defines resectability based on the relationship of the tumor to the celiac axis and the superior mesenteric vessels. For treatment planning, it is of critical importance to use standardized, objective radiologic criteria for preoperative tumor staging. The CT findings defining a potentially resectable pancreatic cancer (American Joint Committee on Cancer [AJCC] Stages I or II) are (1) the absence of extrapancreatic disease, (2) a patent superior mesenteric-portal vein (SMPV) confluence (assuming it is technically possible to resect an isolated involvement of the superior mesenteric vein [SMV] or SMPV confluence), and (3) no direct tumor extension to the celiac axis or superior mesenteric artery (SMA) (Fig. 12.1). A patient is deemed to have locally advanced, unresectable disease (AJCC Stage III) when there is clear evidence on CT scans of encasement of the SMA or celiac axis or occlusion of the SMPV confluence. The accuracy of CT in predicting unresectability is well established; it is not necessary to perform a laparotomy to assess local tumor resectability.[3-5]

The development of multislice or multidetector CT (MDCT) allows imaging of the entire pancreas during the bolus phase of contrast enhancement. In addition, scan data can be processed to display images in three-dimensional and multiplanar formats. MDCT performed with contrast enhancement and a thin-section technique can accurately assess the relationship of the low-density tumor to the celiac axis, SMA, and SMPV confluence. For MDCT scanning at our institution, patients receive 240–280 mL of water or a 2% barium sulfate suspension (Readi-CAT; E-Z-EM, Inc., Westbury, NY) to opacify the stomach and small bowel. Non–contrast-enhanced CT scans are then obtained through the liver and pancreas at 10-mm slice thickness and a 10-mm scan interval to identify large liver metastases and to localize the pancreas. Intravenous (IV) contrast enhancement is achieved with non-ionic contrast material (300–320 mg iodine/mL) administered by an automatic injector at a rate of 3–5 mL/sec for a total of 150 mL. At least two phases of contrast-enhanced helical scanning are performed. The first (arterial) phase begins 25 seconds after contrast injection and is performed during a 20-second breathhold, with imaging done from the diaphragm through the horizontal portion of the duodenum at a slice thickness of 2.5 mm contiguous, reconstructed to 1.25-mm slice thickness for multiplanar reconstructions. Imaging during this phase through the pancreas is done at 35–45 seconds after contrast injection, which, at this rate of contrast injection, optimizes the

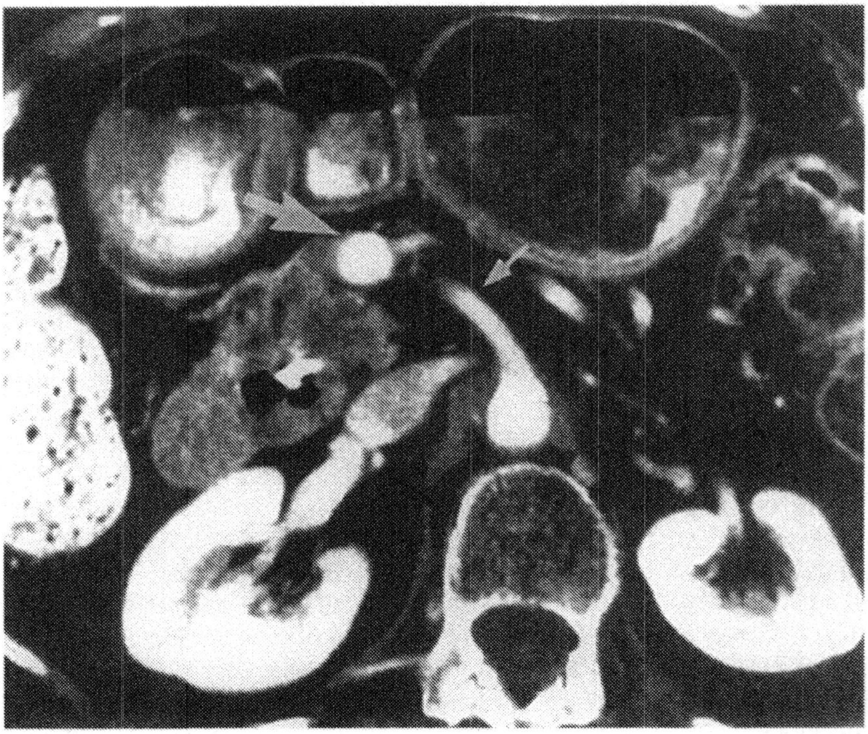

FIGURE 12.1 Contrast-enhanced CT scan demonstrating a resectable adenocarcinoma of the pancreatic head. Note the normal fat plane between the low-density tumor and the superior mesenteric artery (small arrow). The tumor abuts the superior mesenteric vein (large arrow) along its lateral wall and therefore, at the time of surgery, the surgeon should be prepared to resect and reconstruct this segment of superior mesenteric vein.

difference in density between the pancreas and tumor. The second (venous) phase, which is done to look for metastases in the liver and abdomen, begins 55 seconds after the start of IV contrast injection and covers the entire liver and upper abdomen at a 5-mm slice thickness, which is then reconstructed to a 2.5-mm slice thickness.

If a low-density mass is not seen on CT scans, patients with extrahepatic biliary obstruction should undergo diagnostic and therapeutic endoscopic retrograde cholangiopancreatography (ERCP). When possible, ERCP should always be performed after CT, because if ERCP-induced pancreatitis occurs, it may interfere with accurate assessment of the extent of disease. A malignant obstruction can often be accurately differentiated from choledocholithiasis and the long, smooth, tapering bile duct stricture seen in chronic pancreatitis. We routinely place endoscopic stents to prevent cholangitis in patients with extrahepatic biliary obstruction who undergo diagnostic ERCP. We also place endoscopic stents in patients with elevated bilirubin levels in whom surgery is expected to be delayed, including those who are enrolled in preoperative chemoradiation therapy protocols. When ERCP is performed for the sole purpose of placing an endobiliary stent (in patients with an easily visible tumor on CT), the risk of complications can probably be reduced by not cannulating the pancreatic duct.

For the past decade, laparoscopy has been performed in patients who have radiologic evidence of localized pancreatic cancer to detect extrapancreatic tumor not seen on CT scans, thereby limiting laparotomy to those patients who truly have localized disease.[6,7] However, the favorable initial experience with laparoscopy in the frequent identification of subclinical metastatic disease resulted from laparoscopy being done in the absence of high-quality contrast-enhanced CT. Other, more recent studies have suggested that CT occult extrapancreatic disease is found in only 4–13% of patients with tumors otherwise deemed resectable.[8] Therefore, it probably is now inappropriate to perform laparoscopy as a separate staging procedure under general anesthesia in patients with pancreatic cancer. Nonetheless, many surgeons do routinely perform laparoscopy prior to a planned laparotomy when considering major pancreatic resection in patients with presumed localized, resectable pancreatic cancer. Importantly, the rapidly expanding body of literature on laparoscopic staging has drawn attention to the need to avoid nontherapeutic laparotomy. A fortunate consequence of the recent emphasis on minimally invasive surgery is the realization by clinicians that it is no longer acceptable to perform a major laparotomy in patients with presumed pancreatic cancer just to "explore" the possibility of resection. There is now general consensus that resectability be assessed prior to laparotomy.

PRETREATMENT PANCREATIC BIOPSY

In most patients, accurate staging and biliary decompression are achieved with CT and ERCP. EUS-guided fine-needle aspiration (FNA) is currently the procedure of choice for obtaining a cytologic diagnosis of a malignancy.[9] Confirmation of malignancy is required in all patients with locally advanced or metastatic disease prior to treatment with systemic therapy or external-beam radiation therapy (EBRT) and is being done more commonly in patients with localized, potentially resectable disease because of the growing popularity of neoadjuvant therapy. Recent reports of EUS-guided FNA of the pancreas have described its accuracy and safety.[9,10] The most recent experience from our institution involved 233 patients who underwent EUS-FNA of the pancreas.[9] A final diagnosis of cancer was established in 216 patients (93%), 15 patients (6%) were found to have benign disease, and the final diagnosis remained unknown in 2 patients (1%). The sensitivity, specificity, and accuracy of EUS-FNA for diagnosis of a pancreatic malignancy were 91%, 100%, and 92%, respectively. For the 216 patients subsequently proven to have cancer, the results of EUS-FNA were diagnostic in 197 (91%); 96 (90%) of 107 patients with resectable disease, 62 (97%) of 64 with locally advanced disease, and 39 (87%) of 45 with metastatic disease. Four patients (2%) developed a clinically apparent complication that required hospital admission, including 2 patients who required surgery for duodenal perforation. There were no EUS-related deaths.

When FNA material is examined by an experienced cytopathologist, false-positive results should not occur; however, false-negative results may occur, especially when small tumors are involved. Therefore, negative results from EUS-guided FNA should not be considered definite proof that a malignancy does not exist. In a patient who presents with extrahepatic biliary obstruction, a malignant-appearing stricture of the intrapancreatic portion of the common bile duct, and no history of recurrent pancreatitis or alcohol abuse, the absence of a mass on CT or EUS images should not be grounds for ruling out a carcinoma of the pancreas or bile duct. Instead, the results of EUS, with or without FNA, should be considered in the context of the clinical picture and as a complement to CT and ERCP findings. Importantly, high-quality CT imaging should be performed before an FNA is attempted because of the risk of biopsy inducing pancreatitis, which would distort the pancreatic anatomy. Further, FNA biopsy should only be performed if a mass is identified; there is no place for blind biopsy of the pancreas.

The advent of EUS-FNA (combined with high-quality CT and endobiliary stent placement) allows pancreatic cancer to be treated like all other solid tumors; the diagnostic phase is separated from the treatment phase. Patients with suspected pancreatic or periampullary cancer can be accurately staged with contemporary CT imaging, biliary obstruction can be relieved with endobiliary decompression, and the diagnosis can be established endoscopically with EUS-FNA. Patients can then be counseled as to available treatment options and the established short- and long-term benefits of referral to a regional center with expertise in pancreatic surgery.

LOCALIZED RESECTABLE DISEASE

Surgery and Pathology

If the primary tumor cannot be resected completely, surgery for pancreatic cancer (pancreaticoduodenectomy) offers no survival advantage. Patients whose resected tumors show positive margins can expect to survive less than 1 year[11-16] (Table 12.1), a survival duration no different than that seen in patients with locally advanced, unresectable disease who undergo palliative chemotherapy and irradiation.[17,18] Therefore, in contrast to the situation in selected patients with gastric or colorectal cancer, there are no data supporting palliative (incomplete or grossly positive margins [R2]) resection for adenocarcinoma of the pancreas.

The 30-day in-hospital mortality rate is 2% or less in patients who undergo pancreaticoduodenectomy performed by experienced surgeons.[11,19,20] Recently re-

TABLE 12.1 Median Survival Durations for Patients Who Underwent Surgical Resection for Pancreatic Adenocarcinoma and Were Found to Have a Positive Resection Margin[a]

Study Author (Year)	No. of Patients	Margin Status	Median Survival (Months)
Neoptolemos[13] (2001)	101	R1	11
Sohn[11] (2000)	184	R1/2	12
Millikan[14] (1999)	22	R1	8
Nishimura[15] (1997)	70	R1/2	6
Sperti[16] (1996)	19	R1/2	7
Nitecki[12] (1995)	28	R2	9
Willett[14] (1993)	37	R1/2	11

Abbreviations: R2, grossly positive margin; R1, microscopically positive margin.
[a]Many patients received postoperative 5-FU–based chemoradiation therapy.

ported mortality rates from other institutions, including university centers and Department of Veterans Affairs hospitals, range from 7.8% to more than 10%.[21-23] Data from a study conducted by Birkmeyer et al[24] have demonstrated that higher hospital volume is associated with lower surgery-related mortality. The study population consisted of 10,530 Medicare patients older than 65 years who underwent pancreaticoduodenectomy at 1,868 hospitals from 1994 to 1999. The study population was divided into quintiles according to hospital volume: very high volume centers were defined as those that performed greater than 16 pancreatic resections per year; high-volume hospitals, 6–16 per year; median-volume hospitals, 3–5 per year; low-volume hospitals, 1–2 per year; and very low-volume hospitals, less than 1 per year. Twenty-seven (1.4%) very high-volume hospitals performed 2,159 (21%) of the pancreatic resections, and 90 (4.8%) high-volume hospitals performed 2,166 (21%) of the pancreatic resections; 58% of the pancreatic resections were performed at very low, low-, or medium-volume hospitals, where the in-hospital or 30-day mortality was 16.3%, 14.6%, and 11%, respectively. In an analysis of survival duration, after excluding perioperative deaths and adjusting for the case mix, Birkmeyer et al[25] found that patients who underwent surgery at high-volume hospitals were also less likely to experience late mortality. Translating volume-outcome data into public policy has not yet occurred with respect to pancreatic surgery; however, it seems appropriate that this information be made available to patients and that they be given the option of having their surgery at a high-volume center.

The new staging system of the AJCC and International Union Against Cancer is given in Table 12.2.[26] The modifications to the TNM staging system in the 6th edition allow the accurate staging of patients even if they do not undergo pancreatic resection. The T4 (and Stage III) designation is reserved for locally

TABLE 12.2 TNM Staging System

DEFINITIONS			
Primary Tumor (T)			
TX	Primary tumor cannot be assessed		
T0	No evidence of primary tumor		
Tis	In situ carcinoma		
T1	Tumor limited to pancreas and 2 cm or less in greatest dimension		
T2	Tumor limited to pancreas and more than 2 cm in greatest dimension		
T3	Tumor extends beyond the pancreas but without involvement of the celiac axis or the superior mesenteric artery		
T4	Tumor involves the celiac axis or the superior mesenteric artery (unresectable primary tumor)		
Regional Lymph Nodes (N)			
NX	Regional lymph nodes cannot be assessed		
N0	No regional lymph node metastasis		
N1	Regional lymph node metastasis		
Distant Metastasis (M)			
MX	Distant metastasis cannot be assessed		
M0	No distant metastasis		
M1	Distant metastasis		
STAGE GROUPING			
Stage 0	Tis	N0	M0
Stage IA	T1	N0	M0
Stage IB	T2	N0	M0
Stage IIA	T3	N0	M0
Stage IIB	T1–3	N1	M0
Stage III	T4	N0/1	M0
Stage IV	T1–4	N0/1	M1

Adapted from Greene FL, Page DL, Fleming ID, Fritz AG, Balch CN, Haller DG, Morrow M, eds. AJCC Cancer Staging Manual, Sixth Edition: Chapter 18, Exocrine Pancreas. New York: Springer 2002;157–164

advanced unresectable primary tumors in the absence of distant metastases. In addition to TNM staging, when the pancreaticoduodenectomy specimen is evaluated pathologically, the retroperitoneal margin (the soft tissue margin directly adjacent to the proximal 3–4 cm of the SMA, as illustrated in Fig. 12.2) must be evaluated on permanent sections by inking the margin and sectioning the tumor

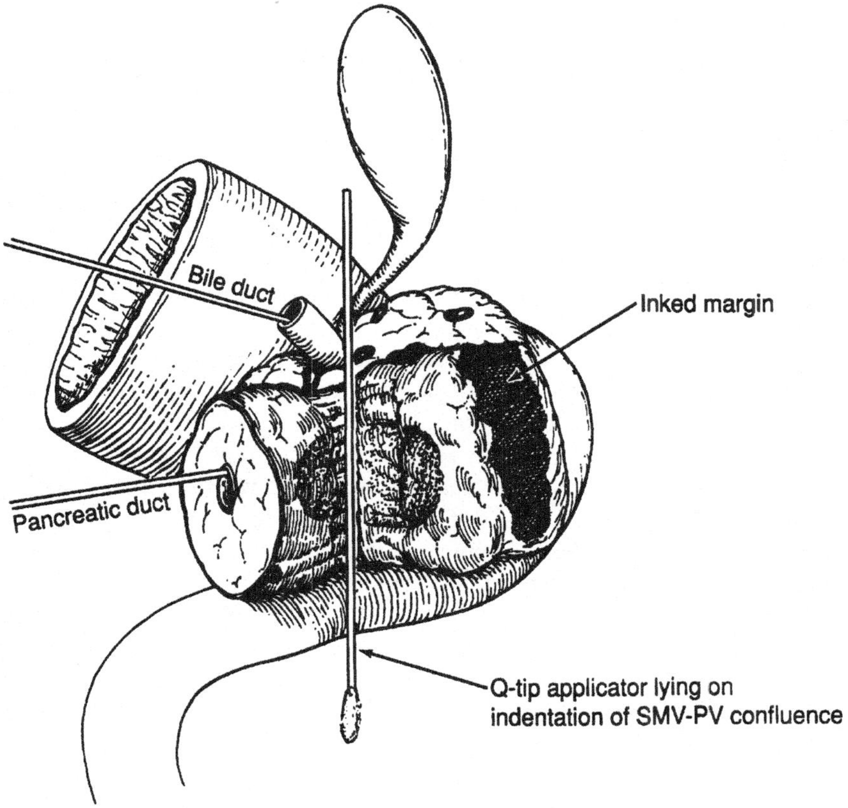

FIGURE 12.2 Illustration of a pancreaticoduodenectomy specimen; the retroperitoneal margin (tissue adjacent to the superior mesenteric artery) is inked for evaluation of margin status. A small probe has been placed in the bile duct and within the pancreatic duct. A white Q-tip applicator stick lies over the indentation from the superior mesenteric-portal vein confluence. Complete permanent-section analysis of the pancreaticoduodenectomy specimen requires that it be oriented to enable the pathologist to accurately assess the retroperitoneal margin of excision and other standard pathologic variables.

perpendicular to the margin. This margin must be evaluated by the pathologist at the time of tumor resection because it is not possible to identify it later. Standardized pathologic assessment of the retroperitoneal margin is mandatory for the conduct of clinical trials that involve pancreaticoduodenectomy. If the patient received preoperative chemoradiation therapy, the grade of the treatment effect is assessed using the grading schema developed by Cleary and reported by Evans et al.[27]

Postoperative Adjuvant Chemoradiation

The Gastrointestinal Tumor Study Group (GITSG) was the first to study whether postoperative adjuvant chemoradiation therapy improved survival in patients with pancreatic adenocarcinoma. In a prospective randomized study of adjuvant chemoradiation therapy (500 mg/m^2/day of 5-fluorouracil (5-FU) for 6 days and 40 Gy of radiation) versus observation alone after pancreaticoduodenectomy, a survival advantage was seen for multimodality therapy (20 months versus 11 months with resection alone).[28,29] However, five (24%) of the 21 patients assigned to the adjuvant chemoradiation arm could not begin chemoradiation until more than 10 weeks after pancreaticoduodenectomy owing to prolonged recovery from surgery. This was despite the fact that the only patients likely to be considered for protocol entry were those who experienced an uncomplicated recovery following surgery and had a good performance status.

Similar findings were reported by Sohn et al[11] from Johns Hopkins University (Table 12.3).[11,28-35] Of 498 evaluable patients who underwent pancreatectomy for adenocarcinoma of the pancreas, 366 (74%) received adjuvant chemoradiation therapy and 132 (26%) declined adjuvant therapy for "various reasons." In all previously reported and currently ongoing postoperative adjuvant trials (with the exception of the Hopkins data), patient enrollment occurred following recovery from surgery; the number of patients not referred for trial entry (due to delayed recovery from surgery) is therefore not known. The very low mortality and morbidity seen for pancreatic surgery at Johns Hopkins University suggests that 26% is the minimum percentage of patients who will not receive adjuvant therapy if a postoperative strategy is used by other less-experienced centers. Adjuvant therapy in the Hopkins study was associated with a statistically significant improvement in survival (19 months versus 11 months, $P < .0001$). The use of an intensified postoperative adjuvant therapy consisting of concurrent 5-FU, leucovorin, dipyridamole, and mitomycin-C, combined with split-course EBRT to 50 Gy, did not improve survival over 5-FU-based chemoradiation.[34,36,37]

The European Organization for Research and Treatment of Cancer (EORTC) recently reported their findings for trial 40891.[31] Between 1987 and 1995, 218 patients were randomized to receive either chemoradiation therapy (40 Gy in a split course and 5-FU given as a continuous infusion at a dose of 25 mg/kg/day during EBRT) or no further treatment following pancreaticoduodenectomy for adenocarcinoma of the pancreas or periampullary region. Eleven patients were deemed ineligible for analysis because of extensive local disease with incomplete resection. Of the remaining 207 patients, 114 (55%) had pancreatic cancer. The median survival was 24.5 months for the entire group that received adjuvant therapy and 19 months for the group that received surgery alone ($P = .2$). For the subset of patients with pancreatic cancer, the median survival was 17.1 months for those who received adjuvant therapy and 12.6 months for those who received surgery alone ($P = .099$). Although these differences were not significant, the wide confidence interval (relative risk, 0.7; 95% CI, 0.5–1.1) for patients with

TABLE 12.3 Recent Chemoradiation Therapy Studies in Patients with Resectable Pancreatic Cancer

Study Author (Year)	No. of Patients[a]	EBRT Dose (Gy)	Chemotherapy Agent(s)	Median Survival (Months)
Preoperative (Neoadjuvant)				
Breslin[47] (2001)	132	30–50.4	5-FU	21
Hoffman[46] (1998)	24	50.4	5-FU + Mito	15.7
Pisters[48] (1998)	20	30	5-FU	25
Postoperative (Adjuvant)				
Neoptolemos[32] (2001)	146	–	5-FU + LV	17.4
Surgery alone	139	–	–	15.9
Nukui[33] (2000)	17	50.4	5-FU + cis + IFN	45
Sohn[11] (2000)	333	40–57.6	5-FU	19
Surgery alone	119	–	–	11
Abrams[34] (1999)	23	50.4–57.6	5-FU + LV	15.9
Klinkenbijl[31] (1999)	60	40	5-FU	17.1
Surgery alone	54	–	–	12.6
Demeure[35] (1998)	30	50.4–54	5-FU	24.2
Surgery alone	31	–	–	16.9
Foo[30] (1993)	29	35–60	5-FU	23
GITSG[28] (1987)	30	40	5-FU	18
Kalser[29] (1985)	21	40	5-FU	20
Surgery alone	22	–	–	11

Abbreviations: EBRT, external-beam radiation therapy; 5-FU, 5-fluorouracil; GITSG, Gastrointestinal Tumor Study Group; LV, leucovorin; Mito, mitomycin C; cis, cisplatin; IFN, interferon-α.

[a]All patients underwent a pancreatectomy with curative intent.

pancreatic cancer does not exclude the possibility of a clinically meaningful improvement in survival in the chemoradiation therapy arm that may not have been apparent owing to the small sample size. Similar to the GITSG trial, patients were considered for enrollment in the EORTC trial after recovering from pancreaticoduodenectomy; despite this selection bias, 21 (20%) of 104 evaluable patients assigned to receive chemoradiation therapy did not receive the therapy because of patient refusal, medical comorbid conditions, or rapid tumor progression. In addition, the retroperitoneal margin of resection was not assessed, and therefore the completeness of surgical resection could not be verified. Although the method of follow-up was not defined (raising a concern about underestimation of the sites of recurrent disease), tumor recurrence in the pancreatic bed was reported as a site of first progression in 20% of patients. This finding combined with the short survival in the observation arm (12 months) suggests that many patients had an incomplete (R2) resection.

Findings from the European Study Group of Pancreatic Cancer (ESPAC)-1 trial were recently reported, and in contrast to previous adjuvant therapy studies, the results suggest no benefit to adjuvant chemoradiation therapy.[13,32] The ESPAC-1 trial used a four-arm, 2 × 2 factorial design to compare (1) adjuvant chemoradiation (40 Gy in a split course and 5-FU), (2) adjuvant chemotherapy (5-FU and folinic acid), (3) chemoradiation therapy followed by chemotherapy, and (4) observation alone following pancreaticoduodenectomy for pancreatic and periampullary carcinomas. Accrual for this study occurred between 1994 and 2000, and 61 medical centers in 11 countries randomized 541 patients. Two-hundred eighty-five patients (53%) were entered into the randomized 2 × 2 factorial design. However, because of the lack of access to EBRT or specific institutional bias, 188 patients were randomized to receive only chemotherapy or no chemotherapy, and 68 patients were randomized to receive either chemoradiation or no chemoradiation therapy. In the latter two nonfactorial groups, patients could receive nonstandardized therapy at the discretion of their treating physicians. For example, patients who were randomized in the nonfactorial design to receive chemotherapy or no chemotherapy could receive EBRT. Importantly, nonrandomized treatments were not standardized. Results from the ESPAC-1 trial suggest that adjuvant chemoradiation therapy provides no survival benefit. Second, adjuvant systemic chemotherapy consisting of 5-FU and leucovorin, which is largely ineffective in patients with measurable metastatic disease, appeared to improve survival. Upon closer examination, however, there was no benefit to chemotherapy in the subset of 285 patients randomized by the 2 × 2 factorial design.

The Radiation Therapy Oncology Group (RTOG) activated the first American phase III cooperative group study of postoperative adjuvant therapy for resected pancreatic adenocarcinoma (RTOG 97-04) since the GITSG trial.[38] Patients were randomly assigned to receive three cycles of weekly gemcitabine or three cycles of infusional 5-FU to be given before and after 5-FU–based chemoradiation therapy. Accrual to this trial is complete, but results are not available.

Investigators at the Virginia Mason Medical Center have reported their findings from a review of their experience with adjuvant EBRT combined with 5-FU, cisplatin, and interferon-α (IFN-α).[33] IFN-α is used in pancreatic cancer because of its ability to function as a radiosensitizer and its use as a systemic agent with possible cytostatic properties. In this study, 33 patients who successfully underwent pancreaticoduodenectomy were then assigned in a nonrandomized fashion to receive either EBRT (45–54 Gy) and concomitant 5-FU or IFN-α-based chemoradiation therapy (45–54 Gy, and concomitant continuous infusion of 5-FU [200 mg/m^2/day], bolus cisplatin [30 mg/m^2/day], and subcutaneous injections of IFN-α [3 million U, q.o.d.]). Although the sample size was small, the 17 patients in the IFN-α regimen had a significantly greater actuarial 2-year survival compared with those receiving EBRT and 5-FU alone (84% versus 54%,

P = .04). The American College of Surgeons Oncology Group currently plans a phase II trial to confirm these favorable results.

Preoperative (Neoadjuvant) Therapy

Because of the risk that a significant percentage of patients who undergo pancreatectomy will not receive intended postoperative adjuvant therapy,[11,31,39,40] and because of published reports of successful pancreatic resection following EBRT,[41,42] preoperative chemoradiation therapy was studied in phase I and phase II trials.[27,43] Theoretical advantages of preoperative chemoradiation over postoperative chemoradiation therapy include (1) the ability to provide immediate systemic therapy for a disease that is systemic at diagnosis in 80% or more of patients with potentially resectable pancreatic cancer; (2) the fact that delayed postoperative recovery has no effect on the delivery of multimodality therapy because chemotherapy and radiation therapy are given first; (3) the high frequency of positive-margin resections supports the concern that the retroperitoneal margin of excision, even when negative, may be only a few millimeters, making surgery alone inadequate local therapy for most patients[11,44]; and (4) the fact that patients found to have disseminated disease on preoperative restaging studies after neoadjuvant therapy will not be subjected to laparotomy.

Repeat (preoperative) staging CT after chemoradiation reveals liver metastases in 15%–25% of patients who receive chemoradiation therapy prior to planned pancreaticoduodenectomy.[2] If these patients had undergone pancreaticoduodenectomy at the time of diagnosis, the liver metastases would likely have been too small to detect intraoperatively; the patients would therefore have undergone a major surgical procedure only to have liver metastases found soon after surgery. In reports of preoperative trials, patients who had disease progression evident at restaging had a median survival of only 7 months.[2] Therefore, a distinct advantage of preoperative over postoperative chemoradiation therapy is that patients who show disease progression following induction chemotherapy and/or chemoradiation are not taken to surgery; such patients thus avoid the lengthy recovery period and the potential morbidity of pancreaticoduodenectomy. As a general oncologic principle, when delivering multimodality therapy, it is beneficial to deliver the most toxic therapy last, thereby avoiding treatment toxicity in patients who experience rapid disease progression not amenable to available therapies.

Despite its potential benefits, preoperative chemoradiation therapy is associated with toxicities. In one study, even though all patients received the intended preoperative treatment with standard-fractionation (5.5 weeks) chemoradiation, the gastrointestinal toxic effects (nausea, vomiting, and dehydration) were severe enough to require hospital admission in one-third of the patients.[45] The Eastern Cooperative Oncology Group (ECOG) multicenter trial documented the need for hospital admission in 51% of patients during or within 4 weeks of completing chemoradiation therapy.[46] Therefore, subsequent pilot, phase I, and phase II studies of preoperative chemoradiation have utilized shorter-course, higher dose-per-fraction radiation regimens termed "rapid fractionation."[47-51] A recent review of the M. D. Anderson Cancer Center experience with preoperative chemoradiation therapy included 132 consecutive patients; 44 received standard-fractionation EBRT (45–50 Gy, 1.8 Gy/fraction per day), and 88 patients received rapid-fractionation EBRT (30 Gy, 3.0 Gy/fraction per day) followed by pancreaticoduodenectomy.[47] The overall median survival from the time of tissue diagnosis was 21 months, and the five-year survival rate was 23% (range, 15%–35%, 95% CI). The dose of preoperative EBRT did not influence survival. The survival of these 132 patients compared favorably with that in other recent series of patients treated by pancreaticoduodenectomy alone or combined with post-operative adjuvant 5-FU-based chemoradiation (Table 12.3). Local (tumor bed) recurrence occurred in only 8 patients (10%), likely due to the protocol-mandated standardization of pretreatment imaging, surgical technique, and chemoradiation. In subsequent reports, the preoperative 30-Gy regimen was noted to be well tolerated, with a toxicity profile that appeared to depend on the radiation sensitizer utilized; hospital admission rates were 4%, 11%, and 43% for patients treated with preoperative radiation therapy (30 Gy) and 5-FU, paclitaxel, and gemcitabine, respectively.[48,50,51]

The small survival advantage seen with 5-FU-based chemoradiation therapy and surgery compared with surgery alone (Table 12.3) probably resulted from improved local-regional tumor control. As patient selection for surgery (pre-operative staging) and surgical techniques improve, the benefit of pre- or post-operative 5-FU and EBRT in terms of local-regional tumor control will likely diminish. In addition, because the rates of response to 5-FU–based systemic therapy are low in patients with measurable metastatic disease, 5-FU–based chemoradiation regimens are unlikely to have a significant impact on the development of distant metastases. Therefore, more effective systemic agents are needed both to maximize radiation sensitization and, most importantly, to treat microscopic extrapancreatic metastatic disease. Current protocol-based preoperative chemotherapy and chemoradiation trials incorporate gemcitabine (2′-deoxy-2′,2′-difluorocytidine, Gemzar) alone or in combination.[52] Gemcitabine is the first-line agent for the treatment of metastatic disease and is also a potent radiation sensitizer. Gemcitabine's inhibitory effect on DNA synthesis, when combined with irradiation, is prolonged in tumors compared with its affect in normal tissues.[53] Such data provide the basis for the ongoing phase I and II studies of this drug-radiation combination in patients with localized pancreatic cancer.[54-56] A phase I study of rapid-fractionation EBRT (30 Gy/2 weeks; 3 Gy/fraction) and concomitant weekly gemcitabine (for 7 weeks) in patients with locally advanced adenocarcinoma of the pancreatic head served as the foundation for a recently reported phase II trial in patients with resectable disease.[49,51] Eighty-six patients received seven weekly infusions of gemcitabine (400 mg/m^2) and 30 Gy of EBRT (3 Gy/fraction, 5 days per week beginning 3 days after the first dose of gemcitabine). All 86 patients completed chemoradiation, and 39% received all scheduled gemcitabine. In contrast to the experience with 5-FU-based chemoradiation, disease progression during the 12- to 14-week preoperative period was less common; 74% of all patients underwent a successful pancreaticoduodenectomy compared with approximately 60% in the trials utilizing 5-FU-based preoperative chemoradiation therapy. In addition, the overall median survival for all 86 patients (including the 26% who did not undergo resection) was 21 months (unpublished data, 2002). Such data strongly suggest a systemic anticancer effect beyond that achieved with previous chemoradiation strategies.

Difficulties associated with the delivery of neoadjuvant therapy include the need for a pretreatment pancreatic biopsy and the frequent need for intermediate-term palliation of jaundice using endoscopically placed biliary stents.[9,20,57] In addition, these stents can occlude during preoperative treatment leading to biliary stent-related morbidity in approximately 15% of patients treated with preoperative chemoradiation therapy.[20] Because of the complexity of patient management introduced by these issues, current neoadjuvant schemas are concentrated in centers already experienced in the multimodality management of pancreatic cancer.

Although postoperative chemoradiation therapy appears to confer a survival advantage compared to pancreaticoduodenectomy alone, at least 30% of eligible patients will not receive the intended therapy owing to a prolonged postoperative recovery. Therefore, future regimens will likely emphasize neoadjuvant therapy and capitalize on our growing understanding of the molecular aspects of metastasis, thereby allowing conventional chemoradiation and surgery to be combined with systemic chemotherapy and novel molecular-based therapies that inhibit essential steps in tumor cell growth.

LOCALLY ADVANCED DISEASE

Published data suggest survival duration is increased in patients who receive chemoradiation therapy for locally advanced pancreatic cancer, but this is limited largely to patients with a good performance status. In the GITSG studies of 5-FU–based chemoradiation therapy in patients with locally advanced pancreatic adenocarcinoma,[17,58] patients were randomly assigned to receive 40 Gy of radiation plus 5-FU, 60 Gy plus 5-FU, or 60 Gy without chemotherapy. Radiation therapy was delivered as a split course, with 20 Gy given over 2 weeks followed by a 2-week rest. 5-FU was delivered IV at a bolus dose of 500 mg/m^2/day for the first 3 days of each 20-Gy cycle and given weekly (500 mg/m^2) following the completion of chemoradiation therapy. The median survival was 10 months in each of the chemoradiation therapy groups and 6 months for the group that received 60 Gy without 5-FU. In subsequent GITSG studies, neither doxorubicin

(Adriamycin)[59] used as a radiation potentiator nor multidrug chemotherapy (streptozocin, mitomycin, and 5-FU [SMF]) alone or continued after chemoradiation therapy[60] was found to be superior to 5-FU-based chemoradiation. Additional chemotherapy after 5-FU–based chemoradiation increased the toxicity without an apparent therapeutic benefit.

More recent trials of chemoradiation therapy for locally advanced pancreatic cancer have investigated continuous-infusion 5-FU in combination with EBRT. The ECOG performed a phase I study to determine the maximal tolerated dose (MTD) of prolonged infusional 5-FU when combined with EBRT to 59.4 Gy in patients with pancreatic or extrahepatic biliary tumors. The MTD of 5-FU was 250 mg/m^2/day, with gastrointestinal toxicity being the dose-limiting factor.[18] A subsequent study conducted in Japan demonstrated the feasibility of utilizing low-dose, continuous-infusion 5-FU (200 mg/m^2/day) given over 5.5 weeks combined with a single course of EBRT to 50.4 Gy for patients with locally advanced pancreatic cancer.[61] This was followed by weekly 5-FU treatments until disease progression was documented. Eighty-five percent of patients completed the chemoradiation therapy. The median survival of patients treated was 10 months, similar to the survival of patients treated with bolus 5-FU and EBRT in the GITSG trials.[17,58] Thus, while infusional 5-FU may provide greater radiosensitivity compared with bolus 5-FU, no clear survival advantage has been established for this approach.

Recent investigations have focused on the combination of gemcitabine with EBRT.[49,55,56,62-64] Several strategies have been investigated including seven-weekly injections of gemcitabine with short-course EBRT (30 Gy), twice-weekly gemcitabine with 50.4 Gy of EBRT, weekly gemcitabine with 50.4 Gy of EBRT, and full-dose weekly gemcitabine with escalating doses of radiation (Table 12.4). Most of these studies showed gastrointestinal toxicity as a dose-limiting factor, but hematologic toxicity has also been observed. At the present time, there is no standard approach for combining gemcitabine and radiation, but several variables appear to be important in predicting the MTD. These include variations in the size of the radiation portal, the dose of radiation per fraction, and whether gemcitabine is administered once or twice weekly.[54] Currently, there is no compelling evidence that survival is better in patients receiving gemcitabine-based chemoradiation therapy than in those given 5-FU-based therapy for locally advanced disease.[65]

Because surgical resection of the primary tumor remains the only potentially curative treatment for pancreatic cancer, preoperative chemoradiation has been studied for its ability to convert locally unresectable pancreatic cancer to resectable disease.[56,62,66-71] Investigators at Duke University re ported that only two (8%) of 25 patients with locally advanced pancreatic cancer treated with 45 Gy of EBRT and 5-FU (with or without cisplatin or mitomycin C) were able to undergo complete resection with negative margins.[66]

TABLE 12.4 Phase I Trials of Gemcitabine in Combination with EBRT for Patients with Localized and Locally Advanced Pancreatic Cancer

Study Author (Year)	No. of Patients	EBRT Dose, Gy (dose per fraction)	Radiation Portal	Gemcitabine Doses MTD	No. with Radiographic Response	Median Survival Months)
Ikeda[63] (2002)	15	50.4 Gy (180 cGy)	1–3 cm margin	250 mg/m² weekly × 6	6	NA
McGinn[55] (2001)	37	Variable[a] MTD = 42 Gy (280 cGy)	1–2 cm margin	1000 mg/m² weekly	2	Phase I study
Pipas[56] (2001)	21	50.4 Gy (180 cGy)	3 cm margin + nodes	50 mg/m² twice weekly	6 PR, 4 MR	Phase I study
Wolff[49] (2001)	18	30 Gy (300 cGy)	3–5 cm margin + nodes	350–400 mg/m² weekly × 7	4 PR	6 months
Blackstock[62] (1999)	17	50.4 Gy (180 cGy)	1–2 cm margin	40–60 mg/m² twice weekly	NA	Phase I study
McGinn[64] (1998)	14	50.4 Gy (180 cGy)	1–2 cm margin	500–700 mg/m² weekly	1	Phase I study

Abbreviations: EBRT, external-beam radiation therapy; NA, not available; PR, partial response; MR, minor response; MTD, maximum tolerated dose.

[a]This trial fixed the dose of gemcitabine at 1000 mg/m², and escalated the radiation dose to the MTD.

Preliminary reports of gemcitabine in combination with radiation have reported sufficient down-staging of locally advanced tumors to occasionally allow for resection with curative intent.[56,62] However, this phenomenon remains uncommon and unlikely to alter the management of the great majority of patients with locally advanced disease. It is also important to acknowledge that, as the definition of locally advanced pancreatic cancer is loosened, results will appear more promising. If one maintains a strict CT definition of locally advanced pancreatic cancer that includes only arterial involvement (low-density tumor inseparable from the SMA or celiac axis on contrast-enhanced CT scans) or SMV or SMPV confluence occlusion, successful down-staging that allows one to proceed to complete surgical resection will be rare with currently available chemotherapy and chemoradiation techniques. One reason for this is that patients with locally advanced disease often have complete encasement of the SMA or celiac axis. In this setting, even the most active chemoradiation regimens that cause marked tumor cell killing would not be expected to result in a margin-negative resection. In contrast, there are patients who have marginally resectable disease, in whom the pancreatic tumor abuts or cuffs a portion of the SMA or other vascular structure. In these patients, sufficient cytoreduction could render a tumor resectable with curative intent.[72]

The use of chemoradiation therapy is justified in fully ambulatory patients with locally advanced disease who have pain but otherwise minimal symptoms. However, reported variations in the estimation of pain relief may be significant in patients receiving chemoradiation or radiation therapy for unresectable pancreatic cancer.[73] It remains unclear whether patients who have received chemoradiation should be treated immediately with further systemic therapy or followed expectantly for clinical and/or radiographic evidence of progressive disease. Recently, investigators at Virginia Commonwealth University reported that 4 months of weekly gemcitabine (3 weeks on, 1 week off) following 5-FU-based chemoradiation therapy is feasible.[74] A total of 23 patients were enrolled in this study, with a median survival of 13 months.

Systemic therapy with gemcitabine alone or in combination also represents a reasonable off-protocol alternative in patients with locally advanced pancreatic cancer. Systemic therapy alone may improve both pain control and performance status[52] and avoids the gastrointestinal toxicity associated with chemoradiation.[49] For those patients with stable or responding disease after 4 to 6 months of systemic therapy, chemoradiation can then be used to maximize local-regional tumor control. This treatment sequence has the advantage of avoiding the toxicity of chemoradiation in those patients who show evidence of progressive disease following systemic therapy. Chemoradiation is thereby applied only to the patients most likely to benefit as defined by the absence of disease progression during systemic therapy; a similar rationale applies to the use of neoadjuvant systemic therapy prior to surgery in patients with potentially resectable pancreatic cancer.

METASTATIC DISEASE

Trials of chemotherapy have usually enrolled two groups of patients: those with locally advanced disease and those with metastatic disease. Median survival duration in such patients may vary from 2 months to 12 months depending on tumor burden and performance status. Using such a heterogeneous population, many phase II trials of chemotherapy have reported survival rates that are quite promising compared to standard treatments. However, if the study population consists of a large proportion of patients with locally advanced disease and good performance status, the favorable survival duration may be largely unrelated to the chemotherapy program being studied. In addition, many early trials of systemic therapy relied heavily on physical examination, liver scan, and ultrasonography to assess response to systemic therapy.[75-78] Current imaging techniques such as high-quality CT and magnetic resonance imaging (MRI) provide better cross-sectional imaging,[79] which may partly explain the substantially lower response rates seen in recent trials of chemotherapy.[52,80-95] Moreover, even with improved imaging, interpreting changes in the primary tumor mass is not an accurate measure of response. A decrease in the primary tumor mass may reflect the resolution of peri-tumoral inflammation rather than malignant cell death. In contrast, the radiographic appearance of a pancreatic mass may be unchanged, even when significant tumor destruction has occurred.

Despite these limitations in the study and delivery of systemic therapy for pancreatic cancer, gemcitabine constitutes the current standard therapy for patients with metastatic pancreatic cancer because of its reproducible clinical benefit and the slight survival advantage it has shown over treatment with bolus 5-FU.[52,80-82] Further investigations of gemcitabine as a treatment for pancreatic cancer have been conducted in an attempt to improve its therapeutic index. A randomized phase II trial in patients with metastatic pancreatic cancer showed that short infusional schedules of gemcitabine (10 mg/m^2/min) may be more effective than the standard 30-minute bolus technique.[96] Preliminary results from this trial further demonstrated that, compared with 2300 mg/m^2 infused over 30 minutes, 1500 mg/m^2 delivered over 150 minutes (10 mg/m^2/min) led to a higher objective response rate (16.2% versus 2.7%) and a trend toward longer survival (6.1 versus 4.7 months). It is anticipated that future clinical studies of gemcitabine alone and in combination with other agents will focus on the delivery of the drug at 10 mg/m^2/min.

Given the growing acceptance of gemcitabine as first-line therapy for advanced pancreatic cancer, gemcitabine-based combinations are under active evaluation. In most trials, gemcitabine has been combined with one other agent such as docetaxel, oxaliplatin, 5-FU with leucovorin, cisplatin, UFT, irinotecan, and epirubicin.[97-110] Table 12.5 summarizes these results. Recently, gemcitabine was also combined with a new multi-targeted antifolate, premetrexed.[111] In addition, regimens consisting of two to four other drugs with gemcitabine are starting to

TABLE 12.5 Selected Trials of Gemcitabine Couplets for Patients with Advanced Pancreatic Cancer

Study Author (Year)	Treatment	No. of Patients	Objective Response Rate (%)	Stable Disease (%)	Median Survival (Months)	1-Year Survival (%)
Louvet[99] (2002)	Gem + Oxaliplatin	64	30.6	36	9.2	36
RochaLima[108] (2002)	Gem + CPT-11	45	20	36	5.7	27
Ryan[97] (2002)	Gem + Docetaxel	34	18	39	8.9	29
Louvet[100] (2001)	Gem + 5-FU/LV	62	22.6	NS	9	32.3
Philip[104] (2001)	Gem + Cisplatin	42	26	38	7.1	19
Stathopoulos[98] (2001)	Gem + Docetaxel	54	13	33	5.6	NS
Brodowicz[105] (2000)	Gem + Cisplatin	16	31	25	9.6	75
Feliu[107] (2000)	Gem + UFT	42	16	39	7	21
Heinemann[106] (2000)	Gem + Cisplatin	41	11	57	8.2	27
Oettle[101] (2000)	Gem + 5-FU/LV	38	5	89	9.3	32
Scheithauer[109] (1999)	Gem + Epirubicin	70	21	41	7.8	21.2

Abbreviations: Gem, gemcitabine; UFT, uracil, fluorouracil, and tegafur; NS, not stated.

appear in the literature. These include a combination of gemcitabine, capecitabine, and docetaxel (GTX)[112], gemcitabine, 5-FU, leucovorin, irinotecan, and cisplatin (G-FLIP)[113]; and gemcitabine, epirubicin, infusional 5-FU, and cisplatin.[114] Results of randomized trials of gemcitabine versus gemcitabine-based combinations of cytotoxic therapy have just recently been reported[82,115] Thus far, just as 5-FU combinations have not been proven to be superior to 5-FU alone, the same is holding true for gemcitabine-based combinations compared with gemcitabine alone. In an Italian study, 107 patients with advanced pancreatic cancer were randomly assigned to receive weekly gemcitabine (1000 mg/m^2 over 7 weeks) or gemcitabine (same dose) combined with cisplatin (25 mg/m^2 weekly for 6 of 7 weeks).[115] The overall response rate in the patients receiving gemcitabine alone was 9.2%, similar to that observed in single-institution phase II trials. Although the patients who received the combination of gemcitabine plus cisplatin had a response rate of 26.4%, unfortunately this did not translate into a statistically significant survival advantage. Patients assigned to receive gemcitabine had a median survival of 20 weeks, whereas those receiving gemcitabine and cisplatin had a median survival of 30 weeks (P = .43). The ECOG compared gemcitabine with or without weekly bolus 5-FU.[82] In this large, cooperative group study, 322 patients with locally advanced (10%) or metastatic disease (90%) were randomized to receive weekly gemcitabine, or weekly gemcitabine and bolus 5-FU. The response rate was slightly higher in the patients receiving the combination therapy (6.9% versus 5.6%) and progression-free survival was also somewhat better in that group (3.4 months versus 2.2 months; P = .02). However, no survival benefit was observed from the addition of 5-FU to gemcitabine (6.7 months for gemcitabine plus 5-FU versus 5.4 months for gemcitabine alone, P = .09).

Whenever possible, patients with a good performance status should be treated with systemic therapy in a clinical trial. Most current multicenter trials require that patients have measurable disease, which may include the primary tumor. Survival duration, time to disease progression, objective response, and clinical benefit are all appropriate endpoints of these studies. Patients whose disease progresses during treatment in a clinical trial that does not include gemcitabine may be considered for gemcitabine-based therapy since some clinical benefit from gemcitabine has been observed for such patients.[116] However, patients who fail to respond to gemcitabine-based therapy are unlikely to receive any meaningful benefit from further conventional chemotherapy and should be offered supportive care. If they maintain an adequate performance status, it may be reasonable for them to participate in a trial of investigational therapy. Second-line treatment with conventional chemotherapy delivered outside of a clinical trial should be discouraged.

CONCLUSIONS

The length and quality of life of patients with localized pancreatic cancer will be maximized by accurate preoperative assessment of resectability, a standardized technique of tumor resection, and the routine use of protocol-based adjuvant or neoadjuvant therapy. Pancreaticoduodenectomy should always be performed as part of a multimodality approach involving chemotherapy or chemoradiation. For patients with locally advanced pancreatic cancer and a good performance status, systemic therapy (gemcitabine alone or in combination) and/or chemoradiation are reasonable treatment alternatives. The care of patients with locally advanced and metastatic pancreatic cancer is greatly complicated by symptoms of biliary and gastric outlet obstruction, pain, anorexia, and fatigue. Palliation must always be the primary goal for this group of patients and is facilitated by a multidisciplinary approach. Symptomatic relief of biliary obstruction and pain should be addressed before consideration is given to systemic therapy. Patients with metastatic disease and a good performance status should be offered gemcitabine-based therapy if a clinical trial is not available. Continued efforts to enroll patients with localized and advanced pancreatic cancer into well-designed clinical trials should remain a high priority for oncologists across all disciplines.

REFERENCES

1. Jemal A, Murray T, Thun M. Cancer statistics, 2003. CA Cancer J Clin 2003;53:7.
2. Evans DB, Abbruzzese JL, Willett CG. Cancer of the pancreas. In: DeVita VT, Hellman S, Rosenberg SA, eds. Cancer, Principles and Practice of Oncology. Philadelphia: Lippincott Williams and Wilkins, 2001:1126–1161.
3. O'Malley ME, Boland GWL, Wood BJ, et al. Adenocarcinoma of the head of the pancreas: determination of surgical unresectability with thin-section pancreatic-phase helical CT. AJR 1999;173:1510–1518.
4. Yeung RS, Weese JL, Hoffman JP, et al. Neoadjuvant chemoradiation in pancreatic and duodenal carcinoma. Cancer 1993;72:2124–2133.
5. Warshaw AL, Gu Z, Wittenberg J, et al. Preoperative staging and assessment of resectability of pancreatic cancer. Arch Surg 1990;125:230–233.
6. Cusheri A. Laparoscopy for pancreatic cancer: Does it benefit the patient? Eur J Surg 1988;14:41–44.
7. Warshaw AL, Tepper JE, Shipley WU. Laparoscopy in the staging and planning of therapy for pancreatic cancer. Am J Surg 1985;151:76–80.
8. Pisters PW, Lee JE, Vauthey JN, et al. Laparoscopy in the staging of pancreatic cancer. Br J Surg 2001;88:325–337.
9. Raut CP, Grau AM, Staerkel GA, et al. Diagnostic accuracy of endoscopic ultrasound-guided fine-needle aspiration in patients with presumed pancreatic cancer. J Gastrointestinal Surg 2003;7:118–128.
10. Suits J, Frazee R, Erickson RA. Endoscopic ultrasound and fine needle aspiration for the evaluation of pancreatic masses. Arch Surg 1999;134:639–643.
11. Sohn TA, Yeo CJ, Cameron JL, et al. Resected adenocarcinoma of the pancreas—616 patients: results, outcomes, and prognostic indicators. J Gastrointestinal Surg 2000;4:567–579.
12. Nitecki SS, Sar MG, Colby TV, et al. Long-term survival after resection for ductal adenocarcinoma of the pancreas. Is it really improving? Ann Surg 1995;221:59–66.

13. Neoptolemos JP, Stocken DD, Dunn AJ, et al. Influence of resection margins on survival for patients with pancreatic cancer treated by adjuvant chemoradiation and/or chemotherapy in the ESPAC-1 randomized controlled trial. Ann Surg 2001;234:758–768.
14. Millikan KW, Deziel DJ, Silverstein JC, et al. Prognostic factors associated with resectable adenocarcinoma of the head of the pancreas. Am Surg 1999;65:618–624.
15. Nishimura Y, Hosotani R, Shibamoto Y, et al. External and intraoperative radiotherapy for resectable and unresectable pancreatic cancer: Analysis of survival rates and complications. Int J Radiat Oncol Biol Phys 1997;39:39–49.
16. Sperti C, Pasquali C, Piccoli A, et al. Survival after resection for ductal adenocarcinoma of the pancreas. Br J Surg 1996;83:625–631.
17. Gastrointestinal Tumor Study Group. A multi-institutional comparative trial of radiation therapy alone and in combination with 5-fluorouracil for locally unresectable pancreatic carcinoma. Ann Surg 1979;189:205–208.
18. Whittington R, Neuberg D, Tester WJ, et al. Protracted intravenous fluorouracil infusion with radiation therapy in the management of localized pancreaticobiliary carcinoma: A phase I Eastern Cooperative Oncology Group trial. J Clin Oncol 1995;13:227–232.
19. Balcom JH, Rattner DW, Warshaw AL, et al. Ten-year experience with 733 resections: Changing indications, older patients, and decreasing length of hospitalization. Arch Surg 2001;136:391–398.
20. Pisters PWT, Hudec WA, Hess KR, et al. Effect of preoperative biliary decompression on pancreaticoduodenectomy-associated morbidity in 300 consecutive patients. Ann Surg 2001;234:47–55.
21. Edge SB, Schmieg RE, Rosenlof LK, et al. Pancreas cancer resection outcome in American university centers. Cancer 1993;71:3502–3508.
22. Wade TP, Kraybill WG, Virgo KS, et al. Pancreatic cancer treatment in the U.S. veteran from 1987 to 1991: Effect of tumor stage on survival. J Surg Oncol 1995;58:104–111.
23. Wade TP, Radford DM, Virgo KS, et al. Complications and outcomes in the treatment of pancreatic adenocarcinoma in the United States veteran. J Am Coll Surg 1994;179:38–48.
24. Birkmeyer JD, Siewers AE, Finlayson EVA, et al. Hospital volume and surgical mortality in the United States. N Engl J Med 2002;346:1128–1137.
25. Birkmeyer JD, Warshaw AL, Finlayson SR, et al. Relationship between hospital volume and late survival after pancreaticoduodenectomy. Surgery 1999;126:178–183.
26. Exocrine Pancreas. In: Greene FL, Page DL, Fleming ID, et al., eds. AJCC Cancer Staging Manual. New York: Springer, 2002:157–164.
27. Evans DB, Rich TA, Byrd DR, et al. Preoperative chemoradiation and pancreaticoduodenectomy for adenocarcinoma of the pancreas. Arch Surg 1992;127:1335–1339.
28. Gastrointestinal Tumor Study Group. Further evidence of effective adjuvant combined radiation and chemotherapy following curative resection of pancreatic cancer. Cancer 1987;59:2006–2010.
29. Kalser MH, Ellenberg SS. Pancreatic cancer: Adjuvant combined radiation and chemotherapy following curative resection. Arch Surg 1985;120:899–903.
30. Foo ML, Gunderson LL, Nagorney DM, et al. Patterns of failure in grossly resected pancreatic ductal adenocarcinoma treated with adjuvant irradiation ±5-fluorouracil. Int J Radiat Oncol Biol Phys 1996;26:483–489.
31. Klinkenbijl JH, Jeekel J, Sahmoud T, et al. Adjuvant radiotherapy and 5-fluorouracil after curative resection for the cancer of the pancreas and peri-ampullary region. Phase III trial of the EORTC Gastrointestinal Tract Cancer Cooperative Group. Ann Surg 1999;230:776–784.

32. Neoptolemos JP, Dunn JA, Stocken DD, et al. Adjuvant chemoradiotherapy and chemotherapy in resectable pancreatic cancer: a randomized controlled trial. Lancet 2001;358:1576–1585.

33. Nukui Y, Picozzi VJ, Traverso LW. Interferon-based adjuvant chemoradiation therapy improves survival after pancreaticoduodenectomy for pancreatic adenocarcinoma. Am J Surg 2000;179:367–371.

34. Abrams RA, Grochow LB, Chakravarthy A, et al. Intensified adjuvant therapy for pancreatic and periampullary adenocarcinoma: Survival results and observations regarding patterns of failure, radiotherapy dose and CA19-9 levels. Int J Radiat Oncol Biol Phys 1999;44:1039–1046.

35. Demeure MJ, Doffek KM, Komorowski RA, et al. Molecular metastases in stage I pancreatic cancer: Improved survival with adjuvant chemoradiation. Surgery 1998;124:663–669.

36. Yeo CJ, Abrams RA, Grochow LB, et al. Pancreaticoduodenectomy for pancreatic adenocarcinoma: Postoperative adjuvant chemoradiation improves survival. Ann Surg 1997;225:621–636.

37. Chakravarthy A, Abrams RA, Yeo CJ, et al. Intensified adjuvant combined modality therapy for resected periampullary adenocarcinoma: acceptable toxicity and suggestion of improved 1-year disease-free survival. Int J Radiation Oncology Biol Phys 2000;48:1089–1096.

38. Regine WF. Postoperative adjuvant therapy: past, present, and future trial development. In: Evans DB, Pisters PWT, Abbruzzese JL, eds. Pancreatic Cancer. New York: Springer-Verlag, Inc, 2001:235–242.

39. Bakkevold KE, Arnesjo B, Dahl O, et al. Adjuvant combination chemotherapy (AMF) following radical resection of carcinoma of the pancreas and papilla of vater-results of a controlled, prospective, randomized multicentre study. Eur J Cancer 1995;29A:698–703.

40. Crucitti F, Doglietto GB, Frontera D, et al. Integrated radiosurgical treatment of resectable pancreatic head carcinoma. Pancreas 1998;16:31–39.

41. Ishikawa O, Ohhigashi H, Teshima T. Clinical and histopathological appraisal of preoperative irradiation for adenocarcinoma of the pancreaticoduodenal region. J Surg Oncol 1989;40:143–151.

42. Pilepich MV, Miller HH. Preoperative irradiation in carcinoma of the pancreas. Cancer 1980;46:1945–1949.

43. Hoffman JP, Weese JL, Solin LJ. A single institutional experience with preoperative chemoradiation for stage I-III pancreatic adenocarcinoma. Am Surg 1993;59:772–780.

44. Willett CG, Lewandrowski K, Warshaw AL, et al. Resection margins in carcinoma of the head of the pancreas: Implications for radiation therapy. Ann Surg 1993;217:144–148.

45. Staley CA, Lee JE, Cleary KA, et al. Preoperative chemoradiation, pancreaticoduodenectomy, and intraoperative radiation therapy for adenocarcinoma of the pancreatic head. Am J Surg 1996;171:118–125.

46. Hoffman JP, Lipsitz S, Pisansky T, et al. Phase II trial of preoperative radiation therapy and chemotherapy for patients with localized, resectable adenocarcinoma of the pancreas: An Eastern Cooperative Oncology Group Study. J Clin Oncol 1998;16:317–323.

47. Breslin TM, Hess KR, Harbison DB, et al. Neoadjuvant chemoradiotherapy for adenocarcinoma of the pancreas: treatment variables and survival duration. Ann Surg 2001;8:123–132.

48. Pisters PWT, Abbruzzese JL, Janjan NA, et al. Rapid-fractionation preoperative chemoradiation, pancreaticoduodenectomy, and intraoperative radiation therapy for resectable pancreatic adenocarcinoma. J Clin Oncol 1998;16:3843–3850.

49. Wolff RA, Evans DB, Gravel DM, et al. Phase I trial of gemcitabine combined with radiation for the treatment of locally advanced pancreatic adenocarcinoma. Clin Cancer Res 2001;7:2246–2253.

50. Pisters PWT, Wolff RA, Janjan NA, et al. Preoperative paclitaxel and concurrent rapid-fractionation radiation for resectable pancreatic adenocarcinoma: toxicities, histologic response rates, and event-free outcome. J Clin Oncol 2002;20:2537–2544.

51. Wolff RA, Evans DB, Crane CH, et al. Initial results of a preoperative gemcitabine (GEM)-based chemoradiation for resectable pancreatic adenocarcinoma. [Abstract]. Proc Am Soc Clin Oncol 2002;21:130a.

52. Burris HAI, Moore MJ, Andersen J, et al. Improvements in survival and clinical benefit with gemcitabine as first-line therapy for patients with advanced pancreas cancer: A randomized trial. J Clin Oncol 1997;15:2403–2413.

53. Lawrence TS, Chang EY, Hahn TM, et al. Radiosensitization of pancreatic cancer cells by 2′,2′-difluoro-2′-deoxycytidine. Int J Radiat Oncol Biol Phys 1996;34:867–872.

54. Crane CH, Wolff RA, Abbruzzese JL, et al. Combining gemcitabine with radiation in pancreatic cancer: understanding important variables influencing the therapeutic index. Semin Oncol 2001;28(suppl 10):1025–1033.

55. McGinn CJ, Zalupski MM, Shureiqi I, et al. Phase I trial of radiation dose escalation with concurrent weekly full-dose gemcitabine in patients with advanced pancreatic cancer. J Clin Oncol 2001;19:4202–4208.

56. Pipas JM, Mitchell SE, Barth RJ, et al. Phase I study of twice-weekly gemcitabine and concomitant external-beam radiotherapy in patients with adenocarcinoma of the pancreas. Int J Radiat Oncol Biol Phys 2001;50:1317–1322.

57. Pisters PWT, Hudec WA, Lee JE, et al. Preoperative chemoradiation for patients with pancreatic cancer: toxicity of endobiliary stents. J Clin Oncol 2000;18:860–867.

58. Moertel CG, Frytak S, Hahn RG, et al. Therapy of locally unresectable pancreatic carcinoma: A randomized comparison of high dose (6000 rads) radiation alone, moderate dose radiation (4000 rads + 5-fluorouracil), and high dose radiation + 5-fluorouracil. The Gastrointestinal Tumor Study Group. Cancer 1981;48:1705–1710.

59. Gastrointestinal Tumor Study Group. Radiation therapy combined with Adriamycin or 5-fluorouracil for the treatment of locally unresectable pancreatic carcinoma. Cancer 1985;56:2563–2568.

60. Gastrointestinal Tumor Study Group. Treatment of locally unresectable carcinoma of the pancreas: Comparison of combined-modality therapy (chemotherapy plus radiotherapy) to chemotherapy alone. J Natl Cancer Inst 1988;80:751–755.

61. Ishii H, Okada S, Tokuuye K, et al. Protracted 5-fluorouracil infusion with concurrent radiotherapy as a treatment for locally advanced pancreatic carcinoma. Cancer 1997;79:1516–1520.

62. Blackstock AW, Bernard SA, Richards F, et al. Phase I trial of twice-weekly gemcitabine and concurrent radiation in patients with advanced pancreatic cancer. J Clin Oncol 1999;17:2208–2212.

63. Ikeda M, Okada S, Tokuuye K, et al. A phase I trial of weekly gemcitabine and concurrent radiotherapy in patients with locally advanced pancreatic cancer. Br J Cancer 2002;86:1551–1554.

64. McGinn C, Smith D, Szarka C, et al. A phase I study of gemcitabine in combination with radiation therapy in patients with localized, unresectable pancreatic cancer. [Abstract]. Proc Am Soc Clin Oncol 1998;17:264a.

65. Crane CH, Abbruzzese JL, Evans DB, et al. Is the therapeutic index better with gemcitabine-based chemoradiation than with 5-fluorouracil-based chemoradiation in locally advanced pancreatic cancer? Int J Radiat Oncol Biol Phys 2002;52:1293–1302.

66. White R, Lee C, Anscher M, et al. Preoperative chemoradiation for patients with locally advanced adenocarcinoma of the pancreas. Ann Surg Oncol 1999;6:38–45.

67. Todd KE, Gloor B, Lane JS, et al. Resection of locally advanced pancreatic cancer after downstaging with continuous-infusion 5-fluorouracil, mitomycin-C, leucovorin, and dipyridamole. J Gastrointest Surg 1998;2:159–166.

68. Kamthan AG, Morris JC, Dalton J, et al. Combined modality therapy for stage II and stage III pancreatic carcinoma. J Clin Oncol 1997;15:2920–2927.

69. Safran H, King T, Choy H, et al. Paclitaxel and concurrent radiation for locally advanced pancreatic and gastric cancer: A phase I study. J Clin Oncol 1997;15:901–907.

70. Jessup JM, Steele G, Mayer RJ, et al. Neoadjuvant therapy for unresectable pancreatic adenocarcinoma. Arch Surg 1993;128:559–564.

71. Jeekel J, Treurniet-Donker AD. Treatment perspectives in locally advanced unresectable pancreatic cancer. Br J Surg 1991;78:1332–1334.

72. Wolff RA. Neoadjuvant chemoradiation for localized adenocarcinoma of the pancreas: great logic, grim reality. [Editorial]. Ann Surg Oncol 2001;8:747–748.

73. Minsky BD, Hilaris B, Fuks Z. The role of radiation therapy in the control of pain from pancreatic carcinoma. J Pain Symptom Manage 1988;3:199–205.

74. Kachnic LA, Shaw JE, Manning MA, et al. Gemcitabine following radiotherapy with concurrent 5-fluorouracil for nonmetastatic adenocarcinoma of the pancreas. Int J Cancer 2001;96:132–139.

75. Bukowski RM, Abderhalden RT, Hewlett JS, et al. Phase II trial of streptozotocin, mitomycin C, and 5-fluorouracil in adenocarcinoma of the pancreas. Cancer Clin Trials 1980:3:321–324.

76. Smith FP, Hoth DF, Levin B, et al. 5-fluorouracil, Adriamycin, and mitomycin-C (FAM) chemotherapy for advanced adenocarcinoma of the pancreas. Cancer 1980;46:2014–2018.

77. Bukowski RM, Abderhalden RT, Hewlett JS, et al. Randomized trial of 5-fluorouracil and mitomycin C with or without streptozotocin for advanced pancreatic cancer: A Southwest Oncology Group Study. Cancer 1983;52:1577–1582.

78. Group GTS. Phase II trials of hexamethylmelamine, dianhydrogalactitol, razoxane, and b-2′-deoxythioguanosine as single agents against advanced measurable tumors of the pancreas. Cancer Treat Rep 1985;69:713–716.

79. Goldberg HI, Margulis AR. Gastrointestinal radiology in the United States: An overview of the past 50 years. Radiology 2000;216:1–7.

80. Casper ES, Green MR, Kelsen DP, et al. Phase II trial of gemcitabine (2′,2′–difluorodeoxycytidine) in patients with adenocarcinoma of the pancreas. Invest New Drugs 1994;12:29–34.

81. Carmichael J, Fink U, Russell RC, et al. Phase II study of gemcitabine in patients with advanced pancreatic cancer. Br J Cancer 1996;73:101–105.

82. Berlin JD, Catalono P, Thomas JP, et al. Phase III study of gemcitabine in combination with fluorouracil versus gemcitabine alone in patients with advanced pancreatic carcinoma: Eastern Cooperative Group Trial E2297. J Clin Oncol 2002;20:3270–3275.

83. Rougier P, De Forni M, Adenis A, et al. Phase II study of Taxotere (RP56976, docetaxel) in pancreatic adenocarcinoma [Abstract]. Proc Am Soc Clin Oncol 1994;13:200.

84. Okada S, Sakata Y, Matsuno S, et al. Phase II study of docetaxel in patients with metastatic pancreatic cancer: A Japanese cooperative study. Cooperative Group of Docetaxel for Pancreatic Cancer in Japan. Br J Cancer 1999;80:438–443.

85. Sugarman SM, Pazdur R, Daugherty K, et al. A phase II trial of topotecan for the treatment of unresectable pancreatic cancer [Abstract]. Proc Am Soc Clin Oncol 1994;13:224.

86. Wagener DJT, Verdonk HER, Dirix LY, et al. Phase II trial of CPT-11 in patients with advanced pancreatic cancer. An EORTC Early Clinical Trials Group study. Ann Oncol 1995;6.

87. Rubin J, Gallagher JG, Schroeder G, et al. Phase II trials of 5-fluorouracil and leucovorin in patients with metastatic gastric or pancreatic carcinoma. Cancer 1996;78:1888–1891.

88. Pazdur R, Meropol NJ, Casper E, et al. Phase II trial of ZD1694 (Tomudex) in patients with advanced pancreatic cancer. Ann Oncol 1996;13:355–358.
89. Thomas E, Dumas P, Ajani JA. Oral etoposide for patients with advanced adenocarcinoma of the pancreas. Invest New Drugs 1999;16:333–335.
90. Mani S, Kruger JW, Sciortino DF, et al. Phase II trial of uracil/tegafur (UFT) plus leucovorin in patients with advanced pancreatic cancer: A University of Chicago phase II consortium study. Ann Oncol 1998;9:1035–1037.
91. Schmidt-Sandte W, Dageforde J, Klapdor R, et al. Trofosfamide in patients with pancreatic cancer. Anticancer Res 1999;19:2485–2487.
92. Maisey N, Chau I, Cunningham D, et al. Multicenter randomized phase III trial comparing protracted venous infusion (PVI) fluorouracil (5-FU) with PVI 5-FU plus mitomycin in inoperable pancreatic cancer. J Clin Oncol 2002;20:3130–3136.
93. Cartwright TH, Cohn A, Varkey JA, et al. Phase II study of oral capecitabine in patients with advanced or metastatic pancreatic cancer. J Clin Oncol 2002;20:160–164.
94. Stehlin JS, Giovanella BC, Natelson EA, et al. A study of 9-nitrocamptothecin (RFS 2000) in patients with advanced pancreatic cancer. Int J Oncol 1999;14:821–831.
95. Konstadoulakis MM, Antonakis PT, Tsibloulis BG, et al. A phase II study of 9-nitrocampthothecin in patients with advanced pancreatic adenocarcinoma. Cancer Chemother Pharmacol 2001;48:417–420.
96. Tempero M, Plunkett W, Ruiz van Haperen V, et al. Randomized phase II trial of dose intense gemcitabine by standard infusion vs. fixed dose rate in metastatic pancreatic adenocarcinoma [Abstract]. Proc Am Soc Clin Oncol 1999;18:273.
97. Ryan DP, Kulke MH, Fuchs CS, et al. A Phase II Study of Gemcitabine and Docetaxel in Patients with Metastatic Pancreatic Carcinoma. Cancer 2002;94:97–103.
98. Stathopoulos GP, Mavroudis D, Tsavaris N, et al. Treatment of pancreatic cancer with a combination of docetaxel, gemcitabine and granulocyte colony-stimulating factor: a phase II study of the Greek Cooperative Group for Pancreatic Cancer. Ann Oncol 2001;12:101–103.
99. Louvet C, Andre T, Lledo G, et al. Gemcitabine combined with oxaliplatin in advanced pancreatic adenocarcinoma: final results of a GERCOR multicenter phase II study. J Clin Oncol 2002;20:1512–1518.
100. Louvet C, Andre T, Hammel P, et al. Phase II trial of bimonthly leucovorin, 5-fluorouracil and gemcitabine for advanced pancreatic adenocarcinoma (FOLFUGEM). Ann Oncol 2001;12:675–679.
101. Oettle H, Arning M, Pelzer U, et al. A phase II trial of gemcitabine in combination with 5-fluorouracil (24-hour) and folinic acid in patients with chemonaive advanced pancreatic cancer. Ann Oncol 2000;11:1267–1272.
102. Cascinu S, Silva RR, Barni S, et al. A combination of gemcitabine and 5-fluorouracil in advanced pancreatic cancer, a report from the Italian Group for the Study of Digestive Tract Cancer (GISCAD). Br J Cancer 1999;80:1595–1598.
103. Hidalgo M, Castellano D, Paz-Ares L, et al. Phase I-II study of gemcitabine and fluorouracil as a continuous infusion in patients with pancreatic cancer. J Clin Oncol 1999;17:585–592.
104. Philip PA, Zalupski MM, Vaitkevicius VK, et al. Phase II study of gemcitabine and cisplatin in the treatment of patients with advanced pancreatic carcinoma. Cancer 2001;92:569–577.
105. Brodowicz T, Wolfram RM, Kostler WJ, et al. Phase II study of gemcitabine in combination with cisplatin in patients with locally advanced and/or metastatic pancreatic cancer. Anti-Cancer Drugs 2000;11:623–628.
106. Heinemann V, Wilke H, Mergenthaler HG, et al. A Phase II trial of gemcitabine and cisplatin in the treatment of advanced or metastatic pancreatic cancer. Ann Oncol 2000;11:1399–1403.

107. Feliu J, Lopez Alvarez MP, Jaraiz MA, et al. Phase II trial of gemcitabine and UFT modulated by leucovorin in patients with advanced pancreatic carcinoma. The ONCOPAZ Cooperative Group. Cancer 2000;89:1706–1713.

108. Rocha Lima CM, Savarese D, Bruckner H, et al. Irinotecan plus gemcitabine induces both radiographic and CA 19-9 tumor marker responses in patients with previously untreated advanced pancreatic cancer. J Clin Oncol 2002;20:1182–1191.

109. Scheithauer W, Kornek GV, Raderer M, et al. Phase II trial of gemcitabine, epirubicin and granulocyte colony-stimulating factor in patients with advanced pancreatic adenocarcinoma. Br J Cancer 1999;80:1797–1802.

110. van Moorsel CJ, Veerman G, Bergman AM, et al. Combination chemotherapy studies with gemcitabine. Semin Oncol 1997;24:17–23.

111. Kindler HL, Dugan J, Hochster H, et al. Clinical outcome in patients with advanced pancreatic cancer treated with premetrexed/gemcitabine. [Abstract]. Proc Am Soc Clin Oncol 2002;21:125.

112. Fine RL, Sherman W, Chabot S, et al. Biochemically synergistic chemotherapy for advanced pancreactic cancer. [Abstract]. Proc Am Soc Clin Oncol 2002;21:144.

113. Kozuch P, Grossbard ML, Barzdins A, et al. Irinotecan combined with gemcitabine, 5-fluorouracil, leucovorin, and cisplatin (G-FLIP) is an effective and non-crossresistant treatment for refractory metastatic pancreatic cancer. Oncologist 2001;6:488–495.

114. Reni M, Passoni P, Panucci MG, et al. Definitive results of a phase II trial of cisplatin, epirubicin, continuous-infusion fluorouracil, and gemcitabine in stage IV pancreatic adenocarcinoma. J Clin Oncol 2001;19:2679–2686.

115. Colucci G, Giuliani F, Gebbia V, et al. Gemcitabine alone or with cisplatin for the treatment of patients with locally advanced and/or metastatic pancreatic carcinoma: a prospective, randomized phase III study of the Gruppo Oncologia dell'Italia Meridionale. Cancer 2002;94:902–910.

116. Rothenberg ML, Moore MJ, Cripps MC, et al. A phase II trial of gemcitabine in patients with 5-FU-refractory pancreas cancer. Ann Oncol 1996;7:347–353.

Chapter 13

Risk-Reducing Salpingo-Oophorectomy in Patients with *BRCA1* and *BRCA2* Mutations

Noah D. Kauff, MD

Richard R. Barakat, MD

Kenneth Offit, MD, MPH

Ovarian cancer remains a relatively uncommon malignancy, affecting approximately 1 in 70 women over the course of a lifetime. However, more than half of the 27,000 women diagnosed with this disease in the United States in 2003 will die of their disease. Because of these observations, and because of the unproven efficacy of screening for early-stage ovarian cancer in the general population,[1] preventive surgery has become an option chosen by many women who are at increased risk for this disease.

For the 90% of ovarian cancers that are of epithelial type, the greatest risk factor for the disease is a family history of ovarian cancer. Despite the well-recognized occurrence of hereditary ovarian cancer, epidemiologic studies have shown that familial clustering is not common. In the large Cancer and Steroid Hormone Study, of 493 patients aged 20–54 years who had ovarian cancer, only 31 (7%) had a first-degree relative who had had ovarian cancer, and only three

(0.6%) had more than one relative affected.[2] Nonetheless, public awareness of the hereditary nature of ovarian cancer is high. In 1989, a popular comedienne, Gilda Radner, died of ovarian cancer. More than 60 million Americans were told about familial ovarian cancer on prime time television programs in the first 6 months of 1990, and a registry of hundreds of families with ovarian cancer was compiled shortly thereafter.[3,4]

The most common hereditary forms of ovarian cancer are hereditary breast-ovarian cancer, site-specific ovarian cancer, and hereditary nonpolyposis colon cancer syndrome.[4] With the discovery of the *BRCA1* and *BRCA2* genes in the mid-1990s, the genetic basis of hereditary breast-ovarian cancer syndrome was confirmed. Inherited mutations of these genes cosegregated with both breast and ovarian cancers in large kindreds.[5,6] However, after 7 years of investigation, the quantitative risk of ovarian cancer associated with germline *BRCA* mutations remains unclear. Studies have documented a lifetime risk (to age 70) of ovarian cancer that ranges from 28%–66% for those with *BRCA1* mutations and 16%–27% for those with *BRCA2* mutations.[5-12] It has been postulated that ascertainment bias, gene-environment interactions, or gene-gene interactions account for these differences.[13]

Even if one assumes the lowest range (1 in 5) of ovarian cancer risk for women carrying *BRCA* mutations, this risk is still more than 10 times greater than the population risk of 1 in 70. This observation, plus the absence of proven efficacy of radiographic and/or serologic ovarian cancer screening, remains a major factor in the decision of many women with *BRCA* mutations to undergo "prophylactic oophorectomy."

In this chapter, we review the retrospective and the prospective evidence for the protective effect of prophylactic oophorectomy. This review supports the rationale for referring to this procedure as *risk-reducing salpingo-oophorectomy* (RRSO). We also review the technical considerations for this procedure in light of our current understanding of the genetics of hereditary ovarian cancer. Finally, we emphasize important psychosocial as well as biologic questions that remain to be addressed for preventive surgical interventions to be most effectively used to decrease the burden of hereditary gynecologic malignancies.

OOPHORECTOMY FOR THE PREVENTION OF OVARIAN CANCER

Retrospective Studies and Decision Analysis

In one of the earliest reports recommending prophylactic oophorectomy in patients with a strong family history of ovarian cancer, Liber,[14] in 1950, described a family in which five sisters and their mother all were diagnosed with histologically confirmed papillary adenocarcinoma of the ovary. The author recommended that family members undergo frequent gynecologic screening and that prophylactic oophorectomy be considered. After that report, there was increasing consideration of risk-reducing oophorectomy for the prevention of subsequent gynecologic cancer in patients with a strong family history of ovarian cancer. At the same time, however, reports emerged of primary peritoneal cancer after "prophylactic" oophorectomy. In 1982, Tobacman and colleagues[15] were the first to report on a series of adenocarcinomas that were histologically indistinguishable from ovarian cancer; these cases occurred after oophorectomy in women with a strong family history of ovarian cancer. After this report, multiple other authors have also documented the occurrence of this entity.[16-18] In 1993, Piver and colleagues[3] reported on one of the largest series to date: six cases of primary peritoneal cancer developing after prophylactic oophorectomy in 324 women with at least two first- or second-degree relatives with ovarian cancer.

In 1995, Struewing and colleagues[19] reanalyzed the data from the cohort that Tabacman et al previously described. These authors analyzed follow-up information on 480 first-degree relatives of probands with breast or ovarian cancer. Eight ovarian cancers occurred during 1600 person-years of observation in the 436 women who had not undergone oophorectomy. Two primary peritoneal cancers occurred during 460 person-years of observation in women who had undergone oophorectomy. Although their study was not powered to show a statistically significant effect of oophorectomy, they found that women in their cohort who had not undergone oophorectomy had a 24-fold increased incidence of gynecologic cancer, compared with a 13-fold increased incidence of "ovarian" cancer in women who had undergone oophorectomy. In 1997, the Cancer Genetics Studies Consortium evaluated all available evidence and concluded: "There is insufficient evidence to recommend for or against prophylactic oophorectomy as a measure for reducing ovarian cancer risk. Women with *BRCA1* mutations should be counseled that this is an option available to them. Those considering prophylactic oophorectomy should be counseled that cancer has been documented to occur after the procedure."[20]

In an attempt to provide guidance to patients and clinicians, several decision analyses were published in the late 1990s. The first of these incorporated the best available evidence regarding the risk of ovarian cancer in patients with a *BRCA1* or a *BRCA2* mutation, the stage distribution and survival of ovarian cancer in *BRCA* mutation carriers, and a presumed efficacy of 50% for prophylactic oophorectomy that was based on the results of Struewing et al.[19] This analysis concluded that prophylactic oophorectomy in a 30-year-old woman with a *BRCA* mutation was associated with a 0.3- to 1.7-year gain in life expectancy.[21] This outcome compared to the 2.8-year gain in life expectancy if a 35-year-old women stops smoking or a 0.9-year gain in life expectancy if a 45-year-old women with node-negative breast cancer receives adjuvant chemotherapy. The authors also noted that oophorectomy could be delayed until age 40 with little loss of the gain in life expectancy. A subsequent study reported that prophylactic oophorectomy was associated with a 0.4- to 2.6-year increase in life expectancy. These authors did not, however, find prophylactic oophorectomy to be cost effective for quality-of-life years saved.[22]

Recently, a large retrospective study of 259 cases and 292 controls concluded that that prophylactic oophorectomy was associated with a hazards ratio of 0.04 (95% confidence interval [CI], 0.01–0.16) for the subsequent development of ovarian or primary peritoneal cancer.[23] The 96% risk reduction reported in this study reflects the exclusion of occult tumors detected at the time of surgery and may also reflect ascertainment biases that are unavoidable in retrospective series. The exclusion of six "occult" ovarian cancers (all stage I) detected at the time of surgery in this series is appropriate because the clinical endpoint of greatest concern to women who are deciding to undergo the procedure is the incidence of advanced-stage cancer after surgery.[24-26]

Prospective Studies

In this setting, a group of investigators at a single institution reported the outcome of 173 women with documented *BRCA1* or *BRCA2* mutations who were older than 35 years and had not undergone a bilateral oophorectomy at the time of genetic testing.[27] Participants were recommended to participate in surveillance for ovarian cancer with annual or biannual gynecologic examinations, twice-yearly transvaginal ultrasonographic examinations, and twice-yearly determinations of serum CA-125 concentration. For women whose childbearing was complete, consideration of salpingo-oophorectomy was recommended. One hundred one women underwent prophylactic salpingo-oophorectomy during prospective follow-up. Three of these women were found to have occult stage I ovarian or fallopian tube cancer at the time of prophylactic salpingo-oophorectomy. As in the previously mentioned retrospective series, these occult stage I cancers were excluded from the statistical analysis of cancer endpoints. Five ovarian or primary peritoneal cancers were diagnosed in the 72 women who elected to undergo surveillance during 139 women-years of follow-up. One peritoneal cancer was diagnosed in the 98 women who chose prophylactic oophorectomy during 191 women-years of follow-up. Cox-regression analysis revealed a trend toward a decreased risk of subsequent *BRCA*-related gynecologic cancer (hazards ratio 0.15, 95% CI 0.02–1.31). We have since expanded this analysis to include an additional 23 participants as well as additional follow-up. Including this additional information, we have now prospectively demonstrated that prophylactic oophorectomy is associated with a significantly decreased risk of subsequent *BRCA*-related gynecologic cancer (hazards ratio 0.11, 95% CI 0.01–0.90).[28]

Questions remain regarding the effect of prophylactic oophorectomy on gynecologic cancer mortality, osteoporosis risk, cardiovascular disease risk, and quality of life. These issues will be best addressed by future prospective studies.

OOPHORECTOMY FOR THE PREVENTION OF BREAST CANCER

Historical and Retrospective Studies

Although he never actually performed the procedure, the German surgeon Albert Schinzinger[29] first proposed a role for oophorectomy as a treatment for breast cancer in 1889. Independent observations by Nunn, Beatson, Gould, and Boyd have also been cited as the first surgical reports of the role of surgery of the ovaries in treating breast cancer (reviewed by Love and Phillips[30]). It was subsequently observed that premenopausal oophorectomy decreased the risk of subsequent breast cancer.[31-33] Oophorectomy has also been documented to decrease the recurrence rate in premenopausal women with breast cancer.[34] Brinton and colleagues[35] observed that prophylactic oophorectomy may also be effective in decreasing the risk of breast cancer in women with a family history of the disease. In 1997, the Cancer Genetic Studies Consortium noted the results of review by Nguyen et al[36] regarding the efficacy of prophylactic oophorectomy for the prevention of breast cancer, but the Consortium stated that these results needed to be confirmed before prophylactic oophorectomy is advocated for this indication.[20]

A retrospective case-control study in 1999 compared the incidence of breast cancer in 43 women who had documented *BRCA1* mutations and had undergone bilateral prophylactic oophorectomy before being diagnosed with breast or ovarian cancer with 79 age-matched women with *BRCA1* mutations who had not undergone bilateral prophylactic oophorectomy.[37] In this series, bilateral prophylactic oophorectomy was associated with an adjusted hazards ratio of 0.53 for the subsequent development of breast cancer (95% CI, 0.33–0.84). The protective effect was noted to be even greater if subjects were followed up for at least 10 years after surgery. In this analysis, the use of hormone replacement after surgery did not negate the protective effect. Rebbeck and colleagues[23] recently updated their case-control series analyzing 99 women with *BRCA* mutations who had undergone oophorectomy and 142 controls. Included in this update were 39 *BRCA2* mutation carriers. These authors again concluded that oophorectomy conferred a significant reduction in subsequent breast cancer risk in carriers of *BRCA* mutations (hazards ratio 0.47, 95% CI, 0.29–0.77).

Prospective Studies

The first prospective report of oophorectomy for the prevention of breast cancer in *BRCA1* and *BRCA2* mutation carriers was published in 2002.[27] One hundred thirty-one women with documented *BRCA* mutations who had both breast and ovarian tissue that was at risk at the time of receipt of genetic test results were followed up for a mean of 24.8 months. Sixty-nine women had prophylactic salpingo-oophorectomy after receiving genetic test results. Sixty-two women elected to undergo ovarian surveillance. All women were recommended to participate in monthly breast self-examination, clinical breast examination two to four times per year, and annual mammography. Eight breast cancers were diagnosed during 120 women years of follow-up in the women who chose ovarian surveillance. Only three breast cancers were diagnosed during 127 women-years of follow-up in the women who had undergone prophylactic salpingo-oophorectomy. The hazards ratio for the development of breast cancer after prophylactic oophorectomy was 0.32 (95% CI, 0.08–1.20).[27]

OOPHORECTOMY FOR THE PREVENTION OF BOTH BREAST AND *BRCA*-RELATED GYNECOLOGIC CANCERS

Decision Analysis

A recent decision analysis using updated estimates of the effect of oophorectomy on both breast and ovarian cancer incidence showed that prophylactic oophorectomy was associated with a significantly increased total life expectancy and quality-adjusted survival.[38] The authors concluded that prospective studies and clinical trials were needed to verify these results and to evaluate the long-term benefits of various preventive strategies.

Prospective Studies

When both breast cancer and *BRCA*-related gynecologic cancer were analyzed together in a recent prospective series, breast or *BRCA*-related gynecologic cancer was diagnosed in four women in the salpingo-oophorectomy group during 186 women-years of follow-up. In the surveillance group, 13 such cancers were diagnosed in 12 women during 135 women-years of follow-up. The estimated time to diagnosis of breast cancer or *BRCA*-related gynecologic cancer according to Kaplan-Meier analysis was significantly longer in the salpingo-oophorectomy group ($P = 0.006$) (Fig. 13.1). To take into account the different proportions in the two groups that had undergone bilateral mastectomy before study entry, a Cox proportional-hazards model for multiple events was used.[39,40] This model allowed adjustment for both differing frequency and differing timing of bilateral mastectomy between the two groups by censoring follow-up data related to breast cancer at the time of bilateral mastectomy. This analysis revealed that the hazards ratio for the development of breast cancer or *BRCA*-related gynecologic cancer after RRSO was 0.25 (95 percent CI, 0.08–0.74).[27] The type of mutation (*BRCA1* vs *BRCA2*) had no significant effect on the time to breast or gynecologic cancer ($P = 0.31$). If the three cases of unsuspected gynecologic cancer detected at the time of risk-reducing surgery were included in the analysis of interval to cancer measured from time of genetic testing, the hazards ratio for the development of breast or gynecologic cancer was 0.37 (95 percent CI, 0.12–0.90). This analysis was recently updated to include a mean of 29.6 months of follow-up. With this increased follow-up, RRSO in carriers of *BRCA* mutations remains

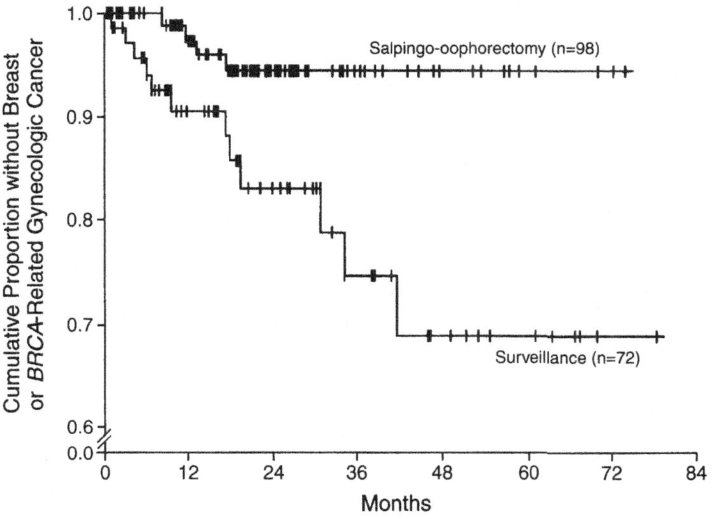

No. at Risk

Salpingo-oophorectomy	98	69	36	17	11	4	0
Surveillance	72	44	28	16	9	5	1

FIGURE 13.1 Kaplan-Meier estimates of time to breast cancer or *BRCA*-related gynecologic cancer in women who chose to undergo risk-reducing salpingo-oophorectomy and women who chose surveillance for ovarian cancer. $P = 0.006$ by the Log-rank test for the comparison between the actuarial mean times to cancer. A Cox proportional-hazards model for multiple endpoints, which took into account the different proportions of women in the two groups with breast tissue at risk, yielded a hazards ratio of 0.25 (95 percent confidence interval, 0.08–0.74) for subsequent breast cancer or *BRCA*-related gynecologic cancer after risk-reducing salpingo-oophorectomy. (Reprinted with permission from reference 27.)

highly protective against subsequent breast or *BRCA*-associated gynecologic cancer (hazards ratio 0.20, 95% CI, 0.07–0.63).[28]

CLINICAL CONSIDERATIONS REGARDING RISK-REDUCING SALPINGO-OOPHORECTOMY

In view if the literature just reviewed, we prefer the term *risk-reducing salpingo-oophorectomy* to the term "prophylactic oophorectomy" for several reasons. First, it is misleading to label a procedure as prophylactic in view of the clearly documented failures of the procedure to prevent peritoneal cancers. Secondly, because of the increased risk for fallopian tube malignancies in patients who are at hereditary risk for ovarian cancer, we believe that it is important to emphasize the importance of the salpingectomy in the discussion of the procedure. RRSO can be performed via laparotomy (an open surgical approach) or laparoscopy (a minimally invasive surgical approach). The appropriate choice of approach is best determined by the patient's prior history, associated comorbid conditions, need for additional procedures (e.g., hysterectomy), and experience of the surgeon. In the absence of contraindications (e.g., multiple prior abdominal surgeries, inability to tolerate pneumoperitoneum, need for concomitant hysterectomy), we generally offer a laparoscopic approach as the least morbid operative procedure, recognizing that the surgery cannot be 100% preventive against subsequent gynecologic malignancies.

Eltabbakh et al[41] reported on one of the first large series of laparoscopic oophorectomy in patients with a family history of ovarian cancer who underwent adnexal surgery for either predicted benign adnexal disease or surgical prophylaxis. Laparoscopic oophorectomy was completed successfully in 60 of 62 (96.8%) patients. In two cases, conversion to laparotomy was required to complete the procedure. Significant complications occurred in one patient (1.6%) who had an operative vascular complication and one patient (1.6%) who had postoperative bleeding requiring transfusion. Ten patients (16%) experienced minor complications, including fever (six patients), ileus (two patients), urinary tract infection (one patient), and urinary retention (one patient). The authors concluded that laparoscopic surgery in women with a family history of ovarian cancer is feasible and safe. The surgical outcome of laparoscopic RRSO has recently been reported in a large series of women with a *BRCA* mutation or a strong family history of cancer.[42] In 131 patients undergoing risk-reducing bilateral salpingo-oophorectomy, nine (6.9%) patients experienced complications, including three uterine perforations and one each of hemorrhage, conversion to laparotomy with wound cellulitis, cystotomy, small bowel obstruction, enterocolitis, and metabolic abnormality. This complication rate is similar to that of other series of laparoscopic gynecologic procedures[43,44] and lower than the 8%–17% complication rate reported with abdominal hysterectomy with concomitant bilateral oophorectomy.[45,46]

DETAILS OF THE SURGICAL APPROACH

Before the patient is brought to the operating room, a consultation that includes a complete history and physical examination should be performed. Details of the medical history that are particularly emphasized include history of prior abdominal surgeries, pelvic infections, diverticulitis, endometriosis, and other infectious or inflammatory processes that could predispose to intra-abdominal adhesions. Other comorbid conditions that could increase a patient's operative risk are also assessed. The patient should be specifically counseled regarding the risks and benefits of the procedure, including the risk of infection, the risk of damage to vascular structures or other intra-abdominal organs, and the possibility of the need for conversion to laparotomy (approximately 1% at the authors' institution). The patient is also counseled regarding the possibility that occult gynecologic malignancy could be diagnosed at the time of risk-reducing surgery. In prior series of risk-reducing oophorectomies in *BRCA* mutation carriers, approximately 2%–4% of risk-reducing oophorectomies were associated with occult malignancy at the time of surgery.[23,27,47] Lastly, the patient is counseled regarding the risks of primary peritoneal cancer after the surgery.

Typically, the night before surgery, the patient undergoes a limited bowel preparation with Fleets Phospho-Soda (C.B. Fleet Co., Lynchburg, VA). This preparation decompresses the bowel, facilitating the surgical exploration. Before surgery, the bladder is also emptied. At our center, laparoscopic RRSO is performed via an open laparoscopy technique. A 1- to 2-cm infraumbilical incision is made and carried through to the underlying fascia. The rectus fascia is grasped and incised. The peritoneum is then visualized and entered under direct vision. A blunt Hasson trocar is placed and anchored. The peritoneal cavity is then insufflated with carbon dioxide.

A suprapubic and a right or left lateral accessory trocar are then placed under direct laparoscopic visualization. Laparoscopic survey of the abdomen and the pelvis is then accomplished. Peritoneal lavage is then performed with washings sent for cytologic evaluation.[48] The right broad ligament inferior to the infundibulopelvic ligament (which contains the ovarian vessels) is then entered. By use of blunt dissection, the ureter is identified. The infundibulopelvic ligament with the ovarian vessels is then divided using an endoscopic stapling device. It is important to divide the infundibulopelvic ligament proximal to its insertion into the ovarian hilum to ensure that no residual ovarian tissue is left behind (Fig. 13.2). The uterine-ovarian vessels and the mesosalpinx (the tissue that carries the blood supply to the fallopian tube) are then skeletonized. Then, the endostapler is used to divide the uterine ovarian ligament and the fallopian tube at their insertion to the uterus (Fig. 13.3).

The free ovary is then placed in the pelvic cul-de-sac while the left ovary and the fallopian tube are excised in a similar fashion. After the ovaries are marked to allow identification of the side of origin by the pathologist, both ovaries and fallopian tubes are placed in an endoscopic bag and removed through the suprapubic incision. A final survey of the abdomen and pelvis is the accomplished to ensure adequate hemostasis and integrity of the ureter, bladder, and bowel. The trocars are removed under direct visualization. Fascial incisions 1 cm or larger are closed. The skin is infiltrated with a long-acting local anesthetic and closed, and the patient is sent to the recovery room.

After a brief period of observation (usually 4 hours), during which the patient demonstrates the ability to void and to tolerate diet, the patient is discharged to home. Approximately 25% of patients require overnight admission for nausea, inability to void, or pain control.[42] A follow-up phone call is made by the nursing staff the following day to assess the patient. If the patient has no complications, she returns for a postoperative visit 2 to 6 weeks after the surgery.

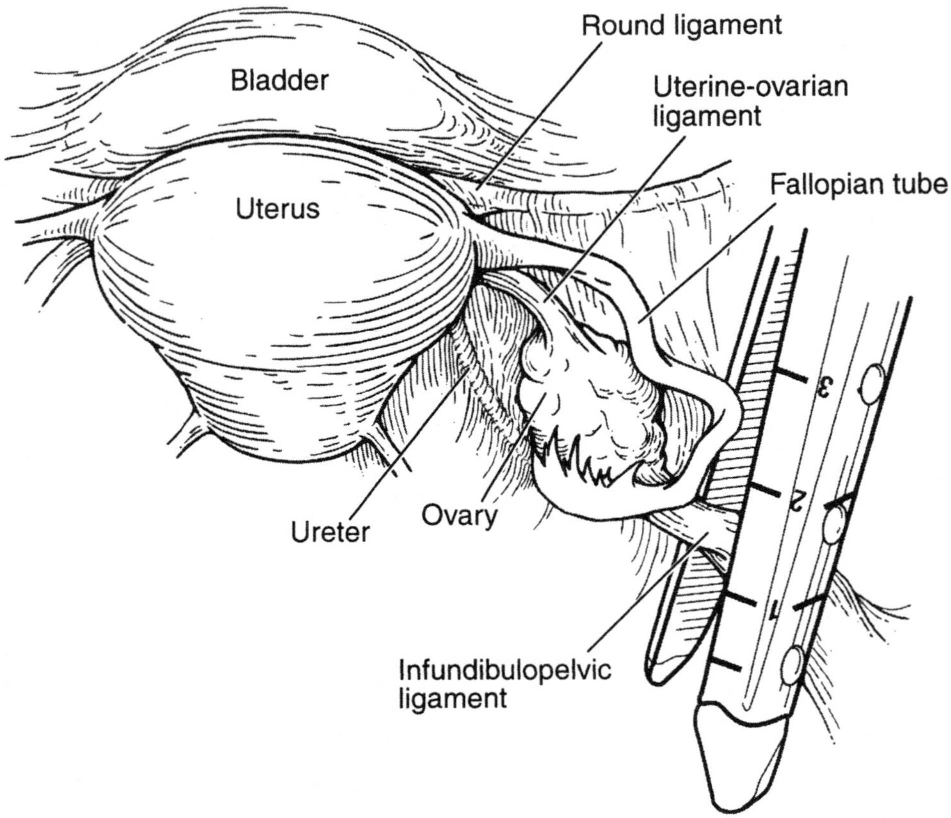

FIGURE 13.2 After the retroperitoneum has been entered and the ureter has been identified, the endoscopic stapler is used to divide the infundibulopelvic ligament (which contains the ovarian vessels) proximal to its insertion into the ovarian hilum. This approach insures that no residual ovarian tissue remains in situ after the procedure.

TECHNICAL SURGICAL CONSIDERATIONS BASED ON THE BIOLOGY OF HEREDITARY OVARIAN CANCER

Several theories exist regarding the origin of primary peritoneal cancer:

1. Undetected occult ovarian cancer was present at the time of surgery.
2. A portion of the ovary (an ovarian remnant) was inadvertently left behind at the time of surgery.
3. The cancer arises de novo from the peritoneal epithelium, which has the same embryologic origin as the ovarian epithelium.

Lu and colleagues[47] reported that unsuspected ovarian carcinomas were found in two of 50 women who underwent RRSO. Both of these tumors were micro-

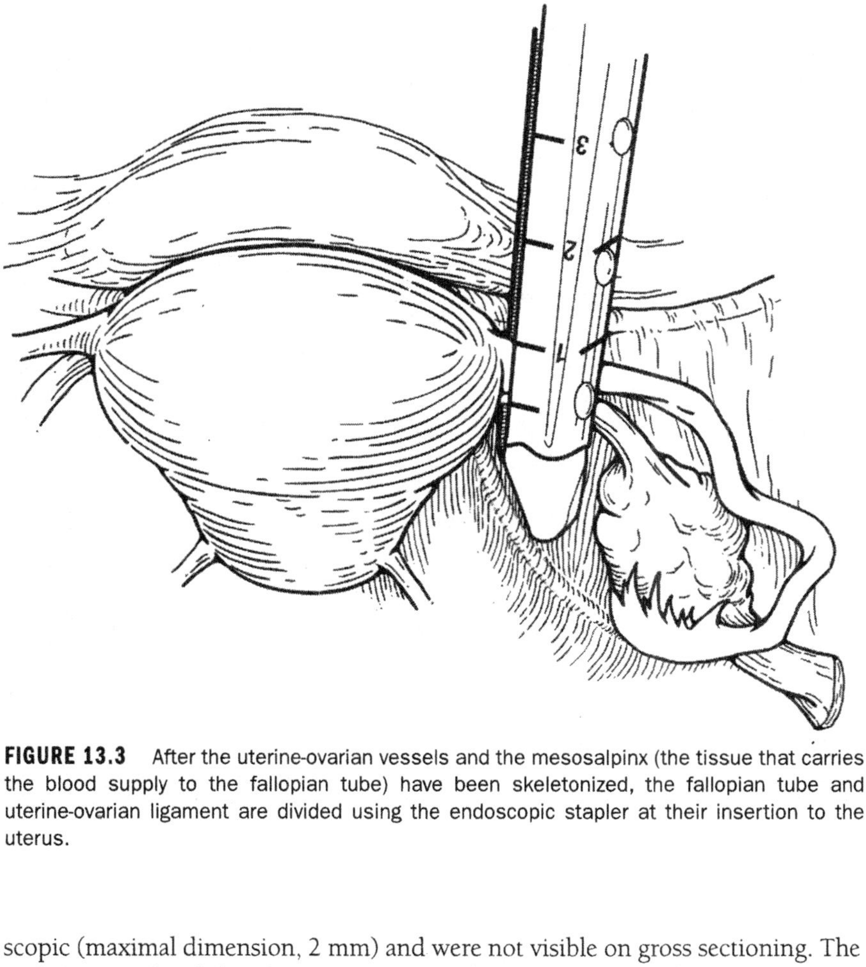

FIGURE 13.3 After the uterine-ovarian vessels and the mesosalpinx (the tissue that carries the blood supply to the fallopian tube) have been skeletonized, the fallopian tube and uterine-ovarian ligament are divided using the endoscopic stapler at their insertion to the uterus.

scopic (maximal dimension, 2 mm) and were not visible on gross sectioning. The authors speculated that these tumors could have been missed if only representative sections were examined. Chen et al[16] reported on a case of papillary serous cancer of the peritoneum after RRSO in women with a strong family history of ovarian cancer. Re-examination of the initial ovarian specimen demonstrated a microscopic focus of adenocarcinoma. Several other series have also identified early and/or occult ovarian or fallopian tube cancers at the time of RRSO.[23,49,50] Figure 13.4 illustrates a microscopic stage I ovarian cancer diagnosed in *BRCA1* mutation carrier at the time of RRSO at the authors' institution. Because of the possibility of metastatic disease arising from unsuspected ovarian cancer at the time of RRSO, careful pathological evaluation with multiple serial sections of the ovaries and fallopian tubes is warranted to rule out occult disease.[47]

Although less widely recognized by nongynecologists, a second possible cause of peritoneal cancer after RRSO is the incomplete removal of the entire ovary at

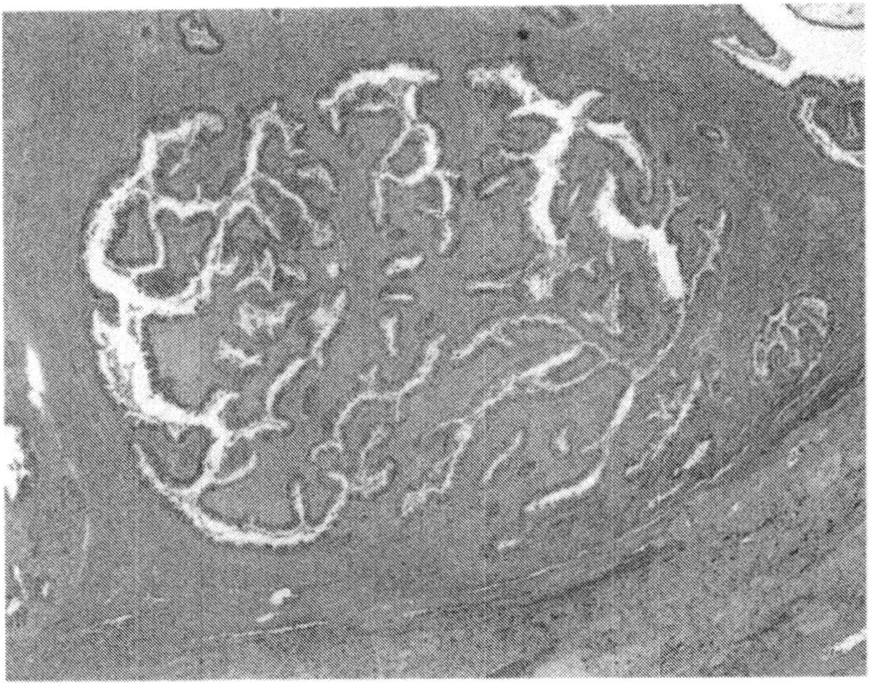

FIGURE 13.4 A hematoxylin and eosin–stained section demonstrating a moderately differentiated serous carcinoma of the ovary diagnosed at the time of risk-reducing salpingo-oophorectomy in a carrier of a *BRCA1* mutation. The tumor measures 5 mm in maximal dimension. Normal ovarian stroma is visible in the lower right of the image (magnification 40×). (Courtesy of Robert A. Soslow, MD.)

the time of risk-reducing oophorectomy. Leaving residual ovarian tissue at the time of oophorectomy is a well-recognized complication of both open and laparoscopic oophorectomy.[51,52] Because this entity is generally diagnosed only in patients with symptoms, the exact incidence is unknown. Risk factors for ovarian remnants include prior abdominal or pelvic surgery, endometriosis, and misapplication of surgical ligatures, linear staples, or bipolar cautery.[52] Several authors have speculated that ovarian cancer can originate in ovarian remnants.[53-57] To minimize this possibility, we believe that it is essential to open the broad ligament in order to facilitate identification of the ureter and allow ligation of the infundibulopelvic ligament sufficiently proximal from the ovary to ensure that no ovarian tissue is left behind. It is important that the surgeon performing a "preventive" oophorectomy is aware of the possibility of an ovarian remnant and is prepared to perform a procedure to minimize this occurrence.

Even if no occult cancer is present at the time of RRSO and the entire ovary and fallopian tube are excised at the time of surgery, histologically documented peritoneal cancer can occur. Several authors have provided strong evidence that primary peritoneal cancer is part of the tumor spectrum in patients with *BRCA1* mutations.[58,59] The risk of this possibility must be discussed with patients considering RRSO surgery.

OTHER CONSIDERATIONS

Estrogens or Anti-Estrogens after Prophylactic Oophorectomy

The role of hormone replacement after RRSO remains unclear. Premenopausal oophorectomy is clearly associated with an early onset of vasomotor and genital symptomatology.[60] It is also a risk factor for osteoporosis[661] and may be a risk factor for cardiovascular disease.[62] Only two studies have provided data on the use of hormone-replacement therapy (HRT) after oophorectomy in women with a family history of cancer. In 1997, Eltabbakh and colleagues[63] reported on 71 women with a family history of ovarian cancer who started HRT after oophorectomy. One patient in this cohort experienced breast cancer 3 years after the initiation of HRT. In a separate study, the use or the lack of use of HRT was not a significant predictor of breast cancer risk after oophorectomy in carriers of *BRCA1* mutations. However, the point estimates for the degree of breast cancer protection were greater for the women in this cohort who were never users of HRT than for the cohort as a whole.[37] Narod et al[64] recently published data that may have bearing on this issue. In this study, *BRCA* mutation carriers with a history of previous breast cancer who had taken tamoxifen and had also undergone oophorectomy experienced an 85% decrease in risk for subsequent breast cancer compared with controls.

Concomitant Removal of the Fallopian Tube and Uterus

Many authors have suggested that carcinoma of the fallopian tube is part of the tumor spectrum in *BRCA1* and *BRCA2* mutation carriers.[65-68] Because of this possibility, we and other authors have advocated that RRSO should include excision of the fallopian tube as close as possible to its insertion onto the uterus.[69]

Whether or not the uterus should be removed at the time of RRSO is more controversial. Concomitant hysterectomy is clearly associated with an increased risk of surgical complications.[45,46] However, many patients undergoing risk-reducing oophorectomy have also been diagnosed with breast cancer and may be taking tamoxifen. Although there were no fatal complications of endometrial cancer or uterine sarcoma in patients taking tamoxifen as part of the National Surgical Adjuvant Breast and Bowel Project P-1 trial,[70] removal of the uterus will eliminate the risk of endometrial cancer as well as the small increased risk of uterine sarcoma in these patients.[71] Additionally, because of the risk of fallopian tube carcinoma arising in the small amount of intramural fallopian tube left by salpingo-oophorectomy, several authors have suggested concomitant hysterectomy at the time of RRSO to address this risk.[72,73] Because the magnitude of increased risk of fallopian tube malignancies in this residual tissue is likely to be very small, a randomized trial to compare the occurrence of peritoneal cancers in patients after RRSO with and without hysterectomy will need to be very large indeed. Additionally, in the series from the Gilda Radner Familial Ovarian Cancer Registry, all six primary peritoneal cancers occurred after hysterectomy with bilateral salpingo-oophorectomy.[3]

It is also not clear whether *BRCA* mutations are independently associated with an increased risk of uterine cancer. In 2001, Levine et al[74] published data based on genotyping of histologically confirmed uterine malignancies in women of Ashkenazi Jewish ancestry. The results of this study indicated that *BRCA1* and *BRCA2* mutations were not associated with an increased risk of uterine cancer. Recently, an analysis from the Breast Cancer Linkage Consortium suggested that a *BRCA1* mutation was associated with a threefold increase in uterine cancer risk.[75] However, Gruber et al raised[76] the possibility that some of these uterine cancers were actually misclassified ovarian cancers. Moreover, a second study published simultaneously with that of the Breast Cancer Linkage Consortium did not demonstrate this increased risk.[77] Additionally, series of papillary serous carcinoma of the endometrium, which are histologically similar to ovarian cancer, have not demonstrated an association with *BRCA* mutations.[74,78]

Whether hysterectomy further reduces the risk of gynecologic cancer in *BRCA* mutation carrier is unknown. Until prospective studies addressing this issue are available, the decision to undergo hysterectomy at the time of RRSO will need to be made individually, with patients balancing considerations of morbidity, mortality, and cancer occurrence.

Peritoneal Lavage Cytology

In the only study to date evaluating peritoneal lavage at the time of RRSO, three of 35 patients who underwent this procedure had malignant cells that were detected on pathology.[48] Two of these women had a histologically confirmed ovarian or tubal carcinoma. In one patient, no additional foci of malignancy were identified, despite hysterectomy, bilateral salpingo-oophorectomy, and complete surgical staging. The patient was treated with systemic chemotherapy and remains without evidence of disease 10 months after surgery. The role of peritoneal lavage at RRSO remains unclear. Until further data become available, surgeons should consider obtaining peritoneal cytology at the time of RRSO.

PATHOLOGICAL EVALUATION OF SALPINGO-OOPHORECTOMY SPECIMENS

Unless gross abnormalities are noted at the time of RRSO, evaluation of frozen-section pathology is not routinely recommend unless it has previously been discussed with the patient and immediate surgical staging (including pelvic and para-aortic lymphadenectomy, omentectomy, and peritoneal and diaphragmatic biopsies) is available. Even if there is a capability for immediate staging, it may be reasonable to defer this procedure until final pathology is available. The significantly greater operative morbidity of surgical staging compared with RRSO may be avoided if the final pathology does not confirm carcinoma. If carcinoma is found, however, it is important to be able to proceed expeditiously to complete staging because early dissemination of ovarian cancer after delayed staging laparotomy has been reported.[79,80]

Occult ovarian and fallopian tube cancers are identified in approximately 2%–4% of risk-reducing surgeries in *BRCA* mutation carriers.[23,27,47] Careful pathological evaluation of the entire ovary and fallopian tube is clearly indicated. Beyond this immediate need, RRSO has also provided ovarian cancer researchers with a unique opportunity to examine possible premalignant alterations in tissue that is at significantly increased risk for cancerous transformation. In 1996, Salazar and colleagues[81] conducted an unblinded study of histologic changes in oophorectomy specimens from 20 women who were at increased risk for developing ovarian cancer and 20 women without known familial predisposition. They examined the incidence of surface epithelial pseudostratification, surface papillomatosis, deep cortical invaginations, epithelial inclusion cysts, and various forms of hyperplasia. They found that a higher proportion of ovaries from women who were at increased hereditary risk had multiple changes than ovaries from women without a familial predisposition. However, several additional studies have not been unable to confirm these findings.[82,83] Immunohistochemical studies have also not shown evidence of p53 overexpression or a difference in ERBB-2 expression in prophylactically removed ovaries from *BRCA1* mutation carriers.[83]

Recently, promising preliminary data was presented from a combined molecular genetic and morphologic analysis of oophorectomy specimens from *BRCA* mutation carriers. Analyzing 39 RRSO specimens and eight stage I ovarian cancers from *BRCA* mutation carriers, the authors suggested that most epithelial ovarian cancers arise within inclusion cysts, that a very limited field of dysplasia precedes the transformation to carcinoma, and that p53 mutation is a very early event in ovarian carcinoma.[84] Although these results need to be confirmed, such studies on histologic and molecular genetic changes in ovaries removed at risk-reducing surgery clearly have a tremendous potential to affect our understanding of carcinogenesis in hereditary and perhaps sporadic ovarian cancer.

Insurance Reimbursement

There is ample documentation in the literature that coverage decisions by health insurers play a significant role in utilization of new technologies.[85,86] There have also been isolated reports that women with familial cancer syndromes are being denied coverage for risk-reducing surgeries.[87,88] In one of the only published studies evaluating health insurance coverage for RRSO, Kuerer and colleagues[88] surveyed medical directors of health plans and found that 10%–11% of private insurers and 48%–50% of governmental carriers had policies specifically denying coverage for risk-reducing surgery in patients with a *BRCA* mutation. An additional 52%–64% of private carriers and 40% of governmental carriers had no identifiable policy regarding coverage of risk-reducing surgery in women with *BRCA* mutations. The authors speculated that without identifiable policies regarding risk-reducing surgery in high-risk individuals, this critical health care decision may be subject to arbitrary criteria that could result in substantial variation in utilization of risk-reducing surgery. We recently looked at the reimbursement experience of women with *BRCA* mutations who underwent RRSO at our institution. Twenty-eight (97%) of 29 prophylactic oophorectomies performed during the study period were reimbursed in full, less applicable co-insurance and deductibles.[89]

Psychosocial Impact of Prophylactic Oophorectomy

Limited information is available regarding the psychosocial impact of RRSO. Several studies have suggested that interest in RRSO correlates with increased levels of anxiety but not with objective risk.[90,91] Two recent retrospective studies have also suggested that women who have undergone RRSO have decreased cancer related anxiety.[92,93] In contrast to these results, a recent retrospective study from Scotland reported that women who underwent RRSO had more adverse physical and emotional symptoms than women who participated in an ovarian cancer screening program. They noted that women who were premenopausal at the time of oophorectomy were particularly vulnerable to psychological distress.[94] In the only prospective study to date assessing the psychologic impact of RRSO, a significant reduction in ovarian cancer anxiety and a high-degree of satisfaction with the procedure were observed.[95] A major limitation of this study is that it involved only 10 patients who were prospectively evaluated. Several groups are now conducting well-designed prospective studies evaluating the psychosocial impact of RRSO. Results from these analyses are expected in the next several years.

CONCLUSION AND CHALLENGES

Despite significant technical advances in surgical procedure and the more precise genetic definition of ovarian risk afforded by *BRCA* testing, important issues remain to be resolved in order to utilize risk-reducing ovarian surgery most effectively. Although recent prospective studies of decreased breast and ovarian cancer incidence after RRSO are encouraging, it remains to be shown whether RRSO will decrease mortality in *BRCA* mutation carriers. It is also unclear whether *BRCA1* and *BRCA2* mutation carriers will experience different levels of risk reduction from this procedure. Studies of gene-environment and gene-

gene interactions may more precisely define cohorts at increased or decreased risk for ovarian cancer. The optimal timing of RRSO, with respect to both reproduction and risk for breast and ovarian cancer and noncancer endpoints, remains to be determined. Improved serum-based (e.g., proteomic) and radiographic screening for ovarian cancer offers the promise of early detection of ovarian, and, perhaps, peritoneal, neoplasms. Finally, studies of the molecular progression of the preinvasive phase of ovarian cancer, in patients and in animal models, offer the promise of novel "chemoprevention" strategies. These biologically targeted prevention approaches will, it is hoped, ultimately render surgical removal of at-risk organs obsolete.

REFERENCES

1. Hensley ML, Castiel M, Robson ME. Screening for ovarian cancer: what we know, what we need to know. Oncology (Huntingt) 2000;14:1601–1607.
2. Schildkraut JM, Thompson WD. Familial ovarian cancer: a population-based case-control study. Am J Epidemiol 1988;128:456–456.
3. Piver MS, Jishi MF, Tsukada Y et al. Primary peritoneal carcinoma after prophylactic oophorectomy in women with a family history of ovarian cancer: a report of the Gilda Radner Familial Ovarian Cancer Registry. Cancer 1993;71:2751–2755.
4. Offit K. Clinical cancer genetics: Risk counseling and management. New York, NY: Wiley-Liss, 1998.
5. Easton DF, Ford D, Bishop DT. Breast and ovarian cancer incidence in BRCA1-mutation carriers. Breast Cancer Linkage Consortium. Am J Hum Genet 1995;56:265–271.
6. The Breast Cancer Linkage Consortium. Cancer risks in BRCA2 mutation carriers. J Natl Cancer Inst 1999;91:1310–1316.
7. Ford D, Easton DF, Bishop DT et al. Risks of cancer in BRCA1-mutation carriers. Breast Cancer Linkage Consortium. Lancet 1994;343:692–695.
8. Whittemore AS, Gong G, Itnyre J. Prevalence and contribution of BRCA1 mutations in breast cancer and ovarian cancer: results from three U.S. population-based case-control studies of ovarian cancer. Am J Hum Genet 1997;60:496–504.
9. Wacholder S, Hartge P, Struewing JP et al. The kin-cohort study for estimating penetrance. Am J Epidemiol 1998;148:623–630.
10. Ford D, Easton DF, Stratton M et al. Genetic heterogeneity and penetrance analysis of the BRCA1 and BRCA2 genes in breast cancer families. The Breast Cancer Linkage Consortium. Am J Hum Genet 1998;62:676–689.
11. Risch HA, McLaughlin JR, Cole DE et al. Prevalence and penetrance of germline BRCA1 and BRCA2 mutations in a population series of 649 women with ovarian cancer. Am J Hum Genet 2001;68:700–710.
12. Satagopan JM, Boyd J, Kauff ND et al. Ovarian cancer risk in Ashkenazi Jewish carriers of BRCA1 and BRCA2 mutations. Clin Cancer Res 2002;8:3776–3781.
13. Begg CB. On the use of familial aggregation in population-based case probands for calculating penetrance. J Natl Cancer Inst 2002;94:1221–1226.
14. Liber AM. Ovarian cancer in a mother and five daughters. Arch Pathol 1950;49:280–290.
15. Tobacman JK, Greene MH, Tucker MA et al. Intra-abdominal carcinomatosis after prophylactic oophorectomy in ovarian-cancer-prone families. Lancet 1982;2:795–797.

16. Chen KT, Schooley JL, Flam MS. Peritoneal carcinomatosis after prophylactic oophorectomy in familial ovarian cancer syndrome. Obstet Gynecol 1985;66: 93S–94S.

17. Kemp GM, Hsiu JG, Andrews MC. Papillary peritoneal carcinomatosis after prophylactic oophorectomy. Gynecol Oncol 1992;47:395–397.

18. White CD. Papillary intraperitoneal neoplasia resembling ovarian carcinoma after removal of benign ovaries. W V Med J 1993;89:282–283.

19. Struewing JP, Watson P, Easton DF et al. Prophylactic oophorectomy in inherited breast/ovarian cancer families. J Natl Cancer Inst Monogr 1995:33–35.

20. Burke W, Daly M, Garber J et al. Recommendations for follow-up care of individuals with an inherited predisposition to cancer. II. BRCA1 and BRCA2. Cancer Genetics Studies Consortium. JAMA 1997;277:997–1003.

21. Schrag D, Kuntz KM, Garber JE et al. Decision analysis: effects of prophylactic mastectomy and oophorectomy on life expectancy among women with BRCA1 or BRCA2 mutations. N Engl J Med 1997;336:1465–1471.

22. Grann VR, Panageas KS, Whang W et al. Decision analysis of prophylactic mastectomy and oophorectomy in BRCA1-positive or BRCA2-positive patients. J Clin Oncol 1998;16:979–85.

23. Rebbeck TR, Lynch HT, Neuhausen SL et al. Prophylactic oophorectomy in carriers of BRCA1 or BRCA2 mutations. N Engl J Med 2002;346:1616–1622.

24. Zhuang SH, Leonard GD, Swain SM. Oophorectomy in carriers of BRCA mutations [letter]. N Engl J Med 2002;347:1037–1038.

25. Whitfield GA. Oophorectomy in carriers of BRCA mutations [letter]. N Engl J Med 2002;347:1039.

26. Kauff ND, Robson ME, Offit K. Re: Oophorectomy in carriers of BRCA mutations [letter]. N Engl J Med 2002;347:1039.

27. Kauff ND, Satagopan JM, Robson ME et al. Risk-reducing salpingo-oophorectomy in women with a BRCA1 or BRCA2 mutation. N Engl J Med 2002;346:1609–1615.

28. Offit K, Kauff N, Scheuer L et al. Risk-reducing salpingo-oophorectomy in women with BRCA1 and BRCA2 mutations Ann Oncol 2002;13 (Suppl 5):9–10.

29. Schinzinger A. Ueber carcinoma mammae. Verhandlungen der Deutschen Gesellschaft fur Chirurgie [abstract]. 18th Kongress, Berlin, April 24–27, 1889. Berlin (Germany): Hirschwald, 1889:28.

30. Love RR, Philips J. Oophorectomy for breast cancer: history revisited. J Natl Cancer Inst 2002;94:1433–1434.

31. Feinleib M. Breast cancer and artificial menopause: a cohort study. J Natl Cancer Inst 1968;41:315–329.

32. Sartwell PE, Arthes FG, Tonascia JA. Exogenous hormones, reproductive history, and breast cancer. J Natl Cancer Inst 1977;59:1589–1592.

33. Brinton LA, Schairer C, Hoover RN et al. Menstrual factors and risk of breast cancer. Cancer Invest 1988;6:245–254.

34. Early Breast Cancer Trialists' Collaborative Group. Ovarian ablation in early breast cancer: overview of the randomised trials. Lancet 1996;348:1189–1196.

35. Brinton LA, Hoover R, Fraumeni JF Jr. Interaction of familial and hormonal risk factors for breast cancer. J Natl Cancer Inst 1982;69:817–822.

36. Nguyen HN, Averette HE, Janicek M. Ovarian carcinoma: a review of the significance of familial risk factors and the role of prophylactic oophorectomy in cancer prevention. Cancer 1994;74:545–555.

37. Rebbeck TR, Levin AM, Eisen A et al. Breast cancer risk after bilateral prophylactic oophorectomy in BRCA1 mutation carriers. J Natl Cancer Inst 1999;91:1475–1479.

38. Grann VR, Jacobson JS, Thomason D et al. Effect of prevention strategies on survival and quality-adjusted survival of women with BRCA1/2 mutations: an updated decision analysis. J Clin Oncol 2002;20:2520–2529.

39. Fine JP, Gray RJ. A proportional hazards model for the subdistribution of a competing risk. JASA 1999;94:496–509.

40. Therneau TM, Grambsch PM. Modeling Survival Data: Extending the Cox Model. New York: Springer-Verlag 2000.

41. Eltabbakh GH, Piver MS, Hempling RE et al. Laparoscopic management of women with a family history of ovarian cancer. J Surg Oncol 1999;72:9–13.

42. Barakat RR, Hensley ML, Bhaskaran D et al. Prophylactic oophorectomy in patients at risk for hereditary ovarian carcinoma [abstract]. Gynecol Oncol 2002;84:482.

43. Bateman BG, Kolp LA, Hoeger K. Complications of laparoscopy—operative and diagnostic. Fertil Steril 1996;66:30–35.

44. Mirhashemi R, Harlow BL, Ginsburg ES et al. Predicting risk of complications with gynecologic laparoscopic surgery. Obstet Gynecol 1998;92:327–331.

45. Kovac SR. Hysterectomy outcomes in patients with similar indications. Obstet Gynecol 2000;95:787–793.

46. Makinen J, Johansson J, Tomas C et al. Morbidity of 10,110 hysterectomies by type of approach. Hum Reprod 2001;16:1473–1478.

47. Lu KH, Garber JE, Cramer DW et al. Occult ovarian tumors in women with BRCA1 or BRCA2 mutations undergoing prophylactic oophorectomy. J Clin Oncol 2000; 18:2728–2732.

48. Colgan TJ, Boerner SL, Murphy J et al. Peritoneal lavage cytology: an assessment of its value during prophylactic oophorectomy. Gynecol Oncol 2002;85:397–403.

49. Colgan TJ, Murphy J, Cole DE et al. Occult carcinoma in prophylactic oophorectomy specimens: prevalence and association with BRCA germline mutation status. Am J Surg Pathol 2001;25:1283–1289.

50. Scheuer L, Kauff N, Robson M et al. Outcome of preventive surgery and screening for breast and ovarian cancer in BRCA mutation carriers. J Clin Oncol 2002;20:1260–1268.

51. Lafferty HW, Angioli R, Rudolph J et al. Ovarian remnant syndrome: experience at Jackson Memorial Hospital, University of Miami, 1985 through 1993. Am J Obstet Gynecol 1996;174:641–645.

52. Nezhat CH, Seidman DS, Nezhat FR et al. Ovarian remnant syndrome after laparoscopic oophorectomy. Fertil Steril 2000;74:1024–1028.

53. Fueyo J, Garces JM, Soriano JC et al. Adenocarcinoma of the ovary in the ovarian remnant syndrome. Rev Clin Esp 1990;186:415–416.

54. Bruhwiler H, Luscher KP. Ovarian cancer in ovarian remnant syndrome. Geburtshilfe Frauenheilkd 1991;51:70–71.

55. Kazadi Buanga J, Laparte Escorza MC, Lopez Garcia G. Ovarian remnant syndrome: a case report of a malignancy. J Gynecol Obstet Biol Reprod 1992;2:769–772.

56. Glaser D, Burrig KF, Mast H. Ovarian cancer in ovarian remnant syndrome? Geburtshilfe Frauenheilkd 1992;52:436–437.

57. Narayansingh G, Cumming G, Parkin D et al. Ovarian cancer developing in the ovarian remnant syndrome: a case report and literature review. Aust NZ J Obstet Gynaecol 2000;40:221–223.

58. Bandera CA, Muto MG, Schorge JO et al. BRCA1 gene mutations in women with papillary serous carcinoma of the peritoneum. Obstet Gynecol 1998;92:596–600.

59. Schorge JO, Muto MG, Welch WR et al. Molecular evidence for multifocal papillary serous carcinoma of the peritoneum in patients with germline BRCA1 mutations. J Natl Cancer Inst 1998;90:841–845.

60. Bachmann G. Physiologic aspects of natural and surgical menopause. J Reprod Med 2001;46[suppl]:307–315.

61. Aitken JM, Hart DM, Anderson JB et al. Osteoporosis after oophorectomy for non-malignant disease in premenopausal women. BMJ 1973;2:325–328.

62. Colditz GA, Willett WC, Stampfer MJ et al. Menopause and the risk of coronary heart disease in women. N Engl J Med 1987;316:1105–1110.

63. Eltabbakh GH, Piver MS, Hempling RE et al. Estrogen replacement therapy following oophorectomy in women with a family history of ovarian cancer. Gynecol Oncol 1997;66:103–107.

64. Narod SA, Brunet JS, Ghadirian P et al. Tamoxifen and risk of contralateral breast cancer in BRCA1 and BRCA2 mutation carriers: a case-control study. Hereditary Breast Cancer Clinical Study Group. Lancet 2000;356:1876–1881.

65. Schubert EL, Lee MK, Mefford HC et al. BRCA2 in American families with four or more cases of breast or ovarian cancer: recurrent and novel mutations, variable expression, penetrance, and the possibility of families whose cancer is not attributable to BRCA1 or BRCA2. Am J Hum Genet 1997;60:1031–1040.

66. Rose PG, Shrigley R, Wiesner GL. Germline BRCA2 mutation in a patient with fallopian tube carcinoma: a case report. Gynecol Oncol 2000;77:319–320.

67. Zweemer RP, van Diest PJ, Verheijen RH et al. Molecular evidence linking primary cancer of the fallopian tube to BRCA1 germline mutations. Gynecol Oncol 2000;76:45–50.

68. Hartley A, Rollason T, Spooner D. Clear cell carcinoma of the fimbria of the fallopian tube in a BRCA1 carrier undergoing prophylactic surgery. Clin Oncol 2000;12:58–59.

69. Eisen A, Rebbeck TR, Weber BL et al. Re: Prophylactic surgery: oophorectomy or adnexectomy? [letter] J Clin Oncol 2000;18:3455.

70. Fisher B, Costantino JP, Wickerham DL et al. Tamoxifen for prevention of breast cancer: report of the National Surgical Adjuvant Breast and Bowel Project P-1 Study. J Natl Cancer Inst 1998;90:1371–1388.

71. Wickerham DL, Fisher B, Wolmark N et al. Association of tamoxifen and uterine sarcoma. J Clin Oncol 2002;20:2758–2760.

72. Paley PJ, Swisher EM, Garcia RL et al. Occult cancer of the fallopian tube in BRCA-1 germline mutation carriers at prophylactic oophorectomy: a case for recommending hysterectomy at surgical prophylaxis. Gynecol Oncol 2001;80:176–1780.

73. Aziz S, Kuperstein G, Rosen B et al. A genetic epidemiological study of carcinoma of the fallopian tube. Gynecol Oncol 2001;80:341–345.

74. Levine DA, Lin O, Barakat RR et al. Risk of endometrial carcinoma associated with BRCA mutation. Gynecol Oncol 2001;80:395–398.

75. Thompson D, Easton DF: Breast Cancer Linkage Consortium. Cancer incidence in BRCA1 mutation carriers. J Natl Cancer Inst 2002;94:1358–1365.

76. Gruber SB, Petersen GM. Cancer risks in BRCA1 carriers: time for the next generation of studies. J Natl Cancer Inst 2002;94:1344–1345.

77. Brose MS, Rebbeck TR, Calzone KA et al. Cancer risk estimates for BRCA1 mutation carriers identified in a risk evaluation program. J Natl Cancer Inst 2002;94:1365–1372.

78. Goshen R, Chu W, Elit L et al. Is uterine papillary serous adenocarcinoma a manifestation of the hereditary breast-ovarian cancer syndrome? Gynecol Oncol 2000;79:477–481.

79. Kindermann G, Maassen V, Kuhn W. Laparoscopic preliminary surgery of ovarian malignancies. Experiences from 127 German gynecologic clinics. Geburtshilfe Frauenheilkd 1995;55:687–694.

80. Lehner R, Wenzl R, Heinzl H et al. Influence of delayed staging laparotomy after laparoscopic removal of ovarian masses later found malignant. Obstet Gynecol 1998;92:967–971.

81. Salazar H, Godwin AK, Daly MB et al. Microscopic benign and invasive malignant neoplasms and a cancer-prone phenotype in prophylactic oophorectomies. J Natl Cancer Inst 1996;88:1790–1791.

82. Stratton JF, Buckley CH, Lowe D et al. Comparison of prophylactic oophorectomy specimens from carriers and noncarriers of a BRCA1 or BRCA2 gene mutation. United Kingdom Coordinating Committee on Cancer Research (UKCCCR) Familial Ovarian Cancer Study Group. J Natl Cancer Inst 1999;91:626–628.

83. Barakat RR, Federici MG, Saigo PE et al. Absence of premalignant histologic, molecular, or cell biologic alterations in prophylactic oophorectomy specimens from BRCA1 heterozygotes. Cancer 2000;89:383–390.

84. Pothuri B, Leitao M, Barakat RR et al. Genetic analysis of ovarian carcinoma histogenesis [abstract]. Gynecol Oncol 2001;80:277.

85. Steiner CA, Powe NR, Anderson GF et al. Technology coverage decisions by health care plans and considerations by medical directors. Med Care 1997;35:472–489.

86. Schoonmaker MM, Bernhardt BA, Holtzman NA. Factors influencing health insurers' decisions to cover new genetic technologies. Int J Technol Assess Health Care 2000;16:178–189.

87. Lynch HT, Severin MJ, Mooney MJ et al. Insurance adjudication favoring prophylactic surgery in hereditary breast-ovarian cancer syndrome. Gynecol Oncol 1995;57:23–26.

88. Kuerer HM, Hwang ES, Anthony JP et al. Current national health insurance coverage policies for breast and ovarian cancer prophylactic surgery. Ann Surg Oncol 2000;7:325–332.

89. Kauff ND, Scheuer L, Robson ME et al. Insurance reimbursement for risk-reducing mastectomy and oophorectomy in women with BRCA1 or BRCA2 mutations. Genet Med 2001;3:422–425.

90. Meiser B, Butow P, Barratt A et al. Attitudes toward prophylactic oophorectomy and screening utilization in women at increased risk of developing hereditary breast/ovarian cancer. Gynecol Oncol 1999;75:122–129.

91. Hurley KE, Miller SM, Costalas JW et al. Anxiety/uncertainty reduction as a motivation for interest in prophylactic oophorectomy in women with a family history of ovarian cancer. J Womens Health Gend Based Med 2001;10:189–199.

92. Hallowell N. A qualitative study of the information needs of high-risk women undergoing prophylactic oophorectomy. Psychooncology 2000;9:486–495.

93. Meiser B, Tiller K, Gleeson MA et al. Psychological impact of prophylactic oophorectomy in women at increased risk for ovarian cancer. Psychooncology 2000;9:496–503.

94. Fry A, Busby-Earle C, Rush R et al. Prophylactic oophorectomy versus screening: psychosocial outcomes in women at increased risk of ovarian cancer. Psychooncology 2001;10:231–241.

95. Tiller K, Meiser B, Butow P et al. Psychological impact of prophylactic oophorectomy in women at increased risk of developing ovarian cancer: a prospective study. Gynecol Oncol 2002;86:212–219.

Chapter 14

Colon Cancer Screening: The Potential Role of Virtual Colonoscopy

Abraham H. Dachman

Seth N. Glick

Hiroyuki Yoshida

Colorectal cancer is the second most common cause of cancer deaths in the United States. Compliance of the population with current screening strategies is poor; thus, the emergence of a new structural examination of the entire colon has attracted the attention of patients and physicians alike. Virtual colonoscopy (also called computed tomographic [CT] colonography) has emerged as a viable alternate test for examining the colon for polyps and masses. The test typically involves supine and prone CT of the cleansed colon, after insufflation of the colon with air or carbon dioxide to patient tolerance, interpreted with specialized software using both two-dimensional and endoluminal three-dimensional images. The academic community has not yet endorsed virtual colonoscopy for mass population screening for colon cancer because of the lack of convincing multicenter trials in a screening setting. Yet, the data to date have been sufficiently convincing to spur academic centers and several community CT screening centers to offer examination for colon cancer screening. Application of the virtual colonoscopy for patients who have undergone an incomplete colonoscopy or who cannot undergo conventional colonoscopy is less controversial. In the setting of an incomplete colonoscopy, the study of choice is often virtual colonoscopy. Nevertheless, the application of this new test for colon cancer screening is a most engaging and potentially powerful application. This essay focuses on the rationale of colon cancer screening and on a comparison of various strategies, including virtual colonoscopy.

INCIDENCE

On the basis of data from the American Cancer Society, approximately 135,400 new cases of colorectal cancer and 56,700 deaths are expected per year. Although the overall incidence of colorectal cancer declined by 9.1% and the mortality declined by 22.6% between 1973 and 1996, it remains the second leading cause of cancer death for men and women. The risk increases with age; in 60- to 64-year-olds, the incidence is 10 times that of 40- to 44-year olds.[1] Both men and women have a 2.45% lifetime risk of colorectal cancer, although the age-adjusted incidence rates are significantly higher in men (51.1. per 100,000) than in women (36.2 per 100,000).

RISK FACTORS

A family history of colorectal cancer in a first-degree relative or a personal history of cancer or polyps, inflammatory bowel disease, or a hereditary syndrome increases the risk of disease. Certain personal habits, such as high fat intake, obesity and inactivity, and consumption of alcohol or red meat are also associated with a higher risk. The role of cigarette smoking is controversial.

RATIONALE FOR COLON CANCER SCREENING

Most, but not all, adenocarcinomas of the colon and rectum are believed to arise in benign adenomatous polyps. This is known as the "adenoma-carcinoma sequence," which was popularized by Day and Morson[2] in the late 1970s. The theory is that of an orderly and temporally consistent progression from normal mucosa to advanced carcinoma.

The prevalence of small, benign adenomas increases with the age of the patient. Some of these adenomas progress and develop varying degrees of cellular atypia or dysplasia. The frequency of dysplasia increased markedly with an increase in the size of the polyp, particularly for those larger than 1 cm. Fewer than 1% of polyps smaller than 1 cm are malignant. Furthermore, a direct correlation has been shown between growth and the probability that the neoplasm harbors malignant foci. This theory could not be directly proved; however, the circumstantial evidence was convincing. Evidence included several observations, including the failure to identify small (<5 mm) pure carcinomas, as well as the combination of benign and malignant elements in adenomatous polyps, with the frequency of associated cancer related to polyp size. Two corollaries to the adenoma-carcinoma sequence are (1) that most colorectal cancers arise in this manner and (2) that the time required for such progression is slow, approximately 10 years or longer. The former was based on the rarity of small carcinomas without benign components, and the latter was extrapolated from demographic data in which the age prevalence for carcinoma rises significantly approximately 10 years after the adenoma prevalence rate sharply increases. This model of colorectal carcinogenesis became generally accepted in the scientific community.

Research in the past decade has accelerated in the study of the genetic factors associated with adenocarcinoma pathogenesis. Most experts estimate that 60% of colorectal cancers are sporadic, 10%–30% are familial, and 5%–10% are associated with hereditary syndromes. The mechanism of pathogenesis included genetic mutations in oncogenes and tumor suppressor genes, such as *APC, p53,* and *SMAD4*.[3-6] The well-known familial adenomatous polyposis is associated with a mutation in the *APC* gene in most patients. In the hereditary nonpolyposis colorectal cancer syndromes, there is a defect in a DNA mismatch repair gene or "caretaker gene."[7]

THE EVOLUTION OF COLON CANCER SCREENING

Given the general acceptance of the adenoma-carcinoma sequence, it is reasonable to assume that, in theory, the early removal of all adenomas should effectively prevent colorectal cancer and eliminate death from this disease. Nevertheless, there were no concentrated efforts to promote any form of screening in the asymptomatic population. This was related to lack of sufficient information on the epidemiology of the disease as well as to lack of agreement pertaining to requisites for screening recommendations.

Existing screening proposals were predominantly centered on cancer detection rather than on benign precursor polyps. It was generally believed that most cancers (> 75%) arose in the distal colon within reach of the flexible sigmoidoscope. Initially screening consisted of a digital rectal examination and, possibly, a rigid sigmoidoscopy or stool testing for occult blood. Even the latter was performed at the time of rectal examination rather than the current more systematic and controlled process. With the addition of flexible sigmoidoscopy, the focus was predominately on the left side of the colon. However, over the next 15–20 years, numerous studies indicated that colorectal cancers and adenomas were more uniformly distributed throughout the colon. These relatively limited screening strategies were not widely adopted. A lack of appreciation and acceptance of the magnitude of an individual's risk and lack of confidence in the effectiveness of screening tests by both patient and primary caregivers were probably major factors. Reimbursement concerns, inconvenience, and the actual test experiences were certainly other factors. In addition to the patient-physician–related factor, policy makers for public health recommendations had specific requirements that had to be met before they endorsed any screening. Considerations such as the cost of mass screening policy implementation, the evaluation and follow-up of false-positive results (including causing unnecessary anxiety for the patient), and the morbidity of invasive follow-up must be calculated. Thus, the decision to advocate screening depends on proof that screening tests and follow-up treatment are effective in reducing morbidity and mortality from a major health care burden and, in addition, meet defined standards of cost-effectiveness. Successful screening requires proof of effectiveness, advocacy by influential groups and providers, availability and access to screening tests, and acceptance by the target population. The last factor is greatly affected by an individual's level of health care motivation and the inconvenience and discomfort of undergoing a screening test, and it may play an important role in the utilization of virtual colonoscopy as a screening tool.

In spite of the acceptance of the adenoma-carcinoma sequence, convincing scientific evidence for screening effectiveness (i.e., that it reduces mortality) did not exist. At the time, the primary screening method for the entire colon was the fecal occult blood test repeated at regular intervals, usually annually. The measure of a truly cost-effective screening test for detecting cancer should show that when cancer is found in asymptomatic individuals, any apparent increase in length of survival is not due to earlier diagnosis (lead time bias) or any shift toward early stage disease is not a function of finding indolent cancers (length time bias). Organizations interested in validating screening procedures imposed strict criteria to determine the scientific studies. The benchmark was the prospective, blinded, randomized, controlled trial. However, the retrospective case-control study was deemed to be a suitable alternative.

In 1992, the first study supporting the effectiveness of colorectal screening was published by Selby et al.[8] This case-control study showed that individuals who had undergone rigid sigmoidoscopy had a reduced odds ratio for the probability of developing fatal cancer within the reach of the sigmoidoscope. The investigators found no difference in screening exposure in those with fatal cancer proximally. It was unclear from the study exactly how such screening produced its effect in the distal colon because no cured cancers were identified in the group that did not have fatal rectal cancer.

Later, in 1993, a randomized trial demonstrated colorectal cancer mortality reduction through screening with fecal occult blood testing.[9] The presumed mechanism of action was a shift in the proportion of earlier stage cancers and, in particular, a marked reduction in the percentage with metastatic disease at diagnosis. The United States Preventative Services Task Force was the first major panel to incorporate the findings of these studies, which supported screening with either sigmoidoscopy or fecal occult blood testing. In 1993, the findings of the multi-institutional National Polyp Study were published.[10] This study assessed the outcome after the surveillance of individuals who had had adenomatous polyps removed at entry. The observed cancer incidence was markedly reduced from the incidences of three published reference groups. Although impressive, this still finding did not demonstrate mortality reduction.

In 1994, a multi-disciplinary panel of experts was convened by the Agency for Health Care Policy and Research to develop recommendations for colorectal cancer screening. Five important conceptual innovations resulted from their proceedings. The first was the relaxation of the stringent evidence-based criteria. Instead of directly linking a specific modality to the existing evidence for screening, it was accepted that if the early detection of cancer reduces mortality, any procedure that reliably detects colon cancer could be assumed to be effective as well. This opened the door to the second major change, the consideration of the double-contrast barium enema and colonoscopy for the general population. Integral to the proposal of such increasingly invasive and expensive procedures was the understanding that screening is not intended to be a one-time event but rather a long-term program of repeated application. If such tests are more thorough and can be performed at longer intervals, their cost and risk are minimized. Thus, this panel became the first to incorporate decision analysis and modeling to assess the overall impact, both favorable and unfavorable, of different screening strategies. As part of this process, cost-effectiveness analysis was also included. It was determined in a study by the Office of Technology Assessment that all the approaches being reviewed were more cost-effective than accepted benchmarks for other medical interventions.

The fourth advance was the refinement of the understanding of cancer risk categories, adding a group termed "above average risk" to the traditional stratification of high and low risk. Decisions regarding who to screen, how to screen, and how often to screen tend to be based on a complex integration of the magnitude of risk, the natural history of the disease, and the diverse characteristics of the screening test or tests. Historically, any form of screening, especially with more aggressive strategies, had been reserved for high-risk groups to limit complication risk and to make resource utilization more efficient. However, it was also appreciated that a high preponderance of the overall tumor burden came from average or above-average risk patients. The latter category included those with a previous history of cancer or large adenoma (especially with more advanced pathology) and those with a first-degree family history, with the relative being under the age of 55 years at diagnosis. Recognizing that risk represented a gradual continuum based on age and other individual variables, the screening recommendations that were proposed were tailored based on the level of screening. Thus, the fifth and most significant conclusion of the panel was the development of recommendations that included a menu of screening options. This was based on the knowledge that all the screening strategies should work to varying degrees and that overall participation in screening could be augmented by enhancing availability and the potential for compliance. Those guidelines were published in 1997 (Table 14.1).[11] Closely following, and to some degree

TABLE 14.1 1997 ACS Screening Guidelines for Patients with Average or Moderate Risk for Colorectal Cancer

Average Risk Patients

Asymptomatic, > 50 years of age:

Initial examination:

1. FOBT and flexible sigmoidoscopy with DRE

OR

2. TCE with DRE (colonoscopy or DCBE)

Follow-up:

1. FOBT yearly, flexible sigmoidoscopy every 5 years

OR

2. Colonoscopy every 10 years or DCBE every 5–10 years

Moderate-Risk Patients

Single small polyp:

Initial examination: colonoscopy
Follow-up: TCE within 3 years from polypectomy,
if normal, return to average-risk guidelines

Large polyp or multiple small polyps:

Initial examination: colonoscopy
Follow-up: TCE within 3 years from polypectomy
if normal, TCE every 5 years

After CRC resection:

Initial examination: TCE within 1 year
Follow-up: TCE in 3 years;
if normal, TCE every 5 years

CRC or adenomatous polyps in first-degree relative:

Initial examination: TCE at age 40

OR

10 years before family case
Follow-up: TCE every 5 years

Abbreviations: CRC, colorectal cancer; DCBE, double-contrast barium enema; DRE, digital rectal examination; FOBT, fecal occult blood test; TCE, total colon examination.
Adapted from Byers et al, CA Cancer J Clin 1997;47:154–160.[12]

influenced by, the Agency for Health Care Policy and Research guidelines were colorectal cancer screening recommendations put forth by the American Cancer Society that were almost identical.[12] At the same time, successful legislative initiatives through which Medicare began providing coverage for the proposed screening modalities were approved. The reimbursement did not include colonoscopy for those at average risk, but this coverage was added in 2001.

Over the past several years, increased media attention to screening—through reports on the subject as well as transmission of the findings of new studies—has provided greater visibility and interest. The National Colorectal Cancer Roundtable, a consortium of medical societies, advocacy groups, government-sponsored organizations, and motivated individuals, was formed to promote awareness and involvement in screening. Research projects have been ongoing to improve compliance, provide a better understanding of the potential implications of the various screening strategies, and increase the knowledge base concerning the epidemiology and genesis of this disease.

CURRENTLY ACCEPTED SCREENING PRACTICES

There currently are several proposed screening choices, including fecal occult blood testing, flexible sigmoidoscopy, or a combination of the two; double-contrast barium enema; and colonoscopy. None of these choices are ideal, and all have strengths and limitations. The fecal occult blood test is inexpensive and amenable for mass screening; however, it is insensitive to adenomatous polyps, and a single application has only fair sensitivity for colorectal cancer, necessitating strict adherence to repeat testing. Patient compliance in placing a stool sample on a card is mediocre and hinders its use. Use by physicians during rectal examination is performed is ideal for processing the specimen and for confirming that proper dietary restrictions that may cause false-positive results were properly observed.

Flexible sigmoidoscopy visualizes less than half of the bowel, but performing colonoscopy after an adenoma is detected improves the sensitivity to approximately 75% of the significant neoplasms. Although it is much safer and less expensive than colonoscopy and does not require sedation, such a regimen overlooks a significant portion of lesions because of their location in the proximal colon. Although in theory the addition of annual fecal occult blood testing should partially compensate for this limitation, there is no evidence whether, or to what degree, the benefits are additive. Furthermore, any improvement is directed toward early cancer detection rather than toward disease prevention.

Because it visualizes the mucosa directly, colonoscopy is the definitive procedure for evaluating the colon and can be both diagnostic and therapeutic. Although the risks of perforation and hemorrhage are relatively low, they are much higher than with any of the screening alternatives. Unlike sigmoidoscopy, colonoscopy also requires more intensive preparation, which many patients find unpleasant. The completion rate for colonoscopy varies from 75% to 99%, depending on the examiner's skills, anatomic variations, prior abdominal surgery, and the patient's reaction to the anesthesia. In either endoscopic scenario, whether sigmoidoscopy or colonoscopy, there may be a significant number of individuals who are averse to having a tube placed in their bowel, and they may be apprehensive regarding the discomfort they may experience. The sensitivity is about 95% for 1-cm lesions.[13] In one study (albeit a small cohort), 6% of 1-cm polyps were missed based on a second colonoscopy performed at the same time as the first.[14]

Double-contrast barium enema is a relatively inexpensive test (equivalent to sigmoidoscopy) and is the safest of all the structural screening examinations. Like colonoscopy, thorough colonic preparation is a requirement, and the test itself, although usually associated with minimal-to-mild discomfort, may be perceived as being painful. A preponderance of literature consisting of observational studies suggests that this test can detect 80%–90% of the large adenomas and 85%–95% of cancers.[15] However, a randomized controlled trial comparing double-contrast barium enema with colonoscopy reported a detection rate of only half the large adenomas.[15] Although this is only a single study and there are a number of limitations, this study has been used to advocate colonoscopy over the double-contrast barium enema. Another important factor in the decline of use of the barium enema is the waning volume of requests and interest of radiologists who perform this procedure. The low reimbursement of the barium enema and its labor-intensive nature have also been deterrents. Radiologists' skills in performing barium enemas have greatly deteriorated because of the decreased number of studies performed as a result of increased utilization of colonoscopy.

The American Cancer Society recommends that patients 50 years of age or older have an initial examination, including a digital rectal examination, fecal occult blood test, and flexible sigmoidoscopy, or a digital rectal examination and a total colon examination. The total colon examination may consist of colonoscopy or a double-contrast barium enema. Follow-up should consist of a fecal occult blood test every year plus a flexible sigmoidoscopy every 5 years, or colonoscopy every 10 years, or a double-contrast barium enema every 5–10 years (Table 14.1).

CT COLONOGRAPHY AND COLON CANCER SCREENING

It is in this context that CT colonography has emerged. The trend in colonic evaluation, particularly for screening, has shifted to total colonic evaluation. All total colonic examinations require a full preparation. In this regard, current research in minimal preparation regimens combined with stool opacification and electronic subtraction may give virtual colonoscopy a distinct advantage from the patient's perspective. Preliminary research in this area is encouraging.[16] The sensitivity of the examinations for cancer, polyps, and flat lesions needs to be determined more definitively, but data to date strongly indicate that in the hands of experts, virtual colonoscopy is as good as or better than the best sensitivity data for barium enema, and the sensitivity for polyps $\gtrsim$ 1 cm is 70%–90%, with by-patient sensitivity in the 70%–100% range. If the higher percentages persist in multicenter trials, the next critical question is whether they be extrapolated to general clinical practice. Some data indicate that the learning curve for virtual colonoscopy is significant and that the sensitivity and specificity of the test in general practice will not be a good as in a research setting. In this regard, research in computer-aided diagnosis and the development of better software for the interpretation of virtual colonoscopic examinations may raise the sensitivity and specificity of the examination for the general practice setting while maintaining or decreasing the interpretation time.[17] Test sensitivity, charge for the examination, and patient acceptance will all affect the ultimate recommendation as to how frequently the examination should be repeated in the screening setting, in contrast to conventional colonoscopy and barium enema.

OBSTRUCTING CANCER AND INCOMPLETE COLONOSCOPY

CT colonography has already achieved a role in the evaluation of patients with incomplete colonoscopy (Fig. 14.1). The patient who is already prepared and has undergone an incomplete colonoscopy can be accommodated for a same-day, unscheduled CT colonography examination, thus eliminating the need for a return visit and repeat preparation. Morrin et al[18] studied 40 patients with the use of CT within 2 hours of an incomplete colonoscopy; the investigators showed the portion of the colon that was not visualized by endoscopy in more than 90% of patients and found a probable cause for the obstruction in 74% of patients. Furthermore, patients preferred CT to colonoscopy. Fenlon et al[19] showed that CT depicted all 29 occlusive carcinomas and also fully evaluated the proximal colon in 26/29 patients. CT also demonstrated two synchronous cancers and 24 polyps in the proximal colon, many of which were subsequently confirmed by endoscopy, although none could be palpated at surgery. Identification of the synchronous cancers in two patients altered the surgical plan. CT was also more accurate than colonoscopy in localizing the cancers, which may be helpful in preoperative planning.

Royster et al[20] reported a 100% sensitivity in detecting masses $\gtrsim$ 2 cm on CT colonography. Several investigators have shown the utility and effectiveness of virtual colonoscopy in imaging of the colon proximal to obstructing lesions. Macari[21] reported on 20 patients with incomplete colonoscopy, 10 of whom had also undergone barium enema. CT found two lesions in the portion of the colon not seen by colonoscopy; these results were confirmed by barium enema. The other eight results were normal on both CT and barium enema.

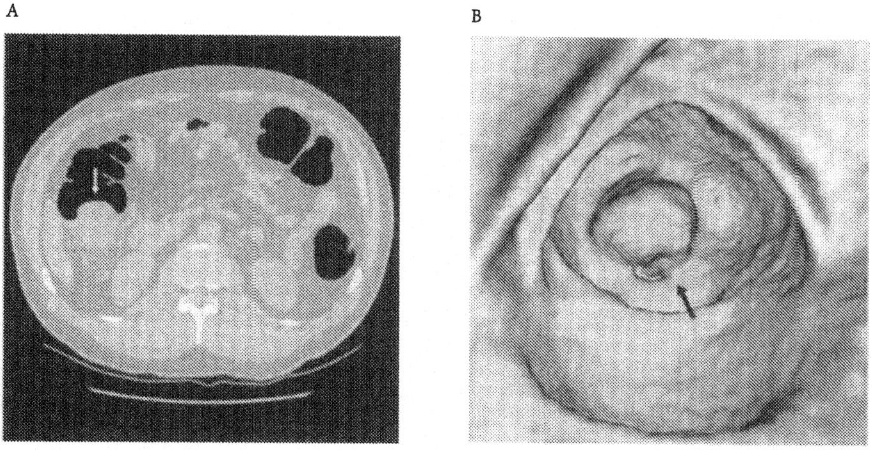

FIGURE 14.1 Right-sided adenocarcinoma. Colonoscopy showed a right-sided mass, which prevented evaluation of the cecum. A, Supine axial image from a virtual colonoscopy showing the mass (*arrow*). B, Endoluminal perspective view shows the same mass.

Neri et al[22] studied 34 patients with CT, both before and after intravenous contrast injection. In 29 patients, surgery showed 30 cancers (including three synchronous cancers). Colonoscopy missed 10 cancers and three synchronous cancers, all of which were detected with CT. The use of intravenous contrast also permitted a definitive search for metastatic disease with a single CT examination.

WHAT SIZE POLYPS SHOULD WE DETECT AND CAN WE DETECT FLAT LESIONS?

Both polyp size and morphology affect the incidence of carcinoma within a polyp. Only 1% of polyps smaller than 1 cm are malignant, whereas about 46% of polyps greater than 2 cm are malignant. Lesions classified histologically as villous have a higher incidence than tubular lesions of carcinoma.

Flat lesions are of concern because they are up to 10 times more likely to harbor high-grade dysplasia.[23] The incidence of flat lesions varies between 8.5% and 40%,[23-26] and in one study, flat and depressed lesions accounted for more than half the early cancerous lesions detected. Data from larger series suggest that the higher frequency of dysplasia is primarily in polyps larger than 1 cm.[24-27] Flat adenomas commonly occur in patients with hereditary nonpolyposis syndrome.[28] In studying the ability of virtual colonoscopy to detect flat lesions, Fidler et al[29] found 22 flat lesions as seen by either conventional colonoscopy or virtual colonoscopy. The sensitivities for detecting all flat lesions and for flat adenomas by each of three independent readers were 43% and 100%, 65% and

100%, and 15% and 13%, respectively. A double reading improved the detection rate to 68% and 100% for all lesions and adenomas, respectively. The essential point is that with proper training, virtual colonoscopy can detect flat adenomas, but this skill requires a careful reading of the axial images on soft tissue windows. This has important implications regarding the method of interpretation and the need for adequate training in a primary two-dimensional reading method.

The decision as to what size lesion to detect is not based solely on the incidence of carcinoma in that lesion. The lesion size that is deemed significant will affect the time between recommended follow-up examination and thus affect the cost-effectiveness of virtual colonoscopy as a screening test for cancer. The controversy is in regard to 5- to 9.9-mm lesions. Most experts agree that lesions less than 5 mm can be ignored because of the low incidence of adenomas in this group and because of the low incidence of carcinoma in 5-mm adenomas. We should recognize that data regarding size of a polyp is often based on visual estimates of the colonoscopist, and only precise measurements using caliper on a fresh gross pathological specimen or use of special calipers placed through an endoscope by the endoscopist will yield accurate measurements. Similarly, the radiologist's measurements are subject to inaccuracy because of the limitation of the scan and inter- and intraobserver variability. Because there is no consensus regarding 5- to 9.9-mm lesions, my recommendation is to report lesions in this range and specify that they are likely to be hyperplastic or benign on the basis of size criteria if they are smaller than 7 mm.

HOW GOOD IS VIRTUAL COLONOSCOPY AT DETECTING CANCER AND POLYPS?

Several articles have attempted to summarize the diagnostic accuracy of virtual colonoscopy, and some investigators have presented a meta-analysis combining data from all published trials. Statisticians at the University of Chicago have argued that a true meta-analysis is not valid because of the tremendous variations in inclusion criteria, the technical parameters of scanning, and the reading techniques between various trials. For this reason, I prefer to summarize the literature. Table 14.2 shows the results of most key publications in the peer-reviewed literature. Inter- and intraobserver variation in reading is also being studied as a function of reading method.[30]

It is important to differentiate between sensitivity by patient and by polyp. In patient assignment to "no need for colonoscopy" versus "need for colonoscopy," only the by-patient results are relevant. The two largest series had a sensitivity of 100% for polyps 1 cm or larger (Fig. 14.2), and most trials had sensitivities ranging from 75% to 100%, with specificities ranging from 74% to 96% (Table 14.2). The retrospective American College of Radiology Imaging Network trial (which included CT performed between 1997 and 1999) had an average sensitivity (as presented at the Radiological Society of North America) of just less than 70%. Results of this trial are in press and will likely underscore the importance of reader

TABLE 14.2 Diagnostic Performance of Virtual Colonoscopy

Source (Total Number of Patients)	Performance of Virtual Colonoscopy: By Patient[a]	By polyp[ab]
Yee et al[31] (*N* = 300)	(*N* = 49 patients) Sensitivity = 100% PPV = 81%	Sensitivity = 93%
Hara et al[32] (*N* = 237)	(*N* = 5 patients) Sensitivity = 100% Specificity = 90%	Sensitivity = 89%[c]
Fletcher et al[33] (*N* = 180)	(*N* = 96 patients) Sensitivity = 85.4% Specificity = 93%	Sensitivity = 75.2%
Fenlon et al[34] (*N* = 100)	(*N* = 15 patients)[d] Sensitivity = 96% Specificity = 96%	(22 polyps) Sensitivity = 91%
Hopper et al[35] (*N* = 100)	Sensitivity = n/a PPV = 92% for ≥ 5 mm	(9 polyps) Sensitivity = 100%
Spinzi et al[36] (*N* = 96)	(*N* = 100 patients)[e] Sensitivity = 80% Specificity = 100%	(13 polyps) Sensitivity = 61.5%
Hara et al[37] (*N* = 70)	Sensitivity = 75% Specificity = 90%	(15 adenomas)[f] Sensitivity = 67-73% (two observers)
Mendelson et al[38] (*N* = 53)[g]	N/A	(11 polyps) Sensitivity = 73%
Pescatore et al[39] (*N* = 50)[h]	(*N* = unknown) Sensitivity = 62%, 37% (two observers) Specificity = 74%	(11 polyps) PPV = 21-31% Sensitivity = 62% NPV = 68-91%
Rex et al[40] (*N* = 46)	(*N* = 10 polyps) Sensitivity = 80% Specificity = 89%	(14 polyps) Sensitivity = 50%
Dachman et al[41] (*N* = 44)	Sensitivity = 83% Specificity = 100%	(6 polyps) Sensitivity = 83%
Macari et al[42] (*N* = 42)	(*N* = 1 patient) Sensitivity = 100% Specificity = 100%	(1 polyp) Sensitivity = 100%
Kay et al[43] (*N* = 38)	(*N* = unknown) Sensitivity = 90% Specificity = 82% (11 polyps ≥ 1 cm)	(11 polyps) Sensitivity = 91%
Morrin et al[18, 44] (*N* = 81)	(*N* = 6 patients) Sensitivity = 86% Specificity = 100%	(12 polyps) Sensitivity = 91%
Royster et al[20,45] (*N* = 20)	(*N* = unknown) Sensitivity = 100%	(22 polyps) Sensitivity = 100%

Abbreviations: CT, computed tomography; n/a, not applicable; PPV, positive predictive value; NPV, negative predictive value.
[a]Number of polyps or patients with polyps shown, if known.
[b]Large masses (≥ 3 cm) and occlusive carcinomas excluded unless indicated.
[c]For single-detector CT (multidetector had an 80% sensitivity for polyps > 1 cm and a patient specificity of 93%).
[d]Personal communication.
[e]Additional data by personal communication.
[f]Data only by adenoma, not for all polyps regardless of histology.
[g]Only patients without intravenous contrast and only polyps 1-2 cm shown.
[h]Includes 2 obstructing carcinomas.

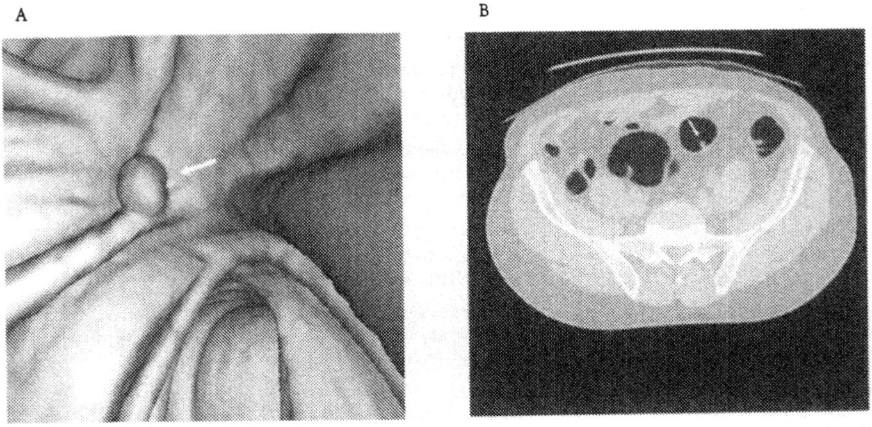

FIGURE 14.2 Adenomatous polyp. A 15-mm polyp is well-seen in-between folds on the three-dimensional endoluminal view (A). Corresponding prone axial image shows the polyp (*arrow*) on the posterior, nondependent surface of a redundant transverse colon dipping into the patient's pelvis.

experience, scan quality control, and changes in technique over the past several years. The by-polyp sensitivity was 90% and 89% in the two largest trials but ranges between 50% and 100% in the literature. However, most recent trials have sensitivities between 73% and 100%.

WHO SHOULD GET A VIRTUAL COLONOSCOPY?

Although several independent CT screening centers around the country have started to offer virtual colonoscopy for colon cancer screening of average-risk or even above-average-risk individuals, general mass screening is premature. The steep learning curve has been sufficiently documented and the examination performance for a screening setting is not well studied, such that only those with extensive research experience in virtual colonoscopy should offer to interpret the examination. Thus, accuracy of interpretation and interpretation time are factors that affect the ability to offer this examination. Recently, our interpretation time has ranged from 5–15 minutes, with only a few examinations requiring a longer interpretation time. However, inexperienced radiologists usually require 15–30 minutes to interpret an examination. There are sufficient data to suggest that virtual colonoscopy is the preferred study for patients who have had an incomplete colonoscopy or who cannot undergo colonoscopy. A virtual colonoscopy performed on the same day as an incomplete colonoscopy has the advantage of not requiring a second preparation. Some retained fluid may have been removed during the colonoscopy, and the patient does not need to spend a second day in the clinic. Colonoscopy may be incomplete as the result of hypotension secondary to the sedation, adhesions from prior surgery, excessive colonic tortuosity, or unusual anatomy, or it may be the result of the skill level of the colonoscopist.

At The University of Chicago, we ask that all patients to also undergo fecal occult blood testing and be informed regarding the pros and cons of virtual colonoscopy before being scheduled. We also require a same-day flexible sigmoidoscopy, performed immediately after the virtual colonoscopy. In doing so, we use an accepted screening strategy recommended by the American Cancer Society and supplement it with a total colonic structural examination in the form of a virtual colonoscopy.

RECENT ADVANCES AND RESEARCH ISSUES

Low-fiber diet preparations are being combined with mild colon cleansing for greater patient acceptance of the preparation regimen. This may be combined with barium or iodinated oral contrast to achieve stool opacification. The stool opacification strategy is combined with a computer-generated "electronic subtraction" of the high-density contrast stool combination, leaving an electronically cleansed colon. In some clinical trials commercially available software is now being used that combines the electronically cleansed colon with a primary three-dimensional interpretation with two-dimensional problem solving. If successful, this strategy would give virtual colonoscopy a significant advantage over conventional colonoscopy in terms of patient acceptance.

To improve the speed and accuracy of interpretation, investigators have developed computer-aided diagnosis programs. These software programs automatically segment the colon from the CT data, analyze the mucosal-gas interface, and perform a shape-based analysis of the mucosal surface to find polyps (Fig. 14.3). In our preliminary trials, we have found the program 100% sensitive for 1-cm polyps, and we have obtained only 2.5 false-positive results per case (case = supine or prone scan).

SUMMARY

Virtual colonoscopy is emerging as an exciting new test to evaluate the colon for polyps and masses. It is probably the best for patients who cannot undergo conventional colonoscopy or have had an incomplete colonoscopy. It will likely be incorporated into a menu of options for colon cancer screening.

ACKNOWLEDGMENTS

The authors thank Angela Green for manuscript preparation. This study was supported in part by a grant from the University of Chicago Cancer Research Center and the Cancer Research Foundation of America.

REFERENCES

1. Ries LAG, Kosary CL, Hankey BF et al. SEER Cancer statistics review, 1973-1996. NIH publication mo. 99-2789. Bethesda, MD: National Cancer Institute, 1999.
2. Day DW, Morson BC. The adenoma-carcinoma sequence. In: Basil C. Morson, ed. The Pathogenesis of Colorectal Cancer. Philadelphia, London, Toronto: WB Saunders, 1978: 58–71.
3. Vogelstein B, Fearon ER, Hamilton SR et al. Genetic alterations during colorectal-tumor development. N Engl J Med 1988;319: 525–532.
4. Fearon ER, Vogelstein B. A genetic model for colorectal tumorigenesis. Cell 1990;61:759–767.
5. Takaku K, Oshima M, Miyoshi H et al. Intestinal tumorigenesis in compound mutant mice of both Dpc4(Smad4) and Apc genes. Cell 1998;92:645–656.
6. Stevenson GW. Colorectal cancer imaging: a challenge for radiologists. Radiology 2000;214:615–621.
7. Kinzler KW, Vogelstein B. Lessons from hereditary colorectal cancer. Cell 1996;87:159–170.
8. Selby JV, Friedman GD, Quesenberry CP et al. A case-control study of screening sigmoidoscopy and mortality from colorectal cancer. N Engl J Med 1992;326:653–657.
9. Mandel JS, Bond JH, Church TR et al. Reducing mortality from colorectal cancer by screening for fecal occult blood. N Engl J Med 1993;328:1365–1371.
10. Winawer SJ, Zauber AG, Ho MN et al. Prevention of colorectal cancer by colonoscopic polypectomy. N Engl J Med 1993;329:1977–1981.
11. Winawer SJ, Fletcher RH, Miller L et al. Colorectal cancer screening: clinical guidelines and rationale. Gastroenterology 1997;112:594–642.
12. Byers T, Levin B, Rothenberger D et al. American Cancer Society guidelines for screening and surveillance for early detection of colorectal polyps and cancer: update 1997. CA Cancer J Clin 1997;47:154–160.
13. Hixson LJ, Fennerty MB, Sampliner RE et al. Prospective blinded trial of the colonoscopic miss-rate of large colorectal polyps. Gastrointest Endosc 1991;37:125–127.
14. Rex DK, Cutler CS, Lemmel GT et al. Colonoscopic miss rates of adenomas determined by back-to-back colonoscopies. Gastroenterology 1997;112:24–28.
15. Glick S. Double-contrast barium enema for colorectal cancer screening: a review of the issues and a comparison with other screening alternatives. AJR Am J Roentgenol 2000;174:1529–1537.
16. Zalis ME, Hahn PF. Digital subtraction bowel cleansing in CT colonography. AJR Am J Roentgenol 2001;176:646–648.
17. Dachman AH. Diagnostic preference of virtual colonoscopy. Abdom Imaging 2002;27:260–267.
18. Morrin MM, Kruskal JB, Farrell RJ et al. Endoluminal CT colonography after an incomplete endoscopic colonoscopy. AJR Am J Roentgenol 1999;172:913–918.
19. Fenlon HM, MacEneaney DB, Nunes DP et al. Occlusive colon carcinoma: virtual colonoscopy in the preoperative evaluation of the proximal colon. Radiology 1999;210:423–428.
20. Royster AP, Fenlon HM, Clarke PD et al. CT colonoscopy of colorectal neoplasms: two dimensional and three dimensional virtual reality techniques with colonoscopic correlation. AJR Am J Roentgenol 1997;169:1237–1242.
21. Macari M, Berman P, Dicher M et al. Usefulness of CT colonography in patients with incomplete colonoscopy. AJR Am J Roentgenol 1999;173:561–564.
22. Neri E, Giusti P, Battolla L et al. Colorectal cancer: role of CT colonography in preoperative evaluation after incomplete colonoscopy. RSNA 2002;223:615–619.
23. Wobler R, Owen D. Flat adenomas of the colon. Hum Pathol 1991;35:685–692.

24. Wolber RA. Flat adenomas of the colon. Hum Pathol 1991;22:70–74.

25. Fujii T, Rembacken BJ, Dixon MF et al. Flat adenomas in the United Kingdom: are treatable cancers being missed? Endoscopy 1998;30:437–443.

26. Adachi M, Muto T, Morioka Y et al. Flat adenoma and flat mucosal carcinoma (IIIb type): a new precursor of colorectal carcinoma? Dis Colon Rectum 1988;31:236–243.

27. Rembacken BJ, Fujii T, Cairns A et al. Flat and depressed colonic neoplasms: a prospective study of 1000 colonoscopies in the UK. Lancet 2000;355:1211–1214.

28. Lynch HT, Smyrk TC, Watson P et al. Hereditary flat adenoma syndrome: a variant of familial adenomatous polyposis? Dis Colon Rectum 1992;35:411–421.

29. Fidler JL, Johnson CD, MacCarty RL et al. Detection of flat lesions in the colon with CT colonography. Abdom Imaging 2002;27:292–300.

30. McFarland EG, Brink JA, Pilgram TK et al. Spiral CT colonography: reader agreement and diagnostic performance with two- and three-dimensional image-display techniques. Radiology 2001;218:375–383.

31. Yee J. Akerkar GA, Hung RK et al. Colorectal neoplasia:performance characteristics of CT colonography for detection in 300 patients. Radiology 2001;219:685–692.

32. Hara AK, Johnson CD, MacCarty RL et al. CT colonography: single- versus multi-detector row imaging. Radiology 2001;219:461–465.

33. Fletcher JG, Johnson CD, MacCarty RL et al. CT colonoscopy: potential pitfalls and problem-solving techniques. AJR Am J Roentgenol 1999;172:1271–1278.

34. Fenlon HM, Nunes DP, Schroy PC III et al. A comparison of virtual and conventional colonoscopy for the detection of colorectal polyps. N Engl J Med 1999;341:1496–1503.

35. Hopper KD, Khandelwal M, Thompson C. CT colonoscopy: experience of 100 cases using volumetric rendering. Proc SPIE 2001;12:489–494.

36. Spinzi G, Belloni G, Martegani A et al. Computed tomographic colonography and conventional colonoscopy for colon diseases:a prospective, blinded study. Am J Gastroenterol 2001;96:394–400.

37. Hara AK, Johnson CD, Reed JE et al. Detection of colorectal polyps with CT colography: initial assessment of sensitivity and specificity. Radiology 1997;205:59–65.

38. Mendelson RM, Foster NM, Edwards JT et al. Virtual colonoscopy compared with conventional colonoscopy: a developing technology. Med J Aust 2000;173:472–475.

39. Pescatore P, Glucker T, Delarive J et al. Diagnostic accuracy and interobserver agreement of CT colonography (virtual colonoscopy). Gut 2000;47:126–130.

40. Rex DK, Cutler CS, Lemmel GT. Colonoscopic miss rates of adenomas determined by back-to-back colonoscopies. Gastroenterology 1997;112:24–28.

41. Dachman AH, Kuniyoshi JK, Boyle CM et al. CT colonography with three–dimensional problem solving for detection of colonic polyps. AJR Am J Roentgenol 1998;171:989–995.

42. Macari M, Milano A, Lavelle M et al. Comparison of time-efficient CT colonography with two– and three–dimensional colonic evaluation for detecting colorectal polyps. AJR Am J Roentgenol 2000;174:1543–1549.

43. Kay CL, Kulling D, Hawes RH et al. Virtual endoscopy—comparison with colonoscopy in the detection of space-occupying lesions of the colon. Endoscopy 2000;32:226–232.

44. Morrin M, Farrell RJ, Kruskal JB et al. Utility of intravenously administered contrast material at CT colonography. Radiology 2000;217:765–771.

45. Royster AP, Fenlon HM, Clarke PD et al. CT colonoscopy of colorectal neoplasms: two-dimensional and three-dimensional virtual-reality techniques with colonoscopic correlation. AJR Am J Roentgenol 1997;169:1237–1242.

Chapter 15

Laparoscopic Colectomy: An Evolving Art

Warren E. Enker

James C. Rosser, Jr.

Earl Noyan

Minimally invasive or laparoscopically assisted colectomy was first introduced in 1991.[1] A century of the advances leading up to the introduction of advanced laparoscopic surgery has been recently reviewed.[2] Despite the rapid development and acceptance of laparoscopic operations for benign colorectal diseases, laparoscopic surgery for cancer has developed slowly because of concern that the technique could adversely affect the risk or the patterns of recurrence. Several single-center reports have advocated the adoption of laparoscopic or laparoscopically assisted colectomy for cancer.[3] In order to study the cancer-related outcomes appropriately, as well as the short- and long-term morbidity, numerous prospective studies have been designed. In the United States, the largest of these is a multicenter trial of laparoscopic colectomy versus open colectomy for colonic cancer (Clinical Outcomes of Surgical Therapy [COST]). The necessary patients have been accrued to the study, and the results of this trial are anxiously awaited. Interim analyses to date have not shown that laparoscopic resections have been associated with any harm in the early years of this trial or in the early period of cancer follow-up.[4]

Questions exist regarding laparoscopic colectomy for cancer. Do laparoscopic surgeons who are performing a laparoscopic colectomy adhere to the principles of surgery for colorectal cancers or, in the name of completing the operation laparoscopically, is the cancer-related outcome ever compromised? In controlled trials, do enthusiasts of laparoscopic colectomy perform as good an anatomic resection of the mesentery for cancer in patients who are randomly assigned to undergo an open colectomy? Are port-site recurrences a real issue in patients undergoing curative resections? Do laparoscopic colectomies utilize or overutilize appropriate operating room resources? Can the surgeon in practice perform a sufficient number of laparoscopic colectomies to be initially credentialed and to remain credentialed over the ensuing years of practice? How is the older but experienced abdominal cancer surgeon, who may be laparoscopically naive, to be adequately and safely trained in advanced laparoscopic operations? How is the recently trained, laparoscopically well-versed surgeon with limited experience in performing colectomies for cancer to be trained and credentialed for cancer surgery? Are laparoscopic colectomies cost-effective in terms of total hospital cost and both physician and hospital reimbursement? Do recent advances in shortening length of stay truly reflect the advantages of minimally invasive surgery (MIS)? What impact do changes in management, such as early feeding, thoracic epidural analgesia, and use of opioid antagonists, have on the reduction of ileus in patients who undergo minimally invasive colectomies? If these changes are equally applied to open colectomy patients, how much sooner can the patients be discharged, and what becomes of the relative benefit of the laparoscopic approach in such an environment?

These and other questions need to be addressed by multicenter, randomized prospective trials if the true status of laparoscopic colorectal surgery for cancer is to be appreciated. The current status and the most widely accepted techniques of laparoscopic colectomy have been recently reviewed.[5] To date, limited progress in answering some of these questions has come from centers where surgeons who are committed to principles of cancer surgery have addressed the efficacy and the cancer-related safety of laparoscopic colectomy. In this article, we systematically review the progress that has been reported in the literature and address some of the progress in education, standardization, and technology that are increasingly important to progress in advanced laparoscopic surgery.

PRINCIPLES OF COLECTOMY FOR COLORECTAL CANCER

Standardized Operations and Surgical and Pathological Quality Assurance

In recent years, the benefits of multidisciplinary therapy for patients with cancer have become obvious. These benefits are often related to patient access to standardized and up-to-date therapy.[6] Nowhere has the importance of standardized operations and surgical and pathological quality assurance been proved more conclusively than in the operative treatment of rectal cancers. The importance of uninvolved—that is, cancer-free—circumferential margins and the resection of all regional disease has been proved repeatedly.[7-10] Recently, attempts to define surgical quality assurance and to document widespread surgeon variability and its impact on outcomes of treatment for rectal and colon cancer have been studied.[11] In a literature review under the auspices of the European Organization for Research and Treatment of Cancer, 122 reports were categorized according to recent definitions of evidence-based analyses, ranked from single-center observations and from multicenter randomized clinical trials. Subjects reviewed included the reported differences in local control and survival rates, factors of influence on local control and survival, long- and short-term morbidity, hospital- and surgeon-related factors, and training and quality assurance.

Local control varied from 1% to 30% and included data from both curative and noncurative operations. Lowest figures for local control were reported from single-center or single-surgeon studies rigorously adhering to standardized operations and ranged from 3.5% to 14%.[12,13]

Survival rates varied from 50% to 85% in patients with curative resections of rectal cancers and from 56% to 76% in those with colonic cancers. Overall survival rates were inversely correlated to local recurrence rates. Because of marked variation in outcomes by surgeon, the surgeons' opinions were considered to be an unreliable predictor of local control and survival.

Only the studies that have reported a standardized operation for rectal cancer have demonstrated optimal results in terms of local recurrence, survival, and optimal quality-of-life (QOL) outcomes. Correlation of surgical outcomes with pathological assessment of the resected specimen has offered both insight and the quality assurance that has eluded numerous investigators who have focused on surgical outcomes alone.[14]

Similarly, optimal outcomes have been reported by investigators that have maintained the principles of radical surgery for the colon, as well as for rectal cancers, even before the current era of adjuvant therapy.[15,16] The principles of radical resection for colon cancer have been described in detail elsewhere.[17-20] The overwhelming volume of surgery performed for colon cancer does not adhere faithfully to these principles. Nationwide, segmental resections, meaning resection of a length of bowel without regard for the anatomically defined resection of the mesentery (based on its total arterial blood supply), are the norm. Survival data from the Surveillance, Epidemiology and End Results group suggest 80%, 60%, and 35%–40% 5-year survival for Dukes A, B, and C tumors, respectively. In contrast, authors who report series of curative resection that adhere to the principles of anatomically defined mesenteric resections report 90%–95%, 85%–87%, and 66%–70% survivals for the same stages in curative resections, defined by the surgeon as leaving behind no grossly visible disease.[20] In advancing the technology from open resection to laparoscopic or laparoscopically assisted resection for colon and rectal cancers, the principles of anatomic resections for the colon and total mesorectal excision (TME) for the rectum need to be faithfully adopted.

As the field of advanced laparoscopic surgery unfolds, these two changes are occurring side by side. For open surgeons, standardization of the resection for colonic and, in particular, for rectal cancer has been implemented widely as a result of studies that have corroborated the initial single-center publications regarding TME.[7,8,10] In the Netherlands, under the auspices of the Dutch Colorectal Cancer Group, surgeons have been taught how to perform TME as part of a national trial, studying the role of radiation therapy and TME versus TME alone.[21] Training programs for standard surgery have also been implemented by the Stockholm Colorectal Cancer Study Group and have improved treatment outcome.[22] In Norway, this change in policy in which TME is used in the surgery for rectal cancer has been implemented nationwide, and recent reports have discussed the surgical quality assurance that has been achieved.[23] At major centers, surgeons who perform TME are more likely to be part of a specialty service, performing anatomically based resections for colonic cancers as well.

Based on this body of knowledge, surgeons in the United States, under the sponsorship of the American College of Surgeons, are learning how to perform standardized operations (e.g., TME) for rectal cancers, putting aside the previous use of conventional blunt dissection or anatomically undefined resections. At the same time, some surgeons are learning how to perform laparoscopic colectomies for cancer, using the same standardized, anatomically based operations that they would have previously performed as open procedures. The progress that has been achieved in standardizing operations for rectal and colon cancers, with definable pathology-based and clinical outcomes criteria now available for surgical quality assurance, makes it essential that current changes to laparoscopic technique faithfully duplicate the proven principles of surgery for colorectal cancer, if the laparoscopic approach to colorectal cancer is to be regarded seriously by the oncologic community. Currently, there is a sense that some of the advocates of laparoscopic surgery (who are not primarily cancer-oriented surgeons) are focused on adopting a laparoscopic approach to colorectal cancer, as long as this approach results in limited morbidity, and national versus optimal long-term oncologic results. Given the progress that we have witnessed in the treatment of colorectal cancer, in which dramatic improvement has occurred because of standardized operations in expert hands, only the best oncologic outcomes achieved laparoscopically can be the acceptable goal.

Progress in Advanced Laparoscopic Surgery

Surgeons today are moving forward slowly to embrace advanced laparoscopic procedures. Only a small percentage of surgeons can routinely offer patients a full and robust menu of minimally invasive options for the most common intra-abdominal surgical procedures.[24] Nowhere is this deficiency more glaring than in the field of colonic and gastrointestinal surgery, leaving a tremendous number of patients without the advantages of a minimally invasive option. The laparoscopic boom began with the laparoscopic cholecystectomy, and the success of this procedure was made possible by mechanical appliances.[25] Further advances will require an unprecedented educational effort to outfit a surgeon with the special skills and knowledge to competently perform advanced procedures in the minimally invasive surgical environment.[26-28]

Securing competence and quality assurance implies that the surgeon blends sophisticated technical skills with sound clinical and intra-operative judgment. For most surgeons, this controlled environment does not yet exist within the laparoscopic arena. Even a very self-assured, highly experienced but laparoscopically naive surgeon may feel compromised when placed in a laparoscopic environment, creating a challenge to quality assurance and patient safety. Under these circumstances, most surgeons would shy away from a procedure rather than put their patients at risk.

Despite a significant corporate investment and a significant increase in the number of preceptorships/mentorships available, only a fraction of surgeons (as few as 15%) are venturing into the laparoscopic "new frontier."[29] The most likely reason for this problem lies in an outdated and misdirected educational strategy.[30-32]

The future of minimally invasive colonic surgery, and of MIS as a whole, lies within the historic framework of traditional surgical education.[33] Surgical educators require a strong training background in traditional techniques as well as many hours of direct supervision before allowing residents to move on to more advanced procedures or techniques. No surgical board would qualify a surgeon without the demonstration of cognitive excellence. No surgical residency would advance a resident who did not participate in an adequate number of cases under the supervision of competent mentors.[34,35]

The challenge is how to advance this tradition of residency education in the continuing medical education arena of MIS and, in particular, MIS colonic and other gastrointestinal procedures. These goals must be accomplished through an educational system that is validated by objective-based metrics and is conveniently and competently delivered to all students through computer-based learning platforms.[36]

Such programs involve standardized progressive skill development with metric evaluation, reinforcement of cognitive data bases via web-based, CD/DVD-ROM tutorials, interactive multimedia-enriched lesson plans that have a large "edutainment" value, and traditional lectures utilizing streaming and videoconferencing technology. Continuity of the educational effort is sustained with the use of web-based and CD/DVD-ROM tutorials that are monitored with metrics and teleproctoring and telementoring. This strategy allows optimum education milestones to be offered cost-effectively to a larger volume of surgeons; at the same time, surgeons must acknowledge that certain standardized, evidence-based procedures, techniques, and strategies are crucial to establishing cost-effective procedural signatures with superior clinical outcomes. These programs, while sounding like they are limited to the peculiar concerns of surgeons, are important to all surgical, radiation, and medical oncologists because they ensure the platform of quality standards that make clinical investigation and clinical outcomes reliable.

Skill Development: The Rosser Minimally Invasive Skills and Suturing Development Program

Several excellent skill development programs have been developed.[36,37] In this section, we highlight the Rosser Minimally Invasive Skills and Suturing Development programs.[38] Endoscopic suturing is the most difficult task to perform in the laparoscopic environment, serving as a goal for laparoscopic training. It requires the possession of an advanced skill set to perform this task on a par with the very best open technique. This program offers the necessary skills in a cost-effective manner, establishing accurate instrument targeting, two-dimension depth perception compensation, bimanual dexterity, and two-hand choreography. This is a highly supervised program focused on efficiency of skill development with an emphasis on nondominant hand development.[24,39] A large database including thousands of surgeons with metric follow-up identifies the participant's skill posture in comparison with his or her peers, represented by a percentile designation.[40] In 150 board-eligible or board-certified surgeons, performance scores on a series of preparatory drills had a high correlation with the ultimate performance of suturing. Suturing skills can be achieved in a very short period.

Objective evaluation of a laparoscopic surgical skill program for residents and senior residents follows.[38] In 291 trained surgeons and 99 residents, there was a high degree of correlation between preparatory drills and suturing skills, regardless of attending or resident status. Age and gender do not correlate with skill development.

A platform to encourage skill development in surgical residency programs, the "Top Gun" competition, is now featured at the annual meetings of the Society of American Gastrointestinal Endoscopic Surgeons, the Society of Laparoscopic Surgeons, and the American College of Surgeons. Almost 50 residencies and postgraduate training programs now use this educational system in one form or the other.

Computer-Assisted Training and Distant Learning

Computer-based instruction enhances cognitive knowledge, speeds up education,[26,36,38,41-46] and helps mature clinical judgment. CD/DVD-ROM instructional tutorials offer a student the presentation of high-quality, consistent information at the convenience of the student, with levels of knowledge transfer similar to those of on-site stand-up tutorials.

Multimedia-enriched computer-assisted instruction can also be used to mature surgical judgment more efficiently,[36] and it allows clinical judgment to be matured outside the surgical suite in a more cost-effective environment. With the development of web-based and CD/DVD ROM tutorials, convenient postcourse instruction can be conducted to continue the learning process after an on-site course.[26,36,41,43-45] Distant learning applications may be deployed globally to expand the education process to include skill as well as cognitive transfer as effectively as on-site programs.

Surgical simulators are another computer-based educational option for future surgical education.[26,27,45,46] Broadband education and clinical telemedicine applications are valuable tools of any cyber-based educational strategy. Teleconferencing and telementoring can allow (1) clinical experience from the surgical suite to be shared and (2) a lecture series to occur in cyberspace.

In addition, surgeons can be guided during their initial procedures and during difficult cases with the assistance of telemonitoring, a technique that involves an experienced surgeon remotely guiding a procedure that is being performed by a surgeon who is inexperienced.

If the proper training protocol is followed, the multimedia-enriched technique is a safe and effective paradigm shift to adapt as an education tool.

Surgical Tactics

Advanced MIS procedures require standardized methodology. In all advanced laparoscopic cancer operations, the laparoscopic surgeon's goal is to duplicate both the standardization and the optimal standards and principles that are performed by the best cancer surgery techniques used in open surgery and then apply laparoscopic technique to minimize morbidity and to enhance recovery.

Room Setup

The concepts of proper room setup strategy must be based on a standardized personnel/equipment organizational format.[48,49] The room is set up to position all personnel on one side of the table, contralateral to the operative site. All of the inanimate equipment is placed on the side of the operative site. This has been called the "flesh and bone; steel and plastic rule." This rule provides a consistent foundation that can be used effectively.

Optical Correctness Optical correctness correlates the direction of movement by laparoscopic instruments to the direction of movement of the instruments on the video monitor.[50] This is established by placing the video camera head, laparoscope, operative site, and video monitor in a linear relationship to one another.[51,52]

Triangle of Success for Trocar Placement The triangle of success theory for trocar placement produces optimal instrument convergence over the operative site, thereby preventing inadvertent collisions of instruments.[53]

The apex of the triangle is the operative site with the base formed by two trocars. The distance between the operative site and the two trocars (20–25 cm) is critical because it dictates the "instrument entry angle" into the abdominal cavity. The distance between the two trocars that form the base of the triangle (10–15 cm) determines the "convergence angle" of the tips of the instruments over the operative area. The proper instrument entry angle and convergence angle of the instruments are very important in determining the operative posture of the hands and arms of the surgeon. The camera port is placed at a 90-degree relationship to the long axis of the triangle of success. Preferably, it should be placed as close to the dominant hand as possible without encouraging the collision of instruments.

Ergonomic Surgeon and Equipment Positioning It is strongly suggested that the surgeon assume a sitting position for laparoscopic procedures. Advanced laparoscopic colonic and intestinal procedures are more time consuming and are more difficult, and sitting is one of the most ergonomically significant benefits that can be deployed. Sitting also allows the surgeon to operate from a very stable platform. When combined with placement of the video monitor at or below eye level, the possibility of chronic musculoskeletal problems, a rapidly increasing healthcare hazard for the surgical community, is decreased.[54,55]

Selective Utilization of Intra and Extracorporeal Techniques

Minimally invasive colonic and gastrointestinal surgeons must be skilled at executing procedures with both extracorporeal and totally intracorporeal techniques. This requirement is not based on surgeon preference but is dictated by the clinical situation, projected operating time, and cost. The extracorporeal approach offers the advantage of faster operative time and decreased cost. The mobilization of the colon is performed intracorporeally. No resection is performed at that time. The specimen is then brought through the abdominal wall, and the resection and anastomosis are performed with standard open techniques. Once the anastomosis is completed, the colon is restored to the abdomen and the abdominal wall is closed. With skill development and proper dissection technique, this can be accomplished very efficiently, with the reduced cost associated with using open instrumentation.

If the patient has a thick abdominal wall or a shortened mesentery, as in Crohn's disease, the extracorporeal route may not be applicable. Then, the totally intracorporeal route may be used. The mobilization takes place in the standard fashion, and the colon is resected and anastomosed by use of laparoscopic stapling techniques within the confines of the pneumoperitoneum. The specimen is removed through an opening in the abdominal wall or, rarely, via the rectum. Some surgeons would resort to hybrid alternatives, such as laparoscopic mobilization and an open resection through a considerably smaller incision. Vithiananthan et al[56] reported smaller incisions and a shorter length of stay (6.1 vs. 11.1 days) with a hybrid approach.

Selection of the Specimen Extraction Site

The appropriate specimen extraction site reduces the morbidity of minimally invasive intestinal procedure when compared with open techniques. A lateral (off the midline) extraction site entails the division of muscle fibers and, once that happens, the morbidity advantages of a minimally invasive approach (ileus and pain) quickly dissipate. The periumbilical region is what is called the primary extraction point, the first specimen removal option. It is the thinnest portion of the abdominal wall. The fascial incision can be extended and the skin incision is smaller, resulting in an excellent cosmetic result.

CREDENTIALING

The strategies that are outlined in this chapter ensure the transfer of knowledge and skills as surgeons advance toward more demanding laparoscopic operations. These educational and credentialing steps have helped to shape a 21st Century credentialing strategy that was debuted at Yale University School of Medicine and is now practiced at Beth Israel Medical Center in New York and its affiliated hospitals. Surgeons requesting first-time privileges must complete the level I Skill and Suturing course, and their percentile ranking is noted. Next, a course with didactic and live animal laboratory must be documented. The MIS director reviews the surgeon's procedure technique. The privilege-requesting surgeon then must choose a partner (a wingman) that is committed to scrubbing with the surgeon for at least five cases. The first two cases are performed with the MIS director in attendance. The next three cases are performed with the wingman, and the MIS director is not in attendance. All cases are videotaped, and after evaluation by the MIS director, a decision is made to allow unrestricted privileges, to be granted by the chairman of surgery. MIS-credentialed surgeons are encouraged to participate in a continuing medical education program that includes skill update seminars and courses and a 12-part lecture series in minimally invasive surgery. The MIS director and other qualified surgeons then handle future mentoring and proctoring needs with telementoring and teleproctoring.[26,36,43,57-59]

Patient Selection Issues

As experience with laparoscopic colectomy builds, it is clear that the optimal patients for laparoscopic colectomy are the same as for open colectomy: thin, no history of prior abdominal surgery, and in good health. Gradually, the criteria for patient selection have broadened to include obese patients and those with a prior history of abdominal surgery. In obese patients, laparoscopic surgeons claim that the anatomic planes may be more easily dissected, whereas in patients who have previously undergone surgery, the laparoscopic dissection of adhesions allows access to the normal anatomy.

Currently, patients with curable primary adenocarcinomas of the large bowel (stages I, II, and III) are best considered candidates for clinical trials in a controlled, randomized setting. Outside of participation in a controlled trial, there are opportunities to perform laparoscopic colectomy in which the benefits of reduced short-term morbidity accrue to the patient. Patients with benign adenomas of the colon and patients with adenomas and in situ carcinomas that may not lend themselves to endoscopic excision are ideal candidates for laparoscopic colectomy. Patients with stage IV disease, in whom a decision has been made to resect the primary disease, are also candidates for laparoscopic colectomy. In such cases, there is no fear that the procedure will adversely affect the natural history of the disease, and patients recovering more rapidly after laparoscopic surgery may move on to systemic or regional chemotherapy that much sooner.

Total abdominal colectomy, as required for premalignant disease (e.g., chronic ulcerative colitis, familial polyposis coli, and, to a lesser extent, Crohn's disease), is the optimal condition by which laparoscopic colectomy may accomplish the same resection as open colectomy, with considerably reduced morbidity. The surgeon considering the options of a lower-abdominal extraction site and the potential for either open or laparoscopic pelvic surgery may choose to reduce such operations to a small, lower abdominal incision and perform the upper abdominal dissections laparoscopically.

Patients with locally advanced (i.e., T4) lesions, those with obvious serosal invasion, or adjacent organ attachment or invasion are best treated with open colectomy, which ensures a minimum of manipulation, adequate margins, and ideal reconstruction of adjacent organs that are in need of resection.

Regarding sites of disease, patients with low-lying rectal cancers that unequivocally require an abdominoperineal resection and patients with either right-sided or sigmoid cancers present the easiest of the operative challenges for laparoscopic colectomy. Patients with lesions of the transverse colon, the flexures, and the descending colon are less ideal for the laparoscopic approach given the origins of the regional blood supply and other considerations of adequate mobilization. Patients with rectal cancers that may lend themselves to a true low anterior resection (TME with a low extraperitoneal anastomosis or a coloanal anastomosis) are not candidates for a purely laparoscopic approach. Hartley and coworkers[60] reported a 50% failure to accomplish such operations laparoscopically, and patients with midrectal cancers deserve every opportunity to receive a sphincter-preserving operation. The subject of laparoscopic surgery for rectal cancer follows. No author has yet to suggest that laparoscopic surgery for rectal cancer interferes with the administration of preoperative neoadjuvant therapy, when indicated.[61]

The physiology of pneumoperitoneum continues to be studied.[62] Patients with serious cardiopulmonary disease or stroke must be carefully considered as candidates for laparoscopic colectomy on an individual basis.

It has been stated by many sources that inexperienced minimally invasive colon surgeons should start their journey by choosing reversal of Hartmann's procedures as their initial efforts. On the contrary, the authors believe that the variability of adhesion deposition, the increased degree of difficulty in the establishment of pneumoperitoneum, and the possibility of bowel injury and additional bowel resection and mobilization make reversal of a Hartmann's resection a poor starting point. If these procedures are going to be attempted, it may be beneficial to use a 2-mm scope as the initial puncture site to evaluate whether the procedure may be attempted laparoscopically. This information is useful and cost-effective.[63]

An extracorporeal right hemicolectomy for benign nondiverticular disease in patients who have not undergone prior abdominal surgery is probably an excellent place to start.

Port-Site Recurrences

Initial reports on port-site recurrences appeared in 1993.[64-66] In their comprehensive review article, Rickard and Bokey[5] reported a wide-ranging incidence for port-site recurrences. These reviewers maintained that the reported incidence of port-site recurrences was the most important factor in preventing the widespread use of laparoscopic surgery for colon cancer. Some good has resulted from the initial case reports of this potentially catastrophic complication. The cautions emanating from these reports undoubtedly catalyzed or facilitated the development of prospective, controlled, randomized surgical trials with long-term follow-up in order to study the natural history of this new modality. More recent reports have demonstrated port-site recurrence rates that are similar to the incidence of wound recurrences after open surgery,[67-69] approximately 1% or less.[70-72] Controlled randomized trials that are currently in progress[4] are structured with built-in safety checks. A disproportionate number of port-site recurrences have not required the early termination of any trials, to date, failing to support initial fears and concerns.

Single-Institution and Retrospective Studies

Most of the early single-center or even multicenter studies of laparoscopic surgery for colorectal cancers are retrospective, whereas some of the prospective studies reported a low volume of patients and are not evaluable for long-term cancer follow-up. Many of the early reports contained patients with benign, as well as malignant, disease. Nevertheless, these studies have played an important role in the initial development of advanced laparoscopic surgery for colorectal cancer by demonstrating feasibility and low short-term morbidity.[73-88] Some authors have attempted to draw conclusions regarding long-term outcomes from their initial patient accrual. These comparisons to historical open colectomy surgical series cannot be used to assess cancer treatment results, requiring instead the development of controlled clinical trials.[89]

Multicenter and Prospective Studies

As of 2001, five randomized, controlled trials have addressed the results of laparoscopic colectomy. All of these are early studies and, with several recent exceptions, they are characterized by the pitfalls of limited volume and follow-up.[5]

Lacy and coworkers[68] initially reported on 25 patients randomized to laparoscopic-assisted colectomy (LAC) and 26 to open colectomy. They observed one death from myocardial infarction in the LAC group but longer operating times for LAC, shorter hospitalization, and more rapid return of bowel function in the LAC group.[68]

When the study was updated at a mean follow-up of 21 months, the LAC group, which had 44 patients, and the open cholectomy group, which had 47 patients, had no differences in total recurrence rates.[90]

Milsom and coworkers[69] randomly assigned 55 patients to LAC and 54 patients to open colectomy. Both benign and malignant diseases were included in this study, which is predominantly a study of feasibility and morbidity. Follow-up at 1.7 and 1.5 years in the LAC and open groups, respectively, was too short for the assessment of recurrence rates. The authors concluded that LAC was as safe as conventional colectomy, and it had faster pulmonary and gastrointestinal recovery than open cholectomy.[69]

Stage et al[91] randomly assigned 34 patients to either LAC or open cholectomy. With five patients excluded from analysis and a failure to analyze the two groups by the principle of intention to treat, the authors risked significant bias. Nevertheless, short-term morbidity was reportedly less in the LAC group.[91]

Wexner et al[92] reported on a prospective trial of patients undergoing total abdominal colectomy. In this report, which appeared early in the course of laparoscopic colectomy, there were no significant differences in early morbidity.

Schwenk et al[93] examined the inflammatory response and concluded that fewer inflammatory consequences occurred after LAC than after open cholectomy. They did not report either survival or recurrence data in their 30 patients.

Numerous prospective randomized trial in progress have been structured with appropriate stratification and sample sizes.[94-97]

In order to observe a 10% difference in 5-year survival, it has been estimated that each arm of a prospective randomized, appropriately stratified study would require the entry of 600 or more patients. The COST study that is currently in progress in the United States will randomly assign 1200 patients and is awaiting the results of a 7-year follow-up before publishing the outcomes.[4]

Studies Reported in 2002

Several long-term prospective series have been the subject of detailed reports in the literature within the past year. From the University of Barcelona, Lacy and coworkers[98] have updated their earlier works to a median follow-up of 43 months (range, 27–85 months). The authors' criteria for eligibility or patient selection included all adenocarcinomas of the colon situated at least 15 cm above the anal verge. Exclusion criteria included cancers within the transverse colon, metastatic disease, adjacent organ invasion, intestinal obstruction, or history of past colon surgery. Patients were stratified according to the location of their primary tumors; proximal or distal to the splenic flexure. Interim analyses were planned for early morbidity, for tumor recurrence, or for port-site metastasis. Both LAC and open cholectomy were performed by a single surgical team. Oral liquids were provided during the first 24 hours and a soft diet thereafter, as tolerated.

Of 442 eligible patients, 223 were excluded for documented reasons, and 219 were randomly assigned to LAC or to open cholectomy. In 64 of the excluded patients, the investigators found distant metastases; in 40 patients, the tumor was located in the transverse colon; and 27 patients had prior colon surgery. Intestinal obstruction was present in 13, and 79 patients refused randomization. In addition, 12 patients (11%) underwent open cholectomy even though they were randomly assigned to the LAC group because the surgeon suspected tumor invasion of adjacent organs. Beyond this information, an overall conversion rate is not provided.

Operative mortality (30-day) included one patient with a myocardial infarct (LAC) and three patients with multisystem organ failure, presumably due to sepsis, in three patients in the open cholectomy group. Short-term morbidity was significantly lower in the LAC group. It is not clear whether this is the case because LAC significantly reduced morbidity or because the morbidity in the open cholectomy group seemed excessive (12% vs 31%). There were more deaths due to multisystem organ failure, as well as what would seem to be a disproportionate incidence of severe complications in the open cholectomy group. Aside from persistent ileus, evisceration, intraperitoneal hemorrhage, anastomotic leakage, abscess, and renal complications were more commonly observed in the open cholectomy group.[98]

LAC was associated with a somewhat longer operating time than open cholectomy (142 vs 118 minutes) but had a lower blood loss (105 vs 193 mL), fewer cases of reinserted nasogastric tube (three vs nine cases), a shorter interval to the start of oral feeding (54 vs 85 hours), and a shorter duration of hospital stay (5.2 vs 7.9 days). For all patients in the study, lymph node metastases, open colectomy, and preoperative serum carcinoembryonic antigen were independent prognostic variables after a multivariate analysis. Lymph node metastasis was the only independent predictor of overall survival. Lymph node metastases and surgical procedure (LAC vs open cholectomy) were independent predictors of cancer-related survival. This discrepancy was due to the superior overall and cancer-related survival of stage III LAC patients when compared with open cholectomy patients. A single port-site metastasis was observed in a curable LAC patient.

The authors refer to the possibility that laparoscopy has an immune protective quality when compared with open laparotomy[99]; this possibility has been previously documented in preclinical laboratory trials[100-102] and in selected clinical trials that measure acute-phase reactants.[103] Aside from the need for independent corroboration of their clinical observations, the mechanism or mechanisms by which immunoprotection is conveyed in any clinical setting has continued to elude most investigators, and it is not even clear that molecular immunology will provide the needed answers to these difficult questions. The authors have demonstrated that in the controlled environment of a single team performing both open and laparoscopic resections for colon cancers, LAC is preferable to open cholectomy in selected patients with curable cancers of stages I–III, as indicated by their own pattern of patient selection. Unlike most other controlled prospective studies, the authors find that survival after LAC is improved. These findings need corroboration in independent trials with strict adherence to cancer principles, as well as elimination of potential biases.

From the Royal Brisbane Hospital, in Queensland, Australia, Lumley and coworkers[104] have reported on the selective use of laparoscopic-assisted resection for patients with colorectal cancer. Since 1991, 750 patients have undergone open resections, and 181 patients were selected for laparoscopic-assisted resections. Most of the open cases involved restorative proctectomy, and the authors clearly preferred laparotomy because of the difficulty of achieving a safe distal rectal transection laparoscopically. Patients whose cancers of rectum required an abdominoperineal resection (APR) were deemed ideal candidates for laparoscopic mobilization of the rectum and perineal excision. As in the Lacy et al[98] study, laparotomy was also preferred in patients with cancers of the transverse colon, palpable cancers, or locally advanced cancers (e.g., T4 lesions, or obstructing or perforated cancers). Patient morphology or a history of prior laparotomy were not necessarily considered contraindications to the laparoscopic approach. Twelve procedures required conversion to open laparotomy (6.6%) for the following indications: failure to make progress, unsuitable pathology, incorrect localization, and laparoscopically unmanageable adhesions. Prospective follow-up of 181 patients is reported, of which 154 were curative resections.

At a median follow-up of 71 months, with more than 90% over 2 years of follow-up, there were 21 recurrences (6%), and most were similar to those observed after open colectomy. There were three local recurrences, and one port-site recurrence after a curative resection (0.6%) and another after a palliative resection.

Two patients died (1%), one of necrotizing fasciitis after a relaparoscopy and six patients experienced a postoperative bowel obstruction due to adhesions. No patient had either pre- or postoperative radiation therapy, and patients with stage C disease (any TN1,2M0) received postoperative adjuvant chemotherapy. Using the Australian Clinico-Pathologic Staging system, the unadjusted 5-year survival figures were 91% for stage A (T1,2N0M0), 83% for stage B (T3,4N0M0), and 74% for stage C (any TN1,2M0). The authors reported a low incidence of both port-site and peritoneal recurrences for stage I–III curable cancers.

The authors commented on the favorable intermediate to long-term results of their patients undergoing curative laparoscopic resection, an overall recurrence rate of 13.6%. In view of the highly selective nature of their series, the authors have elected not to compare their patients' survival to that of historical open controls, because of the high likelihood of bias. They attributed the relatively low rate of conversion to careful preoperative patient selection. The extremely low long-term risk of adhesive obstruction and the low incidence of wound hernias (0.6%) were considered direct benefits of the laparoscopic approach. As with Lacy et al's study,[98] these data will also benefit from corroboration. Localization of the small, early tumor was noted to be a persistent problem that was not solved by on-table colonoscopy.[104]

In the United States, Nelson and Enker[4] have spearheaded a multicenter, prospective, randomized, stratified trial of laparoscopic versus open colectomy for cancer, the COST study.[4] The authors based this trial on the reported experience in previous trials that showed improved short-term morbidity and no adverse cancer-related effects to laparoscopic colectomy.[69,105-107] They have estimated that 1200 patients would need to be enrolled in the study over a 3-year accrual period. The exclusion criteria are very similar to the aforementioned studies from Spain[98] and Australia.[104] Surgery was performed according to uniform guidelines, and quality assurance was maintained by random audit of video-recorded laparoscopic procedures (but, significantly, not of open colectomies). Statistical analysis was in keeping with the intent-to-treat principle, and interim analyses for safety and for outcomes were designated. Quality-of-life, quality-adjusted survival, and cost and cost-effective analyses were prospective features of the study. The study requires a long-term major analysis of survival when all patients have been followed up for 7 years.[108]

Recently, Weeks and coworkers[109] have reported the first data from the COST trial pertaining to short-term QOL outcomes in LAC versus open cholectomy patients.[109]

Since 1994, 37 of the 48 centers involved in the COST trial have prospectively reported on the QOL component for 449 patients with clinically resectable colon cancers. Scores on symptom distress scales, a QOL index and a single-item global rating scale for 2 days, 2 weeks, and 2 months, were evaluated along with duration of hospital analgesic use and length of stay. The conversion rate was 25.7%, and by the intent-to-treat principle, these patients were included in the LAC group for analysis. Only minimal short-term QOL benefits were found with LAC group with colon cancer compared with standard open cholectomy. Patients assigned to undergo LAC required a somewhat shorter duration of both oral and parenteral analgesics while hospitalized, and their mean length of stay was shorter by 0.8 days. Those patients assigned to LAC reported a slightly better QOL on a median global rating scale at 2 weeks (76.9 for LAC vs 74.4 for open cholectomy). Longitudinal rating of overall QOL only approached significance ($P = 0.09$) at 2 weeks after surgery. In this trial, meaningful benefit as well as the patients' own ability to appreciate the benefit were sought rather than proxy measurements of QOL, such as analgesic requirements or length of stay. The authors reported that they did not find this evidence.

In analyzing their data, the authors attempted to define the reasons for failing to observe a QOL advantage for LAC. One of their analyses pertained to the open conversion rate of 25% that did not change over the period of the study. There were no differences in conversion rates between surgeons, and because the study involves laparoscopically experienced surgeons, there was no significant learning curve. The authors indicated that LAC would be especially good if it were applied to patients who could be identified before surgery as low-risk candidates for conversion. However, their conversion rate of 25.7% remains unexplained because the eligibility criteria for this study excluded most patients who would be at high risk for conversion, leaving only locally advanced disease to be discovered intraoperatively in the LAC patients. In fact, their conversion rate for locally advanced cancers was 7.7%, which is consistent with other papers in the literature for that indication alone.[104] The results of the COST trial are eagerly awaited. Interim analyses to date do not suggest any concern about adverse outcome for patients undergoing LAC for cancer.

The COST study is a collaborative, multicenter trial that aims to spell out the current status of LAC and its role in relation to open cholectomy. Well-organized, tightly controlled, prospective, randomized trials of this nature will help define the true indications and roles for LAC. As the laparoscopic and endoscopic and stapling technologies advance, along with advances in imaging, we can expect that the benefits of laparoscopic treatment of colorectal cancer will advance accordingly, on the basis of the scientific foundation provided by dedicated investigators.

Laparoscopic Surgery for Rectal Cancer

As the techniques and the technology of LAC for colon cancer have matured, some members of the laparoscopic community have moved on to apply these methods to the treatment of rectal cancer. Preceding the age of advanced laparoscopic colorectal surgery, the principles of surgery for rectal cancer have been established with the development of TME.[7,10] Laparoscopic surgeons have adopted TME, claiming that the dissection for rectal cancer, between the visceral and the parietal layers of the pelvic fasciae, is enhanced by the magnified images provided by laparoscopy. Several authors have published clinical trials, whereas others have advocated TME by means of video education.

One must assume that in any discussion, the participants are agreed on or are using like definitions. In many publications related to rectal cancer, one cannot make that assumption. Different definitions of the rectum that pertain to rectal cancer have been used in various surgical series. These definitions include the extraperitoneal rectum only, distances of 10 or 12 cm from the anal verge, any cancers distal to the sacral promontory (even if entirely covered by the peritoneum), or cancers whose lowest edge is situated from 0–15 cm from the anal verge.[20] Although the latter is consistent with the American College of Surgeons' database for rectal cancers, the span of 0–15 cm includes some intraperitoneal cancers, creating a potential statistical impression that the local recurrence rates of all rectal cancers may be lower. Most U.S. cooperative groups use an upper limit of 12 cm, based on the patterns of recurrence that have been published.[110] In contrast to local recurrence rates of 30% for adequately operated rectal cancers in the pre-TME era, the local recurrence rates for large bowel cancers greater than 11–12 cm were reported to be 6%, more in keeping with that of adequately operated colonic cancers.

Recent reports regarding the use of laparoscopic surgery for rectal cancer have included broader definitions of the rectum than the standard 0–12 cm that is most commonly utilized by the cooperative groups. Although looser criteria may be understandable because the technical feasibility of laparoscopic surgery for rectal cancer is in its earliest evolution, future studies will depend on the adherence to stricter criteria, if the comparison between open and laparoscopic TME is to be meaningful to surgical and other oncologic investigators. Appropriate stratifications of distance from the anal verge will be essential to the proper structure of any clinical trials regarding laparoscopy and rectal cancer.

Various investigators have reported their early experience with laparoscopic surgery for rectal cancer. Scheidbach and coworkers have recently reported on laparoscopic anterior resection for rectal cancer.[111] They summarized the experience of an ongoing trial initiated by the Laparoscopic Colorectal Surgery Study Group (LCSSG) in 1995. The 273 patients who were reported included 195 who underwent a curative resection for rectal cancer. The male:female ratio was nearly 0.95. The average blood loss was 300 mL, and 12.8% of patients (N = 35) required any transfusion. Ninety-six percent of the anastomoses were performed transanally by use of circular staplers, and about 10% of the patients had a defunctioning stoma, mostly those with low anastomoses. The splenic flexure was mobilized in nearly two of every three patients. Parenteral feeding lasted a mean of 2.4 days (1-7), and oral intake of fluids began on average at 2.9 days (1-7). Solid food was taken on average by 5.5 days (2-12).

Intraoperative complications were reported in 16 patients (5.9%) and included injury to blood vessels or to adjacent loops of large or small bowel.

Ureteral damage was not observed. After surgery, 160 complications were recorded in 99 patients. Wound healing problems were observed in 6.2% of minilaparotomy sites and in 1.5% of trocar sites. Twenty-eight patients required reoperation for bleeding (*N* = 10 [3.7%]), ileus (*N* = 1 [0.4%]), and, notably, for anastomotic leakage (*N* = 17 [6.3%]). There were four deaths, one from peritonitis and three from cardiopulmonary or other perioperative complications.

From the cancer standpoint, the average number of lymph nodes retrieved was 13.8 per specimen; however, the minimum requirements of the International Union Against Cancer for lymph node retrieval was not achieved in 84 patients (43.0%). This study was not controlled for surgeon variability (i.e., for TME), despite its initiation in 1995.[112]

In the median follow-up of 19.2 months, 20 patients have died of disease (14.6%), and 10 patients have experienced a local recurrence (7.3%). No port-site recurrences were observed.

In reviewing their data, Koeckerling and associates[111] noted limited participation in their study—more than 75% of the curative resections were performed in only four hospitals. This is despite the recruitment of more than 2300 patients to the LCSSG multicenter study. The overwhelming concern of the surgeons who chose not to participate was that oncologic surgery should not be performed laparoscopically. The authors reported faster early postoperative recovery, with LAC patients recovering peristalsis in a mean of 3.5 days for laporascopic surgery versus 5.7 days for open colectomy, a 1-day advantage for the initiation of oral solid foods and a shorter hospital stay (14 days for LAC vs 23.8 days for open cholectomy). The unusually long length of stay that the authors attributed to their health insurance system seriously compromises a straightforward clinical analysis of their data. The authors justified their unusual incidence of anastomotic leakage due to their cases of low rectal anastomosis and compared their results with those of other experience in the literature.[113]

The authors concluded that laparoscopic anterior resection for rectal cancer cannot be recommended for general use and that such operations should be performed only in the context of scientifically valid studies. As in other studies, these authors did not mention their definition of the rectum that was used in the LCSSG study. Nevertheless, they concluded that only operations on the upper rectum or the rectosigmoid (that many consider to be the distal sigmoid) may be currently justified, excluding operations on the mid- and lower rectum from attempts at laparoscopic sphincter-preserving operations. This experience has been borne out elsewhere as well. The authors indicated that there are persisting concerns about the oncologic quality of the operations, but they did not indicate whether these are their own concerns or whether they are summarizing the expressed views of others.

Surgeons do appear divided along these lines, and others would disagree with this conservative approach. Poulin and coworkers[114] reported on the prospective follow-up of 80 consecutive unselected patients who underwent a laparoscopic TME for rectal cancer. Patients were operated on between November 1991 and 1999, and they were staged in accordance with the TNM classification. The median follow-up period for curable stages of disease was 31 months. The Kaplan-Meier 5-year survival for stages I, II, and III was 72.1%, and the local recurrence rate was 4.3%. These data are statistically identical to the results reported for open TME in 1995[7] and updated in 2000.[8] These results compared most favorably with the 5-year survival of 42% and the local recurrence rates of 32%–35% in nonstandardized operations.[115] They are also consistent with the successful increase in organ and function preservation, that is, the sphincter and autonomic nerve preservation that is associated with open TME.[116,117] Other studies have reported similar results.[118-124]

Experience with laparoscopic abdominoperineal resection (APR) has found more consistent advocates. Mehigan and Monson[125] have advocated APR to be performed in accordance with the principles of TME. The results of open APR according the principles of TME have been reported previously.[126] The importance of excellence in surgical technique and the advantages of the magnified views facilitate TME with autonomic nerve preservation.[127] Additional advantages in terms of postoperative recovery should accrue because of the absence of any abdominal incision, except for the placement of the stoma site. To avoid any conflict regarding missed opportunities for sphincter-preserving operations, the authors have selected their patients carefully for APR and have included only patients with primary cancers within 1 cm of the sphincter mechanism.[125,128,129]

Tumor-Related Issues

Numerous tumor-related issues are reported to compromise the laparoscopic approach. Identification of the small, early cancer can be a persistent problem,[130] with a discrepancy of up to one flexure noted by some authors.[131] Failure to localize the lesion accurately prolongs laparoscopic colectomy, in some cases leading to conversion to open colectomy.[104] Often, the site of the primary tumor is incorrectly identified by colonoscopy. India ink tattooing has been successful in about 50% of cases, but in the remaining 50% the stain is either inadequate to be viewed laparoscopically or is too scattered or diffuse to help with localization.[132] The value of intraoperative colonoscopy remains controversial. Although some investigators believe that it can make laparoscopic dissection impossible because of colonic distention,[133] others believe that it does help with localization of pathology.[134] Preoperative accuracy may require x-ray imaging at the time of colonoscopy to accurately identify the site of small lesions. The same difficulties may be encountered at open colectomy, but they are easier to resolve in the open setting, hence the likelihood of conversion.

Modifications of Laparoscopic Surgery for Rectal Cancer

Function outcomes after surgery for rectal cancers often depend on restorative operations. Seow-Cheon and colleagues reported that laparoscopically assisted ultra-low anterior resection with colonic J-pouch formation was easier than open surgery and that the incisions were shorter, and the patients required less analgesics. The operation was safe and feasible, but both return of bowel function and length of stay were comparable to those of open conventional surgery.[135] For surgeons who require preserving a tactile sensation, Ichihara and colleagues[136] reported on the advantages of using a Lap-disk for hand-assisted manipulation in low anterior resection. Transection of the rectum with an adjustable linear stapler made the distal staple line equivalent to that obtained by open laparotomy. Others have also advocated either hybrid or hand-assisted laparoscopic operations to overcome these technical issues.[137-139]

Laparoscopic Colectomy Update

A small number of surgeons advocating LAC have recently declared that the 2002 report by Lacy and co-workers[98] supports a claim of superior survival of patients who have undergone laparoscopic, as opposed to open, colectomy for cancer.[140] In Lacy et al's 2002 paper, the survival of stage III patients who underwent laparoscopic resections was statistically superior to that of patients who underwent open colectomy. In an subsequent review and commentary, one reviewer placed much emphasis on the experience of the surgeons as a key factor in accomplishing extraordinary stage-related survival figures; (Dukes A, 100%; Dukes B, 88%; and Dukes C, 84%).[140] However, similar results have also been reported by Lumley et al.[104] So, let us try to understand: What does "experience" really mean? Laparoscopic experience, cancer surgery experience, or both?

In assessing the reviewer's focus, two considerations need be kept in mind as we examine for possible pitfalls. The first is the structure of Lacy et al's trial. Patients with transverse colon cancers or locally advanced lesions that possibly invade adjacent organs (T4), as well as patients with obstructing lesions, were excluded from this trial. Normally, consecutive surgical series of open colectomy do not exclude either transverse or possible T4 lesions, raising concerns about the possibilities of skewed stage and unintended bias. Even obstructing lesions, initially treated by stenting and preparation, are included in open consecutive series. In the absence of rigid stratification, it is essential to await independent clinical corroboration by other investigators before drawing bold conclusions as to the significance of these survival data.

Second, these survival figures, although first being achieved in laparoscopic surgery now, have in fact been previously reported in open resections. Survival figures in the same range, even in rectal cancers, have been reported in consecutive series from specialty services whereby patients undergo surgery in the hands of experienced gastrointestinal cancer surgeons, who perform standardized resections with both surgical and pathological quality assurance.[141]

Now, based on the Lacy et al results, some have digressed into the all-too-common theorizing about the immunologic superiority of laparoscopy, affecting the outcomes of cancer treatment. Despite this wishful thinking, there is little current molecular understanding about any cancer-related immunologic consequences as measured in vivo to support such bold claims. Instead, what we may be observing for the first time is that laparoscopic colectomy may now be achieving the goals of standardization of rational cancer operations, the same goals that have been advocated by, and are in use by, principled, disciplined surgeons in open resections for cancer. What is more likely happening is that the laparoscopic surgeons are now accomplishing a standardized, anatomically defined or radical colectomy, resulting in a complete mesenteric resection. The authors seem to have reached a high level of anatomically based resection standards, as defined by the open literature that precedes laparoscopy. Under such circumstances, superlative survival results are not surprising.

In a further examination of potential pitfalls, and, in view of the well-known laparoscopic interests of the surgical team, one must also feel free to ask whether the same strict operative or anatomically defined standards were followed when the patients underwent open colectomy? In some cases, the open approach may be *more* difficult to accomplish, as in the obese patient. Such a "reverse bias" by a group advocating a specific interest could have also influenced the survival outcomes. Although we laud the results from Barcelona, we enthusiastically await corroborative data from other investigators.

On another note, Lezoche and coworkers[142] have updated their previous work and have reported on laparoscopic versus open left or right colectomy, excluding segmental resections. The randomization was driven by patient choice after they read an informed consent. Follow-up is a mean of 42 months (12–92). The overall conversion rate was 3%. At 48 months, an analysis of cumulative survival reveals excellent cancer-related survival rates, and in this series of 248 randomly assigned patients there were no differences between the laparoscopic and the open colectomy patients. Operations took significantly longer, but hospital stay was significantly shorter.

Similar long-term results were reported by Lechaux et al.[143] In 206 patients who primarily underwent sigmoid resections, there was an 11% rate of conversion (10 for technical failures and 12 for cancer-related reasons). Five-year survival rates were 85% in Dukes A and B combined, 61% for Dukes C, and 8% in stage D patients, and there was one trocar site implant after a curative resection.[143]

In an excellent review article, Ziprin and colleagues[144] reiterate the importance of oncologic principles and put the issue of port-site metastases into proper perspective.

Finally, in a retrospective study, Law and coworkers[145] reported that laparoscopic colectomy is safer in elderly patients, probably because of early resumption of diet and avoidance of the morbidity of severe cardiopulmonary complications (7% vs 22%).

REFERENCES

1. Jacobs M, Verdeja JC, Goldstein HS. Minimally invasive colon resection (laparoscopic colectomy) Surg Laparosc Endosc Percutan Tech 1991;1:144-150.
2. Corman ML, Kaiser AM. History of laparoscopy. Surg Oncol Clin North Am 2001;10:483–492.
3. Ramos JM, Beart RW Jr, Goes R et al. Role of laparoscopy in colorectal surgery: a prospective evaluation of 200 cases. Dis Colon Rectum 1995;38:494–501.
4. Nelson H, Enker WE. Laparoscopic vs. open colectomy for cancer. Society of Surgical Oncology, Denver, Colorado, March 16, 2001.
5. Rickard MJFX, Bokey EL. Laparoscopy for colon cancer. Surg Oncol Clin North Am 2001;10:579–597.
6. Rougier P, Neoptolemos JP. The need for a multidisciplinary approach in the treatment of advanced colorectal cancer: a critical review from a medical oncologist and a surgeon. Eur J Surg Oncol 1997;23:385–396.
7. Enker WE, Thaler HT, Cranor M et al. Total mesorectal excision in the operative treatment of carcinoma of the rectum. J Am Coll Surg 1995;181:335–346.
8. Murali M, Enker WE, Martz JE. Current status of total mesorectal excision and autonomic nerve preservation in rectal cancer. Semin Surg Oncol 2000;19:321–328.
9. Kapiteijn E, Marijnen CAM, Nagtegaal I et al. Preoperative radiotherapy combined with total mesorectal excision for resectable rectal cancer. N Eng J Med 2001;345:638–646.
10. MacFarlane JK, Ryall RD, Heald RJ. Mesorectal excision for rectal cancer. Lancet 1993;341:457–460.
11. Landheer MLEA, Therasse P, van de Velde CJH. The importance of quality assurance in surgical oncology in the treatment of colorectal cancer. Surg Oncol Clin North Am 2001;10:885–914.
12. Arbman G, Nilsson E, Hallbook O et al. Local recurrence following total mesorectal excision for rectal cancer. Br J Surg 1996;83:375–379
13. Konn M, Morita T, Hada R et al. Survival and recurrence after low anterior resection and abdominoperineal resection for rectal cancer: the results of a long-term study with a review of the literature. Surg Today 1993;23:21–30.
14. Birbeck KF, Macklin CP, Tiffin NJ et al. Rates of circumferential resection margin involvement vary between surgeons and predict outcomes in rectal cancer surgery. Ann Surg 2002;235:449–457.
15. Enker WE, Laffer U, Block GE. Enhanced survival of patients with large bowel cancer is based upon wide anatomic resection. Ann Surg 1979;190:350–360.
16. Turnbull RB Jr, Kyle K, Watson FR et al. Cancer of the colon: the influence of "no-touch isolation" technic on survival rates. Ann Surg 1967;166:420–425.
17. Enker WE. Defining the adequate operations for large bowel cancer. Clin Surg Int 1981;1:78–93.
18. Enker WE. Operative treatment for carcinoma of the abdominal colon. In: Block GE, Moossa AR, eds. Operative Colorectal Surgery. Philadelphia: WB Saunders, 1994:193–219.

19. Stearns MW Jr. Adenocarcinomas. In: Stearns MW Jr, ed. Neoplasms of the Colon, Rectum and Anus. New York, J. Wiley & Sons, 1980:79–98.

20. Enker WE, Martz J, Teppez JE et al. Rectal cancer: management of loco-regional primary rectal cancer. In: Kelsen DP, Daly JM, Kern SE, eds. Gastrointestinal Oncology, Principles and Practice. Philadelphia, Lippincott, Williams and Wilkins, 2002:781–824.

21. Kapiteijn E, Klein-Krankenbarg E, Steu W et al. Total mesorectal excision (TME) with or without preoperative radiotherapy in the treatment of primary rectal cancer: prospective randomized trial with standard operative and histopathologic techniques. Dutch ColoRectal Cancer Group. Eur J Surg 1999;165:410–420.

22. Lehander MA, Holm T, Rutqvist LE et al. Effect of a surgical training programme on outcome of rectal cancer in the county of Stockholm. Lancet 2000;356:93–96.

23. Wibe A, Moller B, Norstein J et al. for the Norwegian Rectal Cancer Group. A national strategic change in treatment policy for rectal cancer: implementation of total mesorectal excision as a routine treatment in Norway. A national audit. Dis Colon Rectum 2002;45:857–866.

24. Scott-Conner CE. Integrating advanced laparoscopy into surgical residency training. Surg Endosc 1994;8:1057.

25. Soper NJ, Brunt LM, Kerbl K. Medical progress: laparoscopic general surgery. N Engl J Med 1994;330:409–419.

26. Cuschieri A. Reflections on surgical training. Surg Endosc 1993;7:73–74.

27. Reznick RK. Surgical education: teaching and testing technical skills. Am J Surg 1993;165:358–361.

28. Watson DCT, Matthews HR. Manual skills of trainee surgeons. J R Coll Surg Edinb 1987;32:74–75.

29. Park A, Witzke D, Donnelly M. Ongoing deficits in residence training for minimal invasive training. J Gastrointest Surg 2001;6:501–507.

30. Romeanelli JR, Litwin DEM. Hand-assisted laparoscopic surgery. Probl Gen Surg 2001;18:45–51.

31. Pietrow PK, Albala DM. Hand-assisted urology laparoscopy. Curr Opin Urol 2002;12:233–237.

32. Purohit S et al. Making hand-assisted laparoscopy easier. J Endourol 2001;15:943–945.

33. Lazar HL, DeLand EC, Tompkins RK. Clinical performance versus in-training examinations as measures of surgical competence. Surgery 1989;87:357–362.

34. Squire D, Giachino AA, Profitt AW et al. Objective comparison of manual dexterity in physicians and surgeons. Can J Surg 1989;32:467–470.

35. Schueneman AL, Pickleman J, Hesselein R et al. Neurological predictors of operative skill among general surgery residents. Surgery 1984;96:288–295.

36. Rosser JC, Murayama, M, Gabriel NH. Minimally invasive surgical training solutions for the twenty-first century. Surg Clin North Am 2000;80:1607–1624.

37. Francis NK, Hanna GB, Cuschieri A. The performance of master surgeons on the Advance Dundee Endoscopic Psychomotor Tester. Arch Surg 2002;137:841–844.

38. Rosser JC Jr, Rosser LE, Savalgi RS. Objective evaluation of a laparoscopic surgical skill program for residents and senior surgeons. Arch Surg 1998;133:657–661.

39. Rosser J. CD-ROM multimedia: the step before virtual reality. Surg Endosc 1996; 10:1033–1035.

40. Rosser JC, Rosser LE, Savalgi RS. Skill acquisition and assessment for laparoscopic surgery. Arch Surg 1997;132:200–204.

41. Satava RM. Virtual reality surgical simulator: the first steps. Surg Endosc 1993;7:203–205.

42. Rosser JC Jr, Herman B, Risucci DA et al. Effectiveness of a CD-ROM multimedia tutorial in transferring cognitive knowledge essential for laparoscopic skill training. Am J Surg 2000;179:32–324.

43. Rosser JC, Wood M, Payne JH et al. Telementoring: a practical option in surgical training. Surg Endosc 1997;11:852–855.

44. Satava RM. Virtual reality. Prot Gen Surg 1998;1:75–95.

45. Holden JG, Flach JM, Donchin Y. Perceptual-motor coordination in an endoscopic surgery simulation. Surg Endosc 1999;13:127–132.

46. Taylor HL, Lintern G, Koonce JM. Quasi-transfer as a predictor of transfer from simulator to airplane. J Gen Psychol 1992;120:257–276.

47. Swett HA, Holaday L, Leffell D et al. Telemedicine: delivering medical expertise across the state and around the world. Conn Med 1995;59:593–602.

48. Berguer R. Surgery and ergonomic. Arch Surg 1999;134:1011–1016.

49. Berguer R, Forkey DL, Smith WD. Ergonomic problems associated with laparoscopic surgery. Surg Endosc 1999;13:466–468.

50. Hanna GB, Shimi S, Cushieri A. Influence of direction of view, target-to-endoscope distance and manipulation angle on endoscopic knot tying. Br J Surg 1997;84:1460–1464.

51. Hanna GB, Shimi S, Cushieri A. Task performance in endoscopic surgery is influenced by location of image display. Ann Surg 1998;227:481–484.

52. Emam TA, Hanna G, Cuschieri A. Ergonomic principles of task alignment, visual display, and direction of execution of laparoscopic bowel suturing. Surg Endosc 2002; 16: 267–271.

53. Meng WC, Kwok SP, Leung KL et al. Optimal position of working ports in laparoscopic surgery: an in vitro study. Surg Laparosc Endosc 1996;6:278–281.

54. Patkin M, Isabel L. Ergonomics, engineering and surgery of endosurgical dissection. J R Coll Surg Edinb 1995;40:120–132.

55. Berguer R. The application of ergonomics in the work environment of general surgeons. Rev Environ Health 1997;12:99–106.

56. Vithiananthan S, Cooper Z, Betten K et al. Hybrid laparoscopic flexure takedown and open procedure for rectal resection is associated with significantly shorter length of stay than equivalent open resection. Dis Colon Rectum 2001;44:927–935.

57. Robles AE. Laparoscopy in general surgery: training, credentialing, and safety. Int Surg 1994; 79:266–267.

58. Watts J, Feldman WB. Assessment of technical skills. In: Neufeld VR, Norman GR, eds. Assessing Clinical Competence. New York, Springer, 1985:259–274.

59. Rosser JC Jr, Herman B, Ehrenwerth C. An overview of videostreaming on the Internet and its application to surgical education. Surg Endosc Jun 2001;15: 624–629.

60. Hartley JE, Mehigan BJ, MacDonald AW et al. Patterns of recurrence and survival after laparoscopic and conventional resections for colorectal carcinoma. Ann Surg 2000;232:181–186.

61. Lim CS, Mehigan BJ, Hartley JE et al. Neoadjuvant therapy in the treatment of high risk rectal carcinoma. Surg Oncol 1999;8:1–11.

62. Greene FL. Pneumoperitoneum in the cancer patient: advantages and pitfalls. Semin Surg Oncol 1998;15:151–154.

63. Rosser JC Jr, Palter SF, Rodas EB et al. Minilaparoscopy without general anesthesia for the diagnosis of acute appendicitis. J Soc Laparoendosc Surg 1998;2:79–82.

64. Alexander RJ, Jaques BC, Mitchell KG. Laparoscopically-assisted colectomy and wound recurrence. Lancet 1993;341:249–250.

65. Fusco MA, Paluzzi MW. Abdominal wall recurrence after laparoscopic-assisted colectomy for adenocarcinoma of the colon: report of a case. Dis Colon Rectum 1993;36:858–861.

66. Walsh DC, Wattchow DA, Wilson TG. Subcutaneous metastases after laparoscopic resection for malignancy. Aust NZ J Surg 1993;63:530–534.

67. Fielding GA, Luley J, Nathanson L et al. Laparoscopic colectomy. Surg Endosc 1997;1997:745–749.

68. Lacy AM, Delgado S, Garcia-Valdecasas JC et al. Port-site metastases and recurrence after laparoscopic colectomy: a randomized trial. Surg Endosc 1998;12:1039–1042.

69. Milsom JW, Bohm B, Hammerhofer KA et al. A prospective randomized trial comparing laparoscopic versus conventional techniques in colorectal cancer surgery: a preliminary report. J Am Coll Surg 1998;187:55–57.

70. Reilly WT, Nelson H, Schroeder G et al. Wound recurrence following conventional treatment of colorectal cancer. Dis Colon Rectum 1996;39:200–207.

71. Hughes ES, McDermott FT, Polglase AL et al. Tumour recurrence in the abdominal wound scar after large bowel surgery. Dis Colon Rectum 1983;26:571–572.

72. Hewett P, Baxter P. A survey of recurrence in abdominal incisions after colorectal cancer resection. Pri Intervent 1997.

73. Phillips EH, Franklin M, Carroll BJ et al. Laparoscopic colectomy. Ann Surg 1992; 216:703–707.

74. Corbitt JD Jr. Preliminary experience with laparoscopic-guided colectomy. Surg Laparosc Endosc Percutan Tech 1992;2:79–81.

75. Franklin ME Jr, Rosenthal D, Abrego-Medina D et al. Prospective comparison of open vs. laparoscopic colon surgery for carcinoma: five-year results. Dis Colon Rectum 1996;39:S35–S46.

76. Falk PM, Beart RW, Wexner SD et al. Laparoscopic colectomy: a critical appraisal. Dis Colon Rectum 1993;36:28–34.

77. Delgado F, Bolufer JM, Grau E et al. Laparoscopic colorectal cancer resection: initial follow-up results. Surg Laparosc Endosc Percutan Tech 1999;9:91–98.

78. Kwok SP, Lau WY, Carey PD et al. Prospective evaluation of laparoscopic-assisted large-bowel excision for cancer. Ann Surg 1996;223:170–176.

79. Fleshman JW, Nelson H, Peters W et al. Early results of laparoscopic surgery for colorectal cancer: retrospective analysis of 372 patients treated by the Clinical Outcomes of Surgical Therapy (COST) Study Group. Dis Colon Rectum 1996;39:S53–S58.

80. Bokey EL, Moore JWE, Keating JP et al. Laparoscopic resection of the colon and rectum for cancer. Br J Surg 1997;84:822–825.

81. Lord SA, Larach SW, Ferrara A et al. Laparoscopic resections for colorectal carcinoma: a three-year experience. Dis Colon Rectum 1996;39:148–154.

82. Hoffman GC, Baker JW, Dowey JB et al. Minimally invasive surgery for colorectal cancer; initial follow-up. Ann Surg 1996;223:790–798.

83. Lezoche E, Feliciotto F, Paganini AM et al. Laparoscopic colonic resections versus open surgery: a prospective non-randomized study on 310 unselected cases. Hepatogastroenterology 2000;47:697–708.

84. Molenaar CB, Bijnen AB, de Ruiter P Indications for laparoscopic colorectal surgery: results from the Medical Centre Alkmaar, the Netherlands. Surg Endosc 1998;12:42–45.

85. Croce E, Olmi S, Azzola M et al. Laparoscopic colectomy: indications, standardized technique and results after six years experience. Hepatogastroenterology 2000;47:683–691.

86. Kakisako K, Sato K, Adachi Y et al. Laparoscopic colectomy for Dukes A colon cancer. Surg Laparosc Endosc Percutan Tech 2000;10:66–70.

87. Huscher C, Silecchia G, Croce E et al. Laparoscopic colorectal resection: a multi-center Italian study. Surg Endosc 1996;10:875–879.

88. Chen HH, Wexner SD, Iroatulam AJ et al. Laparoscopic colectomy compares favorably with colectomy by laparotomy for reduction of postoperative ileus. Dis Colon Rectum 2000;43:61–65.

89. Petrelli N. Clinical trial are mandatory for improving surgical cancer care. JAMA 2002;287:377–378.

90. Lacy AM, Garcia-Valdecasas JC, Pique JM et al. Short term outcome analysis of a randomized trial comparing laparoscopic vs open colectomy for colon cancer. Surg Endosc 1995;9:1101–1105.

91. Stage JG, Schulze S, Moller P et al. Prospective randomized study of laparoscopic versus open colonic resection for adenocarcinoma. Br J Surg 1997;84:391–396.

92. Wexner SD, Johansen OB, Nogueras JJ et al. Laparoscopic total abdominal colectomy: a prospective trial. Dis Colon Rectum 1992;35:651–655.

93. Schwenk W, Jacobi C, Mansmann U et al. Inflammatory response after laparoscopic and conventional colorectal resections—Results of a prospective randomized trial. Langenbeck Arch Surg 2000;385:2–9.

94. Hewett P. The Australian laparoscopic assisted resection for adenocarcinoma of the colon trial. Aust NZ J Surg 1997;67:S13.

95. Nelson H, Weeks JC, Wieand HS. Proposed phase III trial comparing laparoscopic-assisted colectomy versus open colectomy for colon cancer. Monogr Natl Cancer Inst 1995;19:51–56.

96. Stead ML, Brown JM, Bosanquet N et al. Assessing the relative costs of standard open surgery and laparoscopic surgery in randomized controlled trial in the United Kingdom. Crit Rev Oncol Hematol 2000:33:99–103.

97. The COLOR Study Group. COLOR: a randomized clinical trial comparing laparoscopic and open resection for colon cancer. Digest Surg 2000;17:617–622.

98. Lacy AM, Garcia-Valdecasas JC, Delgado S et al. Laparoscopy-assisted colectomy versus open colectomy for treatment of non-metastatic colon cancer: a randomized trial. Lancet 2002;359:2224–2229.

99. Hansborough JF, Bender EM, Zapata-Sirvent R et al. Altered helper and suppressor lymphocyte populations in surgical patients: a measure of postoperative immunosuppression. Am J Surg 1984;148:303–307.

100. Vittimberga FJ Jr, Foley DP, Meyers WC et al. Laparoscopic surgery and the systemic immune response. Ann Surg 1998;227:326–334.

101. DaCosta ML, Redmond HP, Finnegan N et al. Laparotomy and laparoscopy differentially accelerate experimental flank tumor growth. Br J Surg 1998;85:1439–1442.

102. Bouvy ND, Marquet RL, Jeekel J et al. Laparoscopic surgery is associated with less tumor growth stimulation than conventional surgery: an experimental study. Br J Surg 1996;84:358–361.

103. Delgado S, Lacy AC, Fillela X et al. Acute phase response in laparoscopic and conventional colectomy in colon cancer: a randomized trial. Dis Colon Rectum 2001;44:638–646.

104. Lumley J, Stitz R, Stevenson A et al. Laparoscopic colorectal surgery for cancer: intermediate to long-term outcomes. Dis Colon Rectum 2002;45:867–874.

105. Fleshman JW, Nelson H, Peters WR et al for the Clinical Outcomes of Surgical Therapy Study Group. Early results of laparoscopic surgery for colorectal cancer. Dis Colon Rectum 1996;39:S53–S58.

106. Mehigan B, Hartley J, MacDonald A et al. Prospective trial of lapaorscopic-assisted vs. conventional resection for colorectal cancer. Dis Colon Rectum 1999;42:A20.

107. Lumley J, Stitz R, Stevenson A Laparoscopic resection for cancer. Dis Colon Rectum 1999;42:A21.

108. Nelson H, Weeks JC, Weiand HS. Proposed phase III trial comparing laparoscopic-assisted colectomy versus open colectomy for colon cancer. Monogr Natl Cancer Inst 1995;19:51–56.

109. Weeks JC, Nelson H, Gelber S et al for the Clinical Outcomes of Surgical Therapy Study Group. Short-term quality-of-life outcomes following laparoscopically-assisted colectomy vs. open colectomy for colon cancer. JAMA 2002;287:321–328.

110. Pilipshen SJ, Heilweil M, Quan SHQ et al. Patterns of pelvic recurrence following definitive resections of rectal cancer. Cancer 1984;53:1354–62.

111. Scheidbach H, Schnieder C, Baerlehner E et al. Laparoscopic anterior resection for rectal cancer. Surg Oncol Clin North Am 2001;10:599–609.

112. Hermanek P, Hermanek PJ. Role of the surgeon as a variable in the treatment of rectal cancer. Semin Surg Oncol 2000;19:329–335.

113. Guillou PJ, Darzi A, Monson JRT. Experience with laparoscopic colorectal surgery for malignant disease. Surg Oncol 1993;2:43–49.

114. Poulin EC, Schlachta CM, Gregoire R et al. Local recurrence and survival after laparoscopic mesorectal resection for rectal adenocarcinoma. Surg Endosc 2002;16:989–995.

115. Havenga K, Enker WE, Norstein J et al. Improved survival and local recurrence after D3 lymphadenectomy in the treatment of primary rectal cancer: an international analysis of 1141 patients. Eur J Surg Oncol 1999;25:368–374.

116. Havenga K, Enker WE, McDermott K et al. Male and female sexual and urinary function after total mesorectal excision with autonomic nerve preservation for carcinoma of the rectum. J Am Coll Surg 1996;182:495–502.

117. Enker WE, Merchant N, Cohen AM et al. Safety and efficacy of low anterior resection for rectal cancer: 681 consecutive cases from a specialty service. Ann Surg 1999;230:544–552.

118. Larach SW, Gallagher JT. Complications of laparoscopic surgery for rectal cancer: avoidance and management. Semin Surg Oncol 2000:18:265–268.

119. Reis Neto JA, Quilici FA, Cordeiro F et al. Laparoscopic total mesorectal excision. JSLS 2002;6:163–167.

120. Bruch HP, Schwandner O, Schiedeck TH et al. Actual standards and controversies on the operative technique and lymph-node dissection in colorectal cancer. Langenbecks Arch Surg 1999;384:167–175.

121. Weiser MR, Milsom JW. Laparoscopic total mesorectal excision with autonomic nerve preservation. Semin Surg Oncol 2000;19:396–403.

122. Hartley J, Mehigan BJ, Qureshi AE et al. Total mesorectal excision: assessment of the laparoscopic approach. Dis Colon Rectum 2001;44:315–321.

123. Hou YK, Chen JB, Tsai CY et al. Lymphovascular clearance in laparoscopic surgery of cancer in the low rectum. Chung Hua I Hsueh Tsa Chih 2001;64:453–458.

124. Zmora O, Wexner SD. Part I. Laparoscopic surgery for colon and rectal cancer. Curr Prob Cancer 2001;25:286–309.

125. Mehigan BJ, Monson JRT. Laparoscopic rectal-abdominoperineal resection. Surg Oncol Clin North Am 2001;10:611–623.

126. Enker WE, Havenga K, Polyak T et al. Abdominoperineal resection via total mesorectal excision and autonomic nerve preservation in low rectal cancer. Symposium on World Progress in Surgery: Clinicopathological Staging and Management of Colorectal Cancer. World J Surg 1997;21:715–720.

127. Enker WE. Total mesorectal excision with sphincter and autonomic-nerve preservation in the treatment of rectal cancer. Curr Tech Gen Surg 1996;5:1–8.

128. Fleshman JW, Wexner SD, Anvari M et al. Laparoscopic vs. open abdominoperineal resection for cancer. Dis Colon Rectum 1999;42:930–939.

129. Darzi A, Lewis C, Menzies-Gow N et al. Laparoscopic abdominoperineal excision of the rectum. Surg Endosc 1995;9:414–417.

130. McDermott JP, Devereaux DA, Caushaj PF. Pitfalls of laparoscopic colectomy in an unselected group of patients. Dis Colon Rectum 1994;37:602–603.

131. Lam DT, Kwong KH, Lam CW et al. How useful is colonoscopy in locating colorectal lesions? Surg Endosc 1998;12:839–841.

132. Kitamura K, Yamane T, Oyama T et al. Rapid accurate method for delineating cancer lesions in laparoscopic colectomy using activated carbon injection. J Surg Oncol 1995;58:31–34.

133. Luck AJ, Thomas ML, Roediger WE et al. Localization of the nonpalpable colonic lesion with intraoperative ultrasound. Surg Endosc 1999;13:526–527.

134. Zmora O, Dinnewitzer AJ, Pikarsky AJ et al. Intraoperative endoscopy in laparoscopic colectomy. Surg Endosc 2002;16:808–811.

135. Pasupathy S, Eu KW, Ho YH et al. A comparison of open versus laparoscopic assisted colonic pouches for rectal cancer. Tech Proctol 2001;5:19–22.

136. Ichihara T, Nagahata Y, Nomura H et al. Laparoscopic lower anterior resection is equivalent to laparotomy for lower rectal cancer at the distal line of resection. Am J Surg 2000;179:97–98.

137. Watanabe Y, Sato M, Kikkawa H et al. Hand-assisted laparoscopic total colorectal resection for familial adenomatous polyposis with coexisting rectal cancer. Surg Endosc 2001;15:445–447.

138. Pietrabissa A, Moretto C, Carobbi A et al. Hand-assisted laparoscopic low anterior resection: initial experience with a new procedure. Surg Endosc 2002;16:431–435.

139. Scott H, Darzi A. Tactile feedback in laparoscopic colonic surgery. Br J Surg 1997;84:1005.

140. Young-Fadok TM. Review of laparoscopy-assisted colectomy vs. open colectomy for treatment of nonmetastatic colon cancer: a randomized trial. Am J Oncol Rev 2002;1:201–203.

141. Murty M, Enker WE, Martz J. Current status of total mesorectal excision and autonomic nerve preservation in rectal cancer. Semin Surg Oncol 2000;19:321–328.

142. Lezoche E, Feliciotti F, Paganini AM et al. Laparoscopic vs. open hemicolectomy for colon cancer: long term outcome. Surg Endosc 2002;16:596–602.

143. Lechaux D, Trebuchet G, LeCalve JL. Five-year results of 206 laparoscopic left colectomies for cancer. Surg Endosc 2002;16:1409–1412.

144. Ziprin P, Ridgway PF, Peck DH et al. The theories and realities of port-site metastases: a critical appraisal. J Am Coll Surg 2002;195:395–408.

145. Law WL, Chu KW, Tung PHM. Laparoscopic colorectal resection: a safe option for elderly patietns. J Am Coll Surg 2002;195:768–773.

Chapter 16

Treatment of AIDS-Related Kaposi's Sarcoma

Bruce Dezube, MD

Kaposi's sarcoma (KS) is the most common tumor arising in human immunodeficiency virus (HIV)–infected patients and is an acquired immune deficiency syndrome (AIDS)–defining illness by the Centers for Disease Control and Prevention guidelines. Recent advances in the elucidation of the pathogenesis of KS are uncovering potential targets for KS therapies. Such targets include the processes of angiogenesis and cellular differentiation and the KS herpesvirus/human herpesvirus 8 (KSHV/HHV8). With the increasing recognition that effective antiretroviral regimens are associated with both a decreased proportion of new AIDS-defining KS cases and a regression in the size of existing KS lesions, most, if not all, KS patients should be advised to take antiretroviral drugs that will maximally decrease HIV-1 viral load. Five agents are currently approved by the United States Food and Drug Administration for the treatment of KS; alitretinoin gel for topical administration and liposomal daunorubicin, liposomal doxorubicin, paclitaxel, and interferon alfa for systemic administration. Many more agents, particularly angiogenesis inhibitors and other pathogenesis-targeted therapies, are in early clinical development. Over the next 5 years, we may see even more of these pathogenesis-targeted therapies in trials and, just as important, we may identify, develop, and validate clinically practical tools for assessing the biologic effects of these therapies.

PATHOGENESIS OF KAPOSI'S SARCOMA: DISCOVERY OF POTENTIAL TARGETS FOR THERAPIES

The pathogenesis of AIDS-related KS is multifactorial and involves the KS KSHV/HHV8, altered expression and response to cytokines, stimulation of KS growth by the HIV-1 *trans*-activating protein Tat, and other factors yet to be described.[1] KSHV/HHV8 is a gamma herpesvirus and is a necessary, but not sufficient, cause of KS. Of note, KSHV/HHV8 *preceded* the arrival of the AIDS virus.[2] The outbreak of KS occurred when HIV eroded the immune system of men already harboring KSHV/HHV8.

KSHV/HHV8 encodes proteins that are homologues of interleukin-6 (IL-6), chemokines of the macrophage inflammatory protein family, cell cycle regulators of the cyclin family, and antiapoptosis genes of the bcl-2 family. Tat promotes the growth of spindle cells of endothelial origin derived from AIDS-KS lesions, but it does so only in the presence of inflammatory cytokines.[3] The synergy between cytokines and the HIV-1 Tat protein, as well as the immunosuppression associated with AIDS, suggests a basis whereby AIDS-related KS is more aggressive than the classic Mediterranean form in which the HIV-1 Tat protein does not play a role.

The remarkable finding that KSHV/HHV8 encodes viral IL-6 and that this IL-6 leads, in turn, to expression of vascular endothelial growth factor (VEGF),[4] provides a missing link in the chain of events by which KSHV/HHV8 creates an inflammatory-angiogenic environment. The creation of this inflammatory-angiogenic state by KSHV/HHV8 is proposed by Mesri[5] as the critical step in the pathogenesis of KS. Although this model is plausible given our current state of understanding of KS pathogenesis, it will no doubt be modified and reworked as our insights in this field improve.

The Model: Creation of an Inflammatory-Angiogenic State

1. Circulating KS progenitors and cells latently infected with KSHV/HHV8 are attracted to inflammatory sites (Fig. 16.1).
2. Exposure to inflammatory cytokines causes differentiation of these latently infected cells into KS-like spindle cells and induces KSHV/HHV8 reactivation.
3. Reactivation of KSHV/HHV8 leads to the expression of potentially pathogenic genes, such as viral IL-6, which can activate VEGF and induce angiogenesis.
4. Viral lytic replication in the same cells activates inflammation, which may also play a proangiogenic role.
5. Creation of this inflammatory-angiogenic environment increases the availability of infectable cells, such as endothelial cells and KS spindle cells, which end up in the development of the KS lesion.

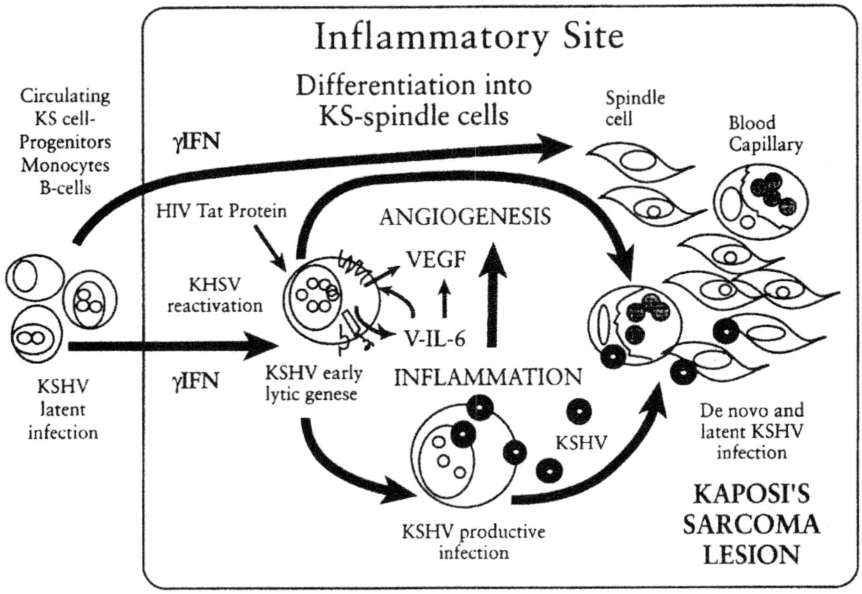

FIGURE 16.1 The creation of the inflammatory-angiogenic environment. Proposed model by which the Kaposi's sarcoma herpesvirus/human herpesvirus 8 (KSHV/HHV8) creates the inflammatory-angiogenic milieu necessary for the growth of Kaposi's sarcoma. (Adapted with permission from Ref. 5.)

6. Cells also become responsive to Tat, the *trans*-activating protein of HIV-1.
7. The HIV-1 Tat protein augments this inflammatory-angiogenic state by increasing the angiogenic activities of basic fibroblast growth factor, interferon gamma, and VEGF; by mimicking the effects of the external matrix protein fibronectin and vitronectin; and by increasing the expression of matrix metalloproteinases.

CLINICAL FEATURES

Cutaneous Involvement

AIDS-related KS has a very variable clinical course, ranging from minimal disease presenting as an incidental finding to explosive growth resulting in significant morbidity and mortality. The skin lesions appear most often on the lower extremities, face (especially the nose), oral mucosa, and genitalia.[6] The lesions are often elliptical and may be arranged in a linear fashion along skin tension lines. The colors associated with these lesions include many hues of pink, red, purple, and brown. More commonly, however, KS lesions are papular, ranging in diameter from several millimeters to several centimeters. Less commonly, KS lesions may be plaque-like, especially on the thighs and soles of the feet, or they may be exophytic and fungating with breakdown of overlying skin. Lymphedema, particularly in the face, genitalia, and lower extremities, may be out of proportion to the extent of cutaneous disease and may be related both to vascular obstruction caused by lymphadenopathy and to cytokines (e.g., VEGF) involved in the pathogenesis of KS. The psychosocial burden associated with KS may be profound and includes emotional distress, guilt, anger, ostracism, and loss of employment.[7]

Extracutaneous Involvement

Extracutaneous spread of KS is common. KS in the oral cavity is particularly common, occurring in approximately one third of patients, and is the initial site of the disease in about 15%. The intraoral site most commonly affected is the palate, followed by the gingiva.[8] Intraoral lesions may become easily traumatized during normal chewing, causing pain, bleeding, ulceration, and secondary infection, and they may interfere with nutrition and speech. The presence or absence of clinical symptoms is often the major determinant of treatment decisions in patients with KS.

Gastrointestinal (GI) involvement is also common in KS and is found in 40% of cases at initial diagnosis and in up to 80% at autopsy. Involvement can occur in the absence of cutaneous disease. GI lesions may cause weight loss, abdominal pain, nausea, vomiting, upper or lower GI tract bleeding, or diarrhea, yet they may be asymptomatic in others.[9,10] Testing the stool for occult blood is an excellent way to screen for GI involvement. For patients with occult blood or GI symptoms, further studies are often recommended. Lesions in the GI tract, often recognized easily by the endoscopist, are typically hemorrhagic nodules, either isolated or confluent, and can be noted in any portion of the tract.[11] Because they tend to be submucosal, biopsies may not demonstrate KS. As with oral lesions, treatment is usually dictated by the presence of symptoms.

Pulmonary involvement is also common and may present as shortness of breath, fever, cough, hemoptysis, or chest pain, or as an asymptomatic finding on chest x-ray study.[12] As many as 15% of patients have no evidence of mucocutaneous KS.[13] Radiographic findings vary greatly and can include nodular, interstitial, or alveolar infiltrates; pleural effusion; hilar or mediastinal adenopathy; or even an isolated pulmonary nodule.[14,15] The pleural effusions of KS are typically serosanguineous and are associated with KS lesions on the visceral pleura that can leak blood into the pleural space.

A presumptive diagnosis of pulmonary KS can usually be made without biopsy if cherry-red, slightly raised lesions are found at bronchoscopy.[16] Biopsy should be avoided because of the risk of hemorrhage posed by these angiogenic lesions. Treatment decisions are usually guided by the presence of respiratory symptoms, the extent of radiographic and bronchoscopic disease,[17] and the exclusion of a concomitant pulmonary infection as the cause of the clinical findings.

Lymph node involvement is not uncommon in KS and may be present in patients with no evidence of mucocutaneous disease. In fact, no organ seems to be spared from involvement with KS, particularly in autopsy series, which describe invasion with tissue replacement in solid organs, such as the liver, pancreas, and heart, as well as in the testes and bone marrow.[11]

Differential Diagnosis

Although a trained observer can often readily make a presumptive diagnosis of KS, a simple skin biopsy can confirm the diagnosis. Early lesions can easily be mistaken as purpura, hematomas, angiomas, dermatofibromas, or nevi. For the biopsy, it is especially important to take samples from lesions that are less typical of KS and are associated with systemic symptoms or appear or progress rapidly in order to rule out bacillary angiomatosis. This condition, which is the most important differential diagnosis of KS, is caused by Bartonella species, a slow-growing, fastidious, gram-negative bacillus, which can be identified by Warthin-Starry silver staining and is readily treated with antibiotic therapy.[18] Skin lesions of bacillary angiomatosis usually appear as numerous high, red, round papules or nodules and may be associated with such symptoms as fever, chills, malaise, headache, or anorexia. KS and bacillary angiomatosis can occur simultaneously.

Exacerbation by Steroids and Opportunistic Infections

Corticosteroid therapy has been associated with the induction of KS and with the exacerbation of preexisting KS in HIV-infected persons,[19] as well as in HIV-negative patients, such as those receiving steroids for organ transplantation, autoimmune disorders, or lymphoproliferative diseases.[20] This association should be emphasized because HIV-infected patients may be treated with corticosteroids for many disorders, including immune thrombocytopenic purpura and *Pneumocystis carinii* pneumonia. Although they are not strictly contraindicated in KS patients, corticosteroids should be used cautiously in this setting. KS lesions may regress on reduction or withdrawal of steroids.[19,20] Opportunistic infections have also been associated with the induction of KS and with the exacerbation of preexisting KS, similar to that described with corticosteroid therapy. High levels of proinflammatory cytokines, which have been demonstrated in the setting of opportunistic infections, may account for these clinical effects on KS.

STAGING AND PROGNOSIS

Initial Evaluation

The initial evaluation of a patient with KS consists of a thorough physical examination, with special attention being paid to those areas typically affected by the disease, such as the lower extremities, face, oral mucosa, genitalia, GI tract, and lungs. Testing the stool for occult blood is an excellent way to screen for GI lesions. Endoscopy can be reserved for patients with occult blood or GI symptoms. In a similar fashion, chest x-ray study is an excellent way to screen for pulmonary lesions. Bronchoscopy can be reserved for those with an abnormal x-ray studies or those with persistent respiratory symptoms when no other cause is found. The potential co-existence of several diseases in patients with KS cannot be overemphasized. The CD4+ T-lymphocyte count and HIV-1 viral load are important both for staging and for treatment decisions.

Staging System

The most commonly used staging system for AIDS-related KS is that developed by the AIDS Clinical Trial Group of the National Institute of Health (Table 16.1).[21] Patients are divided into a good- or poor-risk group according to three parameters: (1) extent of tumor, (2) immune status, and (3) severity of systemic illness. This classification has been shown prospectively to predict survival.[22] When comparing good risk with poor risk groups for each of the three parameters, median survival was 27 months versus 15 months in terms of tumor extent; 40 versus 13 months in terms of immune status; and 22 versus 16 months in terms of systemic illness. Although CD4 cell count and tumor burden provided the most discriminating predictive information, this prospective validation predated the availability of HIV-1 viral load testing, which would be expected to further refine the staging and prognostic criteria for KS.

TREATMENT

The major treatment goals for KS are palliation of symptoms; shrinkage of tumor to alleviate edema, organ compromise, or psychological stress; and prevention of disease progression. Treatment options depend greatly on the tumor (i.e., the extent of disease and the rate of growth), the HIV-1 viral load, and the characteristics of the host (CD4+ T-lymphocyte count, overall medical condition). In terms of the host, it is important to ascertain any impairment in organ function that will increase the potential for drug-related toxicities and to determine whether the patient is taking medications that will increase the likelihood of drug-drug interactions.

Highly Active Antiretroviral Therapy

Most, if not all, KS patients should be advised to take antiretroviral drugs that will maximally decrease HIV-1 viral load. This recommendation is based on the increasing recognition that effective antiretroviral regimens are associated with both a decreased proportion of new AIDS-defining KS cases and a regression in the size of existing lesions. Regression and resolution of not just cutaneous lesions but also visceral ones have been reported in patients taking protease

TABLE 16.1 Staging Classification for AIDS-Related KS

	Good Risk (All of the Following)	Poor Risk (Any of the Following)
Tumor (T)	Confined to skin and/or lymph nodes and/or minimal oral disease (nonnodular KS confined to palate)	Tumor-associated edema or ulceration Extensive oral KS Gastrointestinal KS KS in other nonnodal viscera
Immune system (I)	CD4 cells ≥ 200/μL	CD4 cells < 200/μL
Systemic illness (S)	No history of OI or thrush No "B" symptoms[a] Karnofsky performance status ≥ 70	History of OI and/or thrush B symptoms present[a] Karnofsky performance status < 70 Other HIV-related illness (e.g., neurologic disease, lymphoma)

Abbreviations: AIDS, acquired immune deficiency syndrome; KS, Kaposi's sarcoma; OI, opportunistic infection.

[a]B symptoms are unexplained fever, night sweats, >10% involuntary weight loss, or diarrhea persisting more than 2 weeks

Adapted from Ref. 21.

inhibitor–based therapy.[23-27] Highly active antiretroviral therapy (HAART) prolongs the time to treatment failure of anti-KS therapies.[28] The dramatic impact of HAART on KS is underscored by a large Swiss cohort study of HIV-infected patients. In this cohort, when compared to the relative risk (hazards ratio) of the pre-HAART era between 1992 and 1994, the relative risk of developing KS in the years 1997–1998 (after the introduction of HAART) was 0.08 (95% confidence interval, 0.03–0.22), representing a dramatic reduction in this AIDS-related malignancy.[29] Similarly, in an analysis of 47,936 HIV-positive individuals from North America, Europe, and Australia, the relative risk of developing KS in the years 1997–1999 (1489 cases) when compared with the risk during 1992–1996 (190 cases) was 0.32.[30] Lastly, in pulmonary KS patients, HAART is associated with a reduced risk of death (hazards ratio, 0.09) .[31]

Although the HAART-induced regression of existing KS lesions and the prevention of new lesions have been attributed to the impact of these drugs on the immune system, recent studies suggest that these agents have antineoplastic effects that are independent of their ability to inhibit HIV protease.[32,33] Protease inhibitors block the growth of KS tumors in mouse models and inhibit basic fibroblast growth factor–induced and VEGF-induced angiogenesis in a chorioallantoic membrane assay with a potency similar to that of paclitaxel.

Local Therapy

Alitretinoin gel, 0.1% (9-*cis*-retinoic acid, Panretin) is the only topical, patient-administered therapy approved for the treatment of KS. Alitretinoin is a naturally occurring retinoid that binds both to retinoic acid receptors and to retinoid X receptors. In two phase III studies involving 305 patients, alitretinoin, when compared with vehicle gel, was associated with a shorter time to tumor response, a more prolonged duration of response, and a more prolonged time to disease progression; one of these studies has been published (Table 16.2).[34] Most patients required 4 to 8 weeks of treatment before a response occurred. Responses occurred in patients with a wide range of baseline CD4+ T-lymphocyte counts. Dermal irritation, generally mildly to moderately severe, was common at the site of gel application. Dark-skinned patients may on occasion have undesirable skin lightening after the use of alitretinoin. The gel would not be expected to affect the development of new lesions in untreated areas

Other local treatments include intralesional chemotherapy, radiation therapy, laser therapy, and cryotherapy, all of which can be effective at controlling local tumor growth. Vinblastine is probably the most widely used intralesional agent and has an excellent response rate, approximately 70%.[35] Treated lesions usually fade and regress, although they typically do not resolve completely. Radiation therapy can effectively palliate symptomatic disease that is too extensive to be treated with intralesional chemotherapy, but not extensive enough to warrant systemic therapy.[36] In a series of 36 patients with KS of the feet, a fractionation schedule of three fractions a week at 3.5 Gy/fraction to a total dose of 21.0 Gy yielded an overall response rate of 91% (complete response rate, 80%). Although discomfort from the radiation was common, it usually resolved without intervention within 2 weeks of completion of radiation therapy.[37]

Interferon Alfa

Interferon alfa is a biologic response modifier that can produce clinically significant responses in KS patients, especially those with disease limited to the skin and with relatively modest degrees of immunosuppression.[38] Although low doses of interferon (< 10 million U/m^2 daily) can be used effectively when it is combined with nucleoside reverse transcriptase inhibitors (e.g., zidovudine, didanosine), interferon therapy at higher doses is often associated with significant systemic toxicity that consists of fever, chills, neutropenia, hepatotoxicity, and

TABLE 16.2 Alitretinoin Gel in AIDS-Related Kaposi's Sarcoma

Response Rate (%)	Alitretinoin 0.1% Gel (N = 90)	Vehicle Gel (N = 85)
Clinical complete response	1	1
Partial response	66	28
Stable response	18	24
Time to achieve 50% response rate	98 days (14 weeks)	N/A
Median duration of response	Not reached by 18 weeks	N/A

Abbreviation: AIDS, acquired immune deficiency syndrome.
Adapted from reference 34.

cognitive impairment. In an AIDS Clinical Trial Group study, low-dose (1 million units daily) and moderate-dose (10 million units daily) interferon produced similar response rates when each was combined with didanosine.[39] Poor tumor response and drug-related toxicity are particularly striking in patients with CD4+ T-lymphocyte counts < 200 cells/µL. For some patients with asymptomatic, but relatively disseminated, cutaneous disease, interferon in combination with antiretroviral agents may be a reasonable option before the decision is made to use chemotherapy.

Chemotherapy

Although many chemotherapeutic agents, including bleomycin, vinblastine, vincristine, vinorelbine, and etoposide,[40,41] have been found to be very active against KS, both as single agents or in combination therapy, the current systemic treatments for KS revolve around the newer liposomal anthracyclines, as well as paclitaxel. The liposomal formulation of the anthracyclines provides the theoretical advantage of longer plasma half-life, higher tumor concentrations of drug, and less toxicity in nontarget organs, that is, a better benefit-to-risk ratio than that conferred by conventional chemotherapy.

The two currently approved liposomal anthracyclines, liposomal doxorubicin (Doxil) and liposomal daunorubicin (DaunoXome), have become the first-line chemotherapeutic treatment for patients with disseminated, symptomatic KS. In randomized multicenter trials, each of these liposomal agents has been found to be superior to conventional chemotherapy (bleomycin and vincristine with or without nonliposomal doxorubicin) in terms of response rates and toxicity profiles.[42-44] For example, the response rate to liposomal doxorubicin versus that of the combination of bleomycin and vincristine was 59% and 23%, respectively ($P < 0.001$), most of which were partial responses.[44] The recommended dose of liposomal doxorubicin is 20 mg/m^2 every 3 weeks; the dose of liposomal daunorubicin is 40 mg/m^2 every 2 weeks.

Each of these liposomal compounds can reliably shrink tumors, lessen edema, and cause the color of lesions to fade in 25% to 59% of treated patients, depending on the specific definition of clinical response and other characteristics of the various trials. Moreover, liposomal doxorubicin is effective in 32% of patients whose tumors have progressed while they received conventional doxorubicin, suggesting that the liposomal encapsulation increases the therapeutic effect of doxorubicin.[45] Side effects are, in general, mild. Alopecia and neuropathies, in particular, are unusual with these preparations, when compared with conventional chemotherapies. Further, at higher cumulative doses, these agents have not typically been associated with the cardiomyopathies that have often limited the use of nonliposomal anthracyclines.

Paclitaxel (Taxol), the newest systemic chemotherapeutic agent approved for KS, has shown striking efficacy, even in patients with anthracycline-resistant disease. The response rates in two phase II trials were 71% and 59%.[46,47] The median duration of response, approximately 10 months, is among the longest observed for any regimen reported for this disease.[46] Paclitaxel is well tolerated, but the higher prevalences of alopecia, myalgia/arthralgia, and bone marrow suppression and the need for a 3-hour infusion make paclitaxel less attractive than the liposomal anthracyclines as initial therapy for disseminated disease.

Recommended dosing schedules for paclitaxel are 100 mg/m^2 over 3 hours every 2 weeks or 135 mg/m^2 over 3 hours every 3 weeks. The usual regimens of premedication before paclitaxel therapy include diphenhydramine and ranitidine (or equivalent). Because of the concern about using corticosteroids in these patients, the use of dexamethasone is usually restricted to 20 mg intravenously given just before the paclitaxel or 10 mg administered orally 12 and 6 hours before paclitaxel therapy.

Potential Interaction of Antiretroviral Therapy and Paclitaxel

Drug metabolism of many of the approved antiretroviral agents, particularly protease inhibitors and nonnucleoside reverse transcriptase inhibitors, involves cytochrome P450 metabolic pathways. Taxanes are oxidized to less active metabolites by hepatic cytochrome P450 enzymes. The profound toxicity noted in at least two patients who were receiving paclitaxel has been ascribed to a toxic interaction between this chemotherapeutic agent and antiretroviral drugs.[48] In a pharmacokinetic study in a single male patient, however, the metabolism of paclitaxel given concomitantly with indinavir, ritonavir, saquinavir, or nevirapine

TABLE 16.3 Paclitaxel in AIDS-Related KS

Dose and Schedule	Patients (*N*)	Response Rate (%)	Median Duration of Response (months)	Reference
100mg/m^2 every 2 weeks	56	59	10.4	46
135 mg/m^2 every 3 weeks	28	71	7.4	47

Abbreviatons: AIDS, acquired immune deficiency syndrome; KS, Kaposi's sarcoma.

was not statistically significantly different from that of paclitaxel used as a single agent in historical control subjects.[49] Caution is urged when agents that use the same metabolic pathways are coadministered.

Investigational Agents

Given the highly significant role that angiogenesis plays in the pathogenesis of KS, it is not surprising that many, if not most, of the angiogenesis inhibitors in development have been or are currently being tested in patients with AIDS-related KS. Angiogenesis inhibitors, which have led to durable clinical responses in patients accrued to early trials, include fumagillin,[50] thalidomide,[51] COL-3 (Metastat)[52] and interleukin-12.[53] Many of these agents are being developed clinically as both angiogenesis inhibitors and KS inhibitors. Of note, in the phase I trial of the matrix metalloproteinase (MMP) inhibitor COL-3 in AIDS-related KS, tumor response rate was 44%, and, more importantly, these responses were associated with decreases in MMP-2 levels.[52]

Other potential targets for KS therapies include KSHV/HHV8 and the process of cellular differentiation. In a phase II trial of 9-*cis*-retinoic acid in AIDS-related KS, the oral administration of this differentiating agent led to a tumor response rate of 37%[54]; this agent is currently approved by the U.S. Food and Drug Administration as a topical gel in the treatment of KS.

LONG-RANGE VIEW

Recent advances in the elucidation of the pathogenesis of KS are uncovering many potential targets for KS therapies. Such targets include the processes of angiogenesis and cellular differentiation, cytokine dysregulation, and KSHV/HHV8, each of which is serving as a rationale for ongoing pathogenesis-based clinical trials.

Because of the relative ease in obtaining KS tissue, KS trials provide a perfect opportunity for those interested in angiogenesis to identify, develop, and validate clinically practical tools for assessing the biologic effects of targeted agents against KS and to use these tools to explore correlations with therapeutic efficacy and other patient outcomes. Ongoing trials are already exploring these biologic endpoints, which include changes in MMP-2/MMP-9 levels, changes in VEGF/basic fibroblast growth factor levels, assays for apoptosis (TUNEL assay), measurements of tumor cytokine and receptors in tissues, KS-specific cytotoxic T-lymphocytes, and circulating endothelial precursor cells.

As more drugs and biologic agents are included in our armamentarium, the potential exists for more pharmacokinetic interactions. Ongoing trials are already assessing such interactions between paclitaxel and protease inhibitors.

Given that the pathogenesis of KS involves a blend of virology, immunology, angiogenesis, and inflammation, and given the number of researchers involved in these endeavors, I predict a substantial increase in the understanding of the pathogenesis of this disease. KS will serve as a model of a virally induced neoplastic process.

REFERENCES

1. Martin JN, Osmond DH. Kaposi's sarcoma-associated herpesvirus and sexual transmission of cancer risk. Curr Opin Oncol 1999;11:508–515.
2. Osmond DH, Buchbinder S, Cheng A et al. Prevalence of Kaposi sarcoma associated herpesvirus infection in homosexual men at beginning of and during the HIV epidemic. JAMA 2002;287:221–225.
3. Ensoli B, Gendelman R, Markham P et al. Synergy between basic fibroblast growth factor and HIV-1 Tat protein in induction of Kaposi's sarcoma. Nature 1994;371:674–680.
4. Aoki Y, Jaffe ES, Chang Y et al. Angiogenesis and hematopoiesis induced by Kaposi's sarcoma-associated herpesvirus-encoded interleukin-6. Blood 1999;93:4034–4043.
5. Mesri EA. Inflammatory reactivation and angiogenicity of Kaposi's sarcoma-associated herpesvirus/HHV8: a missing link in the pathogenesis of acquired immunodeficiency syndrome-associated Kaposi's sarcoma. Blood 1999;93:4031–4033.
6. Dezube BJ. Acquired immunodeficiency syndrome-related Kaposi's sarcoma: clinical features, staging, and treatment. Semin Oncol 2000;27:424–430.
7. Holland JC, Tross S. Psychosocial considerations in the therapy of epidemic Kaposi's sarcoma. Semin Oncol 1987;14[2 suppl 3]:48–53.
8. Nichols CM, Flaitz CM et al. Treating Kaposi's lesions in the HIV-infected patient. J Am Dent Assoc 1993;124:78–84.
9. Danzig JB, Brandt LJ, Reinus JF et al. Gastrointestinal malignancy in patients with AIDS. Am J Gastroenterol 1991;86:715–718.
10. Laine L, Amerian J, Rarick M et al. The response of symptomatic gastrointestinal Kaposi's sarcoma to chemotherapy: a prospective evaluation using an endoscopic method of disease quantification. Am J Gastroenterol 1990;85:959–961.
11. Ioachim HL, Adsay V, Giancotti FR et al. Kaposi's sarcoma of internal organs: a multiparameter study of 86 cases. Cancer 1995;75:1376–1385.

12. Aboulafia DM. The epidemiologic, pathologic, and clinical features of AIDS-associated pulmonary Kaposi's sarcoma. Chest 2000;117:1128–1145.
13. Huang L, Schnapp LM, Gruden JF et al. Presentation of AIDS-related pulmonary Kaposi's sarcoma diagnosed by bronchoscopy. Am J Respir Crit Care Med 1996;153:1385–1390.
14. Gill PS, Akil B, Colletti P et al. Pulmonary Kaposi's sarcoma: clinical findings and results of therapy. Am J Med 1989;87:57–61.
15. Garay SM, Belenko M, Fazzini E et al. Pulmonary manifestations of Kaposi's sarcoma. Chest 1987;91:39–43.
16. Judson MA, Sahn SA. Endobronchial lesions in HIV-infected individuals. Chest 1994;105:1314–1323.
17. Gruden JF, Huang L, Webb WR et al. AIDS-related Kaposi sarcoma of the lung: radiographic findings and staging system with bronchoscopic correlation. Radiology 1995;195:545–552.
18. Adal KA, Cockerell CJ, Petri WA Jr. Cat scratch disease, bacillary angiomatosis, and other infections due to Rochalimaea. N Engl J Med 1994;330:1509–1515.
19. Gill PS, Loureiro C, Bernstein-Singer M et al. Clinical effect of glucocorticoids on Kaposi sarcoma related to the acquired immunodeficiency syndrome (AIDS). Ann Intern Med 1989;110:937–940.
20. Trattner A, Hodak E, David M et al. The appearance of Kaposi sarcoma during corticosteroid therapy. Cancer 1993;72:1779–1783.
21. Krown SE, Metroka C, Wernz JC. Kaposi's sarcoma in the acquired immune deficiency syndrome: a proposal for uniform evaluation, response, and staging criteria. AIDS Clinical Trials Group Oncology Committee. J Clin Oncol 1989;7:1201–1207.
22. Krown SE, Testa MA, Huang J. AIDS-related Kaposi's sarcoma: prospective validation of the AIDS Clinical Trials Group staging classification. AIDS Clinical Trials Group Oncology Committee. J Clin Oncol 1997;15:3085–3092.
23. De Milito A, Catucci M, Venturi G et al. Antiretroviral therapy with protease inhibitors in human immunodeficiency virus type 1- and human herpesvirus 8-coinfected patients. J Med Virol 1999;57:140–144.
24. Murphy M, Armstrong D, Sepkowitz KA et al. Regression of AIDS-related Kaposi's sarcoma following treatment with an HIV-1 protease inhibitor. AIDS 1997;11:261–262.
25. Conant MA, Opp KM, Poretz D et al. Reduction of Kaposi's sarcoma lesions following treatment of AIDS with ritonavir. AIDS 1997;11:1300–1301.
26. Aboulafia DM. Regression of acquired immunodeficiency syndrome-related pulmonary Kaposi's sarcoma after highly active antiretroviral therapy. Mayo Clin Proc 1998;73:439–443.
27. Niehues T, Horneff G, Megahed M et al. Complete regression of AIDS-related Kaposi's sarcoma in a child treated with highly active antiretroviral therapy. AIDS 1999;13:1148–1149.
28. Bower M, Fox P, Fife K et al. Highly active anti-retroviral therapy (HAART) prolongs time to treatment failure in Kaposi's sarcoma. AIDS 1999;13:2105–2111.
29. Ledergerber B, Telenti A, Egger M. Risk of HIV related Kaposi's sarcoma and non-Hodgkin's lymphoma with potent antiretroviral therapy: prospective cohort study. Swiss HIV Cohort Study. BMJ 1999;319:23–24.
30. International Collaboration on HIV and Cancer. Highly active antiretroviral therapy and incidence of cancer in human immunodeficiency virus-infected adults. J Natl Cancer Inst 2000;92:1823–1830.
31. Holkova B, Takeshita K, Cheng DM et al. Effect of highly active antiretroviral therapy on survival in patients with AIDS-associated pulmonary Kaposi's sarcoma treated with chemotherapy. J Clin Oncol 2001;19:3848–3851.

32. Sgadari C, Barillari G, Toschi E et al. HIV protease inhibitors are potent anti-angiogenic molecules and promote regression of Kaposi sarcoma. Nature Medicine 2002;8:225–232.

33. Pati S, Pelser CB, Dufraine J et al. Antitumorigenic effects of HIV protease inhibitor ritonavir: inhibition of Kaposi sarcoma. Blood 2002;99:3371–3779.

34. Walmsley S, Northfelt DW, Melosky B et al. Treatment of AIDS-related cutaneous Kaposi's sarcoma with topical alitretinoin (9-cis-retinoic acid) gel. Panretin Gel North American Study Group. J Acquir Immune Defic Syndr 1999;22:235–246.

35. Boudreaux AA, Smith LL, Cosby CD et al. Intralesional vinblastine for cutaneous Kaposi's sarcoma associated with acquired immunodeficiency syndrome: a clinical trial to evaluate efficacy and discomfort associated with infection. J Am Acad Dermatol 1993;28:61–65.

36. Swift PS. The role of radiation therapy in the management of HIV-related Kaposi's sarcoma. Hematol Oncol Clin North Am 1996;10:1069–1080.

37. Gressen EL, Rosenstock JG, Xie Y et al. Palliative treatment of epidemic Kaposi sarcoma of the feet. Am J Clin Oncol 1999;22:286–290.

38. Shepherd FA, Beaulieu R, Gelmon K et al. Prospective randomized trial of two dose levels of interferon alfa with zidovudine for the treatment of Kaposi's sarcoma associated with human immunodeficiency virus infection: a Canadian HIV Clinical Trials Network study. J Clin Oncol 1998;16:1736–1742.

39. Krown SE, Li P, Von Roenn JH et al. Randomized, open-label, phase II AIDS Clinical Trials Group study of two doses of interferon-alfa-2b with didanosine in patients with AIDS-associated Kaposi's sarcoma: efficacy of daily low-dose interferon. J Interferon Cytokine Res 2002;22:295–303.

40. Lee FC, Mitsuyasu RT. Chemotherapy of AIDS-related Kaposi's sarcoma. Hematol Oncol Clin North Am 1996;10:1051–1068.

41. Nasti G, Errante D, Talamini R et al. Vinorelbine is an effective and safe drug for AIDS-related Kaposi's sarcoma: results of a phase II study. J Clin Oncol 2000;18:1550–1557.

42. Gill PS, Wernz J, Scadden DT et al. Randomized phase III trial of liposomal daunorubicin versus doxorubicin, bleomycin, and vincristine in AIDS-related Kaposi's sarcoma. J Clin Oncol 1996;14:2353–2364.

43. Northfelt DW, Dezube BJ, Thommes JA et al. Pegylated-liposomal doxorubicin versus doxorubicin, bleomycin, and vincristine in the treatment of AIDS-related Kaposi's sarcoma: results of a randomized phase III clinical trial. J Clin Oncol 1998;16:2445–2451.

44. Stewart S, Jablonowski H, Goebel FD et al. Randomized comparative trial of pegylated liposomal doxorubicin versus bleomycin and vincristine in the treatment of AIDS-related Kaposi's sarcoma. International Pegylated Liposomal Doxorubicin Study Group. J Clin Oncol 1998;16:683–691.

45. Northfelt DW, Dezube BJ, Thommes JA et al. Efficacy of pegylated-liposomal doxorubicin in the treatment of AIDS-related Kaposi's sarcoma after failure of standard chemotherapy. J Clin Oncol 1997;15:653–659.

46. Gill PS, Tulpule A, Espina BM et al. Paclitaxel is safe and effective in the treatment of advanced AIDS-related Kaposi's sarcoma. J Clin Oncol 1999;17:1876–1883.

47. Welles L, Saville MW, Lietzau J et al. Phase II trial with dose titration of paclitaxel for the therapy of human immunodeficiency virus-associated Kaposi's sarcoma. J Clin Oncol 1998;16:1112–1121.

48. Schwartz JD, Howard W, Scadden DT. Potential interaction of antiretroviral therapy with paclitaxel in patients with AIDS-related Kaposi's sarcoma. AIDS. 1999;13:283–284.

49. Nannan Panday VR, Hoetelmans RM, van Heeswijk RP et al. Paclitaxel in the treatment of human immunodeficiency virus 1-associated Kaposi's sarcoma—drug-drug interactions with protease inhibitors and a nonnucleoside reverse transcriptase inhibitor: a case report study. Cancer Chemother Pharmacol 1999;43;516–519.
50. Dezube BJ, Von Roenn JH, Holden-Wiltse J et al. Fumagillin analog in the treatment of Kaposi's sarcoma: a phase I AIDS Clinical Trial Group study. J Clin Oncol 1998;16:1444–1449.
51. Little RF, Wyvill KM, Pluda JM et al. Activity of thalidomide in AIDS-related Kaposi's sarcoma J Clin Oncol 2000;18:2593–2602.
52. Cianfrocca M, Cooley TP, Lee JY et al. Matrix metalloproteinase inhibitor COL-3 in the treatment of AIDS-related Kaposi's sarcoma: a phase I AIDS malignancy consortium study. J Clin Oncol 2002;20:153–159.
53. Pluda JM, Wyvill K, Little R. Administration of interleukin-12 to patients with AIDS-associated Kaposi's sarcoma: preliminary results of a pilot study. J Acquir Immune Defic Syndr Hum Retrovirol 1999;21:A29.
54. Miles SA, Dezube BJ, Lee JY et al. Antitumor activity of oral 9-cis-retinoic acid in HIV-associated Kaposi's sarcoma. AIDS 2002;16:421–429.

Chapter 17

Current Status of Targeted Therapy in Chronic Myeloid Leukemia

Charles L. Sawyers

Neil Shah

The signal transduction inhibitor imatinib mesylate (STI571; Gleevec) has revolutionized the treatment of Philadelphia chromosome–positive leukemias. Imatinib mesylate is a small-molecule inhibitor with activity against Bcr-Abl, the deregulated tyrosine kinase responsible for the initiation and maintenance of chronic myeloid leukemia (CML) in its chronic phase. Clinical trials have demonstrated the ability of imatinib mesylate to induce hematologic and cytogenetic remissions in patients in all stages of CML. Although remissions in patients with chronic-phase disease are durable with 18 months of follow-up, relapse commonly occurs in patients in more advanced stages of disease. Studies investigating the molecular mechanisms of resistance to this novel compound have progressed rapidly and point to the continued importance of Bcr-Abl in disease maintenance, even in its latest stages. This chapter summarizes the rationale leading to the development of imatinib mesylate as a treatment for CML; the clinical results from phase I, II, and III studies; and recent work aimed at elucidating the nature of imatinib resistance. We conclude by offering our view of the future of targeted therapy for CML, including the possibility of combination therapy with signal transduction pathway inhibitors.

INTRODUCTION TO CHRONIC MYELOID LEUKEMIA

CML is a proliferative clonal disorder of hematopoietic stem cells that results primarily in the expansion of mature myeloid cells but also expansion of the erythroid compartment and increase in platelets in the peripheral blood.[1,2] The median age at presentation is about 53 years, but all age groups can be affected, including children. The most common symptoms at presentation are fatigue, anorexia, and weight loss, but about half of patients are asymptomatic at the time of diagnosis. The disease in these cases is suspected solely on the basis of an elevated white blood cell count. Splenomegaly is the most common abnormal physical finding and is detected in approximately 50% of patients. CML typically progresses from the initial stage, termed chronic phase, to a rapidly fatal blast crisis after a median duration of 5 to 6 years. Often, the blast crisis phase is preceded by an accelerated phase in which the white blood cell count becomes difficult to control with standard outpatient oral chemotherapy. In contrast to the normal maturation of blood cells that occurs during the chronic phase, blast crisis cells exhibit a maturation defect in which the bone marrow and the peripheral blood become populated predominantly by myeloblasts or lymphoblasts similar to those found in patients with acute leukemias.

The cytogenetic hallmark of CML is the Philadelphia chromosome translocation, which fuses the Bcr gene on chromosome 22 to the Abl gene on chromosome 9. The resulting *Bcr-Abl* fusion gene encodes a cytoplasmic protein with constitutive tyrosine kinase activity.[3] Various in vitro and mouse models have established that *Bcr-Abl* is an oncogene and is sufficient on its own to produce a CML-like disease in mice within weeks.[4,5] The *Bcr-Abl* oncogene is expressed at all stages, but blast crisis is characterized by multiple additional genetic and molecular abnormalities. Similarly, mouse models of CML can give rise to leukemias that are histologically similar to blast crisis and are characterized by additional cytogenetic or molecular abnormalities.

Before imatinib mesylate was developed, the standard treatments for CML included allogeneic stem cell transplantation for appropriate patients with human leukocyte antigen–matched donors, interferon-α–based therapy, or oral chemotherapy with agents such as hydroxyurea. Allogeneic transplantation is the only known curative therapy, but its utility is complicated by the high rate of mortality and morbidity from transplant-related complications and the lack of suitable donors for many patients. Interferon-α controls the blood counts in most patients and induces cytogenetic remissions in about 20%, but it is associated with significant toxicity, that although not life-threatening, can substantially alter quality of life. Importantly, patients who achieve a cytogenetic remission with interferon-α–based therapy have a substantial survival benefit. Hydroxyurea is very effective at controlling the blood counts of patients CML and has minimal side effects, but it does alter disease progression to blast crisis.

STRATEGIES TO TARGET BCR-ABL

Because the Bcr-Abl kinase is present in essentially all cases of CML and because it plays a causative role in the genesis of the disease, it provides an ideal drug target for the treatment of Philadelphia chromosome–positive leukemias. Before the development of imatinib mesylate, the concept of targeted therapy against Bcr-Abl was explored through the use of antisense RNA or ribozymes, which could specifically bind or cleave the Bcr-Abl fusion messenger RNA (mRNA). Although these approaches showed some feasibility in in vitro models, substantial technical barriers were encountered that preclude meaningful in vivo application. Currently, it appears unlikely that these technologies can be successfully applied to clinical situations unless critical issues, such as the efficient delivery of the targeted agent to all tumor cells, can be overcome.

Immunologic strategies to target Bcr-Abl have also been considered, primarily because of the clear evidence from allogeneic transplantation studies that a graft-versus-leukemia phenomenon plays a critical role in maintaining remissions. One line of investigation is based on the in vitro isolation and expansion of leukemia-specific cytotoxic T-cell clones from patients and donors. An alternative approach is based on the notion that CML cells express the tumor-specific Bcr-Abl fusion protein; therefore, tumor-specific peptides spanning the Bcr-Abl junction could theoretically elicit a tumor-specific immune response. Such peptides have been shown to induce T-cell immune responses, and recent evidence demonstrates that one such peptide could be detected on primary cells isolated from CML patients. Moreover, these patients mounted a cytotoxic T-lymphocyte response directed at the junction peptide that also killed autologous CML cells.[6-8]

ISOLATION OF IMATINIB MESYLATE AS A KINASE INHIBITOR

An alternative strategy for targeting Bcr-Abl is through a more traditional small-molecule pharmacologic approach. Imatinib mesylate is a 2-phenylamino pyrimidine that was originally isolated in a high throughput drug screen for small-molecule inhibitors of the platelet-derived growth factor receptor tyrosine kinase.[9] It was subsequently shown to have potent inhibitory activity against two other tyrosine kinases, Abl and c-Kit, which have become the primary targets of clinical relevance in CML and gastrointestinal stromal tumors, respectively. Imatinib mesylate inhibits all three kinases by targeted the adenosine triphosphate–binding site of the kinase domain. The molecular details of this inhibition were revealed by the determination of the crystal structure of the Abl kinase domain complexed with imatinib mesylate.[10] This study revealed that imatinib mesylate interacts with the inactivated Abl kinase, a more unique conformation than its activated form, and that it is this characteristic that confers drug specificity. Once it was recognized that imatinib mesylate had activity against Abl, preclinical studies were performed that showed activity against Bcr-Abl–expressing tumor cell lines and bone marrow cells isolated from patients with CML.[11,12]

CLINICAL TRIALS OF IMATINIB MESYLATE

Chronic-Phase Trials

On the basis of the preclinical data showing relatively specific activity of imatinib mesylate against Bcr-Abl–expressing CML cells and a favorable preclinical toxicology profile, a phase I clinical trial of oral imatinib mesylate was initiated in June 1998. Eligibility was initially restricted to patients with chronic-phase CML who had not achieved a cytogenetic response to standard therapy with interferon and were not candidates for allogeneic bone marrow transplantation. The trial was intentionally designed to test the drug in patients with chronic-phase rather than blast crisis because Bcr-Abl is the only known molecular abnormality in these patients, thereby allowing a more controlled clinical test of the hypothesis that ABL-directed kinase inhibitor therapy might be effective. The original study design was a standard-dose escalation format with safety as the primary endpoint, beginning at 25 mg per day and then increasing to a maximum tolerated dose. This approach was abandoned after the 1000-mg-per-day cohort because dramatic clinical responses were observed at all dose cohorts beginning with 300 mg and above. Retrospectively, it was learned that a dose of 300 mg per day gave pharmacokinetic profiles that correlated with consistent inhibition of Bcr-Abl kinase activity in circulating blood cells. The clinical results at this dose and greater showed a hematologic response in 53 of 54 patients with chronic-phase CML.[13] Additionally, patients treated with imatinib had a major cytogenetic response rate of 31% despite having failed to achieve a cytogenetic response with interferon-α-based regimens (Table 17.1). The drug had an excellent toxicity profile, with the most common side effects being mild nausea, myalgias, edema, and diarrhea.

These exciting results rapidly led to a phase II study in which 454 patients with chronic-phase CML who had not responded to interferon or were intolerant of interferon because of severe side effects were treated with 400 mg per day of imatinib mesylate. At 18 months of follow-up, the hematologic response rate was 95%, and the major cytogenetic response rate was 60% (Table 17.1).[14] Eleven percent of patients showed disease progression at 18 months, a finding that compares extremely favorably with historical data from patients treated with interferon or hydroxyurea. Again, the drug was extremely well tolerated. These data led to the approval of imatinib mesylate for the treatment of interferon-refractory CML by the U.S. Food and Drug Administration in May 2001.

TABLE 17.1 Hematologic and Cytogenetic Response Rates (Percent) to Imatinib

	Study	Disease Status	Number of Patients	Hematologic Response Rate	Major Cytogenetic Rate
Phase 1	13	CP IFN failure	54	98	31
Phase 1	16	MBC	38	55	11
		ALL (10), LBC (10)	20	70	15
Phase 2	14	CP IFN failure	454	95	60
Phase 2	17	AP	181	82	24
Phase 2	18	MBC	229	52	16
Phase 3	15	CP no previous tx	553 (imatinib)	94	83
		CP no previous tx	553 (IFN/Ara-C)	55	20

AP, acute phase; CP, chronic phase; MBC, myeloid blast crisis; ALL, acute lymphoblastic leukemia; LBC, lymphoid blast crisis; IFN, interferon; tx, treatment.

Data from a randomized study comparing the activities of imatinib mesylate and interferon-α plus cytarabine in newly diagnosed patients with CML now provides strong evidence for the use of imatinib as front-line therapy. In this trial of 1106 patients, the major cytogenetic response rate in the imatinib-treated patients was 83% at 1 year versus 20% in the interferon/cytarabine arm (Table 17.1). In addition, time to progression, although low for both groups, was significantly reduced in the imatinib-treated patients. Because of crossover provisions in the trial design and the availability of imatinib mesylate off study, it is unlikely that this trial will be capable of comparing survival in the imatinib versus the interferon/cytarabine arms.[15]

Accelerated Phase and Blast Crisis Trials

Once the remarkable activity of imatinib mesylate in patients with chronic-phase CML became apparent, the phase I study was amended to test the efficacy of imatinib in patients in the blast crisis phase of CML as well as in patients with Philadelphia chromosome–positive acute lymphoid leukemia (ALL). In addition to providing insight into the activity of imatinib in advanced-stage CML, this trial provided an important opportunity to examine the question of whether such genetically complex tumors still require the expression of the Bcr-Abl tyrosine kinase even at late stages of the disease. Remarkably, 55% of patients with myeloid blast crisis CML and 70% of patients with ALL or lymphoid blast crisis CML had some form of hematologic response to the drug, a finding that is significantly better than historical data on induction chemotherapy regimens used for acute leukemias, and it has substantially less toxicity.[13,16] Major cytogenetic responses also occurred in 11%–15% of patients, and these responses are extremely rare with chemotherapy (Table 17.1). However, the major complication was a high relapse rate that approached 100% in lymphoid disease and 70% in myeloid disease within 6 months of initiation of treatment. In addition, there was an increase in the frequency of drug-induced cytopenias compared with patients with chronic-phase CML, presumably because the number of Philadelphia chromosome–negative cells in these patients is significantly reduced.

Two multicenter phase II studies on advanced-stage CML, one in accelerated phase and one in myeloid blast crisis, were conducted to further explore the utility of imatinib in these patients (Table 17.1). The hematologic response rate in 181 patients with accelerated-phase CML was 82%, and the major cytogenetic response rate was 24%.[17] The median time to disease progression was greater than 12 months in patients treated with 600 mg, and the overall survival was 74% at 1 year. In patients in myeloid blast crisis, the overall hematologic response rate was 52%, but only 31% had sustained responses lasting for more than 4 weeks.[18] The major cytogenetic response rate was 16%. Median survival was 6.9 months, with 32% of patients surviving for 1 year. In both studies, patients who began treatment with 600 mg of imatinib daily fared better than those treated with 400 mg per day. Although this dose comparison was not conducted in a randomized fashion, imatinib mesylate was approved for clinical use in accelerated-phase and blast crisis at a dose of 600 mg by the U.S. Food and Drug Administration on the basis of the strength of this data. Although imatinib is an active single agent for these patients, it is clear that imatinib monotherapy is not sufficient to achieve long-term disease control in these patients. Current clinical studies for the treatment of advanced-stage disease are focused on the use of imatinib in conjunction with other agents, guided in part by laboratory studies that have defined the reasons for imatinib failure.

USE OF MOLECULAR ASSAYS TO FOLLOW PATIENTS TREATED WITH IMATINIB MESYLATE

Although the very high rate of complete cytogenetic response in patients with chronic-phase CML is wonderful news, it raises new issues about how to monitor patients receiving treatment who have no measurable disease that can be detected by standard assays, such as bone marrow cytogenetics. Where do these patients lie in the disease burden schema pictured in Figure 17.1? Fluorescence in situ hybridization is one technology currently in use at most centers that allows the number of Philadelphia chromosome–positive cells to be easily measured in peripheral blood or bone marrow without the need to grow cells and prepare metaphase spreads. Typically, these assays can examine about 250 cells with a background level (false-positive rate) of between 5% and 10%. Therefore,

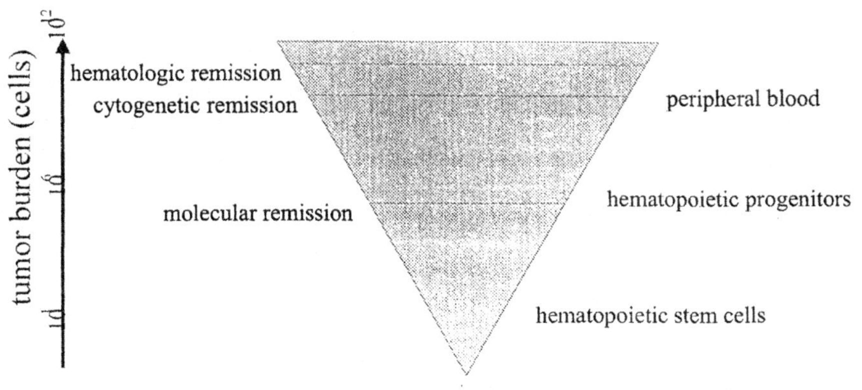

FIGURE 17.1 Relative disease burden in patients with hematologic, cytogenetic, and molecular remissions. The illustration depicts the disease burden in chronic myeloid leukemia (CML) as in inverted triangle beginning with a pleuripotent hematopoietic stem cell that expands and differentiates. Based on estimates of the total number of CML cells in a patient with an elevated leukocyte count at diagnosis, a considerable number of tumor cells may be present in patients who have hematologic or cytogenetic remissions. Quantitative polymerase chain reaction assays are typically sensitive over a range of six orders of magnitude and therefore may offer a much more useful measure of disease burden. The diagram also makes the point that CML cells can exist even in patients in molecular remission.

the sensitivity of fluorescence in situ hybridization is somewhat better than that of cytogenetic analysis (which typically examines 20 metaphases). Most imatinib-treated patients who achieve complete cytogenetic remissions also have no detectable Ph^+ cells by fluorescence in situ hybridization; therefore, alternative assays need to be used to quantify minimal residual disease in these patients.

The solution, almost certainly, will be the use of quantitative polymerase chain reaction (PCR)-based assays, which can reliably measure the level of *Bcr-Abl* mRNA in circulating blood cells. Many iterations of such assays have been developed in academic laboratories and validated in studies of patients with CML who were treated with allogeneic stem cell transplantation or interferon-based regimens. These studies have established that molecular remissions, defined as no detectable *Bcr-Abl* mRNA, can be obtained in a significant fraction of allotransplant recipients but only rarely in interferon-treated patients, and that increasing levels of *Bcr-Abl* mRNA over time in such patients correlate with subsequent cytogenetic and hematologic relapse.[19,20] Early results using similar assays applied to imatinib-treated patients indicate that a subset of patients who experience complete cytogenetic remissions appear to have molecular remissions, whereas others have clearly measurable disease burdens that can vary by several orders of magnitude.[21] There is currently no consensus on the frequency of molecular remissions, largely because of differences in the types of patients analyzed and in the sensitivity of the assays used to measure *Bcr-Abl* mRNA. In addition, there is limited information on the prognostic significance of a *Bcr-Abl* mRNA PCR result in these patients, although one would assume that rising levels of *Bcr-Abl* transcripts over time would predict for eventual relapse. Because such a large number of CML patients reach a state of complete cytogenetic remission, it is imperative that such assays be standardized so that clinical results from different groups can be compared. In addition to academic laboratories, many commercial diagnostic laboratories offer quantitative *Bcr-Abl* testing, but it is essential that clinicians become educated about this topic because it seems likely that PCR-based assays will have a strong impact on clinical decision making in the very near future.

MECHANISMS OF RESISTANCE TO IMATINIB MESYLATE IN PATIENTS

Resistance to STI571 needs to be classified into at least two distinct clinical scenarios, for which the mechanisms of resistance may be quite different. These groups include patients who fail to respond to initial imatinib treatment (up-front resistance) versus those who experience relapse after having an initial response to imatinib.

Up-Front Resistance

The frequency of up-front resistance varies dramatically depending on the stage of disease (chronic, accelerated, or blast crisis) and on whether remissions are measured at the hematologic, cytogenetic, or molecular level. In patients with chronic-phase CML, fewer than 10% have up-front hematologic resistance. However, 20%–40% of such patients have cytogenetic resistance, meaning that a major cytogenic response is not observed in the first year of treatment. The fact that these cytogenetic nonresponders have good hematologic disease control indicates that imatinib is clearly exerting a therapeutic effect, but the reason for the failure to convert from a hematologic to a cytogenetic response is unknown. One possibility is that progenitor cells in the bone marrow, which are measured in karyotype assays, may be less sensitive than mature blood cells to imatinib, raising the question of whether dose escalation could be effective. Indeed, dose increases of imatinib from 400 mg to either 600 or 800 mg can induce cytogenetic remissions in some patients, a finding that is consistent with the notion that higher drug levels are required to block Bcr-Abl kinase activity in the progenitor cell compartment in some patients. For patients who do not respond to higher doses, the same mechanism could apply, or there may be Bcr-Abl–independent signals that are responsible for the continued survival of these cells. The molecular basis for these responses has not been defined and requires careful analysis to determine the level of Bcr-Abl inhibition by imatinib mesylate in different cellular compartments and at distinct stages of differentiation. Similar reasoning can also be applied to accelerated phase and blast crisis patients with up-front hematologic resistance, which occurs more commonly than in chronic phase. Again, it will be important to know whether these patients do not respond because of ineffective inhibition of Bcr-Abl or because of the presence of secondary mutations that allow the leukemia cells to proliferate independent of Bcr-Abl. Another extension of this line of reasoning is to patients with chronic-phase CML who do not achieve molecular remissions.

Acquired Resistance

Much more information is available on the mechanism of imatinib resistance in patients who initially respond to treatment but subsequently experience relapse while still taking the drug. In an initial study of 11 such patients with blast crisis CML or Philadelphia chromosome–positive ALL, Bcr-Abl kinase activity was reduced in leukemia cells during the time of response to imatinib but was reactivated in all patients at the time of relapse.[22] Three patients had amplification of the Bcr-Abl gene, and six patients had an identical single nucleotide change that led to a single amino acid substitution in the kinase domain of Bcr-Abl (threonine to isoleucine at position 315, T315I). This T315I amino acid change prevented imatinib from binding to Bcr-Abl and inhibiting its kinase activity. The mechanism for this effect was immediately apparent because of the prior solution of the crystal structure of imatinib bound to imatinib, which noted that threonine 315 forms a hydrogen bond with the drug.[10] In the mutant Bcr-Abl allele, the bulkier isoleucine prevents imatinib binding due to steric hindrance at the drug binding pocket and inability to form the hydrogen bond (Fig. 17.2). These findings of Bcr-Abl gene amplification[22-26] and Abl kinase domain mutation[27-29]

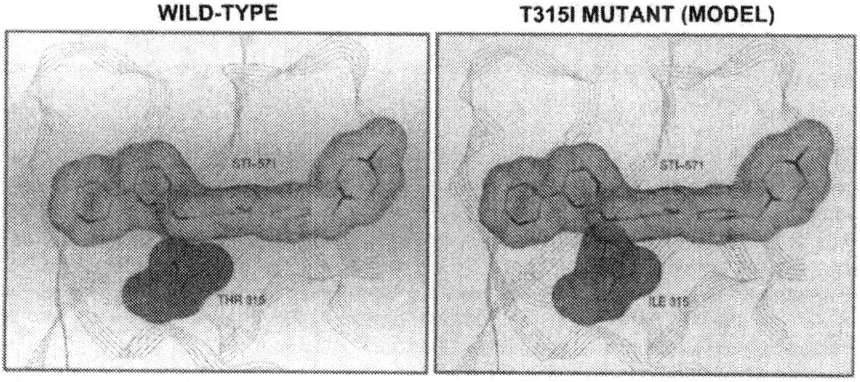

FIGURE 17.2 Model of the STI-571–binding pocket of wild-type (*left*) and T315I mutant (*right*) Abl in complex with STI-571. (Reprinted with permission from Gorre et al.[22])

were confirmed by several other small studies, including a study in which additional single nucleotide changes were identified in patients with acquired imatinib resistance. The most comprehensive report to date estimated that mutations can be detected in a very high fraction of patients with CML who experience relapse after an initial response to therapy, including patients in chronic phase, accelerated phase, or blast crisis.[30] This study reported 15 different nucleotide changes that encoded for 13 different amino acid substitutions within the kinase domain, three of which accounted for more than 60% of the cases (Fig. 17.3). All the mutations studied to date were shown to confer resistance to imatinib in in vitro models, providing strong evidence that these mutations play a causal role in clinical imatinib resistance. When these mutations were examined in the context of the Abl/imatinib crystal structure, two potentially distinct mechanisms for confering drug resistance became apparent. Three of the 13 amino acid substitutions occur at sites of contact with the drug (as demonstrated by the T315I substitution in Fig. 17.2) and are presumed to directly interfere with imatinib

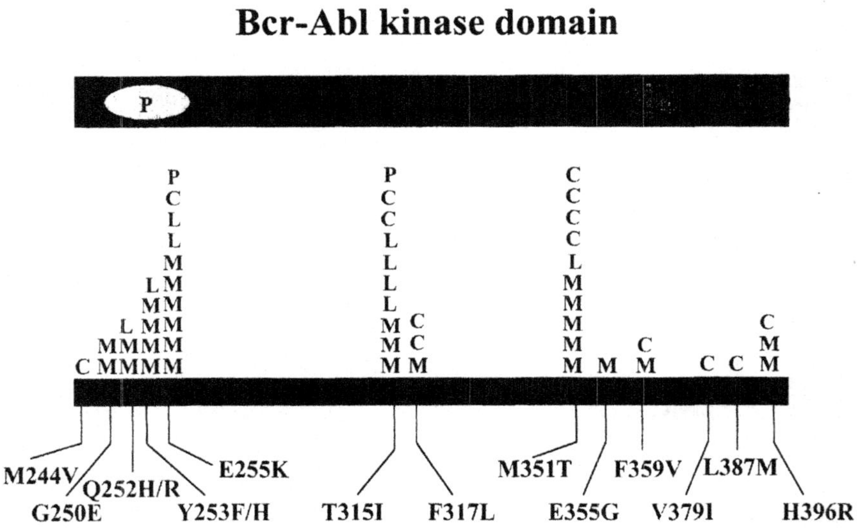

FIGURE 17.3 Summary of imatinib-resistant Bcr-Abl kinase domain mutations. Schematic representation of the Bcr-Abl kinase domain. P-loop (P), catalytic domain (C), and activation loop (A) are depicted. Each letter represents a patient in whom the corresponding mutation was detected (*lower*). Relapsed chronic-phase patients are represented by the letter "C" (*exception:* see below). Relapsed myeloid blast crisis patients are indicated by the letter "M." Patients with relapsed lymphoid blast crisis are represented by the letter "L." "P" indicates mutations detected before imatinib treatment in patients with myeloid blast crisis who exhibited primary resistance to treatment. V379I was detected in a single chronic-phase patient who had persistence of the Philadelphia chromosome and sustained hematologic response. Note that kinase domain is not drawn to scale. (Adapted with permission from Shah et al.[30])

binding. However, the other 10 amino acid changes did not occur at drug contact sites. Rather, these residues were located in two regions of the kinase domain (the phosphate binding loop and the activation loop) that must undergo substantial torsional change in order to bind imatinib. Mutations affecting these residues presumably cause drug resistance by altering the ability of the kinase to undergo these structural changes.

Perhaps the most surprising result from the studies of imatinib mesylate resistance is that blast crisis cells, which have numerous additional genetic abnormalities affecting oncogenes and tumor suppressor genes, default to Bcr-Abl reactivation as the primary mechanism to bypass imatinib mesylate. Although there has been no direct evidence for Bcr-Abl–independent and/or cell autonomous mechanisms of imatinib mesylate resistance in patients, these possibilities cannot be ruled out until more comprehensive analyses are performed on larger numbers of patients. In a gene expression profiling study using bone marrow samples from 19 imatinib mesylate–treated, Philadelphia chromosome–positive ALL patients, 56 genes were reported to have differential expression patterns in cells from patients who had acquired resistance to imatinib mesylate versus in cells from those who were sensitive to the drug.[31] Among those genes with greater mRNA levels in the resistant cells were Bruton's tyrosine kinase and two adenosine triphosphate synthetases. The authors suggested that up-regulation of an alternative pathway in which Bruton's tyrosine kinase plays a role could be a mechanism of resistance to imatinib mesylate independent of Bcr-Abl.[31] However, the authors also noted that a significant fraction of the patients in whom relapse was associated with these gene expression changes also had Bcr-Abl kinase domain mutations. As mentioned in the discussion of up-front imatinib resistance, it will be important to rule out ineffective blockade of Bcr-Abl kinase activity before invoking a role for alternative signaling pathways that drive the proliferation of Philadelphia chromosome—positive leukemias in the presence of imatinib mesylate.

CLINICAL MANAGEMENT OF PATIENTS WHO DO NOT RESPOND TO IMATINIB THERAPY

Most patients who do not respond to imatinib mesylate therapy are those with advanced-stage CML at the time of treatment initiation. The failure rate of imatinib in patients with chronic-phase CML remains low (<15% at 18 months in patients who did not respond to interferon), but several more years of follow-up are required before the full magnitude of the problem will be known. Until these data become available, we can only speculate about whether imatinib mesylate is capable of eliminating all Philadelphia chromosome–positive cells in any CML patients. One strategy for addressing this question is to examine the status of the stem cell compartment in patients who have no measurable disease, that is, those with complete cytogenetic or even molecular remissions. On the basis of this approach, several groups have reported that imatinib induces growth arrest but not apoptosis in CD34-positive progenitor cells.[32,33] In addition, small numbers of Philadelphia chromosome–positive cells can be detected in the CD34 fraction or in colony-forming cells or long-term culture initiating cells propagated from the CD34 fraction, in patients with complete cytogenetic or molecular remissions.[34] The clinical significance of these observations remains to be determined, but the probability of residual disease must be considered, even in patients with molecular remissions.

What are the treatment alternatives for patients who fail to respond to imatinib today? In the absence of definitive clinical trial data, no firm recommendations can be made. For suitable patients with an human leukocyte antigen–matched donor, allogeneic stem cell transplantation should be immediately considered because it offers a possibility for cure. If this choice is not feasible, a commonly used option is to escalate the dose of imatinib to 800 mg, given in divided doses of 400 mg twice daily. As mentioned in the discussion of upfront cytogenetic resistance, this manipulation can often convert cytogenetic nonresponders to responders. Similar success with dose escalation has been achieved in some (but not all) patients with acquired cytogenetic or hematologic relapse. It is interesting to note that some of the Bcr-Abl mutants isolated from imatinib-resistant patients confer relative, but not absolute, drug resistance and remain sensitive to imatinib in vitro at drug concentrations that can easily be achieved in patients treated with 800 mg per day.[30,35] These findings raise the possibility that PCR-based mutation detection assays could be developed to identify, in advance, those patients who are most likely to respond to dose escalation. Mutation assessment in patients with CML may also have a role in assessing prognosis. In a small study of patients with chronic-phase CML who failed to achieve cytogenetic responses, mutations were detected in a subset of patients and correlated with subsequent disease progression.[30] Other approaches for the management of imatinib failure include the addition of interferon to imatinib therapy for cytogenetic nonresponders or the addition of chemotherapy to imatinib therapy for advanced-stage patients before imatinib failure occurs.

TARGETING CML WITH COMBINATIONS OF SIGNALING PATHWAY INHIBITORS

A critical question for the future is how to exploit the knowledge of imatinib mesylate resistance mechanisms to improve patient care. Although it is logical to examine combinations with chemotherapy, one can envision a different approach in which various signal transduction pathway inhibitors are combined, because Bcr-Abl remains the target of interest. Presumably, candidate compounds used in combination with imatinib mesylate should not rely on exactly the same molecular features of Bcr-Abl that imatinib mesylate exploits. Instead, one might develop compounds that target Bcr-Abl by binding to the kinase domain in a different manner[36] or by inhibiting other necessary functions of the protein, such as dimerization. Alternatively, one might exploit drugs that trigger Bcr-Abl protein degradation, such as geldanamycin and 17-AAG (Fig. 17.4).[37,38] Recent evidence indicates that imatinib-resistant mutants of Bcr-Abl isolated from patients with acquired resistance to imatinib mesylate have enhanced sensitivity to geldanamycin and 17-AAG, in comparison with wild-type Bcr-Abl.[39] Clinical trials to examine the activity of 17-AAG in patients with imatinib resistance are underway. Finally, compounds that target known downstream effectors of Bcr-Abl, such as the Ras or PI3-kinase/Akt pathway, could be used in combination with imatinib mesylate. Two leading possibilities that might be tested in clinical trials are the Raf kinase inhibitor BAY43-9006[40] and the MEK inhibitor CI-1040,[41] both of which are in early-phase clinical testing for a range of cancers.

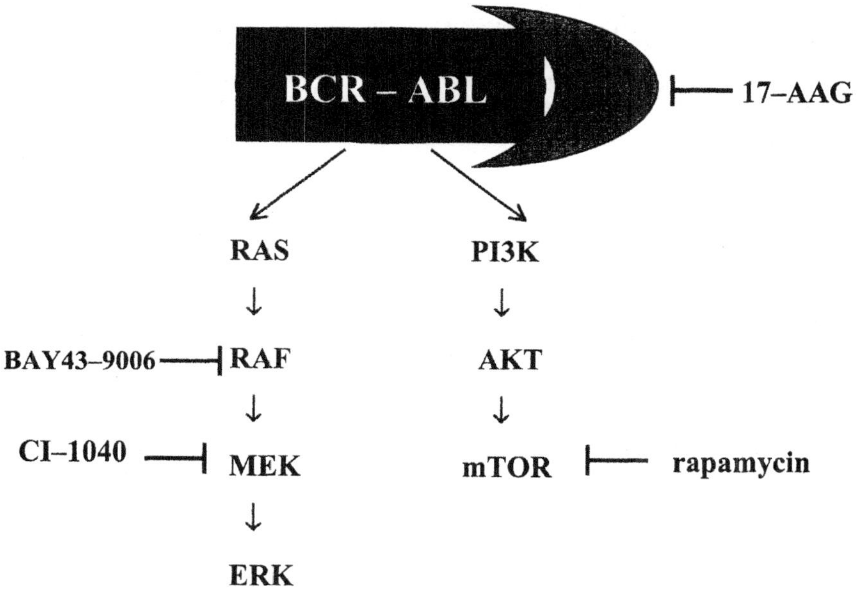

FIGURE 17.4 Alternative strategies to target the Bcr-Abl pathway in chronic myeloid leukemia. The illustration depicts aspects of the Bcr-Abl signal transduction pathway that might be targeted by signal transduction inhibitors currently under clinical investigation for other indications. 17-AAG is a geldanamycin derivative that binds Hsp90 and promotes the degradation of Hsp90 client proteins, such as Bcr-Abl. BAY43-9006 and CI-1040 are small-molecule inhibitors of Raf kinase and MEK kinase, respectively. Rapamycin is a natural-product drug that inhibits the mTOR kinase, which can function downstream of a pathway involving phosphatidylinositol 3-kinase (PI3K) and Akt.

The early lessons learned from studies of imatinib mesylate resistance are likely to have implications for other clinical settings in which imatinib mesylate has utility, such as the gastrointestinal stromal tumors that contain activating mutations in the c-kit kinase. Similarly, the increasing clinical application of other inhibitors against kinase targets, such as the epidermal growth factor receptor, may lead to similar mechanisms of resistance. Although concerns about resistance are a sobering reminder of the difficulties in treating cancer, it is instructive to compare the early results with imatinib mesylate with those of antiretroviral drugs, such as AZT in the treatment of the human immunodeficiency virus. In a remarkably parallel sequence of events, the excitement over the dramatic clinical activity of AZT was followed 2 years later by reports of clinical resistance caused by mutations in reverse transcriptase.[42] It seems clear that we can learn from the infectious disease experience, in which a cocktail of inhibitors targeted against the primary molecular lesion has been extraordinarily successful at extending life.

ACKNOWLEDGMENT

This chapter was supported by grants from the Leukemia and Lymphoma Society (C.L.S. and N.S.) and the National Cancer Institute (C.L.S.). C.L.S. is a Doris Duke Distinguished Clinical Scientist and Investigator of the Howard Hughes Medical Institute.

REFERENCES

1. Sawyers CL. Chronic myeloid leukemia. N Engl J Med 1999;340:1330–1340.
2. Faderl S, Talpaz M, Estrov Z et al. The biology of chronic myeloid leukemia. N Engl J Med 1999;341:164–172.
3. Konopka JB, Watanabe SM, Singer JW et al. Cell lines and clinical isolates derived from Ph1-positive chronic myelogenous leukemia patients express c-abl proteins with a common structural alteration. Proc Natl Acad Sci USA 1985;82:1810–1814.
4. Daley GQ, Van Etten RA, Baltimore D. Induction of chronic myelogenous leukemia in mice by the P210bcr/abl gene of the Philadelphia chromosome. Science 1990;247:824–830.
5. Heisterkamp N, Jenster G, ten Hoeve J et al. Acute leukaemia in bcr/abl transgenic mice. Nature 1990;344:251–253.
6. Pinilla-Ibarz J, Cathcart K, Korontsvit T et al. Vaccination of patients with chronic myelogenous leukemia with bcr-abl oncogene breakpoint fusion peptides generates specific immune responses. Blood 2000;95:1781–1787.
7. Bertazzoli C, Marchesi E, Passoni L et al. Differential recognition of a BCR/ABL peptide by lymphocytes from normal donors and chronic myeloid leukemia patients. Clin Cancer Res 2000;6:1931–1935.
8. Sun JY, Krouse RS, Forman SJ et al. Immunogenicity of a p210(BCR-ABL) fusion domain candidate DNA vaccine targeted to dendritic cells by a recombinant adeno-associated virus vector in vitro. Cancer Res 2002;62:3175–3183.

9. Buchdunger E, Zimmermann J, Mett H et al. Selective inhibition of the platelet-derived growth factor signal transduction pathway by a protein-tyrosine kinase inhibitor of the 2-phenylaminopyrimidine class. Proc Natl Acad Sci USA 1995;92:2558–2562.

10. Schindler T, Bornmann W, Pellicena P et al. Structural mechanism for STI-571 inhibition of Abelson tyrosine kinase. Science 2000;289:1938–1942.

11. Buchdunger E, Zimmermann J, Mett H et al. Inhibition of the Abl protein-tyrosine kinase in vitro and in vivo by a 2-phenylaminopyrimidine derivative. Cancer Res 1996;56:100–104.

12. Druker BJ, Tamura S, Buchdunger E et al. Effects of a selective inhibitor of the Abl tyrosine kinase on the growth of Bcr-Abl positive cells. Nat Med 1996;2:561–566.

13. Druker BJ, Talpaz M, Resta DJ et al. Efficacy and safety of a specific inhibitor of the BCR-ABL tyrosine kinase in chronic myeloid leukemia. N Engl J Med 2001;344:1031–1037.

14. Kantarjian H, Sawyers C, Hochhaus A et al. Hematologic and cytogenetic responses to imatinib mesylate in chronic myelogenous leukemia. N Engl J Med 2002;346:645–652.

15. Druker BJ. STI571 (Gleevec/Glivec, imatinib) versus interferon (IFN) + cytarabine as initial therapy for patients with CML: results of a randomized study. ASCO Plenary Session 2002.

16. Druker BJ, Sawyers CL, Kantarjian H et al. Activity of a specific inhibitor of the BCR-ABL tyrosine kinase in the blast crisis of chronic myeloid leukemia and acute lymphoblastic leukemia with the Philadelphia chromosome. N Engl J Med 2001;344:1038–1042.

17. Talpaz M, Silver RT, Druker BJ et al. Imatinib induces durable hematologic and cytogenetic responses in patients with accelerated phase chronic myeloid leukemia: results of a phase 2 study. Blood 2002;99:1928–1937.

18. Sawyers CL, Hochhaus A, Feldman E et al. Imatinib induces hematologic and cytogenetic responses in patients with chronic myelogenous leukemia in myeloid blast crisis: results of a phase II study. Blood 2002;99:3530–3539.

19. Branford S, Hughes TP, Rudzki Z. Monitoring chronic myeloid leukaemia therapy by real-time quantitative PCR in blood is a reliable alternative to bone marrow cytogenetics. Br J Haematol 1999;107:587–599.

20. Hochhaus A, Lin F, Reiter A et al. Quantitative molecular methods to monitor the response of CML patients to interferon-alpha. Bone Marrow Transplant 1996;17[suppl 3]: S41–S44.

21. Barbany G, Hoglund M, Simonsson B. Complete molecular remission in chronic myelogenous leukemia after imatinib therapy. N Engl J Med 2002;347:539–540.

22. Gorre ME, Mohammed M, Ellwood K et al. Clinical resistance to STI-571 cancer therapy caused by BCR-ABL gene mutation or amplification. Science 2001;293:876–880.

23. Sirulink A, Silver RT, Najfeld V. Marked ploidy and BCR-ABL gene amplification in vivo in a patient treated with STI571. Leukemia 2001;15:1795–1797.

24. Weisberg E, Griffin JD. Mechanism of resistance to the ABL tyrosine kinase inhibitor STI571 in BCR/ABL-transformed hematopoietic cell lines. Blood 2000;95:3498–3505.

25. Mahon FX, Deininger MW, Schultheis B et al. Selection and characterization of BCR-ABL positive cell lines with differential sensitivity to the tyrosine kinase inhibitor STI571: diverse mechanisms of resistance. Blood 2000;96:1070–1079.

26. le Coutre P, Tassi E, Varella-Garcia M et al. Induction of resistance to the Abelson inhibitor STI571 in human leukemic cells through gene amplification. Blood 2000;95:1758–1766.

27. Branford S, Rudzki Z, Walsh S et al. High frequency of point mutations clustered within the adenosine triphosphate-binding region of BCR/ABL in patients with chronic myeloid leukemia or Ph-positive acute lymphoblastic leukemia who develop imatinib (STI571) resistance. Blood 2002;99:3472–3475.

28. Shah NP, Sawyers CL. Recent success with the tyrosine kinase inhibitor STI-571: lessons for targeted therapy of cancer. Curr Opin Investig Drugs 2001;2:422–423.
29. von Bubnoff N, Schneller F, Peschel C et al. BCR-ABL gene mutations in relation to clinical resistance of Philadelphia-chromosome-positive leukaemia to STI571: a prospective study. Lancet 2002;359:487–491.
30. Shah NP, Nicoll JM, Nagar B et al. Multiple BCR-ABL kinase domain mutations confer polyclonal resistance to the tyrosine kinase inhibitor imatinib (STI571) in chronic phase and blast crisis chronic myeloid leukemia. Cancer Cell 2002;2:117.
31. Hofmann WK, de Vos S, Elashoff D et al. Relation between resistance of Philadelphia-chromosome-positive acute lymphoblastic leukaemia to the tyrosine kinase inhibitor STI571 and gene-expression profiles: a gene-expression study. Lancet 2002;359:481–486.
32. Graham SM, Jorgensen HG, Allan E et al. Primitive, quiescent, Philadelphia-positive stem cells from patients with chronic myeloid leukemia are insensitive to STI571 in vitro. Blood 2002;99:319–325.
33. Holtz MS, Slovak ML, Zhang F et al. Imatinib mesylate (STI571) inhibits growth of primitive malignant progenitors in chronic myelogenous leukemia through reversal of abnormally increased proliferation. Blood 2002;99:3792–3800.
34. Bhatia R, Holtz MS, Natcher K et al. Persistence of malignant stem cells in CML patients in complete cytogenetic remission following Gleevec treatment. Blood 2003 (in press).
35. Roumiantsev S, Shah NP, Gorre ME et al. Clinical resistance to the kinase inhibitor STI-571 in chronic myeloid leukemia by mutation of Tyr-253 in the Abl kinase domain P-loop. Proc Natl Acad Sci USA 2002;99:10700–10705.
36. Nagar B, Bornmann WG, Pellicena P et al. Crystal structures of the kinase domain of c-Abl in complex with the small molecule inhibitors PD173955 and imatinib (STI-571). Cancer Res 2002;62:4236–4243.
37. Blagosklonny MV, Fojo T, Bhalla KN et al. The Hsp90 inhibitor geldanamycin selectively sensitizes Bcr-Abl-expressing leukemia cells to cytotoxic chemotherapy. Leukemia 2001;15:1537–1543.
38. Nimmanapalli R, O'Bryan E, Bhalla K. Geldanamycin and its analogue 17-allylamino-17-demethoxygeldanamycin lowers Bcr-Abl levels and induces apoptosis and differentiation of Bcr-Abl-positive human leukemic blasts. Cancer Res 2001;61:1799–1804.
39. Gorre ME, Ellwood-Yen KB, Chiosis G et al. BCR-ABL point mutants isolated from patients with STI571-resistant chronic myeloid leukemia remain sensitive to inhibitors of the BCR-ABL chaperone heat shock protein 90. Blood 2002;100:3041–3044.
40. Hilger RA, Kredtke S, Hedley D et al. Inhibition of ERK phosphorylation and clinical outcome in patients treated with the Raf kinase inhibitor BAY 43-9006 [abstract 1916]. American Society of Clinical Oncology 2002.
41. Mitchell DY, Reid JM, Parchment RE et al. Pharmacokinetics (PK) and pharmacodynamics (PD) of the oral MEK inhibitor, CI-1040, following multiple dose administration to patients with advanced cancer [abstract 320]. American Society of Clinical Oncology 2002.
42. Larder BA, Kemp SD. Multiple mutations in HIV-1 reverse transcriptase confer high-level resistance to zidovudine (AZT). Science 1989;246:1155–1158.

Chapter 18

Value of Adjuvant Interferon-Alfa-2b Therapy in High-Risk Melanoma: The Case In Favor

John M. Kirkwood

Vernon K. Sondak

Frank G. Haluska

Joseph G. Ibrahim

The clinical and pathological staging of melanoma (as well as most forms of carcinoma and sarcoma) has advanced significantly over the past several decades, with the adoption of the TNM (tumor, node, metastasis) staging system that is based on clinical outcomes data from thousands of patients. For example, the current American Joint Committee on Cancer (AJCC) staging system for melanoma is based on complete information from 17,600 patients.[1] This extensive database provides precise estimates of a patient's probability of survival at 5 and 10 years based on data collected at initial diagnosis. Most importantly, these prognostic data can be used to guide treatment decisions.

Patients with T4 primary tumors without nodal involvement (i.e., AJCC stage IIB) and patients with nodal involvement (i.e., AJCC stage III) at initial diagnosis are at high risk for disease recurrence and death from their disease after definitive surgery. The risk of disease-related mortality in these patients reflects the fact that their disease may have already spread to distant sites at the time of diagnosis. Therefore, despite resection of regional lymph nodes in patients with clinical or pathological evidence of nodal metastasis, these patients remain at significant risk of recurrence. Therefore, systemic therapy has been pursued to improve the cure rate in these patients. The available prognostic data on melanoma indicate that 30%–50% of patients with T4 primary tumors (i.e., stage IIB/C) and 40%–70% of patients with stage III melanoma have a recurrence and ultimately die of melanoma within 5 years of surgery.[1] Put into perspective, this prognosis is similar to comparable stages of colorectal cancer, in which the 5-year survival rates for T4N0 and stage III disease are approximately 30%–50%.[2] In melanoma, as in breast and colorectal cancer, the number of involved lymph nodes is one of the most important prognostic factors for patients with stage III disease.[3,4] These data suggest that most patients with T4N0 or stage III disease have distant spread already at the time of definitive surgery that cannot be treated effectively with local or regional therapy.

ADJUVANT THERAPY

The ultimate goal of adjuvant therapy is to prolong survival by reducing the risk of recurrence and thus increasing the fraction of patients who are cured. Although reducing the rate of recurrence should theoretically result in an improvement in overall survival, in clinical practice, these two endpoints have not always shown a consistent correlation. In the case of melanoma, many oncologists (and most patients) would argue that improvement in relapse-free survival is also meaningful and justifies the use of adjuvant therapy even if overall survival is not significantly prolonged. The reason for this is that melanoma recurrence is associated with substantial morbidity, and distant metastatic disease is associated with a high probability of disease-related mortality. Therefore, with a disease with no uniformly effective treatment options for distant metastatic disease, preventing recurrence may have greater clinical relevance than for malignancies that are more responsive to systemic therapy.

The benefit of adjuvant therapy is typically expressed as the reduction in the risk of relapse or death as determined by either a proportional hazard model or Kaplan-Meier estimates of survival rates at discrete time points. Of these methods, the proportional hazards model is preferred because it provides a more comprehensive assessment of the risk of an event during the entire follow-up period. The difference between the hazard ratio and 1.0 is the proportional risk reduction. For example, a hazard ratio of 0.75 denotes a 25% risk reduction. Depending on how the calculation is performed, the hazard ratio may also be expressed as a number greater than 1.0. For example, a hazard ratio of 1.33 also denotes a 25% risk reduction (by dividing the hazard ratio into 1.0). Hazard ratios were calculated in this way in the U.S. cooperative group trials discussed later in this chapter.

DEFINING ACCEPTABLE MEASURES OF EFFICACY

Evidenced-based medicine has set high standards for trials of adjuvant therapy based on prolongation of relapse-free and overall survival. The standard agreed on in the regulator forum is that the benefit in terms of these rigorous endpoints must be statistically significant and clinically meaningful. However, in the realm of clinical practice, there is little consensus as to what constitutes a clinically meaningful benefit, and quality-of-life considerations may weigh more heavily for some. Therefore, other endpoints may be relevant. For example, quality-adjusted survival (QAS) can be assessed to consider quality-of-life data, and distant relapse-free survival has been proposed as an alternative to overall survival in diseases such as melanoma, in which distant metastatic disease is associated with a high mortality rate.

What Is the Standard for an Effective Adjuvant Therapy?

Tamoxifen for patients with high-risk resected breast cancer is arguably the most successful adjuvant therapy available. The most recent data from the Early Breast Cancer Trialists' Collaborative Group (EBCTCG), on the basis of combined analysis of 55 adjuvant trials involving 30,000 women, showed that 5 years of tamoxifen therapy (20 mg/day) reduces the risk of recurrence by 47% and the risk of mortality by 26% over 10 years of follow-up ($P_2 < .00001$) in patients who were estrogen receptor positive or unknown.[5] These benefits are based on a proportional hazards model. A similar benefit has been achieved with polychemotherapy regimens in breast cancer, but with substantially more toxicity.[6] A reduction in the risk of recurrence was seen primarily within the first 5 years, and this led to a steady increase in the overall survival benefit over 10 years. Moreover, tamoxifen is extremely well tolerated with long-term use, although it is associated with an increased risk of endometrial cancer.

The experience with adjuvant tamoxifen in breast cancer sets a high standard against which adjuvant therapies can be compared, but it may be an unrealistic benchmark for more refractory diseases, given that breast cancer is generally very responsive to both hormonal manipulation and chemotherapy. In addition, hormonal therapy is well tolerated when compared with many other systemic therapies, such as the cytokine therapies that have been widely used in the treatment of melanoma. In colon cancer, for example, adjuvant therapy with 5-fluorouracil plus leucovorin is the current standard of care for patients with stage III (Dukes' stage C) disease, and the benefits are more modest. Randomized trials have demonstrated a 15% to 20% reduction in both the risk of recurrence and of mortality over 3 to 5 years with standard 5-fluorouracil/leucovorin regimens.[2,7] Although adjuvant therapy has not demonstrated a consistent benefit for patients with stage II (Dukes' B2) colon cancer,[7] most otherwise healthy patients with high-risk primary or node-positive colon cancer are offered adjuvant therapy in the United States today.

Based on our clinical experience in the adjuvant treatment of melanoma, we consider a ≥ 10% improvement in relapse-free survival and overall survival at 5 or more years to be clinically meaningful. Melanoma-free survival at 5 years may be a reasonable estimation of the cured fraction, but few randomized trials have been reported at more than 5 years of follow-up. One can also look at prolongation of the median relapse-free and overall survival. In this context, prolongation of the median by at least 1 year is, in our estimation, a clinically meaningful benefit. Finally, it should be possible to demonstrate an increase in quality-adjusted survival. Based on the patient preference studies described later, benefits of this magnitude are also meaningful to the patient.

Importance of a Meta-Analysis

Demonstrating the clinical benefit of adjuvant therapy typically requires large, adequately powered trials and sufficient lengths of follow-up to detect enough events to show meaningful differences between treatment groups. Moreover, interpreting the results of any one trial can often be difficult because so many factors can affect the outcome. Therefore, it may be necessary to interpret the data from a large number of trials (controlling for heterogeneity between trials) to arrive at a consensus. For example, despite the highly significant clinical benefit of adjuvant tamoxifen in estrogen receptor–positive breast cancer cited earlier, this benefit was not demonstrated in a compelling manner until the EBCTCG conducted a combined analysis of many separate trials involving thousands of patients treated over the past 20 years. In fact, many individual trials of adjuvant tamoxifen did not demonstrate a significant benefit. Therefore, meta-analysis of large databases populated with mature data can sometimes reveal clinical benefit where individual trials have not.

ADJUVANT THERAPY FOR MELANOMA

In this context, we discuss the data demonstrating the clinical benefit of adjuvant therapy with interferon alfa (IFN-α) in patients with high-risk melanoma. This includes patients with stage IIB/C disease who have deep (> 4 mm) primary tumors (with or without ulceration) but no lymph node involvement and patients with stage III regional nodal disease. Patients with stage IIB disease (i.e., nonulcerated primary tumors, as determined by the revised AJCC staging system) have an intermediate prognosis, with a 67% 5-year survival rate.[1] In contrast, patients with stage IIC disease (i.e., ulcerated T4 primary tumor) have only a 45% 5-year survival rate. In patients with nodal metastases, those with a single microscopic metastasis have a relatively favorable prognosis, with a 5-year survival rate of nearly 70%. At the opposite end of the spectrum, patients with four or more involved nodes or macroscopic nodal metastases and an ulcerated primary tumor have a dismal prognosis (5-year survival rates < 30%). Most adjuvant studies of IFN-α therapy have enrolled patients who, according to the current AJCC staging system, would be classified as having stage IIB/C and stage III melanoma. It is important to keep in mind that in the absence of surgical staging of regional lymph nodes, the lines between these two groups of patients are blurred because approximately 35% of patients with T4 primary tumors have occult nodal metastases at presentation.[8-10]

Metastatic melanoma is generally considered to be refractory to chemotherapy. Consequently, immunotherapy has become the mainstay of systemic treatment for melanoma. Indeed, the only agents approved for the treatment of melanoma over the past 25 years are IFN-α-2b and interleukin-2. Single-agent dacarbazine was approved for metastatic melanoma 26 years ago, but it would not likely be approved today on the basis of the available data. In patients with metastatic disease, interleukin-2 was approved because of the durability of complete responses achieved with this agent.[11] In the adjuvant setting, various IFN-α regimens have been investigated; however, the only regimen that has been demonstrated to improve relapse-free and overall survival is the high-dose regimen.

Evidence Supporting the Efficacy of Adjuvant IFN-α Therapy

Initial clinical trials that we and others conducted more than 20 years ago demonstrated that IFN-α-2b is able to induce objective antitumor responses in approximately 20% of patients with melanoma, and that higher doses were consistently associated with higher response rates and more durable responses.[12] The application of IFN-α-2b therapy to high-risk melanoma was subsequently tested in three prospective multicenter, national, cooperative group trials enrolling nearly 1800 patients.

The high-dose IFN-α-2b regimen, which consists of 20 MU/m^2/day intravenously × 5 days per week for 4 weeks, followed by 10 MU/m^2/day by subcutaneous injection three times per week for 48 weeks, was first approved for use in the United States in 1996 on the basis of results of the Eastern Cooperative Oncology Group (ECOG) trial E1684. In this trial, 287 patients were randomly assigned to high-dose IFN-α-2b for 1 year (N = 137) or observation (N = 143), and all patients underwent wide local excision of their primary tumor and complete regional lymph node dissection. When reported on in 1996 at a mature median follow-up of 6.9 years,[13] this study demonstrated that treatment with high-dose IFN-α-2b significantly prolonged both relapse-free and overall survival. Median relapse-free survival was 1.72 years in the high-dose IFN-α-2b arm, versus 0.98 years in the observation arm (one-sided log-rank $P = 0.0023$). The hazard ratio was 1.43 (95% CI, 1.08, 1.89) for the intent-to-treat population, indicating a 30% reduction in the risk of recurrence. The Kaplan-Meier estimate of the 5-year relapse-free survival rate was 37% in the IFN-α-2b arm, versus 26% in the observation arm (i.e., an 11% absolute reduction or a 42% relative reduction in the rate of recurrence). In addition, median overall survival was prolonged by 1 year in the high-dose IFN-α-2b arm (3.82 vs 2.78 years in the observation arm; $P_1 = .0237$). The hazard ratio for overall survival was 1.32 (95% CI, 0.98, 1.77), indicating a 24% reduction in the risk of mortality. The estimated 5-year survival rate was 46% for patients treated with IFN-α-2b, compared with 37% in the observation arm (i.e., a 9% absolute reduction or a 24% relative reduction in the risk of mortality at 5 years). Of note, despite the use of one-sided log-rank statistics in this trial, both the relapse-free and the overall survival benefits remain significant by Kaplan-Meier analysis when two-sided statistic tests are applied ($P = .005$ and $P = .047$, respectively).

Intergroup Trial E1690

After E1684 was conducted, a larger adjuvant trial was conducted by the Intergroup. Intergroup trial E1690 was conducted to confirm the efficacy of high-dose IFN-α-2b versus observation and to investigate the activity of a low-dose regimen (3 MU subcutaneously three times a week for 2 years).[14] This trial accrued 642 patients with melanoma and was powered from a cure-rate model that used interim data from E1684. However, unlike E1684, this trial did not require patients to undergo regional lymphadenectomy after wide local excision of their primary tumor. Consequently, in 163 (25%) patients who were clinically node negative at study entry (T4N0), only 24% of these patients received elective lymph node dissection, and only 5% were evaluated by sentinel lymph node biopsy. Therefore, 71% of these patients were not surgically staged.

The results of this trial were reported at a median follow-up of 52 months (4.3 years) and showed a marginally significant reduction in the risk of recurrence for patients treated with high-dose IFN-α-2b when compared with observation (hazard ratio = 1.28; 95% CI, 1.0–1.65; $P_2 = .054$) in the intent-to-treat analysis, although a Cox model adjusting for significant prognostic factors demonstrated a significant relapse-free survival benefit ($P_2 = .03$).[14] Thus, hazard analysis suggested a 22% reduction in the risk of recurrence, whereas Kaplan-Meier analysis estimated a 5-year relapse-free survival rate of 44% for patients treated with high-dose IFN-α-2b when compared with 35% in the observation arm (a 9% absolute reduction in the risk of recurrence), which is similar to the results of E1684. However, unlike E1684, there was no difference in overall survival between treatment groups. The estimated 5-year survival rates were 52% in the high-dose IFN-α-2b arm, compared with 55% in the observation arm. This study also showed that the low-dose regimen had no significant impact on either relapse-free or overall survival when compared with observation. Other studies have also found no significant clinical benefit associated with various low-dose IFN-α regimens in high-risk resected melanoma, including the European Organization for Research and Treatment of Cancer trial 18871 of IFN-α-2a (1 MU/day subcutaneously for 1 year)[15] and the World Health Organization trial 16 of IFN-α-2a (3 MU subcutaneously three times a week for 3 years).[16]

The outcome of E1690 led to a great deal of speculation as to why an overall survival benefit was not demonstrated despite the improvement in relapse-free survival. It is noteworthy that patients in both arms of E1690 had a better outcome than patients in E1684; however, the differences between trials are particularly striking when one compares the observation arms. Patients in the E1690 observation arm had a 5-year relapse-free survival rate of 35%, compared with only 26% in E1684, but more importantly, 55% of patients in the E1690 observation arm survived 5 years compared with only 37% of patients in E1684. In fact, the median survival in the E1690 observation arm was 6.0 years, compared with only 2.8 years in E1684 (Fig. 18.1). Patients treated with IFN-α-2b in E1690 also had a better outcome than those in E1684, but to a lesser extent than the observation group. This disparity between trials is not easily explained, but it may be related to subtle differences in eligibility criteria and enrollment between the two studies.

Notable differences between these two trials include a higher proportion of patients with T4N0 disease (25% vs 11%) and a lower proportion of patients with recurrent disease (51% vs 65%) at study entry in E1690 compared with E1684. Moreover, the possibility exists for an imbalance between treatment groups with respect to the proportion of node-positive patients in the T4N0 subgroup because most of these patients were not surgically staged at randomization. All of these factors and the opportunity for patients in the E1690 observation arm to have received adjuvant high-dose IFN-α-2b therapy off protocol for local recurrence could have affected the outcome of this trial. However, regardless of these caveats, the results of this trial called into question the survival benefit of high-dose IFN-α-2b .

Intergroup Trial E1694

Just as the results of E1684 were emerging in the mid-1990s, a third adjuvant trial of high-dose IFN-α-2b was initiated. Intergroup trial E1694 is the largest of the three adjuvant trials coordinated by the ECOG. In contrast with the first two trials, high-dose IFN-α-2b was considered the control arm in this trial, which was designed to investigate the efficacy of the GMK vaccine targeting the GM_2 ganglioside antigen.[17] The E1694 trial accrued 880 patients by October 1999 but was closed by the independent Data Safety Monitoring Committee in June 2000 on the basis of an interim analysis indicating that high-dose IFN-α-2b was

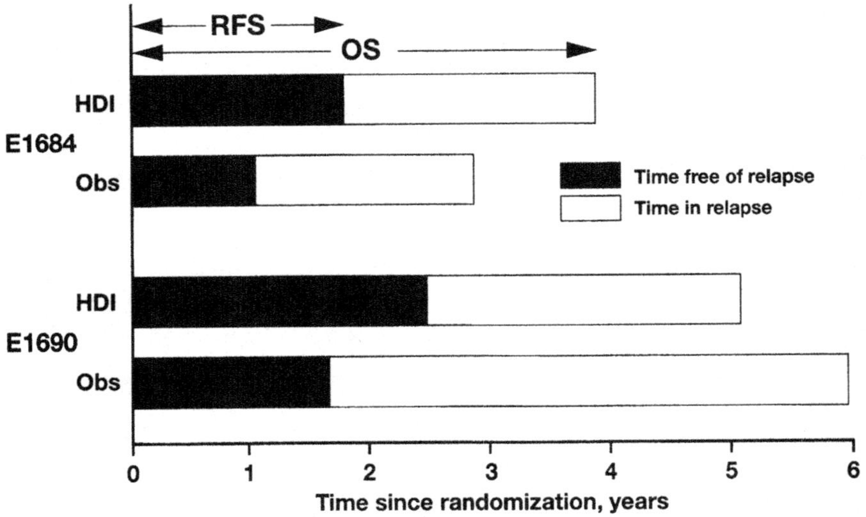

FIGURE 18.1 Comparison of median relapse-free survival (RFS) and overall survival (OS) for the high-dose interferon-α-2b (HDI) and observation (Obs) arms of E1684 and E1690.

significantly more effective than the vaccine in preventing both recurrence and mortality. This trial was first reported at a median follow-up of 16 months, and at that time IFN-α-2b demonstrated a significant relapse-free survival benefit (hazard ratio, 1.47; 95% CI, 1.14, 1.90; $P_2 = 0.003$) and overall survival benefit (hazard ratio, 1.52; 95% CI, 1.07, 2.15; $P_2 = .018$) for patients treated with high-dose IFN-α-2b compared with GMK (eligible population).[17] A Cox regression analysis, adjusting for prognostic variables, also demonstrated a significant survival benefit. As demonstrated by the hazard analysis, the risk of recurrence was reduced by 32%, and the risk of mortality was reduced by 34% for patients treated with IFN-α-2b. The estimated 2-year relapse-free survival rates were 62% in the IFN-α-2b arm, compared with 49% in the GMK arm, and the estimated 2-year survival rates were 78% and 73%, respectively. The short median follow-up drew criticism when the Data Safety Monitoring Committee took action to close and unblind the trial in accordance with predefined early stopping rules. However, the analysis has recently been updated at a median follow-up of 2.1 years, and the results remain significant and consistent with the initial results.[16]

This trial is the largest to date and should be viewed as a confirmatory trial of the significant relapse-free and overall survival benefits of high-dose IFN-α-2b. There is no evidence that patients in the GMK arm had a worse-than-expected outcome, either because of imbalances in prognostic factors or because they were treated with the vaccine. In fact, patients in the GMK arm who exhibited elevated titers of anti-GM_2 antibodies showed a trend toward improved relapse-free and overall survival compared with nonresponders.[17] Therefore, there is no evidence to suggest that the effect of the vaccine was contrary to the initial hypothesis. Furthermore, the survival curves for the GMK arm have closely matched those for the observation arms of E1684 and E1690, and no significant imbalances in recognized prognostic factors have emerged. Therefore, the only reasonable explanation for the improved relapse-free and overall survival of patients treated with IFN-α-2b is a beneficial effect of IFN-α-2b, not a detrimental effect of the vaccine.

The relapse-free and overall survival benefits of high-dose IFN-α-2b demonstrated in each of these three trials are summarized in Table 18.1.[13,14,17,18]

Long-Term Follow-Up for E1684

Long-term follow-up for E1684 has added new fuel to the controversy over the survival benefit of high-dose IFN-α-2b therapy. Recently, the data from trial E1684 were updated to a median follow-up of 12.6 years and were presented to the U.S. Food and Drug Administration Oncologic Drugs Advisory Committee in February 2002. The updated analysis of the original trial data showed that the continuous relapse-free survival benefit has maintained statistical significance over long-term follow-up (P_2 = .02). However, the statistical significance of the overall survival benefit has not been similarly maintained (P_2 = .18), although the IFN-α-2b arm continues to have a survival benefit. Unfortunately, disease-specific survival data are not maintained in the cooperative group databases. Therefore, competing causes of death cannot be ruled out and are likely to be a factor in this overall survival analysis, given the median age of the patient population. Several patients in the IFN-α-2b arm died after 10 years, whereas no late deaths occurred in the observation arm. Thus, the Kaplan-Meier survival curves begin

TABLE 18.1 Reduction in the Risk of Recurrence and Mortality for Patients Treated With Interferon-α-2b

Trial	Proportional Hazards Model		Kaplan-Meier Estimate of Impact Upon Recurrence and Survival Rates	
	RFS	OS	RFS	OS
E1684 (HDI vs Obs)	30%	24%	11% (5 years)	9% (5 years)
E1690 (HDI vs Obs)	22%	0%	9% (5 years)	0% (5 years)
E1694 (HDI vs GMK)	32%	34%	13% (2 years)	5% (2 years)
Meta-analysis[a]	16%	10%	—	—

RFS, relapse-free survival; OS, overall survival; HDI, high-dose Interferon-α -2b; Obs, observation.

[a]Includes data from all available trials of both high-dose interferon alfa and low-dose interferon alfa regimens.

Data from Kirkwood et al[13,14,17] and Wheatley et al.[18]

to converge between 10 and 12 years after randomization. However, the survival curves remain divergent for 10 years (9 years beyond the completion of therapy), and at all points along the curve out to 10 years, the proportion of surviving patients is approximately 10% higher in the high-dose IFN-α-2b arm than in the observation arm. It is also noteworthy that because all patients in E1684 underwent complete lymphadenectomy at randomization, relapse-free survival in this study population should represent "distant disease-free" survival, which has been proposed as an appropriate surrogate for overall survival by cooperative groups in Europe. Nevertheless, these results and the results of E1690 have cast doubts on the overall survival benefit of adjuvant high-dose IFN-α-2b therapy both in Europe and in the United States (as reflected in the discussions before the Oncologic Drugs Advisory Committee).

Wheatley Meta-Analysis

Wheatley and colleagues[18] recently conducted the first systematic meta-analysis of the adjuvant trials of IFN-α in melanoma in an attempt to reconcile some of the inconsistencies between studies and to begin to reach a consensus. They performed a meta-analysis of published data from 10 randomized trials of IFN-α versus control (i.e., no IFN-α) that enrolled approximately 3700 patients. The analysis combined the efficacy data from studies of both high-dose and low-dose IFN-α regimens but did not include data from the largest trial of high-dose IFN-α-2b, namely E1694. Nevertheless, this meta-analysis demonstrated that adjuvant IFN-α therapy significantly reduced the risk of recurrence by 16% (hazard ratio = 0.84; 95% CI 0.77–0.92; *P* = .0001) and reduced the risk of mortality by 10% (hazard ratio = 0.90; 95% CI 0.82–1.0; *P* = .05) compared with control (Table 18.1).[13,14,17,18] A strong trend toward a dose response favoring higher doses of IFN-α was also observed. Therefore, this analysis confirmed that adjuvant therapy with IFN-α significantly reduces the risk of recurrence and death, but the overall survival benefit of IFN-α therapy in this tabulation remains equivocal because of the borderline significance of the log-rank statistic.

To place these results in proper perspective, it is important to recognize the limitations of this analysis. Given that the analysis included several studies of low-dose IFN-α regimens (1–3 MU administered by several treatment schedules), which clearly do not provide a durable or significant clinical benefit in patients with high-risk melanoma (i.e., stages IIB/C and III),[16,19-21] and did not include any of the published data from the largest positive trial (E1694), the analysis underestimates the true benefit of IFN-α therapy. Moreover, the database is still small. With these limitations in mind, it seems short-sighted to dismiss the statistical significance of the overall survival benefit based on a 95% confidence interval that reaches but does not cross the 1.0 value. Perhaps the more important number is the estimated 10% reduction in the risk of mortality, which is borne out by the data from E1684 at 7 years' median follow-up. This evidence provides substantial reason to believe that high-dose IFN-α therapy does confer a significant and clinically meaningful overall survival benefit in addition to the documented improvement in relapse-free survival. Given that this is the only regimen shown to provide a significant clinical benefit in randomized, multicenter, cooperative group trials, it should be held as the standard against which other regimens are compared.

IMPEDIMENTS TO ACCEPTANCE OF HIGH-DOSE IFN-α-2B THERAPY AS THE STANDARD

Perhaps the greatest impediment to the acceptance of high-dose IFN-α-2b as the standard of care for adjuvant therapy in patients with high-risk melanoma is the toxicity profile. High-dose IFN-α-2b therapy is associated with a constellation of constitutional symptoms (i.e., flu-like symptoms), fatigue, anorexia, myelosuppression, elevated liver enzyme levels, and neurologic symptoms, which affect most patients to some extent.[13,14,17,22-26] The incidence and the severity of these adverse events are clearly dose related, and some adverse events, particularly fatigue and depression, occur more frequently and may become more severe with longer duration of therapy. However, the more acute flu-like symptoms (e.g., fever, chills/rigors, nausea/vomiting, arthralgia, and myalgia) often diminish with continued therapy. In the pivotal trial E1684, 66% of patients treated with high-dose interferon had at least one grade 3 adverse event, and 14% of patients had a grade 4 event.[27] Consequently, many patients find it very difficult to tolerate this therapy, and many oncologists are hesitant to expose their patients to a regimen that they believe is highly toxic. In many practices, only half to two thirds of patients who are eligible for adjuvant therapy elect to receive it after reviewing all of the efficacy and safety data. Some patients elect not to receive it primarily because of concerns about side effects. Reasons cited for not wanting to receive adjuvant therapy are fear that it will affect their ability to work and concerns among elderly patients about quality of life. In addition, many patients are fearful of self-injection. One key to overcoming this impediment is to better understand, anticipate, and proactively intervene to manage toxicity. Although it is unreasonable to expect that all patients will choose to receive adjuvant high-dose IFN-α-2b therapy (or any adjuvant therapy, no matter how firmly established it is), it is important to educate patients about the management of toxicity to help alleviate some of the fear and help them make an objective informed decision.

Most IFN-α–related side effects can be managed with appropriate supportive care (Table 18.2).[22,26] For example, an important strategy for managing constitutional symptoms is evening or bedtime administration of IFN-α along with prophylactic acetaminophen administration. Nausea and vomiting, when encountered, also respond well to antiemetics (e.g., chlorpromazine and metoclopramide). These measures and careful attention to fluid balance can alleviate

TABLE 18.2 Supportive Care for Interferon Side Effects

Symptoms	Care Measures and Interventions
Flu-like symptoms	• Bedtime administration with acetaminophen • Antiemetics • Adequate fluids
Fatigue	• Psychosocial support • Behavioral modifications and light exercise • Improved nutrition • Thyroid replacement therapy if hypothyroid • Megestrol acetate • Methylphenydate (in severe cases) • Activating SSRIs (fluoxetine or paroxetine, 20 mg/day)
Anorexia	• Small frequent meals • Megestrol acetate (800 mg/day) • Dronabinol (2.5–5.0 mg t.i.d. after meals)
Depression	• Psychosocial support or psychotherapy • Activating SSRIs (fluoxetine or paroxetine, 20 mg/day)

SSRI, selective serotonin reuptake inhibitor; t.i.d., three times per day.
From Kirkwood et al.[26]

much of the discomfort from flu-like symptoms. Fatigue may be a byproduct of other syndromes, such as hypothyroidism, which can be managed with appropriate therapy. Likewise, if the patient experiences anorexia, poor nutrition may be a factor in fatigue and may require nutritional counseling. If the cause of fatigue is not otherwise known, behavioral and pharmacologic interventions can be implemented.[22,28,29] Many interventions for fatigue are behavioral, but if support groups, behavior modification, and light exercise do not help minimize fatigue, pharmacologic agents can be prescribed. For example, stimulants (e.g., methylphenydate),[30,31] progestational agents (e.g., megestrol acetate),[32] and antidepressants have shown some promise in relieving cancer-related fatigue. Antidepressants, particularly selective serotonin reuptake inhibitors, can improve depression associated with IFN-α therapy and may be effective when they are used prophylactically.[33-38] Anorexia can be caused by a variety of factors, such as dysgeusia, nausea, gastrointestinal dysmotility, dry mouth, food aversion, pain, depression, fatigue, and lack of social interaction and support. Therefore, appetite may be improved by addressing the underlying cause.[22] In addition, patients may benefit from nutritional counseling and appetite stimulants, such as megestrol acetate.[39] If patients experience clinically significant myelosuppression or elevated liver enzyme levels, dose modifications are appropriate. With close attention to the known side effects of IFN-α therapy and with appropriate interventions and dose modifications, most patients are able to tolerate the full year of high-dose therapy.

PATIENT PREFERENCES

Given the concerns about the tolerability of the high-dose IFN-α-2b regimen, numerous studies have been conducted to assess quality-of-life issues and patient preferences. The question that these studies have sought to address is whether the relapse-free and overall survival benefits of adjuvant therapy outweigh the decrease in quality of life during therapy. A series of studies have been conducted using the Quality-Adjusted Time Without Symptoms or Toxicity (Q-TWiST) methodology to weigh patient preferences and to estimate the QAS benefit of high-dose IFN-α-2b therapy based on data from the ECOG and Intergroup trials.[40-42] The patient preference study by Kilbridge and colleagues[41] collected data from melanoma patients regarding the utility scores they would assign to treatment-related toxicity and posttreatment outcomes (i.e., disease-free health, recurrence, and death). This study also collected data on what degree of clinical benefit patients would require in order to accept IFN-α–related toxicity. The outcome of this patient preference study indicated that on average, patients rated quality of life with melanoma recurrence much lower (i.e., lower utility scores) than even severe treatment-related toxicity. Patients were willing to tolerate severe toxicity for a 10% improvement in 5-year disease-free survival in the absence of any defined overall survival benefit. These results suggest that patients place high value on remaining free of recurrence. The most recent of these studies went one step further by using the utility scores provided by melanoma patients themselves to calculate a QAS benefit based on data from E1684 and E1690.[42] Based on the utility scores these trials provided, 77% of patients would receive a benefit in terms of QAS, which was statistically significant for 16% of patients, whereas 23% of patients would experience a decrease in QAS. This study also formulated a decision rule to help identify patients who would not accept the anticipated level of toxicity and for whom treatment with IFN-α-2b might detract from QAS. This information is useful and may help patients who face difficult treatment decisions.

COST-EFFECTIVENESS

The cost-effectiveness of adjuvant therapy with the high-dose IFN-α-2b regimen has also been studied to determine how this regimen compares with other established cancer therapies. Hillner et al[43] published an economic analysis of data from E1684 and showed that the projected incremental cost (in 1996 dollars) per life-year gained in the IFN-α-2b arm ranged from $32,600 after 7 years to $13,700 after 35 years. The authors concluded that the cost-effectiveness and cost-utility ratios for adjuvant IFN-α-2b therapy were comparable to those of other cancer treatments and were within the benchmark set by adjuvant therapy for breast and colon cancer.

ALTERNATIVE REGIMENS

Although adjuvant therapy with high-dose IFN-α-2b may not be optimal, no alternative regimen or agents have demonstrated a significant and durable clinical benefit in terms of either relapse-free or overall survival when compared with observation in patients with stage IIB/C and stage III disease. Numerous intermediate and low-dose IFN-α regimens have been investigated, but none has been shown to be effective. The greatest downfall of these alternative IFN-α regimens has been the lack of durability of the clinical benefit. Although there have been hints of a relapse-free survival benefit while patients remain on therapy, the Kaplan-Meier curves converge relatively quickly once therapy is discontinued. This was seen clearly in the WHO16 trial of low-dose IFN-α-2a (3 MU three times a week for 3 years), which represents the longest duration of therapy tested to date. The curves seemed to separate between 1 year and 3 years, but in the final analysis, there was no benefit in terms of either relapse-free or overall survival.[16] Preliminary results from the European Organization for Research and Treatment of Cancer trial 18952 also suggest that longer therapy duration (i.e., 2 years versus 1 year) with intermediate doses of IFN-α (5–10 MU) may be effective when compared with observation, but it is too early to tell whether the benefit will be durable. These studies have raised the question, how long is enough?

In contrast, high-dose IFN-α-2b has yielded early and continuous benefit for many years after therapy is completed. Indeed, the early separation of the relapse-free and overall survival curves in the ECOG and Intergroup trials has led to the hypothesis that 1 month of intravenous induction therapy with 20 MU/m^2/day of IFN-α-2b for 5 days per week may be necessary and sufficient. This hypothesis is currently being tested in patients with intermediate-risk disease (E1697 Intergroup trial and the Sunbelt Melanoma trial).

Vaccines have also failed thus far to demonstrate a significant benefit as adjuvant therapy for high-risk melanoma. This is illustrated most dramatically in E1694. The GMK vaccine (GM_2-KLH-QS21 conjugate developed by Progenics) was selected by the Intergroup as the most promising candidate (among all whole-cell and defined-antigen vaccines available at the time) for testing in a randomized phase III trial derived on studies conducted at Memorial Sloan Kettering Cancer Center.[44,45] However, the Melacine vaccine has subsequently shown some promise in the adjuvant setting for patients with intermediate-risk melanoma (T3N0M0) and appears to provide a significant relapse-free survival benefit in a subset of patients with specific human leukocyte antigen serotypes.[46,47] Given the limited success achieved with vaccines to date, the approach being taken in many vaccine trials is to evaluate their efficacy in patients with intermediate-risk disease (e.g., stage IIA).

Many other alternative regimens are currently under investigation. Adjuvant therapy with granulocyte macrophage colony stimulating factor is being studied in Intergroup trial E4697 in patients with high-risk regional nodal disease and limited resectable distant metastases. However, it will be several years before the outcome of this trial is known. In addition, the S0008 Intergroup trial is testing an intensive biochemotherapy regimen as adjuvant therapy for high-risk melanoma. The regimen, which consists of cisplatin, vinblastine, and dacarbazine in combination with high-dose intravenous interleukin-2 and subcutaneous IFN-α, was pioneered at the University of Texas, M.D. Anderson Cancer Center for the treatment of advanced metastatic melanoma. This trial is currently comparing three cycles of biochemotherapy with the standard high-dose IFN-α-2b regimen in patients with stage III melanoma.

CONCLUSIONS

Based on available data, the approved high-dose IFN-α-2b regimen meets the standard of an effective adjuvant therapy for patients with high-risk resected melanoma. This regimen clearly reduces the risk of recurrence and provides a significant survival benefit. In light of the grave prognosis associated with recurrence in distant metastatic sites, adjuvant therapy with IFN-α-2b should be the standard of care for patients with stage IIB/C or stage III melanoma because of the high risk of recurrence in these patient populations. However, the decision to undergo adjuvant therapy must be made by the individual patient on the basis of a balanced discussion of all the data regarding the risk of recurrence and mortality and the risks and benefits of adjuvant therapy. Select subgroups of patients within these staging categories have a lower risk of death than others from melanoma and may view the potential benefits and side effects of adjuvant IFN-α-2b therapy in a different light than patients with a worse prognosis. Once a patient has made the decision to undergo adjuvant IFN-α-2b therapy, it is imperative that the clinical team manage toxicity so as to maximize the therapeutic effect and reduce the affect of treatment on the patient's quality of life.

Issues of Informed Consent

To ensure that patients are able to make an independent informed decision about whether to receive adjuvant therapy, it is critical that they receive a balanced presentation of the risks and benefits of high-dose IFN-α-2b therapy that is based on all available data. Unfortunately, this may not be happening in all treatment centers, which is cause for concern. Although the known side effects of IFN-α-2b therapy may cause some patients to refuse adjuvant therapy (particularly if they perceive their risk of recurrence to be low), the patient preference study described in this chapter suggests that most patients would choose high-dose IFN-α-2b therapy regardless of the possibility of severe toxicity, if it would lower their risk of recurrence by 10%. The efficacy data are highly consistent with this level of risk reduction. Therefore, it is hard to reconcile the tremendous disparity between treatment centers with respect to the frequency with which patients refuse adjuvant therapy. In fact, at some centers, virtually every patient "refuses" adjuvant therapy. This suggests that the efficacy and safety data are not being presented in a uniform manner.

Because the available data are complex, the oncologist often becomes the interpreter with the power to influence how the data are communicated and ultimately perceived by the patient. This provides both an opportunity and an obligation to scrutinize the available data and distill it down to a language that is comprehensible by the patient, thus allowing an appropriately informed choice. Currently available adjuvant therapy for melanoma is far from optimal; thus, clinical trials should continue to search for better and/or less toxic alternatives. At the present time, some fully informed patients may elect to forego adjuvant therapy with high-dose IFN-α-2b, and such patients are proper candidates for clinical trials, including trials with a no-treatment or inactive treatment control arm. However, the existence of clinical trials is not adequate justification for an incomplete discussion of available therapeutic options, and high-dose IFN-α-2b remains the standard for off-protocol treatment of otherwise healthy patients who are seeking adjuvant therapy for high-risk melanoma.

REFERENCES

1. Balch CM, Buzaid AC, Soong SJ et al. Final version of the American Joint Committee on Cancer staging system for cutaneous melanoma. J Clin Oncol 2001;19:3635–3648.
2. Van Cutsem E, Dicato M, Wils J et al. Adjuvant treatment of colorectal cancer (current expert opinion derived from the Third International Conference: Perspectives in Colorectal Cancer, Dublin, 2001). Eur J Cancer 2002;38:1429–1436.
3. Gershenwald JE, Thompson W, Mansfield PF et al. Multi-institutional melanoma lymphatic mapping experience: the prognostic value of sentinel lymph node status in 612 stage I or II melanoma patients. J Clin Oncol 1999;17:976–983.
4. Buzaid AC, Ross MI, Balch CM et al. Critical analysis of the current American Joint Committee on Cancer staging system for cutaneous melanoma and proposal of a new staging system. J Clin Oncol 1997;15:1039–1051.
5. Tamoxifen for early breast cancer: an overview of the randomised trials. Early Breast Cancer Trialists' Collaborative Group. Lancet 1998;351:1451–1467.
6. Polychemotherapy for early breast cancer: an overview of the randomised trials. Early Breast Cancer Trialists' Collaborative Group [see comments]. Lancet 1998;352:930–942.
7. Mamounas E, Wieand S, Wolmark N et al. Comparative efficacy of adjuvant chemotherapy in patients with Dukes' B versus Dukes' C colon cancer: results from four National Surgical Adjuvant Breast and Bowel Project adjuvant studies (C-01, C-02, C-03, and C-04). J Clin Oncol 1999;17:1349–1355.
8. McMasters KM, Reintgen DS, Ross MI et al. Sentinel lymph node biopsy for melanoma: how many radioactive nodes should be removed? Ann Surg Oncol 2001;8:192–197.
9. Morton DL, Thompson JF, Essner R et al. Validation of the accuracy of intraoperative lymphatic mapping and sentinel lymphadenectomy for early-stage melanoma: a multicenter trial. Multicenter Selective Lymphadenectomy Trial Group. Ann Surg 1999;230:453–463.

10. Reintgen D, Cruse CW, Wells K et al. The orderly progression of melanoma nodal metastases. Ann Surg 1994;220:759–767.

11. Atkins MB, Lotze MT, Dutcher JP et al. High-dose recombinant interleukin 2 therapy for patients with metastatic melanoma: analysis of 270 patients treated between 1985 and 1993. J Clin Oncol 1999;17:2105–2116.

12. Legha SS. The role of interferon alfa in the treatment of metastatic melanoma. Semin Oncol 1997;24:S24–S31.

13. Kirkwood JM, Strawderman MH, Ernstoff MS et al. Interferon alfa-2b adjuvant therapy of high-risk resected cutaneous melanoma: the Eastern Cooperative Oncology Group Trial EST 1684. J Clin Oncol 1996;14:7–17.

14. Kirkwood JM, Ibrahim JG, Sondak VK et al. High- and low-dose interferon alfa-2b in high-risk melanoma: first analysis of Intergroup Trial E1690/S9111/C9190. J Clin Oncol 2000;18:2444–2458.

15. Kirkwood JM. Adjuvant IFN alpha2 therapy of melanoma. Lancet 1998;351:1901–1903.

16. Cascinelli N, Belli F, MacKie RM et al. Effect of long-term adjuvant therapy with interferon alpha-2a in patients with regional node metastases from cutaneous melanoma: a randomised trial. Lancet 2001;358:866–869.

17. Kirkwood JM, Ibrahim JG, Sosman JA et al. High-dose interferon alfa-2b significantly prolongs relapse-free and overall survival compared with the GM2-KLH/QS-21 vaccine in patients with resected stage IIB-III melanoma: results of Intergroup trial E1694/S9512/C509801. J Clin Oncol 2001;19:2370–2380.

18. Wheatley K, Hancock B, Gore M et al. Interferon-α as adjuvant therapy for melanoma: a meta-analysis of the randomised trials [abstract 1394]. Proc Am Soc Clin Oncol 2001;20:349a.

19. Cameron DA, Cornbleet MC, Mackie RM et al. Adjuvant interferon alpha 2b in high risk melanoma: the Scottish study. Br J Cancer 2001;84:1146–1149.

20. Kleeberg UBEB, Chartier C et al. EORTC 18871 adjuvant trial in high risk melanoma patients: IFN vs IFN vs Iscador vs observation [abstract]. Eur J Cancer 1999;35:264.

21. Kirkwood JM, Ibrahim J, Lawson DH et al. High-dose interferon alfa-2b does not diminish antibody response to GM2 vaccination in patients with resected melanoma: results of the Multicenter Eastern Cooperative Oncology Group phase II Trial E2696. J Clin Oncol 2001;19:1430–1436.

22. Kiley KE, Gale DM. Nursing management of patients with malignant melanoma receiving adjuvant alpha interferon-2b. Clin J Oncol Nurs 1998;2:11–16.

23. Caraceni A, Gangeri L, Martini C et al. Neurotoxicity of interferon-α in melanoma therapy: results from a randomized controlled trial. Cancer 1998;83:482–489.

24. Greenberg DB, Jonasch E, Gadd MA et al. Adjuvant therapy of melanoma with interferon-alpha-2b is associated with mania and bipolar syndromes. Cancer 2000;89:356–362.

25. Quesada JR, Talpaz M, Rios A et al. Clinical toxicity of interferons in cancer patients: a review. J Clin Oncol 1986;4:234–243.

26. Kirkwood JM, Bender C, Agarwala S et al. Mechanisms and management of toxicities associated with high-dose interferon alfa-2b therapy. J Clin Oncol 2002;20:3703–3718.

27. Schering-Plough. Package Insert, Intron® A Interferon alfa-2b, recombinant for Injection. Kenilworth, NJ: Schering-Plough, 1999.

28. Portenoy RK, Itri LM. Cancer-related fatigue: guidelines for evaluation and management. Oncologist 1999;4:1–10.

29. Clark PM, Lacasse C. Cancer-related fatigue: clinical practice issues. Clin J Oncol Nurs 1998;2:45–53.

30. Meyers CA, Weitzner MA, Valentine AD et al. Methylphenidate therapy improves cognition, mood, and function of brain tumor patients. J Clin Oncol 1998;16:2522-2527.
31. Weitzner MA, Meyers CA, Valentine AD. Methylphenidate in the treatment of neurobehavioral slowing associated with cancer and cancer treatment. J Neuropsychiatry Clin Neurosci 1995;7:347–350.
32. Mantovani G, Maccio A, Massa E et al. Managing cancer-related anorexia/cachexia. Drugs 2001;61:499–514.
33. Hauser P, Soler R, Reed S et al. Prophylactic treatment of depression induced by interferon-α. Psychosomatics 2000;41:439–441.
34. Schramm TM, Lawford BR, Macdonald GA et al. Sertraline treatment of interferon-alfa-induced depressive disorder. Med J Aust 2000;173:359–361.
35. Valentine AD, Meyers CA. Successful treatment of interferon-alpha-induced mood disorder with nortriptyline. Psychosomatics 1995;36:418–419.
36. Valentine AD, Meyers CA, Kling MA et al. Mood and cognitive side effects of interferon-α therapy. Semin Oncol 1998;25:39–47.
37. Valentine AD, Meyers CA, Talpaz M. Treatment of neurotoxic side effects of interferon-α with naltrexone. Cancer Invest 1995;13:561–566.
38. Musselman DL, Lawson DH, Gumnick JF et al. Paroxetine for the prevention of depression induced by high-dose interferon alfa. N Engl J Med 2001;344:961–966.
39. Nelson KA. Modern management of the cancer anorexia-cachexia syndrome. Curr Pain Headache Rep 2001;5:250–256.
40. Cole BF, Gelber RD, Kirkwood JM et al. Quality-of-life-adjusted survival analysis of interferon alfa-2b adjuvant treatment of high-risk resected cutaneous melanoma: an Eastern Cooperative Oncology Group study. J Clin Oncol 1996;14:2666–2673.
41. Kilbridge KL, Weeks JC, Sober AJ et al. Patient preferences for adjuvant interferon alfa-2b treatment. J Clin Oncol 2001;19:812–823.
42. Kilbridge KL, Cole BF, Kirkwood JM et al. Quality-of-life–adjusted survival analysis of high-dose adjuvant interferon alfa-2b for high-risk melanoma patients using intergroup clinical trial data. J Clin Oncol 2002;20:1311–1318.
43. Hillner BE, Kirkwood JM, Atkins MB et al. Economic analysis of adjuvant interferon alfa-2b in high-risk melanoma based on projections from Eastern Cooperative Oncology Group 1684. J Clin Oncol 1997;15:2351–2358.
44. Livingston PO, Wong GYC, Adluri S et al. Improved survival in stage III melanoma patients with GM2 antibodies: a randomized trial of adjuvant vaccination with GM2 ganglioside. J Clin Oncol 1994;12:1036–1044.
45. Helling F, Zhang S, Shang A et al. GM2-KLH conjugate vaccine: increased immunogenicity in melanoma patients after administration with immunological adjuvant QS-21. Cancer Res 1995;55:2783–2788.
46. Sondak VK, Liu PY, Tuthill RJ et al. Adjuvant immunotherapy of resected, intermediate-thickness, node-negative melanoma with an allogeneic tumor vaccine: overall results of a randomized trial of the Southwest Oncology Group. J Clin Oncol 2002;20:2058–2066.
47. Sosman JA, Unger JM, Liu PY et al. Adjuvant immunotherapy of resected, intermediate-thickness, node-negative melanoma with an allogeneic tumor vaccine: impact of HLA class I antigen expression on outcome. J Clin Oncol 2002;20:2067–2075.

Chapter 19

Value of Alpha Interferon in Adjuvant Therapy for Melanoma: The Case Against

Lynn E. Spitler

A new staging system for melanoma went into effect in 2002 with the publication of the Sixth Edition of the American Joint Committee on Cancer (AJCC) Cancer Staging Manual.[1] This new staging system is important because it allows precise determination of the prognosis for individual patients with melanoma and has been validated in more than 17,000 patients with melanoma (Table 19.1).[2,3] Under the new staging system, survival curves correlate well with stage of disease, and subgroupings within each stage allow further refinement of prognosis. This allows the physician to determine with precision which patients are at high risk for recurrence and to counsel patients about their prognosis and therapeutic options.

On the basis of this important information, the dilemma being faced by the treating physicians and patients with melanoma is what, if any, surgical adjuvant therapy they should choose. The problem arises in part because studies of adjuvant therapy for melanoma are not as advanced as those on other cancers, and no therapeutic agent has yet been identified that shows unequivocal efficacy combined with an acceptable safety profile. In breast cancer, for example, tens of thousands of women have participated in randomized controlled clinical trials of

TABLE 19.1 Staging of Malignant Melanoma

Stage		Characteristics	5-Year Survival
I		No nodal or distant metastases and	
	A	Primary tumor ≤ 1 mm in thickness without ulceration	95%
	B	Primary tumor ≤ 1 mm in thickness with ulceration or level IV or V or primary tumor 1.01–2 mm in thickness without ulceration	90%
II		No nodal or distant metastases and	
	A	Primary tumor 1.01–2 mm in thickness with ulceration or primary tumor 2.01–4 mm in thickness without ulceration	78%
	B	Primary tumor 2.01–4 mm in thickness with ulceration or primary tumor > 4 mm in thickness without ulceration	64%
	C	Primary tumor > 4 mm in thickness with ulceration	45%
III			
	A	1–3 nodes with micrometastasis and no ulceration of the primary tumor	67%
	B	1–3 nodes with micrometasis and ulceration of the primary tumor or 1–3 nodes with macrometastasis and no ulceration of the primary tumor or in transit met(s)/satellite(s) without metastatic nodes with or without ulceration of the primary	52%
	C	1–3 nodes with macrometastasis and ulceration of the primary tumor or 4 or more nodes with micro- or macrometastasis with or without ulceration of the primary tumor or satellite or in-transit metastases with metastatic nodes with or without ulceration of the primary	27%
IV			
	M1a	Skin and/or subcutaneous metastasis, normal LDH	19%
	M1b	Lung metastasis, normal LDH	7%
	M1c	Other visceral metastasis or any distant site of metastasis and elevated LDH	9%

Abbreviations: LDH, lactate dehydrogenase.
Modified from Balch et al.[2]

tamoxifen as surgical adjuvant therapy, and this agent offers a clear survival benefit with acceptable toxicity. A meta-analysis of 28 randomized trials of tamoxifen as surgical adjuvant therapy in 16,581 patients with stage I and II breast cancer showed a reduction of 16% (± 3%) in the odds of death in women of all ages who were assigned to receive tamoxifen. The analysis also showed a clear reduction of mortality in women 50 years of age and older for whom tamoxifen reduced the annual odds of death during the first 5 years by about 20% ($P < 0.0001$).[4]

Clinical trials of adjuvant therapy for melanoma have focused mainly on patients with stage III disease, probably because these patients have a poor prognosis (< 50% 5-year survival) and are represented in greater numbers than patients with stage IV disease that was surgically excised, who have an even worse prognosis. In the United States and Canada, but not in other countries, high-dose interferon (HDI) is approved for adjuvant therapy for "high-risk" melanoma, although many patients refuse this therapy after being informed of the risk/benefit ratio. There is no approved adjuvant therapy for patients in other categories, so such patients can receive standard therapy (observation) after surgery, participate in a clinical trial, or receive off-label treatment. It is clear that alternative therapies with greater efficacy and less toxicity are needed, but, so far, all phase 3 trials of alternative treatments have failed to show a difference between the control and treatment arms, i.e., they have been negative studies.

INTERFERON

The results of multicenter randomized controlled trials for interferon for the adjuvant treatment of melanoma have been the subject of several reviews.[5-8] The reviews included between 8 and 12 of the following trials: Austrian,[9] Eastern Cooperative Oncology Group (ECOG) 1684,[10] ECOG 1690,[11] ECOG 1694,[12,13] EORTC 18871,[14] EORTC 18952,[14] French,[15] NCCTG 83705,[16] Scottish MG,[17] UKCCCR,[18] and WHO 16.[19,20] The trials varied in terms of the product used (interferon-α2b [Intron® A] or interferon α2a [Roferon®]), dose (high or low), duration of interferon administration, and stage of disease.

Even though the trials were heterogeneous and the reviews each included different trials, the conclusions of the reviews were remarkably similar in the following ways: They agreed that the administration of interferon alfa (IFN-α) as adjuvant therapy for melanoma does prolong disease-free survival (DFS) but not overall survival (OS):

1. "In our review, results from included RCTs (randomized clinical trials) demonstrated no clear benefit of IFN-α therapy on OS in melanoma patients."[8]
2. "With mature data on OS of some trials using this schedule still pending, high-dose IFN-α does prolong DFS but not OS in patients with stage IIB-III melanoma. Given the toxicity of this treatment, the standard use of adjuvant high-dose IFN-α currently cannot be recommended." [7]

3. "For DFS, there was clear benefit for IFN: odds ratio (OR) = 0.84, 95% confidence interval (CI) = 0.77-0.92, $P = .0001$. The advantage was less clear for OS (OR = 0.76, CI = 0.82-1.00, $P = .05$) and the upper CI is compatible with no survival benefit . . . decisions on the use of IFN for melanoma will need to be based on considerations such as the relative importance of benefits on DFS compared to OS, patient quality of life and financial cost."[21]
4. ". . . all estimates of odds ratios are < 1.0, indicating survival benefit. However, only one of these estimates appears to be significantly different from 1.0 [Kirkwood et al[10]]. The upper bounds of all other 95% confidence intervals include 1.0. The estimate of odds ratio for all studies is 0.88 (95% CI: 0.77, 1.03; $P = .065$)."[5]

HIGH-DOSE INTERFERON

The only drug approved for the postsurgical adjuvant treatment of melanoma in the United States and Canada is interferon-α2b. The labeled indication on the package insert states: "INTRON®A Interferon alfa-2b, recombinant for injection is indicated as adjuvant to surgical treatment in patients 18 years of age or older with malignant melanoma who are free of disease but at high risk for systemic recurrence within 56 days of surgery." The meaning of "high risk" is not defined on the product label, so it is not clear exactly what this approval covers. However, the clinical trials on which this approval was based included patients with primary melanoma > 4 mm in thickness (stage II, T4) and melanoma metastatic to regional nodes (part of the stage III classification). One assumes that this is the population that the approval covers, but that has not been made clear. The clinical trials did not include patients with in transit or satellite metastases (another part of the stage III classification) or patients with stage IV disease that has been surgically excised, who are also at very high risk for recurrence.

HDI is an imperfect solution for adjuvant therapy for melanoma because most studies show improvement in DFS, but survival benefit in the treated patients is controversial and toxicity is considerable. The details of the clinical trials of HDI supporting this conclusion have been extensively reported and debated and are summarized in Table 19.2.

Clinical Benefit, Overall Survival

E1684[10] The ECOG completed a prospective, randomized, controlled study of interferon-2αb versus observation as surgical adjuvant therapy in 287 patients with melanoma. As reported, with a median follow-up time of 6.9 years, the median OS was increased by 1 year in the treatment arm as compared with the ob-

TABLE 19.2 ECOG Trials of HDI as Adjuvant Therapy of Melanoma

Trial	Design	Outcome	Toxicity	Comments
E1684[10]	252 eligible patients (280 ITT) randomly assigned to high-dose interferon or observation; 11% node negative.	Publication reports significant improvement in disease-free survival in patients receiving high-dose interferon. Survival at 5 years: 46% in patients receiving interferon, 37% in observation group. Median follow-up = 6.9 years.	67% of patients had severe (grade 3) toxicity at some point during the year of treatment, 9% had life-threatening toxicity, and two had lethal hepatic toxicity.	The most important prognostic indicator for this patient population, number of positive nodes,[3,67] was not recorded; therefore, it is not known whether the treated and observation patient populations were balanced with regard to this indicator. The overall survival benefit was lost with longer follow-up (median, 145 months; $P = .09$)[7]
E1690[11]	608 eligible patients (642 ITT) randomly assigned to high-dose or low-dose interferon or observation; 25% had nodes clinically or pathologically negative.	Significant improvement in disease-free survival in patients receiving high-dose interferon but no difference in overall survival ($P = 0.99$). Median follow-up = 4.3 years.	The manuscript does not state the percentage of patients with grade 3 or 4 toxicity but states that "Treatment with HDI was associated with significant toxicity consistent with the adverse events that have been reported by others and those observed in trial E1684." There were no treatment-related deaths in the HDI arm.	Patients randomly assigned to the observation who experienced relapse and then received interferon-containing salvage therapy had an apparent postrelapse survival advantage compared with patients who did not receive interferon-containing salvage therapy, indicating that interferon treatment is beneficial when it is given immediately after lymphadenectomy or after relapse.
E1694[12]	774 eligible patients (880 ITT) randomly assigned to high-dose interferon or GMK melanoma vaccine; no observation group: 23% had nodes clinically or pathologically negative.	Significant improvement in disease-free and overall survival in patients receiving high-dose interferon as compared with those receiving vaccine. Median follow-up = 16 months.	The manuscript does not state what percentage of patients had grade 3 or 4 toxicity but does state there were no treatment-related deaths.	Median follow-up relatively short.

Abbreviations: ECOG, Eastern Cooperative Oncology Group; HDI, high-dose interferon; ITT, intent-to-treat.

servation arm, and the 5-year survival was increased by 9% from 37% in patients randomly assigned to observation to 46% in patients receiving HDI (*P* = .0237, one-sided log-rank test). The analysis performed by the U.S. Food and Drug Administration (FDA) also concluded that the improvement in median OS was 12 months (3.8 years vs 2.8 years) but the *P* value did not meet the standard measure of significance (*P* = .06 unstratified log-rank test, two-sided log-rank test; *P* = .045 stratified log-rank test). In a later analysis by Cole et al[22] using the same data set, there was an improvement of 7.0 months of OS, and the difference between the treatment arm and observation arm did not reach the level of statistical significance when a two-sided test was applied (*P* = .07). Similarly, Lens and Dawes[8] reviewed this trial and calculated the number needed to treat for OS and found that it did not reach statistical significance. Recent long-term follow-up data at a median follow-up of 145 months shows no OS benefit, with 95 deaths in the control arm and 93 deaths in the HDI arm (*P* = .09).[7]

E1690[11] In follow-up, a large, prospective, randomized trial was performed on 608 eligible patients who were randomly assigned to one of three arms: HDI, low-dose interferon, or observation. There was no survival benefit in patients receiving HDI compared with those receiving low-dose interferon (LDI) or observation (*P* = 0.99). In Europe, after the publication of these data, reimbursement for HDI as surgical adjuvant therapy for melanoma was no longer offered, and the use of this modality virtually ceased. Another observation in this study was that patients who were randomly assigned to the observation arm who experienced relapse and then received interferon-containing salvage therapy had an apparent postrelapse survival advantage compared with those who did not receive interferon-containing salvage therapy, indicating that timing of the interferon treatment is not important—it can be given immediately after lymphadenectomy or after relapse.

E1694[12] The study included 774 eligible patients who were randomly assigned to HDI or to the GM2/KLH vaccine with QS 21 (called GMK). There was progression-free and OS benefit in patients receiving HDI compared with those receiving GMK vaccine, but the median follow-up was only 16 months, and there was no untreated control group. Because there was no untreated control arm, it is not possible to rule out the possibility that the GMK vaccine had a deleterious effect on survival. It is noteworthy that the adjuvant was changed from bacille Calmette-Guérin (BCG), which was used in the phase II trial,[23] to QS21 in the phase III trial. This could have produced a higher level of gamma G immunoglobulin antibodies, which might have adversely affected the outcome.

The value of HDI in improving OS was discussed in detail at the meeting of the Oncologic Drugs Advisory Committee on February 27, 2002. Although the committee did not vote on the issues, the consensus was that HDI has not been shown to provide benefit in OS and that phase III trials of adjuvant therapy for high-risk melanoma are not required to include a HDI treatment arm. It would not be appropriate to include quotes on this subject by the committee members out of context, but the transcript of their deliberations is available on-line.[24]

Toxicity

- 67% of the patients in E1684 had grade 3 toxicity; 9% had grade 4 toxicity, and two deaths occurred as a result of hepatotoxicity.[10]
- Comparable figures are not given for E1690 or E1694, except to state that no deaths occurred as a result of toxicity.[11,12]
- The product label includes toxicity data only from 143 patients included in the first trial (E1684); it has not been updated with data from the other trials or with phase IV data.
- The manufacturer states that they are not collecting postmarketing toxicity data.
- The FDA prepared a lengthy and detailed analysis of the results of the trials on the use of interferon as adjuvant therapy for melanoma, but this analysis does not include any mention of toxicity.[5]
- The toxicity of the regimen must be viewed in the context of the patients' clinical status. Although these patients are at high risk for recurrence, they have been treated with surgery, the best treatment available for melanoma, and they are clinically tumor free at the time of treatment with HDI; therefore, some may already have been cured of their disease by surgery.

Here is as description written by a patient taking interferon and published in "Rays of Wisdom," a publication of the American Melanoma Foundation: ". . . most of the time I make it into the bathroom before my world spins to black. The cool of the porcelain feels good against my cheek, and I rest there, on the floor, dizzy from the exertion that has gotten me here. And now, the next decision comes. Do I use the sink to pull myself off the floor, knowing the explosive and instant pain it will bring, or do I stay resting, soothing my face on the coolness, and moving as little as possible?" This patient had a recurrence of her melanoma, and the same publication states, "When her doctor prescribed more interferon, Linn told him, unequivocally, that she would rather die."

LOW-DOSE INTERFERON

The use of LDI for patients with stage II melanoma has been approved by the European Medicine Evaluation Agency, but not by the U.S. FDA. The approval was based on two trials. Low-dose interferon was evaluated in a large, randomized study on adjuvant therapy in 499 patients with stage II melanoma (primary melanoma greater than 1.5 mm in thickness with clinically negative nodes).[25] The results in this patient population seemed promising; even though the low-dose regimen does not seem effective in higher-risk patients; there was benefit in progression-free survival in the patients who were randomly assigned to LDI. There was also benefit in terms of OS at a median follow-up of 5 years, but not at a median follow-up of 8 years.[7,15] In a second randomized trial of LDI in 311 patients with resected primary stage II melanoma, prolonged DFS was also demonstrated.[9] The results of the LDI on OS in this trial are unknown. A third trial included patients with stage II and III disease who were randomly assigned to LDI or observation; this trial demonstrated no difference between the treatment arms.[17]

ALTERNATIVE APPROACHES

Negative Phase 3 Trials

Numerous therapeutic agents other than interferon have completed randomized phase 3 trials as adjuvant therapy for melanoma, and none of the trials have shown a survival benefit (Table 19.3).

These trials included evaluation of four vaccines. In one study, 217 eligible subjects with stage III melanoma were randomly assigned to receive vaccinia melanoma oncolysate or vaccinia alone. There was no difference in the DFS

TABLE 19.3 Agents that Have Been Tested as Adjuvant Therapy for Melanoma in Randomized Trials and Have Been Shown Not to Affect Overall Survival

Agent	Reference, Comments
Vaccinia melanoma oncolysate (VMO)	Wallack et al[26]
Vaccina melanoma cell lysate (VMCL)	Hersey et al[27,28]
Melacine	Sondak et al[29]; subjects of specified HLA type had improved disease-free survival.[30]
GMK vaccine	Kirkwood et al[12]
Dacarbazine (DTIC)	Hill et al[31]
Bacille Calmette-Guérin (BCG)	Pinsky et al[33]; Cunningham, T.J. et al[32]
Levamisole	Quirt et al[34]; Spitler et al[35]; the study by Quirt et al reported clinical benefit in the treated patients, and on this basis, levamisole was approved as adjuvant therapy for melanoma in Canada but is no longer available.

Abbreviation: HLA, human leukocyte antigen.

(*P* = 0.61) or the OS (*P* = 0.79).[26] In a similar study using different melanoma cell lines, 675 eligible patients with stage IIB and III melanoma were randomly assigned to vaccinia melanoma cell lysate or observation. After a median follow-up of 8 years, the median OS was 88 months in the control arm and 151 months in the treated arm (*P* = 0.068).[27,28] The Southwest Oncology Group (SWOG) conducted a randomized trial (SWOG-9035) of Melacine versus observation in 600 eligible patients with stage II melanoma.[29] The results showed no difference in the DFS rates in the treatment arms; there were 65 deaths in the vaccine arm and 71 deaths in the treatment arm. A further analysis of this study was performed on the basis of the patients' human leukocyte antigen (HLA) type.[30] There were 97 vaccine-treated patients and 78 observation patients whose HLA type matched ≥ two of the M5 HLA class I antigens, and these vaccine-treated patients had a significantly better relapse-free survival than the observation patients (5-year relapse-free survival was 83% vs 59%; *P* = 0.0002). Finally, a combined intergroup protocol by three cooperative groups (E1694/S9512/C50981) was conducted in which 774 eligible patients with high-risk melanoma were randomly assigned to the GM2/KLH vaccine with QS 21 (called GMK) versus high-dose interferon.[12] The results showed that patients receiving the HDI had better OS and DFS than in patients who received the vaccine.

Other agents that have been tested and failed as adjuvant therapy for high-risk melanoma include dacarbazine (DTIC)[31] and BCG.[32,33] In a large, prospective, randomized trial, levamisole was reported to be effective in the adjuvant therapy of high-risk melanoma,[34] and on the basis of that study, levamisole was approved for this purpose in Canada, but not in the United States. A similar, prospective, randomized, placebo-controlled trial failed to show a benefit of le-vamisole in the adjuvant treatment of melanoma, but the dose used was slightly different.[35] The manufacturer has ceased production of levamisole, so it is no longer available in the United States.

Vaccines

Numerous vaccines have completed phase 2 trials with encouraging results, but as of August 2002, only three of them (a multiepitope peptide vaccine, Melacine, and the GMK vaccine) were in phase 3 trials open to patient accrual (Table 19.4). CancerVax was developed by Donald Morton at the John Wayne Cancer Institute and consists of an irradiated live-cell preparation of three allogeneic melanoma cell lines chosen for their high content of immunogenic melanoma–associated and common tumor–associated antigens, administered with BCG as an adjuvant.[36] In phase 2 clinical trials conducted worldwide, the vaccine has been administered to more than 1600 patients with advanced-stage melanoma, and the results document the safety of the vaccine and its potential efficacy, as shown by a significant increase in 5-year survival rates and in OS time when compared with historical controls.[37,38] CancerVax is now in phase 3 trials in separate

TABLE 19.4 Noninterferon Agents in Phase 2 or 3 Clinical Trials as Adjuvant Therapy for Malignant Melanoma

Agent	Stage	Phase	Comments
[a]Peptide vaccine, GM-CSF vs placebo	III, IV	3	Randomized intergroup trial (E1697)
[a]GMK vs observation	II	3	EORTC trial
[a]Melacine + LDI vs HDI	III	3	
CancerVax vs observation	III	3	Study on indefinite hold for patient accrual.
CancerVax vs observation	IV	3	Study on indefinite hold for patient accrual.
Melacine(®) vs observation	II	3	Study not yet open for accrual.
[a]Biochemotherapy vs HDI	III	3	Bedikian[68]
TriGem + HDI vs HDI	III	3	Study not yet open for accrual.
[a]GM-CSF	II(T4), III, IV	2	
[a]Peptide vaccine + adjuvants	IIB, IIC, III, IV	2	Conducted by Dr. J. Weber, pers. comm. 2002
[a]Peptide vaccine + Montanide ISA-51	I-IV	2	Patients must be HLA-A1, A3, or 0201 positive.[69] Accrual for types HLA-A24 and HLA-A31 is closed.
[a]Autologous tumor cells plus autologous dendritic cells	III, IV	2	Conducted by Dr. R.O. Dillman, pers. comm. 2002
[a]Neoadjuvant biochemotherapy	III, IV	2	

Abbreviations: GM-CSF, granulocyte macrophage colony stimulating factor; LDI, low-dose interferon; HDI, high-dose interferon; EORTC, European Organization for Research and Treatment of Cancer; HLA, human leukocyte antigen.
[a]Study open to accrual.

studies in patients with stage III and in those with stage IV disease that has been surgically excised. These studies have been placed on indefinite hold for patient accrual by the FDA because of manufacturing issues.

Analysis of tumor-infiltrating lymphocytes obtained from patients with melanoma led to the cloning of the genes that encode proteins recognized by T cells with antitumor activity and to the subsequent identification and synthesis of the relevant peptides. This led to the synthesis of peptides designed to have increased binding to the HLA-A2 molecule. The combination of these synthetic peptides resulted in the multiepitope peptide vaccine. The peptides included in this vaccine are gp 100 209-217 210M, MART-1 26-35 27L, and tyrosinase 368-376 370D. A trial (E1697) has been initiated that will include 600 patients with known HLA-A2 status. Eligibility is restricted to melanoma patients with locoregional recurrence after prior adjuvant interferon therapy, local recurrence after adequate surgical excision of the primary tumor, mucosal melanoma, stage IV melanoma, satellite or intransit disease, stage III disease with gross extracapsular extension, recurrence in a previously resected nodal basin, four or more involved lymph nodes, matted lymph nodes, or an ulcerated primary melanoma and any involved lymph nodes, and to those who are medically unfit for HDI. Patients must not have received prior treatment with granulocyte macrophage colony stimulating factor (GM-CSF) and must be rendered surgically free of disease. Eligible patients who are HLA-A2 positive will be randomly assigned to control (placebo), multiepitope peptide vaccine, GM-CSF, or GM-CSF and multiepitope peptide vaccine. Patients who are HLA-A2 negative will be randomly assigned to GM-CSF or placebo. Accrual to this study is slow, probably because of the restrictive eligibility criteria.

Melacine consists of lysed cells from two human melanoma cell lines combined with an adjuvant, DETOX, which consists of monophosphoryl lipid A and mycobacterial cell wall skeleton. The vaccine induced an increase in precursors of cytolytic T cells and objective responses in some patients with advanced melanoma.[39,40] This led to the design of a phase 3 randomized trial in patients with stage II melanoma, described earlier, in which there was no difference in outcome between patients randomized to the treatment or control arms, i.e. it was a negative study. The subgroup analysis showing clinical benefit for vaccinated patients who were positive for HLA-A2, HLA-C3, or both, prompted the owner, Corixa Corporation, to propose a second randomized pivotal trial of Melacine as adjuvant therapy for patients with stage II melanoma who exhibited those HLA types.[24] Melacine is also being evaluated in a phase III randomized multicenter trial of Melacine and LDI versus HDI as adjuvant therapy for patients with stage III melanoma (study #6875-01).

GM2 is a ganglioside that is overrepresented on melanoma cells and thus can be used in a vaccine in an effort to stimulate an immune response to melanoma. A double-blind, randomized trial was conducted of a GM2 ganglioside vaccine, administered with bacille Calmette-Guérin (GM2/BCG) versus BCG alone as adjuvant therapy in 122 patients with stage III melanoma.[23] The results showed improved survival in patients with GM2 antibodies over patients who did not have these antibodies. In a subsequent phase I trial, it was shown that conjugating the GM2 ganglioside with keyhole limpet hemocyanin and administering to it the QS-21 as adjuvant resulted in serologic responses against GM2 that were strikingly superior, quantitatively and qualitatively, to any seen with previously tested GM2 vaccines.[41] The resulting vaccine is named GMK, and it was evaluated in the randomized trial described earlier, which showed that patients receiving HDI had a better OS and DFS than patients who received the vaccine.[12] The GMK vaccine is also being tested in Europe in ongoing studies by the EORTC in a randomized trial of the vaccine versus observation as adjuvant therapy for patients with stage II melanoma.[42]

Some vaccines have completed successful phase 2 trials but have not progressed to phase 3 trials and are not currently available. One of these is a polyvalent, shed-antigen vaccine prepared from material shed into the culture medium by three allogeneic and one xenogeneic melanoma cell line adapted to long-term growth in serum-free medium.[43] A double-blind, prospectively randomized, placebo-controlled trial of this vaccine was initiated.[44] Thirty-eight patients with resected melanoma to regional nodes (stage III) were randomly assigned in a 2:1 ratio to vaccine or placebo. With a median follow-up of 2.5 years, there was a statically significant prolongation of time to disease progression, but not of OS. Unfortunately, the study was stopped because of poor patient accrual.[45]

In another approach, patients were immunized with haptenized autologous tumor cells.[46] Autologous tumor cells were conjugated to the hapten dinitrophenol and administered with BCG to patients who had been sensitized to dinitrophenol alone. In 214 patients with stage III disease who were rendered tumor free by surgery, with a median follow-up time of 4.4 years, the overall 5- year survival was 47% in patients treated with the vaccine with BCG, a result believed comparable to those obtained with HDI.[47,48] Unfortunately, there are no clinical trials of this vaccine currently under way.[49]

TriGem is an antiidiotypic monoclonal antibody that mimics the disialoganglioside GD2. It was evaluated in a multicenter evaluation in 69 patients with stage III melanoma, of whom 25 also received HDI. At a median follow-up of 2 years, the data suggested a clinical benefit of TriGem.[50]

Numerous other vaccines are in phase 1 clinical trials aimed at defining the safety and immunogenicity of these vaccines in patients with melanoma, but it will be some time before these products will be ready for phase 2 testing for the adjuvant therapy for melanoma. Two centers where these studies are being conducted are the University of Wisconsin (M.R. Albertini, personal communication, 2002) and the Memorial Sloan-Kettering Cancer Center.

GM-CSF (Leukine, Sargramostim)

Many lines of evidence suggest that GM-CSF might have activity in the adjuvant therapy for cancer. Activated macrophages distinguish tumor cells from normal cells and kill only the tumor cells.[51] GM-CSF, which is approved for marketing for hematopoietic reconstitution and reversal of iatrogenic neutropenia, also has activity as a macrophage activator. GM-CSF stimulates peripheral blood monocytes in vitro to become cytotoxic for human melanoma cells.[52,53] Further, in vivo administration of low doses of GM-CSF also results in monocyte activation, as shown by enhanced cytotoxicity.[54,55] GM-CSF also serves as the principal mediator of proliferation, maturation, and migration of dendritic cells,[56-58] antigen-presenting cells that play a major role in the induction of primary and secondary T-cell immune responses. Finally, GM-CSF increases production of angiostatin by the macrophages.[59,60]

We conducted a trial of GM-CSF as a surgical adjuvant treatment in patients who were at very high risk for recurrence of melanoma.[61] The patient population included 48 patients with stage III disease who were at very high risk for recurrence (more than four positive nodes) or with stage IV disease who were rendered clinically disease free by surgery before enrollment. The OS and the DFS were significantly prolonged in patients who received GM-CSF compared with matched historical controls. This means that the patients recieving GM-CSF had a longer median time to disease progression and a longer survival than the matched controls. At 2 years, the survival in the control group was 15%, and in the treatment group, it was 64%. The median survival was 37.5 months in the study patients, versus 12.2 months in the matched controls ($P < 0.001$).

We have initiated a second trial to further evaluate this therapy in an expanded patient population. Eligible patients are those with stage II (T4), III, or IV melanoma that has been surgically excised. An interim analysis of this study was presented at the 4th International Conference on Adjuvant Therapy of Melanoma held at the Royal College of Physicians in London, March 2002.[62] Fifty patients were included in the analysis, and the results suggested a survival benefit for the patients treated with GM-CSF as compared with 1000 matched patients from the AJCC database who had been treated with surgery alone (Fig. 19.1).

A prospective randomized trial to definitively evaluate efficacy of this approach has been initiated by a consortium of cooperative groups. This trial includes vaccine arms and is described in the Vaccines section.

Other Biologic Approaches

Other biologic approaches for adjuvant therapy of melanoma are being pursued, including monoclonal antibodies, gene transfer, cellular therapies, and antiangiogenesis (Table 19.5). These agents are earlier in the course of development than other agents discussed in this chapter, but most have completed phase 1 trials that have shown safety and potential efficacy.

Chemotherapy

In a series of phase 2 trials in patients with stage III node-positive melanoma, investigators found that patients receiving vindesine alone or in combination with DTIC or LDI had a statistically significant benefit when compared with the

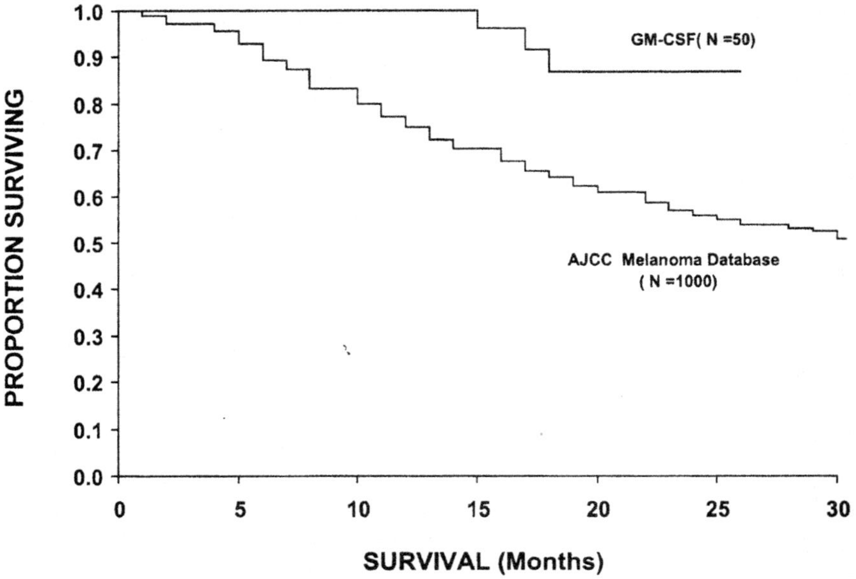

FIGURE 19.1 Survival in patients with high-risk melanoma treated with granulocyte macrophage colony stimulating factor (GM-CSF) or surgery alone (American Joint Committee on Cancer [AJCC] Melanoma Database).

untreated concurrent controls or the AJCC stage III patients enrolled in the Aim High trial, which was conducted in the United Kingdom.[63,64] Because of reports of the efficacy of biochemotherapy, especially CVD (cisplatin, vinblastine, dacarbazine) therapy for patients with metastatic melanoma[65], a phase III randomized trial has been initiated consisting of biochemotherapy with CVD, interleukin-2, and interferon versus HDI for adjuvant therapy for melanoma patients with lymph node metastases that have been surgically resected (MDA-DM-95196, MDA-ID-95196, NCI-G96-1089). A pilot phase II study of neoadjuvant biochemotherapy was performed in 48 patients with stage III melanoma. The patients were given two cycles of biochemotherapy consisting of cisplatin, vinblastine, DTIC (CVD), interleukin-2, and interferon before and after lymph node dissection.[66] At a median follow-up of 31 months, 38 or the 48 patients (79%) were alive, and 31 patients (65%) remained free of disease progression.

SUMMARY AND CONCLUSIONS

The FDA approved HDI for adjuvant therapy for high-risk melanoma on the basis of a trial (E1684) in which the survival benefit to patients did not reach the usually accepted level of statistical significance. Long-term follow-up of these patients showed less difference (not statistically significant, even by the one-tailed test used

TABLE 19.5 Biologic Agents in Development as Adjuvant Therapy for Melanoma

Monoclonal Antibodies

- Ch14.18: monoclonal antibody to the ganglioside GD2[70]
- R24: monoclonal antibody to the disialoganglioside GD3[71,72]
- ch14.18-IL-2: a fusion protein of the anti GD-2 antibody with IL-2[73,74]
- Anti-CTLA4: antibody to the cytotoxic T lymphocyte antigen 4[75]
- TriGem: anti-idiotype antibody that mimics the disialoganglioside GD2[50,76] (phase 3 trial planned)
- BEC2: anti-idiotypic antibody that mimics the GD3 disialoganglioside[77] (phase 3 trial planned in small-cell lung cancer)

Gene Transfer

- GM-CSF into melanoma cells[78-80]
- IL-2 into melanoma cells[81,82]
- IL-4 into melanoma cells [Maio, 2002 #751
- IL-12 gene into autologous fibroblasts [Kang, 2001 #752]
- IL-2 gene in a monkey fibroblast cell line (Vero)[83]
- gp75 (TRP-1) xenogeneic DNA vaccine
- Tyrosinase human vs xenogeneic DNA vaccine

Cellular Therapies

- Autologous dendritic cells pulsed with peptides representing epitopes of melanoma-associated antigens[84-87]
- Autologous dendritic cells pulsed with tumor lysates[88]
- Autologous dendritic cells transduced with autologous tumor RNA[89]
- Autologous tumor cells plus autologous dendritic cells administered as a vaccine[90]

Antiangiogenesis

- Thalidomide with temozolomide, [91–93] REVIMID

Abbreviations: GM-CSF, granulocyte macrophage colony stimulating factor; IL, interleukin.

in the original analysis) in survival between treated and control subjects. A large, randomized, follow-on study (E1690) showed no survival benefit. Four reviews that analyzed results from eight to 12 randomized trials of interferon as adjuvant therapy for melanoma each concluded that survival benefit was not demonstrated. At its meeting on February 27, 2002, the Oncologic Drugs Advisory Committee also concluded that a survival benefit of HDI had not been demonstrated. However, a consensus supports the notion that HDI therapy increases DFS. What price is paid for such an increase? HDI is toxic, but detailed information on its toxicity is lacking. The product label describes only the toxicity observed in the 143 patients treated in E1684. The follow-on publications provide minimal information regarding toxicity. The manufacturer has not conducted postmarketing surveillance regarding toxicity. Finally, the analysis prepared by the FDA for the meeting that occurred on February 27, 2002 did not consider the issue of toxicity. No report indicates how many HDI-treated patients have committed suicide or required psychiatric hospitalization, although most physicians who care for these patients know of such untoward events. Detailed information regarding toxicity is essential for the physicians who advise patients with high-risk melanoma concerning the risk/benefit ratio of HDI use to prolong DFS.

As with HDI, no randomized trial of alternative therapies for the adjuvant treatment of melanoma has shown survival benefit. These include four recent trials of vaccines and earlier trials of DTIC, BCG, and levamisole. Nonetheless, several agents (vaccines, GM-CSF, and biochemotherapy) that have completed phase 2 trials show promise, and some of these have advanced to phase 3 trials. Additional agents are being evaluated in phase 1 and 2 trials. HDI provides an imperfect solution for the adjuvant therapy of melanoma. Trials of alternative agents are needed to find more effective and less toxic therapies.

REFERENCES

1. Greene FL, Page DL, Fleming ID et al, eds. American Joint Committee on Cancer Cancer Staging Manual, 6th ed. New York: Springer-Verlag 2002.
2. Balch CM, Buzaid AC, Soong SJ et al. Final version of the American Joint Committee on Cancer staging system for cutaneous melanoma. J Clin Oncol 2001;19:3635–3648.
3. Balch CM, Soong SJ, Gershenwald JE et al. Prognostic factors analysis of 17,600 melanoma patients: validation of the American Joint Committee on Cancer melanoma staging system. J Clin Oncol 2001;19:3622–3634.
4. Effects of adjuvant tamoxifen and of cytotoxic therapy on mortality in early breast cancer: an overview of 61 randomized trials among 28,896 women. Early Breast Cancer Trialists' Collaborative Group. N Engl J Med 1988;319:1681–1692.
5. FDA: Issues in the clinical development of investigational agents being evaluated for the post-surgical adjuvant treatment of high-risk (stages IIb and III) melanoma. http://www.fda.gov/ohrms/dockets/ac/02/briefing/3838bl.htm. February 27, 2002.
6. Wheatley K, Ives N. Adjuvant interferon for melanoma. Ann Oncol 2002;13:1319–1920.
7. Punt CJA, Eggermont AMM. Adjuvant interferon-alfa for melanoma revisited: news from old and new studies. Ann Oncol 2001;12:1663–1666.
8. Lens MB, Dawes M. Interferon alfa therapy for malignant melanoma: a systematic review of randomized controlled trials. J Clin Oncol 2002;20:1818–1825.
9. Pehamberger H, Soyer HP, Steiner A et al. Adjuvant interferon alfa-2a treatment in resected primary stage II cutaneous melanoma. Austrian Malignant Melanoma Cooperative Group [see comments]. J Clin Oncol 1998;16:1425–1429.
10. Kirkwood JM, Strawderman MH, Ernstoff MS et al. Interferon alfa-2b adjuvant therapy of high-risk resected cutaneous melanoma: the Eastern Cooperative Oncology Group Trial EST 1684 [see comments]. J Clin Oncol 1996;14:7–17.
11. Kirkwood JM, Ibrahim JG, Sondak VK et al. High- and low-dose interferon alfa-2b in high-risk melanoma: first analysis of Intergroup Trial E1690/S9111/C9190. J Clin Oncol 2000;18:2444–2458.

12. Kirkwood JM, Ibrahim JG, Sosman JA et al. High-dose interferon alfa-2b significantly prolongs relapse-free and overall survival compared with the GM2-KLH/QS-21 vaccine in patients with resected stage IIB-III melanoma: results of Intergroup Trial E1694/S9512/C509801. J Clin Oncol 2001;19:2370–2380.
13. Kirkwood JM, Ibrahim J, Lawson DH et al. High-dose interferon alfa-2b does not diminish antibody response to GM2 vaccination in patients with resected melanoma: results of the Multicenter Eastern Cooperative Oncology Group Phase II Trial E2696. J Clin Oncol 2001;19:1430–1436.
14. Eggermont AMM, Kleeberg UR, Ruiter DJ et al. The European Organization for Research and Treatment of Cancer Melanoma Group Trial experience with more than 2000 patients, evaluating adjuvant therapy treatment with low or intermediate doses of interferon alpha-2b. Am Soc Clin Oncol 2001 Educational Book. Alexandria, VA, 2001:88–93.
15. Grob JJ, Dreno B, Delaunay M et al. Long-term results of adjuvant therapy with low dose IFN-g2A in resected primary melanoma thicker than 1.5 mm without clinically detectable node metastases. Proc ASCO 1998:1983a.
16. Creagan ET, Dalton RJ, Ahmann DL et al. Randomized, surgical adjuvant clinical trial of recombinant interferon alfa-2a in selected patients with malignant melanoma. J Clin Oncol 1995;13:2776–2783.
17. Cameron DA, Cornbleet MC, Mackie RM et al. Adjuvant interferon alpha 2b in high risk melanoma: the Scottish study. Br J Cancer 2001;84:1146–1149.
18. Hancock BW, Wheatley K, Harrison G et al. Aim high: adjuvant interferon in melanoma (high risk), a United Kingdom Co-ordinating Committee on Cancer Research (UKCCCR) randomized study of observation vs. adjuvant low dose extended duration interferon alfa-2a in high risk resected malignant melanoma [abstract]. Proc Am Soc Clin Oncol 2001;20:1393.
19. Cascinelli N, Bufalino R, Morabito A et al. Results of adjuvant interferon study in WHO melanoma programme. Lancet 1994;343:913–914.
20. Cascinelli N, Belli F, MacKie RM et al. Effect of long-term adjuvant therapy with interferon alpha-2a in patients with regional node metastases from cutaneous melanoma: a randomised trial. Lancet 2001;358:866–869.
21. Wheatley K, Hancock B, Gore M et al. Interferon-alpha as adjuvant therapy for melanoma: a meta-analysis of the randomised trials. Proc ASCO 2001:1394a.
22. Cole BF, Gelber RD, Kirkwood JM et al. Quality-of-life-adjusted survival analysis of interferon alfa-2b adjuvant treatment of high-risk resected cutaneous melanoma: an Eastern Cooperative Oncology Group study. J Clin Oncol 1996;14:2666–2673.
23. Livingston PO, Wong GY et al. Improved survival in stage III melanoma patients with GM2 antibodies: a randomized trial of adjuvant vaccination with GM2 ganglioside. J Clin Oncol 1994;12:1036–1044.
24. FDA: Oncologic Drugs Advisory Committee, Trial design considerations and appropriate patient populations for studies of investigational agents for adjuvant therapy of melanoma given the availability of an approved agent for this indication. http://www.fda.gov/ohrms/dockets/ac/02/transcripts/3838t1.htm, February 27, 2002
25. Grob JJ, Dreno B, de la Salmoniere P et al. Randomised trial of interferon alpha-2a as adjuvant therapy in resected primary melanoma thicker than 1.5 mm without clinically detectable node metastases. French Cooperative Group on Melanoma. Lancet 1998;351:1905–1910.
26. Wallack MK, Sivanandham M, Balch CM et al. Surgical adjuvant active specific immunotherapy for patients with stage III melanoma: the final analysis of data from a phase III, randomized, double-blind, multicenter vaccinia melanoma oncolysate trial. J Am Coll Surg 1998;187:69–77; discussion 77–79.

27. Hersey P, Coates A, McCarthy WH et al. Adjuvant immunotherapy of patients with high risk melanoma using vaccinia viral lysates of melanoma: results of a randomized trial. J Clin Oncol 2002;20:4181–4190.

28. Hersey P, Coates A, McCarthy WH et al. Adjuvant immunotherapy of patients with high risk melanoma with vaccinia viral lysates of melanoma. 4th International Conference on The Adjuvant Therapy of Malignant Melanoma. Royal College of Physicians, London, United Kingdom, 2002:15 (I-25a).

29. Sondak VK, Liu PY, Tuthill RJ et al. Adjuvant immunotherapy of resected, intermediate-thickness, node-negative melanoma with an allogeneic tumor vaccine: overall results of a randomized trial of the Southwest Oncology Group. J Clin Oncol 2002;20:2058–2066.

30. Sosman JA, Unger JM, Liu PY et al. Adjuvant immunotherapy of resected, intermediate-thickness, node-negative melanoma with an allogeneic tumor vaccine: impact of HLA class I antigen expression on outcome. J Clin Oncol 2002;20:2067–2075.

31. Hill GJ, Moss SE, Golomb FM et al. DTIC and combination therapy for melanoma: III. DTIC (NSC 45388) Surgical Adjuvant Study COG PROTOCOL 7040. Cancer 1981;47:2556–2562.

32. Cunningham TJ, Schoenfeld D, Nathanson L et al. A controlled ECOG study of adjuvant therapy (BCG, BCG-DTIC) in patients with stage I and II malignant melanoma, Second International Conference on the Immunotherapy of Cancer; Present Status of Trials in Man. Bethesda, MD, 1980.

33. Pinsky CM, Hirshaut Y, Wanebo HJ et al. Randomized trial of Bacillus Calmette-Guerin (percutaneous administration) as surgical adjuvant immunotherapy for patients with stage-II melanoma. Ann NY Acad Sci 1976;277:187–194.

34. Quirt IC, Shelley WE, Pater JL et al. Improved survival in patients with poor-prognosis malignant melanoma treated with adjuvant levamisole: a phase III study by the National Cancer Institute of Canada Clinical Trials Group [see comments]. J Clin Oncol 1991;9:729–735.

35. Spitler LE. A randomized trial of levamisole versus placebo as adjuvant therapy in malignant melanoma. J Clin Oncol 1991;9:736–740.

36. Morton DL, Foshag LJ, Hoon DS et al. Prolongation of survival in metastatic melanoma after active specific immunotherapy with a new polyvalent melanoma vaccine [published erratum appears in Ann Surg 1993;217:309]. Ann Surg 1992;216:463–482.

37. Morton DL. Current Status of Vaccines for Melanoma. Baltimore, MD, Lippincott Williams & Wilkins, 2000.

38. Chan AD, Morton DL. Active immunotherapy with allogeneic tumor cell vaccines: present status. Semin Oncol 1998;25:611–622.

39. Mitchell MS, Kan-Mitchell J, Kempf RA et al. Specific immunotherapy for melanoma: phase I trial of allogeneic lysates and a novel adjuvant. Cancer Res 1988;48:5883–5893.

40. Mitchell MS, Harel W, Kempf RA et al. Active-specific immunotherapy for melanoma. J Clin Oncol 1990;8:856–869.

41. Livingston PO, Adluri S, Helling F et al. Phase 1 trial of immunological adjuvant QS-21 with a GM2 ganglioside-keyhole limpet haemocyanin conjugate vaccine in patients with malignant melanoma. Vaccine 1994;12:1275–1280.

42. Eggermont AM. Phase III randomized study of postoperative GM2-KLH and QS21 vaccination versus observation in patients with primary cutaneous stage II melanoma. http://www.cancer.gov/clinical_trials/view_clinicaltrials.aspx?version=health+professional&args=8;a66fcf71-4563-4bda-8cfa-eb848d77dcd1, 2002

43. Bystryn JC, Oratz R, Roses D et al. Relationship between immune response to melanoma vaccine immunization and clinical outcome in stage II malignant melanoma. Cancer 1992;69:1157–1164.

44. Bystryn JC, Zeleniuch-Jacquotte A, Oratz R et al. Double-blind trial of a polyvalent, shed-antigen, melanoma vaccine. Clin Cancer Res 2001;7:1882–1887.

45. Livingston P. The unfulfilled promise of melanoma vaccines. Clin Cancer Res 2001;7:1837–1838.

46. Berd D, Murphy G, Maguire HC Jr et al. Immunization with haptenized, autologous tumor cells induces inflammation of human melanoma metastases. Cancer Res 1991;51:2731–2734.

47. Berd D. Autologous, hapten-modified vaccine as a treatment for human cancers. Vaccine 2001;19:2565–2570.

48. Berd D. M-Vax: an autologous, hapten-modified vaccine for human cancer. Expert Opin Biol Ther 2002;2:335–342.

49. AVAX Technologies I. 2002. http://www.avax-tech.com/mvax.html.

50. Safa M, Lutzky J, Chatterjee M et al. Trigem anti-idiotype (Anti-Id) monoclonal antibody (MAb) treatment for stage III melanoma: results of a multicenter phase II trial. Proc Am Soc Clin Oncol 2001;20:1008a.

51. Fidler IJ, Kleinerman ES. Lymphokine-activated human blood monocytes destroy tumor cells but not normal cells under cocultivation conditions. J Clin Oncol 1984;2:937–943.

52. Grabstein KH, Urdal DL, Tushinski RJ et al. Induction of macrophage tumoricidal activity by granulocyte-macrophage colony-stimulating factor. Science 1986;232:506–508.

53. Thomassen MJ, Barna BP, Rankin D et al. Differential effect of recombinant granulocyte macrophage colony- stimulating factor on human monocytes and alveolar macrophages. Cancer Res 1989;49:4086–4089.

54. Wing EJ, Magee DM, Whiteside TL et al. Recombinant human granulocyte/macrophage colony-stimulating factor enhances monocyte cytotoxicity and secretion of tumor necrosis factor alpha and interferon in cancer patients. Blood 1989;73:643–646.

55. Chachoua A, Oratz R, Hoogmoed R et al. Monocyte activation following systemic administration of granulocyte-macrophage colony-stimulating factor. J Immunother Emphasis Tumor Immunol 1994;15:217–224.

56. Young JW, Szabolcs P, Moore MA. Identification of dendritic cell colony-forming units among normal human CD34+ bone marrow progenitors that are expanded by c-kit-ligand and yield pure dendritic cell colonies in the presence of granulocyte/macrophage colony-stimulating factor and tumor necrosis factor alpha [published erratum appears in J Exp Med 1996;183:1283]. J Exp Med 1995;182:1111–119.

57. Szabolcs P, Moore MA, Young JW. Expansion of immunostimulatory dendritic cells among the myeloid progeny of human CD34+ bone marrow precursors cultured with c-kit ligand, granulocyte-macrophage colony-stimulating factor, and TNF-alpha. J Immunol 1995;154:5851–5861.

58. Szabolcs P, Avigan D, Gezelter S et al. Dendritic cells and macrophages can mature independently from a human bone marrow-derived, post-colony-forming unit intermediate. Blood 1996;87:4520–4530.

59. Kumar R, Dong Z, Fidler IJ. Differential regulation of metalloelastase activity in murine peritoneal macrophages by granulocyte-macrophage colony-stimulating factor and macrophage colony-stimulating factor. J Immunol 1996;157:5104–5111.

60. Dong Z, Kumar R, Yang X et al. Macrophage-derived metalloelastase is responsible for the generation of angiostatin in Lewis lung carcinoma. Cell 1997;88:801–810.

61. Spitler LE, Grossbard ML, Ernstoff MS et al. Adjuvant therapy of stage III and IV malignant melanoma using granulocyte-macrophage colony-stimulating factor [see comments]. J Clin Oncol 2000;18:1614–1621.

62. Spitler LE, Weber R, Rose M et al. Adjuvant Therapy of Stage II (T4), III and IV Malignant Melanoma using GM-CSF. 4th International Conference on The Adjuvant Therapy of Malignant Melanoma. London, March 15–16, 2002 10 (I-08).

63. Retsas S, MacRae K, Henry K. Adjuvant treatment for clinically apparent regional lymph node metastases [>N1b] from melanoma: single-institution experience from a cohort of 318 patients. 4th International Conference on The Adjuvant Therapy of Malignant Melanoma. Royal College of Physicians, London, March 15–16, 2002 I-26.

64. Retsas S, Quigley M, Pectasides D et al. Clinical and histologic involvement of regional lymph nodes in malignant melanoma: adjuvant vindesine improves survival. Cancer 1994;73:2119–2130.

65. Legha SS, Ring S, Eton O et al. Development of a biochemotherapy regimen with concurrent administration of cisplatin, vinblastine, dacarbazine, interferon alfa, and interleukin-2 for patients with metastatic melanoma. J Clin Oncol 1998;16:1752–1759.

66. Gibbs P, Anderson C, Pearlman N et al. A phase II study of neoadjuvant biochemotherapy for stage III melanoma. Cancer 2002;94:470–476.

67. Balch CM, Soong SJ, Murad TM et al. A multifactorial analysis of melanoma: III. Prognostic factors in melanoma patients with lymph node metastases (stage II). Ann Surg 1981;193:377–388.

68. Bedikian AY. Phase III randomized adjuvant study of interferon alfa-2b (IFN-A) Alone vs biochemotherapy using cisplatin, vinblastine, dacarbazine (DTIC), IFN-A, and interleukin-2 (IL-2) in melanoma patients with regional lymph node metastases. http://www.cancer.gov/clinical_trials/view_clinicaltrials.aspx?version=health+professional&args=4;e14d7b24-9181-4fa6-b429-50ef712e4fe7, 2002.

69. Rosenberg SA. Phase II randomized study of gp100:209-217 (210M) or gp100:17-25 antigen and tyrosinase:368-376 (370D), tyrosinase:240-251 (244S), tyrosinase:206-214, or tyrosinase-related protein-1 (ORF3):1-9 peptide emulsified in Montanide ISA-51 in patients with melanoma at high risk for recurrence. http://www.cancer.gov/clinical_trials/view_clinicaltrials.aspx?version=health+professional&args=2;feedefa3-7625-401b-bc66-b8eaf9ec8521, 2002.

70. Kendra K, Malkovska V, Allen M et al. In vivo binding and antitumor activity of Ch14.18. J Immunother 1999;22:423–430.

71. Maguire HC Jr, Berd D, Lattime EC et al. Phase I study of R24 in patients with metastatic melanoma including evaluation of immunologic parameters. Cancer Biother Radiopharm 1998;13:13–23.

72. Nasi ML, Meyers M, Livingston PO et al. Anti-melanoma effects of R24, a monoclonal antibody against GD3 ganglioside. Melanoma Res 1997;7[suppl 2]:S155–S162.

73. Lode HN, Xiang R, Duncan SR et al. Tumor-targeted IL-2 amplifies T cell-mediated immune response induced by gene therapy with single-chain IL-12. Proc Natl Acad Sci USA 1999;96:8591–8596.

74. Lode HN, Reisfeld RA. Targeted cytokines for cancer immunotherapy. Immunol Res 2000;21:279–288.

75. Fallarino F, Fields PE, Gajewski TF. B7-1 engagement of cytotoxic T lymphocyte antigen 4 inhibits T cell activation in the absence of CD28. J Exp Med 1998;188:205–210.

76. Foon KA, Lutzky J, Baral RN et al. Clinical and immune responses in advanced melanoma patients immunized with an anti-idiotype antibody mimicking disialoganglioside GD2. J Clin Oncol 2000;18:376–384.

77. McCaffery M, Yao TJ, Williams L et al. Immunization of melanoma patients with BEC2 anti-idiotypic monoclonal antibody that mimics GD3 ganglioside: enhanced immunogenicity when combined with adjuvant. Clin Cancer Res 1996;2:679–686.

78. Soiffer R, Lynch T, Mihm M et al. Vaccination with irradiated autologous melanoma cells engineered to secrete human granulocyte-macrophage colony-stimulating factor generates potent antitumor immunity in patients with metastatic melanoma. Proc Natl Acad Sci USA 1998;95:13141–13146.

79. Kusumoto M, Umeda S, Ikubo A et al. Phase 1 clinical trial of irradiated autologous melanoma cells adenovirally transduced with human GM-CSF gene. Cancer Immunol Immunother 2001;50:373–381.

80. Rankin EM, Spits H, Orsini D et al. A phase 1 study of vaccination with autologous, GM-CSF-transduced and irradiated tumour cells in patients with advanced melanoma. Proc Am Soc Clin Oncol 1995;14:226.

81. Belli F, Arienti F, Sule-Suso J et al. Active immunization of metastatic melanoma patients with interleukin-2-transduced allogeneic melanoma cells: evaluation of efficacy and tolerability. Cancer Immunol Immunother 1997;44:197–203.

82. Osanto S, Schiphorst PP, Weijl NI et al. Vaccination of melanoma patients with an allogeneic, genetically modified interleukin 2-producing melanoma cell line. Hum Gene Ther 2000;11:739–750.

83. Rochlitz C, Dreno B, Jantscheff P et al. Immunotherapy of metastatic melanoma by intratumoral injections of Vero cells producing human IL-2: phase II randomized study comparing two dose levels. Cancer Gene Ther 2002;9:289–295.

84. Gajewski TF, Fallarino F, Ashikari A et al. Immunization of HLA-A2+ melanoma patients with MAGE-3 or MelanA peptide-pulsed autologous peripheral blood mononuclear cells plus recombinant human interleukin 12. Clin Cancer Res 2001;7:895s–901s.

85. Panelli MC, Wunderlich J, Jeffries J et al. Phase 1 study in patients with metastatic melanoma of immunization with dendritic cells presenting epitopes derived from the melanoma-associated antigens MART-1 and gp100. J Immunother 2000;23:487–498.

86. Banchereau J, Palucka AK, Dhodapkar M et al. Immune and clinical responses in patients with metastatic melanoma to CD34(+) progenitor-derived dendritic cell vaccine. Cancer Res 2001;61:6451–6458.

87. Schuler-Thurner B, Schultz ES, Berger TG et al. Rapid induction of tumor-specific type 1 T helper cells in metastatic melanoma patients by vaccination with mature, cryopreserved, peptide-loaded monocyte-derived dendritic cells. J Exp Med 2002;195:1279–1288.

88. Nestle FO, Alijagic S, Gilliet M et al. Vaccination of melanoma patients with peptide- or tumor lysate-pulsed dendritic cells. Nat Med 1998;4:328–332.

89. Nair SK, Morse M, Boczkowski D et al. Induction of tumor-specific cytotoxic T lymphocytes in cancer patients by autologous tumor RNA-transfected dendritic cells. Ann Surg 2002;235:540–549.

90. Dillman RO, Schiltz PM, Selvan R et al. Patient-specific cancer vaccine of cultured autologous tumor cells and autologous dendritic cells. J Immunother 2001;24:S5.

91. Hwu WJ. New approaches in the treatment of metastatic melanoma: thalidomide and temozolomide. Oncology (Huntingt) 2000;14:25–28.

92. Hwu WJ, Krown SE, Panageas KS et al. Temozolomide plus thalidomide in patients with advanced melanoma: results of a dose-finding trial. J Clin Oncol 2002;20:2610–2615.

93. Hwu WJ, Krown SE, Panageas KS et al. Treatment of Meatastic melanoma in the brain with temozolomide and thalidomide. Lancet Oncol 2001;2:634–635.

Indexes

SUBJECT INDEX

A

B

D

E

F

G

H

I

K

L

M

N

O

R

S

T

U

V

W

Y

INDEX OF TABLES

9 780763 720643

Printed in Dunstable, United Kingdom

88177729R00248